CATHOLIC HEALTH CARE ETHICS

CONTRIBUTORS

Rev. David Beauregard, O.M.V., Ph.D.
Former Academic Dean
Our Lady of Grace Seminary
Boston, Massachusetts

†Rev. Dennis A. Brodeur, Ph.D.
Former Senior Vice President,
  Stewardship
SSM Healthcare
St. Louis, Missouri

Grattan T. Brown, S.T.D.
Assistant Professor of Theology
Belmont Abbey College
Belmont, North Carolina

E. Christian Brugger, D.Phil
Associate Professor of Philosophy
  and Theology
Director of Integrative Research
Institute for the Psychological Sciences
Arlington, Virginia

Greg F. Burke, M.D., F.A.C.P.
Geisinger Medical Center
Danville, Pennsylvania

Nicholas P. Cafardi, J.D.
Joseph Katarincic Chair in Legal
  Process and Civil Procedure
Duquesne University School of Law
Pittsburgh, Pennsylvania

Peter J. Cataldo, Ph.D.
Former Director of Research
The National Catholic Bioethics Center
Philadelphia

Helen Stanton Chapple, Ph.D., R.N.,
  M.A., C.C.R.N., C.T.
Resident Faculty
Center for Health Policy and Ethics
Creighton University Medical Center
Omaha, Nebraska

James M. DuBois, Ph.D., D.Sc.
Director, Center for Health Care Ethics
Mäder Professor of Health Care Ethics
Saint Louis University
Saint Louis, Missouri

Edward J. Furton, M.A., Ph.D.
Director of Publications
Staff Ethicist
The National Catholic Bioethics Center
Philadelphia

David M. Gallagher, Ph.D.
Thomistic Seminar
The Witherspoon Institute
Princeton, New Jersey

T. Murphy Goodwin, M.D.
Professor and Director
Division of Maternal–Fetal Medicine
Co-director of the Institute for Maternal
  and Fetal Health
University of Southern California
Los Angeles, California

Suzanne Gross, F.S.E.
Administrator, Franciscan
  Home Care and Hospice Care
Pro-Life Program Coordinator
  for the Diocese of Hartford
Chairman of the Board of the
  Physician's Health Alliance
Meriden, Connecticut

John M. Haas, Ph.D., S.T.L.
President
The National Catholic Bioethics Center
Philadelphia

Marie T. Hilliard, J.C.L., Ph.D., R.N.
Director of Bioethics and Public Policy
The National Catholic Bioethics Center
Philadelphia

Rev. Thomas Knoblach, Ph.D.
Consultant for Health Care Ethics Diocese
  of St. Cloud
St. Cloud, Minnesota

Rev. Germain Kopaczynski,
  O.F.M.Conv., Ph.D., S.T.D.
Former Director of Education and
  Staff Ethicist
The National Catholic Bioethics Center
Philadelphia

Erica Laethem, Be.L., Ph.D. (cand.)
Athenaeum Pontificium Regina
  Apostolorum
Rome

Matthew P. Lomanno
Lecturer in Humanities
Saint Anselm College
Manchester, New Hampshire

William E. May
Michael J. McGivney Professor of
  Moral Theology
John Paul II Institute for Studies on
  Marriage and Family
Washington, D.C.

Gerald J. McShane, M.D.
Director, OSF Medical Group
OSF Health Care System
Peoria, Illinois

†Rev. Albert S. Moraczewski, O.P.,
  Ph.D., S.T.M.
President Emeritus
The National Catholic Bioethics Center
Philadelphia

Kevin J. Murrell, M.D.
FIAMC Representative
Catholic Medical Association
Augusta, Georgia

Stephen R. Napier, Ph.D.
Staff Ethicist
The National Catholic Bioethics Center
Philadelphia, Pennsylvania

Marie T. Nolan, M.P.H., Ph.D., R.N.
Director of Ph.D. Program
Associate Professor
Johns Hopkins University School of
  Nursing
Baltimore, Maryland

Daniel O'Brien, Ph.D.
Vice President for Ethics
Ascension Health
St. Louis, Missouri

Rev. James A. O'Donohoe, J.C.D.
Former Ethicist
Covenant Health Systems
Lexington, Massachusetts

Sheila O'Friel, D.C.
Former Chair
Carney Hospital Ethics Committee
Boston, Massachusetts

Edmund D. Pellegrino, M.D.
Chairman
President's Council on Bioethics
Professor Emeritus of Medicine and
  Medical Ethics
Georgetown University Medical Center
Washington, D.C.

Joseph J. Piccione, J.D., S.T.D.
Corporate Ethicist
OSF Healthcare System
Peoria, Illinois

John B. Shea, M.D., F.R.C.P.
Member, Canadian Catholic Bioethics
  Institute
Toronto

Rev. Joseph Tham, L.C., M.D., Ph.D.
Professor of Bioethics
Athenaeum Pontificium Regina
  Apostolorum
Rome

Patrick Yeung Jr., M.D.
Assistant Professor
Department of Obstetrics & Gynecology
Duke University Medical Center
Diplomate of the American Board of
  Obstetrics & Gynecology
Durham, North Carolina

CATHOLIC HEALTH CARE ETHICS

A MANUAL FOR PRACTITIONERS

Second Edition

Edited by Edward J. Furton
with Peter J. Cataldo and Albert S. Moraczewski, O.P.

Foreword by Edmund D. Pellegrino, M.D.

THE NATIONAL CATHOLIC BIOETHICS CENTER

Cover Design
Thomas Gannoe and Nicholas Furton

Cover Image
The Carl Zeiss Universal Fluorescence Microscope image, courtesy of the of the Optical Microscopy
Division of the National High Magnetic Field Laboratory's "Museum of Microscopy,"
http:/microscopy.fus.edu, Michael W. Davidson, Director
Used with permission

Second Edition
ISBN 978-0-935372-54-0

Unless otherwise noted, quotations from Scripture are from the *Revised Standard Version, Catholic Edition*, prepared by the Catholic Biblical Association of Great Britain © 1965, 1966 National Council of the Churches of Christ in the United States of America; quotations from official Church documents are from the Vatican English translation, published online at www.vatican.va © Libreria Editrice Vaticana; and quotations from the Catechism are from the *Catechism of the Catholic Church*, 2nd ed. © 1994, 1997 United States Catholic Conference, Inc. / Libreria Editrice Vaticana.

Library of Congress Cataloging-in-Publication Data

Catholic health care ethics : a manual for practitioners / edited by Edward J. Furton with Peter J. Cataldo and Albert S. Moraczewski ; foreword by Edmund D. Pellegrino. -- 2nd ed.
     p. ; cm.
  Includes bibliographical references and index.
  ISBN 978-0-935372-54-0 (alk. paper)
 1. Medical ethics--Religious aspects--Catholic Church--Handbooks, manuals, etc. 2. Medical ethics committees--Decision making--Handbooks, manuals, etc. I. Furton, Edward James. II. Cataldo, Peter J., 1956- III. Moraczewski, Albert S., 1920-2008. IV. National Catholic Bioethics Center.
  [DNLM: 1. Catholicism. 2. Ethics, Medical. 3. Bioethical Issues. W 50 C3629 2009]
  R724.C38 2009
  174.2'08822--dc22
                    2009026859

In Memory of

Father Albert S. Moraczewski, O.P.

1920–2008

CONTENTS

PART I   FOUNDATIONAL PRINCIPLES

PART III   BEGINNING-OF-LIFE ISSUES

PART V   SELECTED CLINICAL ISSUES

PART VI   INSTITUTIONAL ISSUES

APPENDICES   SELECTED CHURCH DOCUMENTS

FOREWORD

by Edmund D. Pellegrino, M.D.

The National Catholic Bioethics Center was established in 1973 as The Pope John XXIII Medical-Moral Research and Education Center. Since then, and now under its current name, the center has been an authoritative and authentic guide to Catholic medical moral teaching. Through its publications, consultations, and twenty-two bishops' workshops to date, it has engaged the major issues of contemporary bioethics from a consistent Roman Catholic perspective.

The present volume continues that tradition. It was originally intended as a guide for ethics committees and their members. In actual fact, it is a comprehensive, up-to-date compendium of Roman Catholic ethics and morals that has become an invaluable *vade mecum* for all Catholic individuals and institutions seeking to understand and apply the Roman Catholic perspective in their daily lives.

The book appears at a time both propitious and troublesome for Catholic and Christian ethics and bioethics. Never have Roman Catholic health professionals been more urgently in need of a reliable moral compass to navigate the shoals of secularization, postmodernism, and antirationalism in ethics. Never, on the other hand, has there been a more urgent exposure of the inadequacies of ethics without a metaphysical, theological, and reasoned foundation, just those features which Roman Catholic ethics so well synthesizes.

The secularization of contemporary bioethics has been rapid and deep. In the late sixties and early seventies of the twentieth century, bioethics still drew heavily on religious traditions, Christian and Jewish. But as American society became increasingly pluralistic morally and culturally, the clarity and stability of religiously based moral norms fell into disfavor. Philosophical ethics entered the field and formalized it, through the application of established philosophical systems to the complex dilemmas emerging from medical progress. This appealed to a wider audience than religiously inspired ethicists, especially among physicians and other health professionals.

As the number and complexity of ethical issues in biomedicine proliferated, however, bioethics expanded beyond philosophy and theology. Today it embraces the social and behavioral sciences, law, economics, and politics. Today bioethics is a multidisciplinary enterprise attempting to accommodate to a society progressively more diverse and individualistic in its interpretations of moral truth. In the process, bioethics has become overtly and militantly secular and has turned increasingly to political liberalism for its norms and for resolution of ethical differences.

The result has been a flight from traditional moral norms to what "works," that is, what resolves conflicts. The search for the right and the good in ethical decisions has been openly and frankly abandoned.[1] Normative ethics has been supplanted by procedure, psychology, and social construction. Ethical principles are scorned as rigid, tyrannical, and outmoded. Norms have been replaced by paradigm cases, stories, and consensus committees.

In all of this, contemporary bioethics has followed the lead of contemporary moral philosophy. Moral skepticism, denial of any cognitive content to moral judgment, and erosion of the normative claims of ethics are the result. Normative judgments have become attitudes, values, perspectives, or consensus statements subject only to social and historical construction. The gap between this state of affairs and the traditional Roman Catholic perception of ethics and moral philosophy could not be more extreme. As a result, secular bioethics is becoming less and less receptive to dialogue with the Roman Catholic moral tradition. This is one of the reasons for Pope John Paul II's encyclical *Fides et ratio*, which stresses the importance of dialogue with contemporary philosophy including the postmodern version.

In some paradoxical ways, however, the engagement with postmodernism may represent the most timely opportunity for genuine dialogue. This is because the major thrust of postmodernism is to challenge the reliance of secular ethics and postenlightenment philosophy on unaided or autonomous human reason. By eroding reason itself, secular philosophy faces two alternatives: one is the direction of the relativism, nihilism, and chaos; the other is the recovery, partial at least, of metaphysics and religion as the grounding for moral norms.

To the postmodern critique, Roman Catholic bioethics can offer the alternatives of a grasp of moral truths, an articulated system of moral philosophy based in an explicit philosophical anthropology, an ethic formulated in terms of principles deducible from the nature of man, and a set of specific ethical action guidelines for specific moral confrontations like abortion, euthanasia, assisted suicide, cloning, stem-cell research, etc.

But this synthesis is increasingly challenged even by those who themselves come from a religious tradition. For example, in *Christian Bioethics*, a journal dedicated to "non-ecumenical studies in medical morality," the Roman Catholic tradition was soundly criticized by a Greek Orthodox Christian, a Jew, and an avowed pagan for its insistence on a synthesis of faith and reason.[2] Each singled out Pope John Paul II, and St. Thomas Aquinas especially, for their willingness to enter into a serious dialogue with the modern and the classical worlds of philosophy. Like the postmodernists, these ethicists assailed the use of reason in moral discourse and accused Roman Catholicism of secularizing itself by its attempts to present reasoned arguments for its beliefs.

These trends to secularization, deconstruction, and derationalization of bioethics underscore the need for an informed body of Catholic health care professionals who know the origins and foundations of their own faith and its place in bioethical decisions and policies. All Catholic health care professionals share the responsibility to give witness to Church teachings on bioethical questions in their work and daily lives. This manual provides a guide to action and to understanding the reasons for those actions if they are to be consistent with Roman Catholic teaching in bioethics.

This book begins with a clear statement of the foundations for Church teaching and authority and with the principle which derives from those foundations. Specific and practical discussion follows on a wide range of concrete ethical issues and problems from the beginning and procreation of human life to its ending, from organ transplantation and genetics to organizational ethics and ethics committees as they should function in Catholic health care institutions. The book closes with a selection of documents drawn from magisterial teaching on the most important topics.

With this volume available, no Catholic health care professional can afford to disclaim knowledge of Church teaching when asked by Catholics and non-Catholics, nor easily have a legitimate excuse for lapses in making ethical decisions relevant to clinical practice. In Catholic hospitals at least, in service programs, and in seminars and conferences aimed at familiarizing the staff with Church teaching, using this and related texts would be one way to define and maintain Catholic character. For a Roman Catholic health professional to be unfamiliar with the relevant contents of this manual would be to fail to meet a rudimentary requirement for authenticity as a Catholic and Christian.

Notes

[1] See Anna Smith Iltis, "Bioethics as Methodological Case Resolution: Specification, Principlism and Casuistry," *Journal of Medicine and Philosophy* 25.3 (June 2000): 277–279.

[2] In the December 1999 issue of *Christian Bioethics* (5.3), see Michael Rie, "What Is Christian About Christian Bioethics?" 263–266; H. Tristram Engelhardt, Jr. "Can Philosophy Save Christianity? Are the Roots of the Foundations of Christian Bioethics Ecumenical? Reflection on the Nature of a Christian Bioethics," 203–212; and Ruiping Fan, "The Memoirs of a Pagan Sojourning in the Ruins of Christendom," 232–237.

PREFACE TO THE NEW EDITION

The work of an editor usually begins with a blank page. A new volume requires laying out the structural plan, finding experts who can address the key questions, reviewing manuscripts, dunning authors who fall behind, and then editing and laying out the work as a whole. All of that was required here, but I had the distinct advantage of having a first edition produced by Peter Cataldo and Rev. Albert Morczewski, O.P. Their labors remain very much in evidence, and it has been a pleasure to begin from such an outstanding starting-point. The first edition was brilliantly conceived and superbly executed.

Nonetheless, the need for a revision had become obvious. Nothing stands still for long in the world of bioethics. The first edition appeared in 2001, and much has changed. Cloning and embryonic stem cell research were then still in their infancy. No one had yet heard of induced pluripotent stem cells. The mapping of the human genome was in process but had not yet been completed. The death of Terri Schiavo was still a future event and John Paul II had not responded to this tragedy with his critical remarks on the provision of food and water. Joseph Ratzinger was head of the Congregation for the Doctrine of the Faith and was yet to ascend the chair of St. Peter. Brain death was then the most controversial issue under the heading of the determination of death, but now we face new concerns over donation after cardiac death. Many other important events have transpired since the publication of the first edition. As a result of this sea of change, virtually every article in the original needed updating if it was to continue to serve Catholic heath care ethics committees.

But as Dr. Edmund Pellegrino notes in his Foreword, this work is much more than a volume for ethics committees. It is a compendium of Catholic moral teaching on virtually every subject that confronts those facing serious health care decisions. We hope that a wide range of readers, Catholic and non-Catholic alike, will find answers to their questions here. The National Catholic Bioethics Center has a reputation for being a trustworthy voice in the exposition of the moral teachings of the Roman Catholic Church. Every effort has been made to ensure that the highest respect for both faith and reason is reflected in the work of the authors published here.

Among articles either new or substantially revised are "Ordinary and Extraordinary Means," "The Natural Moral Law," "Health Care Ethics Committees," "Diocesan Health Care Ethics Committees," "Human Cloning," "Stem Cell Research," "Determining Death," "Palliative Care, Pain Management, and Human Suffering," "Assessing Benefits and Burdens," "Health Care Proxies and Advance Directives," "Vaccination Refusals," "Human Experimentation and Research," "Triage and the Duty to Care," "Cooperating with Non-Catholic Partners," and "State Mandates." Other entries, such as "Nutrition and Hydration" and "The Persistent Vegetative State," have had significant new material added that reflects recent developments in Church teaching. For topics that remain the subject of debate, we have tried to do justice to both sides by printing contrasting essays. This is especially evident in "Pregnancy Prevention in Sexual Assault," where the advent of Plan B, and recent scientific studies, have produced considerable disagreement among Catholic scholars. Also, the appendices have been updated to include new documents of the Roman Catholic Church in medical ethics.

Nearly all of the editorial summaries have been revised to better reflect the material in the various articles. The reader who wants to get a quick overview of a particular topic can turn to these summaries for a sense of what to expect. The print size has been increased and the pages redesigned to ensure a more easy-to-read format. After much consideration, we decided to forgo the three-ring binder format and to print the volume in the traditional way. We have chosen a strong case stitching that should enable the book to hold up to many years of use. We have likewise abandoned the difficult section numbering and redone the index. The bibliographies have been moved to the end of the volume.

I would like to say a special word in memory of Father Albert Moraczewski, O.P, the first president and founder of The National Catholic Bioethics Center, who along with Peter Cataldo edited the first edition. Fr. Albert passed away on May 1, 2008, Ascension Thursday, and has been much missed. His influence remains strong in this work, as is evident from a glance at the table of contents, a testament to his wide-ranging interests. A man of strong scholarly instincts and jovial personality, Father Albert exemplified all that is best in the Thomistic tradition and the Dominican Order. He took care to examine all sides of an issue, was willing to take an adventurous stand when he had principle on his side, and held all with whom he debated and disagreed in high regard. Everyone who knew Father Albert was obliged to think deeply about the moral issues that now dominate so much of medicine and the life sciences. All of us here at the NCBC enjoyed his company and his wit.

I would like to thank all of my colleagues here at the NCBC for their understanding, support, and contributions, in particular, Marie Hilliard, Stephen Napier, Rev. Alfred Cioffi, Rev. Tad Pacholczyk, and especially John Haas, president of the Center and publisher of this volume. I also owe an enormous debt of gratitude to my staff, Rebecca Robinson, production manager, and Susan Gallen and Melanie Anderson, production editors.

No doubt another editor will take up the task of revising this volume in the not-too-distant future. Although the moral principles that guide our tradition remain the same, change in this field is relentless. There will always be new challenges requiring new applications of these timeless truths.

EDWARD J. FURTON
Editor
Director of Publications and Staff Ethicist
The National Catholic Bioethics Center

PREFACE TO THE 2001 EDITION

Among various religious groups and other institutions, the Catholic Church probably has the longest record of reflecting on the moral aspects of medicine.[1] In the wake of the revelations of the Nuremberg trials after World War II, the world became aware of severe ethical violations associated with the "medical experimentations" of the Nazi physicians. No longer could it be assumed that if a person were a physician, the medical behavior of that individual could be trusted to be honorable. Suddenly it became necessary to scrutinize carefully the research carried on in the name of medicine. Medical practice, too, soon fell under the same shadow of suspicion.

Coupled with this recognition was the rapid and extraordinary development of medical technology during and following upon the hostilities of World War II: for example, a plethora of antibiotics were introduced; transplantation of a variety of organs and tissues became possible; to limit fertility a large choice of anovulants became available; as a means in the management of infertility, in vitro fertilization and other technological reproductive methods became possible; and life support technology and procedures that could keep a person alive almost indefinitely were introduced into medical practice. These developments and others brought to the fore new ethical questions, and older ones were cast in new terms.

In modern times, the Catholic Church has begun to address these issues, such as human reproduction.[2] Pope Pius XII addressed a number of other medical topics, such as euthanasia, responsibilities of the pharmacist, moral aspects of genetics, removal of a healthy organ, antibiotics, and tissue transplantation.[3] Pope Paul VI took on the difficult task of making a definitive judgment about contraception in *Humanae vitae*, while John Paul II declared in *Veritatis splendor* that some moral methodologies were not compatible with the Faith.[4] John Paul II also addressed some fundamental questions regarding human life in his *Evangelium vitae*.[5] The instruction *Donum vitae*, issued by the Congregation for the Doctrine of the Faith (1987) and approved by John Paul II, stipulated the principles by which the morality of various reproductive methodologies could be evaluated.[6]

In the late 1960s, the Catholic Hospital Association (now known as the Catholic Health Association of the United States–CHA) initiated a study to determine the best way in which it could deal with the newer ethical challenges which modern medical technology was presenting to the Catholic Church. After several years of study, CHA concluded that, all things considered, what was needed was a daughter organization which could undertake systematic and sustained studies of these new ethical issues. Thus was born in 1972 in St. Louis, Missouri, the Pope John XXIII Medical-Moral Research and Education Center, officially known since 1998 as The National Catholic Bioethics[1] Center and now located in Philadelphia, Pennsylvania.

The NCBC has the mandate to study these issues with particular attention to the needs of the bishops, Catholic health care institutions, and health care professionals in light of the Catholic Church's moral tradition and relevant teachings. Where such teachings are lacking or insufficient because of the nature of the rapidly developing medical knowledge and technology, the NCBC seeks to help develop appropriate moral analyses of the issues, subject, of course, to any subsequent teaching of the magisterium.

---

[1]The term "bioethics" is used because in contemporary usage it is a broader term than "medical-moral," for it covers topics such as biological and psychological research (e.g., the Human Genome Project), legislation on health care matters, medical insurance, and institutional alliances.

The genesis of this ethics manual is rooted in the above history. The purpose of the manual is to provide a handy reference source for ethics committees in Catholic health care facilities as well as for Catholic health care personnel working in other contexts. In particular, the NCBC is committed to providing in this manual reliable statements of Catholic moral principles and ethical analyses which are consonant with Catholic teaching. In addition to various papal documents, such as the *Catechism of the Catholic Church* (approved by Pope John Paul II on June 25, 1992), a sure guide for ethics committees is the *Ethical and Religious Directives for Catholic Health Care Services* (*ERDs*), approved by the full body of bishops at their annual meeting in November 1994, issued by the National Conference of Catholic Bishops, and revised in 2001. Whenever appropriate, specific directives from the *ERDs* are cited in the text of the manual.

The manual begins with an explanation of the central moral tenets and principles of the Catholic moral tradition and Catholic teaching that are directly relevant to questions and issues faced by ethics committees. The primary purpose of an ethics committee is education. A complete education includes a grounding in the foundations of Catholic moral tradition and Catholic teaching. The contents then progress to the areas of ethics committee processes and to specific ethical questions and issues addressed by ethics committees. The structure of the volume should allow the user to apply what is learned about the moral foundations to the specific issues that are presented.

Several appendices are included which provide key Church documents relevant for Catholic bioethics and to which frequent references are made in the manual. A detailed index and comprehensive bibliography are also provided. Our decision to use multiple authorship was made in order to have experienced persons write on topics about which they have both theoretical and practical knowledge.

This volume is the result of dedicated efforts by a number of individuals whom we gratefully acknowledge. The manual originated from an earlier interdisciplinary research task force. We are grateful to several individuals who assisted in different ways with that effort: Jeanne Burke, Donald Powers, Barbara Sullivan, and Sister Margaret Mary Turner, R.S.M. (formerly with the NCBC). We are very thankful to a number of individuals for their work with the manuscript: Doris Amirault (formerly with the NCBC) for her preparation of the typescript for many of the chapters, Veronica McLoud Dort for copy editing,

The Dominican nuns at the Monastery of Our Lady of the Rosary (Buffalo, New York) for proofreading, and Dale O'Leary for formatting the text and assisting in numerous publication details. We thank Thomas Gannoe for his work on the design of the cover, and Brother Ignatius Perkins, O.P., and Susan Jordan for the production and marketing of the manual. Finally, we are grateful and fortunate to have received valuable advice and comments on the content and structure of the manual from our other NCBC colleagues John M. Haas, Germain Kopaczynski, O.F.M. Conv., and Edward J. Furton.

The publisher (John M. Haas) and editors welcome any comments or suggestions the readers desire to make directed to improve the usefulness of the manual.

PETER J. CATALDO
ALBERT S. MORACZEWSKI, O.P.
Editors

Notes

[1] Stanley L. Jaki, *The Road of Science and the Ways to God* (Chicago: University of Chicago Press, 1978), 304–307. Russell E. Smith, ed., *Conserving Human Life* (Braintree, MA: Pope John XXIII Medical-Moral Research and Education Center, 1989). Christopher J. Kauffman, *Ministry and Meaning: A Religious History of Catholic Health Care in the United States* (New York: Crossroad, 1995). Benedict M. Ashley, *Living the Truth in Love: A Biblical Introduction to Moral Theology* (New York: Alba House, 1996).

[2] Pius XI, *Casti connubii* (On Christian Marriage) (December 31, 1930). Pius XII, "The Immorality of Euthanasia," discourse to the delegates of the International Union of Catholic Women's Leagues (September 11, 1947), in *The Human Body*, ed. Monks of Solesmes (Boston: St. Paul Editions, 1960), 90–91.

[3] Pope Pius XII, in *The Human Body*, ed. Monks of Solesmes: "Immorality of Euthanasia"; "The Responsibility of the Pharmacist," discourse to Catholic pharmacists (September 2, 1950), 128–130; "Moral Aspects of Genetics," discourse to those attending the "Primum Symposium Geneticae Medicae" (September 7, 1953), 246–260; "Removal of a Healthy Organ," discourse to delegates at the Twenty-Sixth Congress of Urology (October 8, 1953), 277–281; "Antibiotics," discourse to specialists in biology (May 12, 1955), 329–330; and "Tissue Transplantation," discourse to a group of eye specialists (May 14, 1956), 373–384.

[4] Paul VI, *Humanae vitae* (July 25, 1968). John Paul II, *Veritatis splendor* (August 6, 1993).

[5] John Paul II, *Evangelium vitae* (March 25, 1995).

[6] Congregation for the Doctrine of the Faith, *Donum vitae* (February 22, 1987).

Part I

Foundational Principles

CHAPTER 1

The Human Person and the Church's Teaching Authority

Rev. Albert S. Moraczewski, O.P.

Life as a Gift from God

Basic to an understanding of Catholic bioethics is the acceptance of the truth that all existing beings come from God. All beings are created and continue to be sustained by God's creative power. Nothing would exist except that God has willed it to be: "Let there be light ... God looked at everything he had made, and he found it very good" (Gen. 1:3, 31). In particular, God created man in a manner distinct from the remainder of creation: "God created man in his image; in the divine image He created him; male and female He created them" (Gen. 1:27). Therein lies the foundation of human dignity and worth.

> Of all visible creatures only man is "able to know and love his creator" [*Gaudium et spes*, n. 12]. He is "the only creature on earth that God has chosen for its own sake" [*Gaudium et spes*, n. 24], and he alone is called to share, by knowledge and love, in God's own life. It was for this end that he was created, and this is the fundamental reason for his dignity. (*CCC*, n. 356)

To say that life is a *gift* is to acknowledge that life has been received from someone other than the individual who lives. It is something to which the recipient has no right; it is not something which the recipient can merit. Furthermore, a person cannot grant life to himself. That is obvious. It is also clear that life proximately comes from other human beings, specifically, the parents who may or may not even be known to the one generated. Today, the parents may not even be known to one another if certain forms of reproductive technology have intervened. In the latter case, the involvement of other human beings may have been required in order to utilize technological intervention such as in the case of in vitro fertilization.

Notwithstanding intermediate human causes, ultimately, however, human life is a gift from God. The power of living beings to pass on life to offspring of their own kind comes from God, who in creation gave the requisite specific powers and properties to each kind of creature so that they could develop and function according to their respective roles under Divine Providence. God imparted to human beings, in particular, a spiritual soul, which made them to be "in the image" of God; as Genesis 2:7 tells it, "The Lord God ... blew into his nostrils the breath of life." This was not said of any other creature which God fashioned.

The Church teaches that the human spiritual soul is created directly by God for each individual human being:

> The Church teaches that every spiritual soul is created immediately [that is, without any intermediate agent, angelic or demiurgic] by God—it is not "produced" by the parents—and also that it is immortal: it does not perish when it separates from the body at death, and it will be reunited with the body at the final resurrection. (*CCC*, n. 366)

While the human parents, each in their respective manner, contribute to the making of the individual child's body, it is God who directly infuses the soul of each individual human being when the material component is ready for the reception of a spiritual soul. This process should not be imagined as if one were pouring something into a vessel or plugging a lamp into an electric outlet. Rather it is a creative act of God—which of its very nature is mysterious to us and beyond our comprehension, that is, the bringing into existence of a being from absolute nothingness. It is the act of God who brings forth within the very core of the material reality a spiritual soul which becomes the principle of life, of unity, and of specificity of that bodily being and so constitutes a human person.

As a consequence of this special gift—the spiritual soul—each person has an inherent dignity and sacredness which is independent of human society's recognition. That dignity transcends the individual's age, condition, sex, socioeconomic status, religion, health, or stage of development. Upon this truth, namely, the *inherent* dignity and sacredness of human life, rests the principles of medical ethics and morals. That is the reason that humans are to be treated differently from animals. Human reason transcends the limitations of the here and now, of the particular and the concrete, and thus is able to formulate universal principles for moral conduct.

> Man participates in the wisdom and goodness of the Creator who gives him mastery over his acts and the ability to govern himself with a view to the true and the good. The natural law expresses the original moral sense which enables man to discern by reason the good and the evil, the truth and the lie. (*CCC*, n. 1954)

> The natural law, the Creator's very good work, provides the solid foundation on which man can build the structure of moral rules to guide his choices. It also provides the indispensable moral foundation for building the human community. Finally, it provides the necessary basis for the civil law with which it is connected, whether by a reflection that draws conclusion from its principles or by additions of a positive and juridical nature. (*CCC*, n. 1959)

The inherent dignity which humans have received from the Creator is a gift which came along with the gift of human life. Humans recognize in each other a reciprocal right to the respect owed them by virtue of that original gift. In the area of medical matters, the appropriate mutual respect is guided by the natural law concretized in medical ethics.

The Body–Soul Unity of the Human Person

The human person is a composite, but a unique type of composite. There is a material "component"—which is obvious to all. And there is a spiritual "component"— which is not immediately obvious; self-reflection is needed to perceive it. The two components coexist, but not as two things, each with their independent existence, such as would be the case of an automobile and the driver in it. The human person exists as one reality, having one

interdependent existence of the two components which *together* constitute the one living human body, the one existing human person.

The human person is not the body taken by itself, nor is it the soul taken by itself.

> The human person, created in the image of God, is a being at once corporeal and spiritual. The biblical account expresses this reality in symbolic language when it affirms that "then the Lord God formed man of dust from the ground, and breathed into his nostrils the breath of life; and man became a living being." Man, whole and entire, is therefore *willed* by God. (*CCC*, n. 362, original emphasis)

The human body shares in the dignity of "the image of God": it is a human body precisely because it is animated by a spiritual soul, and it is the whole human person that is intended to become, in the body of Christ, a temple of the Spirit:

> Man, though made of body and soul, is a unity. Through his very bodily condition he sums up in himself the elements of the material world. ... For this reason man may not despise his bodily life. Rather he is obliged to regard his body as good and to hold it in honor since God has created it and will raise it up on the last day. (*CCC*, n. 364)

Although man is made in the image of God and has a spiritual and therefore an immortal soul, death is a reality. Death was not part of God's "original" plan for man. Man was designed for eternal life with God ... and still is.

> As a consequence of original sin, man must suffer "bodily death, from which man would have been immune had he not sinned." (*CCC*, n. 1018)

> Jesus, the Son of God, freely suffered death for us in complete and free submission to the will of God, his Father. By his death he has conquered death, and so opened the possibility of salvation to all men. (CCC, n. 1019)

At death, what is seen and buried is *not* the human body which before was alive. What is seen now is a collection of tissues and organs, loosely bound together but rapidly disintegrating, falling apart, because the principle of life which held them together—the human spiritual soul—is no longer present and acting on that matter. The soul is no longer exercising its unifying power over the material principle. Strictly speaking, that matter, that corpse, *is* not a human body but *was* a human; to have a human body requires the soul to give that matter the specificity, unity, and life which characterizes the human person. When that principle of unity is no longer present and acting on the matter, that condition is called death.

> By death the soul is separated from the body, but in the resurrection God will give incorruptible life to our body, transformed by reunion with our soul. Just as Christ is risen and lives forever, so all of us will rise at the last day. (*CCC*, n. 1016)

The human person (the body–soul composite), as such, no longer exists after death except in a residual sense. While the human soul continues to exist because it is a spiritual being and has no parts into which it could disintegrate, by itself it is not the person. (Of course, God could annihilate it—and so it would cease to exist in any case—but there is no evidence that God has ever annihilated anything He has created.) But the human soul exists in a sort of attenuated existence, because of its very nature it demands union with its material principle to which it has an enduring and everlasting relationship.

It should be noted that the soul does not preexist its union with the material principle. But once having been joined, as it were, to such a material principle it will exist forever. Initially after death it exists "alone," but at the general resurrection it once again is united to the material principle (from which it was separated at death) to reconstitute that specific human person. "The Church teaches that ... [the soul] is immortal: it does not perish when it separates from the body at death, and it will be reunited with the body at the final resurrection" (*CCC*, n. 366).

Teaching Authority of the Bible and the Church

How do we know what is true and what is good? How do we know what is morally right behavior, whether in medicine or in any other area of human life? In the Gospel according to St. Matthew (19:16) the question is asked, "Teacher, what good must I do to have eternal life?" Jesus answers the question, "If you wish to enter into life, keep the commandments ... [and] if you wish to be perfect ... come follow me" (Matt. 19:17, 21). After quoting and briefly reflecting on these words, Pope John Paul II states in his encyclical *Veritatis splendor* (The Splendor of Truth):

> *People today need to turn to Christ once again in order to receive from him the answer to their questions about what is good and what is evil.* Christ is the Teacher, the Risen One who has life in himself and who is always present in his Church and in the

world. It is He who opens up to the faithful the book of the Scriptures and, by fully revealing the Father's will, teaches the truth about moral action.[1]

Yes, for Christians the example and teaching of Christ is the right path to follow, and indeed the only secure path. Jesus said, "I am the way and the truth and the life" (John 14:6). The sacred Scriptures, particularly the New Testament, contain his words, his acts. In addition, He taught that the moral law which Moses promulgated was also part of his teaching, as is indicated in the opening paragraph of this chapter: "Keep the commandments" (Matt. 19:17). But he also gave a definitive and authentic interpretation of these same commandments, both by his teaching—"You have heard that it was said ... But I say to you ..." (see Matt. 5:21–48)—and by his example, such as the way of keeping the Sabbath holy.

Jesus no longer walks among us in a visible fashion, but he did not leave us orphans (see John 14:18). He did two things to realize this: (1) he appointed and taught selected followers (the Twelve) who would have a universal mandate to carry on his mission: "Go, therefore, and make disciples of all nations, baptizing them in the name of the Father, and of the Son, and of the Holy Spirit, teaching them to observe all that I have commanded you" (Matt. 28:19–20). And (2) he promised not to abandon them: "And behold, I am with you always, until the end of the age" (Matt. 28:20). His presence is continued in this world by his spirit which he had promised them (John 14:16: "I will ask the Father and He will give you another Advocate to be with you always, the Spirit of truth"). His spirit is the Holy Spirit, which made his presence manifest on Pentecost when, with a mighty rush of wind and tongue-like flames, the Spirit of Jesus descended upon the apostles (see Acts 2:1–4). That Spirit dwells in the Church to this day and, indeed, will continue to do so until the end of time.

It is the Church to which Jesus sent his Holy Spirit that teaches us today the truth which Jesus gave to the apostles:

> The law of Christ, the New Law, the Gospel, therefore, is more than a set of rules. It is Jesus' own teaching brought alive in our hearts by the Holy Spirit and confirmed by him through the teaching of the shepherds of the Church commissioned by him to keep us on the straight and narrow path. Theologians seek to formulate and systematize this teaching to help us further, but their human systems are trustworthy only when conformed to the teaching of our God-commissioned pastors. The holy, orthodox faith alone can find a way

through the thicket of error and confusion produced by human pride, one-sided subjective thinking, human stupidity, and the cunning lies of the Accuser.[2]

This is the reason why Church teaching is the sure guide for Catholics (and for others, too, who wish to follow the Lord Jesus) in making moral choices in matters of medical ethics. The magisterium of the Church has given sure guidance in a number of specific medical-moral issues, especially since the reign of Pope Pius XI (1922–1939), and amply continued by Pius XII (1939–1958). While Pope John XXIII did not address many issues in medical morals, some of his teachings on larger social issues had significant impact on raising the level of consciousness on medical issues. Pope Paul VI is known in the medical field and in marriage teaching, particularly for his encyclical *Humanae vitae* (Of Human Life), which was promulgated in 1968 and taught that the use of contraceptive devices (mechanical or chemical), which separated the unitive and the procreative meanings of the conjugal act, was immoral. Having less than a month in the papal office, Pope John Paul I did not have the opportunity to issue any teachings bearing on bioethics.

His successor, Pope John Paul II (1978–2005), was vigorous in his defense of human life and the sacredness of human procreation. In addition, he had to face a number of new bioethical problems such as cloning, partial-birth abortions, physician-assisted suicide, in vitro fertilization, and others. In his first encyclical, *Redemptor Hominis* (The Redeemer of Man, 1979), John Paul II asserted one of his basic messages. While technology is good in making human life more secure and enjoyable, it has to submit to the judgment of ethics in order to make sure that its methods and products do in fact promote the authentic good of human beings and human society. Thus, John Paul II writes,

> The essential meaning of this "kingship" and "dominion" . . . over the visible world, which the Creator himself gave man for his task, consists in the priority of ethics over technology, in the primacy of the person over things, and in the superiority of spirit over matter.[3]

The doctrine of the Catholic Church holds that the bishops are the legitimate descendants, as it were, of the apostles who had received their commission to preach the Good News directly from Jesus Christ. They in turn commissioned others to continue proclaiming the Good News beyond the confines of Palestine to "all nations." As the preaching of the Gospel was extended in space,

so too was it extended in time. This commission was understood by successive generations of teachers and preachers to continue until the Lord chose to end time and inaugurate the new era where the Kingdom of God (the Reign of God) would finally become fully manifest and clothed with the Glory of God.

In the meanwhile, the faithful together with the commissioned teachers, preachers, and leaders had to continue preaching and living the Gospel truth, directed, fortified, and guarded by the Spirit of truth which Jesus had promised his Church. As the Church expanded its geographical and temporal borders and, in the process, absorbed a wide variety of people and cultures with their own history and experiences, the relatively simple moral problems which plague all human beings assumed a number of forms and complexity. Problems that arose with explorations and conquests of new lands in the thirteenth to the eighteenth centuries required careful analyses to determine the Christian way of dealing with them. As trade and commerce developed and money took on new functions and meanings, the Church had to discover what the Gospel had to say to those involved in such matters. More recently, warfare has taken on such enormous destructive power over land and people that the older principles of legitimate self-defense and separation of civilian populations from soldiers are no longer clear in their applications.

Now, technology has marched in with a plethora of new challenges. Perhaps nowhere have new technological "advances" raised more serious challenges to the Gospel than in the medical field, which touches human life and procreation so intimately. The popes saw that human life was being devalued both by the "hardening of hearts" following the terribly destructive World War II and by the dehumanization associated with some applications of modern technology, such as birth-control devices, and the consequent mentality, and several of them issued statements of their own or approved declarations made by the Congregation for the Doctrine of the Faith. Thus, Pope Paul VI issued his encyclical *Humanae vitae* (1968) to clarify the teaching and remove any doubts with regard to moral dimensions of human procreation. Probably in response to the U.S. Supreme Court decision of January 1973, *Roe v. Wade*, which legalized abortion in the United States, the CDF (with the approval of Pope Paul VI) issued the *Declaration on Procured Abortion* in 1974, which clearly and unequivocally condemned elective abortion.

With the rapid development of technological means of generating human life, the CDF with the approval of Pope John Paul II issued a clear judgment about the role of technology in human procreation in *Donum vitae* (1987).

It outlines the essential elements for morally acceptable means of bringing new human life into this world. Human procreation is to take place (1) within a marriage, (2) through a conjugal act (i.e., intercourse of a man and woman married to each other) in which fertilization and gestation take place within the body of the woman, (3) who then gives birth to the child.

With the increasing control of human beings over life and the use of modern developments in life-support systems, it becomes possible to maintain life where before the individual would have readily succumbed to life-threatening diseases and injuries. These advances in medical technology give the medical profession unprecedented control over human life while at the same time creating excruciating conscience problems about whether and when life-support interventions should be initiated, withheld, or terminated. Thus the Church, in its traditional respect for life, has had to face the problem arising from the development of life-supporting technologies that seemed to prolong unnecessarily the dying process to the extent that the patient experienced additional suffering even when there was no reasonable hope for a recovery. Families, too, frequently found that such technological improvement imposed suffering and often great financial losses on them. Pope Pius XII initiated a response to these issues by recalling the long-developing tradition with regard to life-saving interventions and making a distinction between what has become known as the "ordinary and extraordinary means of sustaining life": "Normally one is held to use only ordinary means—according to the circumstances of persons, places, times, and culture—that is to say, means that do not involve any grave burden for oneself or another."[4] This statement of papal teaching was amplified and clarified by the *Declaration on Euthanasia* (1980), issued by the CDF and approved by Pope John Paul II. This document noted that the use of "ordinary" and "extraordinary" had caused some confusion, since the medical use of these terms is notably different. Hence, the words "proportionate" and disproportionate" were suggested as a substitute without any change in meaning.

However, as clear as these various teachings may have been, there were some Catholic theologians who disagreed with some of the Vatican statements, especially in the area of human sexuality. Parallel to the increase of scientific knowledge and technological applications to everyday human life, there seems to have been a gradual deterioration of faith. Theories, philosophical and scientific, have brought into question the validity of our knowledge, the capacity of humans to know the truth

in general—whatever truth might be, it was said—and of objective moral truth in particular. Statements by the Church, and indeed by most establishments, are today often greeted with opposition, resistance, and defiance. Teachings and proclamations by the Church are subject to a "hermeneutic of suspicion." Although this is done by the more educated and sophisticated members of the Church, in general the faithful become contaminated with the virus of dissent.[5] John Paul II also issued important statements on the topics of neurological criteria for the determination of death, nutrition and hydration, and the persistent vegetative state.

In spite of such opposition, the Church leaders, the Pope, and bishops united to him (that is, the magisterium of the Church) continue to reflect on the various moral issues which have inundated our culture and to offer appropriate teaching and guidance. They are aided in this task by theologians and other scholars who strive to remain faithful to the mission of the Church and to its moral tradition and teachings. The challenge that the teachers of the Church have is to apply long-accepted moral principles to the complexities of technological development in the field of medicine. Starting from principles found in the Church's moral tradition, the theologians apply these to the specific problem at hand. Before addressing these specific topics in an official document, the magisterium generally seeks the opinion of a variety of persons knowledgeable on the topic and waits until major theologians have discussed, debated, and decided on their respective conclusions. The magisterium will then exercise its pastoral charism to decide its response to a vexing question in order to safeguard the faith and morals of the Church. Employing the best of its collective human skills, the magisterium, after pondering the range of theological responses coming from the faithful and the theologians (who are, of course, part of the faithful), relies on he Holy Spirit to guide its decisions and declarations.

Notes

[1] John Paul II, *Veritatis spendor* (August 6, 1993), n. 8 (original emphasis).

[2] Benedict M. Ashley, *Living the Truth in Love: A Biblical Introduction to Moral Theology (*New York: Alba House, 1996), 458–459.

[3] John Paul II, *Redemptor hominis* (March 4, 1979), n. 16.

[4] Pius XII, Address before the International Congress of Anesthesiologists (November 24, 1957), in *The Pope Speaks* 4.4 (Spring 1958): 393–398.

[5] See William E. May, "The Magisterium and Bioethics," *Ethics & Medics* 12.8 (August 1987): 1–3.

✠

Editorial Summation: All being and life are radically dependent on God's creative act, which is the cause and enduring source of being. God creates the body and soul of every person, and together these confer human dignity. The conscientious Catholic wants to do what is morally right in the eyes of God. Many Catholics know, but some may not accept, the teachings of the Church on matters of morality, but Jesus is the ultimate font of truth: "I am the Way, and the Truth, and the Life" (John 14:6). He instructed his disciples to "observe all that I have commanded you" (Matt. 28:19–20). He gave them the security of knowing that He would not abandon his Church: "And behold I am with you always, until the end of the age" (Matt. 28:20). Jesus would bring this about by sending the Holy Spirit: "I will ask the Father, and He will give you another Advocate—to be with you always, the Spirit of truth" (John 14:16). That same Spirit of truth is with Jesus's Church to this day. The Church, in its official teaching, is guided by the Holy Spirit. That does not mean that every statement or teaching of the magisterium enjoys the charism or gift of infallibility. That charism is reserved for certain conditions, among which is when the Pope intends to address in a binding way the universal Church on a teaching of revealed truth which pertains to faith (what to believe) and morals (how to behave). Other teachings enjoy the guidance of the Holy Spirit, but without the guarantee of infallibility; these are nonetheless authoritative. While there may be a diversity of theological opinion on a number of moral issues, the secure course is to follow what the Church teaches through its pastoral charism.

CHAPTER 2

The Moral Fonts of Action and Decision Making

Peter J. Cataldo

Human Nature: The Basis of Morality

Chapter 1 showed that the human person possesses a specific rational nature by which an individual is able to be and to function as a human being. It is because of this nature—endowed with an intellect and free choice—that human acts necessarily possess a specific moral character and identify the person acting as a moral agent. Those human acts performed knowingly and willingly have a moral dimension, whereas those human acts which are done without knowledge or without free choice of the will, such as scratching one's head or sneezing, do not necessarily have a moral aspect. There is no truly human act which falls outside the parameters of ethical identification and evaluation. Every human act and every general human endeavor is directed toward what is understood as, or appears in some sense to be, suitable, preferable, or fulfilling relative to some aspect of human nature; that is, every human act appears to the agent to be good. Everything—from talking on a telephone, to an alcoholic's drinking (distinguishing between the initial drinking and that which proceeds from the addiction), to receiving or performing heart bypass surgery—is inescapably moral in the sense that these actions are all attempts to fulfill the various ends of human nature. In each of these situations, the actions have the appearance of being good, of being desirable and suitable. That is why the person is able to act at all. Any number of factors can influence how something has the appearance of being good, from familial and societal conditions to neurochemical elements and events of the brain. However, all individuals who act knowingly and freely have the capacity to ask and answer the question whether their acts truly fulfill their human nature and are morally good. Indeed, ethics in general should but does not always ask what kinds of actions are truly good and what actions are only apparently good but actually immoral.

The view that there are human actions which are inherently good or immoral as they either fulfill or contradict a stable human nature is contrary to the common assumption that there is an ethically neutral zone in human affairs in which science, technology, and medicine in particular are situated. In this view there are supposedly many human acts that are neither good nor bad. The fact that this position is false is evident from the very attempt to be ethically neutral, because the attempt is itself a value-laden act. The attempt to be ethically neutral would not be possible were it not for the fact that ethical neutrality is perceived and pursued as something more suitable and preferable than not being ethically neutral. Ethical neutrality is regarded as something good for human beings to pursue just as much as any other good might be considered. Because being ethically neutral is actually just one more perceived good among others in human action, the claim to be ethically neutral is self-refuting. The attempt necessarily brings about the precise opposite of what is sought from the perspective of ethical neutrality, namely, a specific value over others that is thought to be conducive to human flourishing.

Hence, the attempt to be ethically neutral is really to be ethically particular. This is often evident when the prohibition of certain procedures in a Catholic hospital is characterized as "bad medicine," or interference with treatment and the physician–patient relationship, or as an imposition of Catholic values on others. One of the assumptions behind the objection is that the patient's desire for the procedure is an ethically neutral matter, and therefore, any prohibition of it is a deprivation of something to which the patient is reasonably entitled. In reality this is a conflict between two different and opposing views of what is considered to be ethical medicine. One view is that the patient's medical needs are independent of any other considerations and thus the response to those needs is an ethically neutral matter; the other is that the patient's needs must also be viewed in light of specific ethical principles. The fact that the patient or caregiver may find acceptable something considered unacceptable by the Catholic hospital means that the patient or caregiver is advancing an ethical view different from that of the hospital. It does not mean that the view of the patient or caregiver is ethically neutral (and, therefore, supposedly better medicine) while the hospital's view is not. Ultimately, the patient seeks the procedure that the hospital disallows because he or she considers it more suitable to, and compatible with, a human good, whereas the hospital disallows the procedure because it is viewed as being contrary to human good. Both hospital and patient or caregiver arrive at different views of what constitutes good medicine from the same starting point, that is, human nature. But because they hold to differing views of human nature, they arrive at conflicting views of what should be allowed and what should not.

The centrality of human nature for ethics shows that the charge of "interference" cannot be made on the basis of ethical neutrality, because such neutrality, as we have seen, does not exist. Health care is always provided according to a particular vision of what is good for the patient as a human person. Every health care provider, Catholic and non-Catholic alike, individual or institutional, determines what is health care and delivers that care consistent with a certain view of human well-being. This view can be explicit or implicit, but in either case it is present and at work. The vision of human good in Catholic health care excludes certain options, such as abortion or direct sterilization, but the vision of what is good for the patient in many non-Catholic institutions includes these procedures as options. The fact that Catholic health care excludes these options while many non-Catholic health care institutions include them is a function of two different views of serving the human good of the patient. It certainly is not a matter of interference. The current debate about Catholic interference in the practice of medicine is instructive for our purposes because it is an example of how the moral dimension of human acts (and in particular acts of health care) is inescapable.

Structure of the Moral Act

As morality cannot be properly understood apart from the structure of human nature, so too does the individual moral act have a specific structure rooted in human nature. Before considering the process of moral decision making that concludes in a moral act, we first need an understanding of the structure of the moral act itself.

The Catholic moral tradition has identified three basic factors that shape the morality of an act: the *object*, the *intention*, and the *circumstances* of the act. The primary determinant or source of the moral status of an act is the act's "moral object."[1] The *object* of a moral act is the specific kind of action or behavior chosen. The moral status of an act's object is independent of the person choosing. The object is the substance of an act and is a datum as objective as any physical aspect of the act. The moral object of an act provides the basis on which moral acts are distinguished from one another. The object defines the substance of the act as being, for example, an act of charity, self-defense, adultery, theft, or life conservation. Depending on its definition, the object of an act is something that either truly fulfills and completes human nature or detracts from, and is contrary to, its integral unity.

Unlike the object of an act, intention is a factor that is dependent on the will of the one acting. Intention is the subjective act of moving or tending toward an ultimate end or toward one end for the sake of another. The will's tending toward such intermediate ends is another way of stating that the will intends specific means for the attainment of ends. Intention answers the question, "Why is this act being done?" For example, one can intend the end of providing for the material needs of one's family by knowing and tending toward that end. Such an end can then be achieved in any number of ways, each being intended as an intermediate step or means to the desired end.

Circumstances include the manner in which the act is carried out; for example, the time, place, or instruments used. The circumstances of the moral act are not part of the substance of the act; they do not enter into the definition of what the act is. For example, the deliberate taking of another's property is not a circumstance of the act of theft, nor is it a circumstance of fornication that the man and woman are both unmarried. The quality of being another's property or being unmarried belongs to the very substance and identity of either act. However, in the case of theft, the time of day or the instruments used are properly understood to be circumstances of the theft. Likewise, where and when an act of fornication takes place are circumstances of the act.

The distinctions between object, intention, and circumstances indicates that the reality of a moral act is complex and not reducible to one single factor. In taking account of this reality, the Catholic moral tradition bases moral evaluation on all three factors of the moral act. Every truly good human act possesses a moral integration of object, intention, and circumstances, that is, all three must be good. For example, helping to restore the health of another is a moral object good in kind. Intending this end for the sake of the other's well-being and not for vainglory is a good intention. Administering a dose of medication in the right amount, at the right time, and in the right way are all circumstances proportionate to the object of restoring health. If any of the three moral sources is defective, the action in question cannot be good. Thus, acts are immoral insofar as this integration is fractured in some way.[2]

The Process of Making a Moral Decision

Having explained (1) that all truly human acts (i.e., acts involving knowledge and free choice) have a moral dimension, and (2) the nature of the moral act, we can now address the process of moral decision making that leads to a moral act. Just as the moral basis of action is not reducible to one thing, so also does the process of engaging in a moral act have many components. Chapter 1 showed that human action cannot be explained simply in terms of deterministic physiological and biochemical processes. Human nature is endowed with intellect and will, which are two powers that cannot be explained by neurochemical causes. It is precisely through the interaction of the powers of intellect and free will in the process of moral decision making that means and ends are ordered to each other and moral goods are freely desired. This integrated process has been traditionally divided into deliberation, judgment, and choice.[3]

The first step in the process of moral decision making is *deliberation*. The person uses the power of intellect to initiate a search or discovery of the various means (within the relevant circumstances) that are suitable for attaining the intended end. Not only is the suitability of certain means for reaching the end taken into account on their own merits, but the different relationships of specific acts (means) to the end are also compared and weighed. Hence, good deliberation includes a consideration of whether the various means are morally right actions, and how the circumstances will affect the act.

Moreover, one who deliberates well is able to make a correct determination of certain circumstances pertaining to the deliberation itself. This person deliberates neither too slowly nor too quickly with respect to what should be done. If quick action is required, then deliberation is not delayed. If there is more time to act, then the person who deliberates well knows this and allows for a proportionate deliberation. Consider, for example, the situation of a toddler who is at imminent risk of burning himself on a barbecue grill. A nearby parent of the child knows that the danger must be eliminated. He or she knows that preventing this harm is something good, as it will preserve the well-being of the child. Assuming there is no one in the vicinity to assist, the parent could deliberate (either implicitly or explicitly) about different means to the intended end, including rolling the grill away from the child, dropping the valuable bowl that the parent is holding and grabbing the child, or holding onto the bowl while grabbing the child. Dropping the bowl would ensure that the child is safely pulled away and would probably save critical seconds of time. When something must be done, the parent does not dwell on the probable damage to the bowl, but rushes to pull the child away from danger. In contrast to the quick deliberation in this case, consider the case of applying to colleges. Here the deliberation about the various means to the end of attending college is complex and can take place over an extended period of time.

The next step in the process of decision making is to bring deliberation to a close. Deliberation proposes several options for action, but only one option at a time can be done. Thus, a *judgment* is needed to decide which means will be acted on. This is an intellectual judgment or determination that a certain means is the best under the existing circumstances. However, not only does a person make a practical judgment of the intellect that an act ought to be done, but the person also needs to adhere to that judgment. At the same time that the person intellectually judges what ought to be done, there is a volitional response corresponding to the judgment. At one and the same time the will is moved so that the person becomes committed to the judgment. Philosophically, this conjoined activity between intellect and will is known as the act of *choice*. Following the act of choice, what has been judged and chosen must be executed. The intellect is the power which *directs and commands* the execution and implementation of the means toward the end. The will is the principal cause by which the other various powers of human nature are *used* to bring about what is directed by the intellect.

It will be helpful to see how deliberation, judgment, and choice function together in ordinary and emergency clinical examples. Consider first a routine case of a radiologic examination of a suspected broken limb. The radiologic technologist first deliberates about the various ways in which the limb can be x-rayed so that the best x-ray may be obtained under the circumstances. The technologist will deliberate about possible views (e.g., upright, flat, anterior, or posterior lateral), possible positions of the patient's limb on the x-ray table, and techniques to be used (i.e., adjustments to the technical settings of the x-ray machine). After considering and weighing these means, a judgment is made about the best view, position, and technique to obtain the desired information about the condition of the fractured limb. This judgment is then adhered to by the will, and the various powers of the technologist are directed and commanded to bring about the end of producing the requisite x-ray films. The case of an emergency appendectomy, on the other hand, involves a "fast-track" decision process. The emergency room physician must be able to execute deliberation, judgment, and choice with celerity so that surgery may be performed on the ruptured appendix.

A Catholic health care ethics committee is, among other things, responsible for moral decisions that are made about patient care. It is not sufficient for the committee to proceed simply on the basis of the details of each case. The committee must also have a foundational knowledge about the structure of a moral act and the various elements of our human nature that make any particular moral decision possible. Without this foundation, any evaluation of a decision will be incomplete.

Notes

[1] John Paul II, *Veritatis splendor* (August 6, 1993), nn. 78–79.

[2] See *Catechism of the Catholic Church*, nn. 1750–1756.

[3] See Vernon J. Bourke, *Ethics: A Textbook in Moral Philosophy* (New York: Macmillan, 1951).

Editorial Summation: Human beings are endowed with a rational nature that has the faculties of intellect, by which truth can be known, and free choice, by which the good can be chosen without being determined internally or externally. All truly human acts, that is, those which proceed from appropriate knowledge and free choice, are either morally good or evil; there is no morally neutral ground in this sphere. A moral act has a structure; it is composed of three parts or components: the moral object, the intention, and the circumstances. (1) The *moral object* specifies the moral act. It answers the question, "What is being done?" It is the specific, physical act which is deliberately selected for execution and possesses an objective moral quality, for example, not simply the taking of someone's purse but the taking of property that does not belong to the taker. (2) The *intention* answers the question, "Why is this act being done?" It is a subjective element that is the reason this particular act is selected for execution. (3) The *circumstances* are those factors which "stand round the act," as it were, and do not pertain to its essential nature. They answer the questions where, when, and how about the act and the persons involved in the act. For a moral evaluation that finds the entire act good, all three components must be good. Traditionally, the process by which a moral act is executed involves three integrated components: deliberation, judgment, and choice. Deliberation is a search for and identification of relevant options as means to achieve the desired act. Judgment is a decision among the various options for suitably achieving the goal desired. Choice adheres to that decision.

CHAPTER 3

Selected Moral Principles

A. Totality and Integrity

Rev. Germain Kopaczynski, O.F.M. Conv.

Good sense and sound medicine concur in the judgment that the part exists for the sake of the whole:

> All persons served by Catholic health care have the right and duty to protect and preserve their bodily and functional integrity. The functional integrity of the person may be sacrificed to maintain the health or life of the person when no other morally permissible means is available.[1]

This passage from the *Ethical and Religious Directives for Catholic Health Care Services* conveys not only Christian ethical reflection but also a Christian anthropology.

Stewardship of Human Life

Human beings are made in the image of God. From that source derives our inestimable dignity. God has created us intelligent and free. Part of that exercise of intelligence and freedom is found when men and women exercise care for themselves, and for those who may be entrusted to their care, as created in God's image.

This is the foundation of the Catholic teaching: we are meant to exercise responsible stewardship for all that we have received from God, including our physical health. We are not absolute masters but responsible stewards; in the difference between those two terms is found differing views of the human person. The text from St. Paul's First Letter to the Corinthians is most instructive in this regard: "Do you not know that your body is a temple of the holy Spirit within you, whom you have from God, and that you are not your own? For you have been purchased at a great price. Therefore glorify God in your body" (6:19–20).

It is as responsible stewards that we are to make health care decisions. Because we are made in God's image, the human person has a great dignity that cannot be attacked, degraded, or harmed, be it at the very beginning or at the very end of life. The introduction to part five of the *ERDs* restates the thought of St. Paul on the matter in these words:

> The truth that life is a precious gift from God has profound implications for the question of stewardship over human life. We are not the owners of our lives, and hence, do not have absolute power over life. We have a duty to preserve our life and to use it for the glory of God; but the duty to preserve life is not absolute, for we may reject life-prolonging procedures that are insufficiently beneficial or excessively burdensome. Suicide and euthanasia are never morally acceptable options.

The Catholic tradition in health care attempts to exercise this responsible stewardship at every stage of life. This is seen especially in the principles we elaborate by the use of our human reason. The principle of totality and integrity is most helpful in understanding Catholic teaching on procedures that involve inflicting harm on some part of the body for the sake of the good of the whole. Acts undertaken in the spirit of stewardship are legitimate; those undertaken with a spirit of absolute autonomy are illicit.[2]

Sacrificing for the Good of the Whole

Church teaching on matters pertaining to integrity and totality owes much to the thought of St. Thomas Aquinas (a thirteenth-century doctor of theology) who wrote in his masterpiece of theology, "A member of the human body is to be disposed of according as it may profit the whole. ... [If] a member is healthy and continuing in its natural state, it cannot be cut off to the detriment of the whole."[3] Surgery to save the life of someone who is sick is an honorable and noble use of human reason and medical skill; mutilation of a healthy human being is not, since it harms the integral human being God has fashioned in his own image.

Two popes of the last century did much to build on the foundations erected by St. Paul and St. Thomas. Pope Pius XI speaks of the limitations we must keep in mind regarding stewardship and totality,[4] while Pope Pius XII shows how far we can go in applying the principle to health care decisions. Indeed, in a 1952 address to the First International Congress of the Histopathology of the Nervous System, Pius XII speaks of the duty to intervene "as often as, and to the extent that the good of the whole demands, to paralyze, destroy, mutilate and separate the members."[5]

Taken together, the popes give a lesson in authentic Christian anthropology, telling us we are indeed responsible stewards, never absolute masters. In Pius XII, we find the emphasis being placed on the *principle of totality*, ordered toward the preservation of the physical whole of the human body, while Pius XI stresses the *principle of integrity*, perhaps best understood as being respectful of the hierarchical ordering of the members of the body.

The task for members of ethics committees will be to ensure that the complementarity of the approaches of the two popes be kept in mind. Though mutilation of the human body is always to be lamented, when it does take place, we should be sure that it is always merely physical, never moral, that is, we must not harm our moral life. This can be done to the extent that safeguards are in place to guarantee that mutilating surgery is both justified (because we are responsible stewards), and restricted (because we are not absolute masters of the human condition).

When a part or a function of the body becomes harmful to the whole body—a cancerous breast, for example—steps may be taken to control the damage, even to the point of removing the breast in order to preserve the life of the person. The part in this case must be sacrificed for the good of the whole.

May healthy organs ever be excised? Pius XII spells out instances when this may be legitimately done: First, when the preservation of the organ may cause grave injury or even threaten the life of the individual; second, when a reasonable hope exists that such surgery is the only means of avoiding the contemplated serious future damage; and third, when such excision of the organ or suppression of its function will either diminish substantially or eliminate totally the risk to the person. Pius XII writes,

It can [also] happen that the removal of a healthy organ and the paralyzing of its function remove from the evil—cancer, for example—the possibility of extending further, or else change the effect of this evil on the body. If there is no other alternative available, in both cases a surgical operation on the healthy organ is permissible.[6]

After granting that the above is a legitimate extension of the meaning of the principle of totality, Pius XII goes on to observe that the principle may not be extended to directly contraceptive measures. Why?

Considerations allied with Christian anthropology have led Catholic teaching to give special consideration to the generative organs, ordained as they are both to the good of the individual and to the good of society. Since standard medical practice ought to preserve functional integrity whenever possible, this ought to hold no less for the generative faculty. Yet when the generative organs in men or women become diseased and pose a direct threat to the life of the individual, they may either be functionally suppressed or removed.

Helpful to keep in mind in this regard is a distinction made by Jesuit Thomas O'Donnell:

Therapeutic procedure: A procedure is said to be therapeutic when a generative organ is removed or its function is suppressed insofar as the organ, precisely as part of the body, is destructive of the good of the whole body. An example of this would be the removal of a cancerous uterus.

Contraceptive procedure: A procedure is said to be contraceptive when a generative organ is removed or its function is suppressed insofar as the organ is a medium of generation, and for the purpose of destroying its generative function. An example of this would be sterilization in the presence of some cardiac disease.[7]

This helps explain the wording of directive 53 of the *ERDs*:

Direct sterilization of either men or women, whether permanent or temporary, is not permitted in a Catholic health care institution. Procedures that induce sterility are permitted when their direct effect is the cure or alleviation of a present and serious pathology and a simpler treatment is not available.[8]

One further question under the heading of totality and integrity concerns organ donation: may individuals offer body parts such as kidneys to help others? For serious reasons, yes. The bishops speak of this possibility in directive 30 of the *ERDs*:

The transplantation of organs from living donors is morally permissible when such a donation will not sacrifice or seriously impair any essential bodily function and the anticipated benefit to the recipient is proportionate to the harm done to the donor. Furthermore, the freedom of the prospective donor must be respected, and economic advantages should not accrue to the donor.

The bishops add in a note: "While the donation of a kidney represents loss of biological integrity, such a donation does not compromise functional integrity since human beings are capable of functioning with only one kidney."[9] Here the mutilation is justified by the good of charity.

Perhaps it is not an exaggeration to say that one of the most important duties of those serving on ethics committees in Catholic health facilities is to help individuals weigh the advantages and the disadvantages of such serious, loving, and at times perilous courses of action.

Notes

[1] U.S. Conference of Catholic Bishops, *Ethical and Religious Directives for Catholic Health Care Services*, 4th ed. (Washington, D.C.: USCCB, 2001), n. 29.

[2] Thomas J. O'Donnell, S.J., writes, "If the procedure is strictly an act of wise administration and the proper exercise of stewardship, it is morally right; but if it is an act of ownership and a usurpation of God's absolute prerogative, and in violation of the immanent teleology of the body and its parts, it is morally wrong." *Medicine and Christian Morality*, 3rd ed. (New York: Alba House, 1996), 75.

[3] Thomas Aquinas, *Summa theologiae*, II-II, Q. 65.1.

[4] See Gerald Kelly, "Pope Pius XII and the Principle of Totality," *Theological Studies* 16 (1955): 373–396.

[5] Pius XII, Address to the First International Congress of Histopathology (September 13, 1952), in *Papal Teachings: The Human Body*, ed. Monks of Solesmes (Boston: Daughters of St. Paul, 1960), 194–208.

[6] Pius XII, Address to the Delegates at the Twenty-Sixth Congress of Urology (October 8, 1953), in *Human Body,* ed. Monks of Solesmes, 278.

[7] O'Donnell, *Medicine*, 84–85.

[8] For more on this line of reasoning, see Congregation for the Doctrine of the Faith, "Responses to Questions Proposed concerning 'Uterine Isolation' and Related Matters" (July 31, 1993), in *L'Osservatore Romano*, English ed. (August 3, 1994), 2.

[9] USCCB, *Ethical and Religious Directives*, note 16, 40.

✠

Editorial Summation: The Catholic moral tradition has developed the principle of totality and integrity as a guide to evaluate the morality of medical treatments in certain life-threatening situations, namely, those in which a part or function of the body must be deliberately harmed for the good of the whole. A part or function of the body may be sacrificed if this is the only way that the health or integral function of the whole body can be preserved. The principle of totality and integrity does not justify sterilization, because the direct purpose of this procedure is not the health of the whole body, but the elimination of the generative function. Actions that have as their direct purpose the suppression or eradication of some serious pathology but indirectly result in sterility are permitted. Organ donation and organ transplantation are justifiable under the principle of totality and integrity. While organ donation is not done for the sake of the health of the donor, nevertheless it is an act of charity that can be acceptable so long as no essential bodily function of the donor is sacrificed. Thus, one kidney may be donated when the remaining kidney is sufficient for organic function.

B. Ordinary and Extraordinary Means

Grattan T. Brown

The distinction between ordinary or proportionate and extraordinary or disproportionate means is used in judging whether it is morally acceptable to refrain from or cease medical intervention. A patient has an obligation to use ordinary or proportionate means of preserving his or her life but may choose not to use extraordinary or disproportionate means. This principle applies to a wide range of medical practices but most frequently to means of "life support," which in some circumstances gives a patient the necessary time to heal, but in others actually prolongs the dying process while offering little or no benefit. Centuries ago, theologians developed this distinction to understand whether a refusal to accept a life-preserving treatment constitutes a failure in the duty to preserve one's life. While recently developed medical interventions are much more effective than those of the past, the basic moral question remains the same.

People sometimes speak of ordinary and extraordinary means, and at other times of proportionate and disproportionate means. These sets of terms are typically used interchangeably, and what difference there is between them is not yet fully settled. What can be said is that each set of terms clarifies a different aspect of the same principle, and so it seems appropriate to use them interchangeably. The terms "ordinary" and "extraordinary" highlight the fact that some means lie beyond what is morally necessary for a patient to pursue.

This terminology, however, can become confusing when means rightly judged to be extraordinary in one case or in one historical period are rightly judged to be ordinary in another. For example, the pain associated with amputation made it an extraordinary treatment until effective means of anesthesia reduced that burden. The term "proportionate" clarifies why some means are ordinary, namely, their benefit is proportionate to the burden. Likewise, some means are extraordinary because their benefit is disproportionate to the burden. The term "disproportionate," however, can suggest unreasonable or perhaps even irrational, and hence immoral. Yet disproportionate means can be morally good, though not obligatory.[1]

Theological and Philosophical Context

Christian tradition places this principle within a theological and philosophical framework. Man is created in God's image and shares in God's dignity. Thus, each human life has paramount dignity and merits utmost care, but humans are mortal and may be allowed to die in certain circumstances. The patient has a duty to care for and preserve his or her own life, and caregivers have a duty to assist with medical expertise and intervention. These duties, however, are not absolute, and patients, their families, and caregivers may sometimes forgo measures that prolong life. The principle of ordinary/proportionate and extraordinary/disproportionate means guides judgment regarding when life-preserving means should be used and when they need not be.

The Christian definition of "human person" as the union of a body and an immortal soul provides a philo-

sophical context for interpreting this principle. Although modern scientific knowledge may make traditional understandings of "soul" difficult to understand, this definition of the person still provides an alternative to a purely material conception of the human person. Further, it implies that the bodily and spiritual dimensions of the human person exist for each other. Thus, the spiritual gifts of intelligence and choice enable the rational care of the body, and bodily health promotes such spiritual activities as thinking, communicating, maintaining friendships, and working. One implication of this union is that the body never represents mere "biological life" as long as the person lives, even when the person is unable to perform spiritual activities, as in a persistent vegetative state.

The principle of ordinary/proportionate and extraordinary/disproportionate means steers a reasoned middle course between the extremes of vitalism and relativism. Vitalism assumes that human life is of absolute value, maintains a duty to try to preserve life until death has passed, and thus admits no circumstances for refraining from or ceasing life support. On the other hand, relativism here assumes that human life possesses no inherent value, carries no obligation for its preservation, and thus can be abandoned simply at will. In contrast, the principle of ordinary/proportionate and extraordinary/disproportionate means accords with the above theological and philosophical framework, excludes the direct killing or mutilating of the person, and relates the benefits and burdens of treatment to the circumstances of the patient, especially the patient's medical condition.

The Principle in Practice

Ordinary/proportionate means of medical care are those that are proven to be successful, are customarily used, and in the judgment of the patient offer reasonable hope of benefit without imposing disproportionate burdens. Accordingly, extraordinary/disproportionate means of medical care are those that are not proven to be successful, are not customarily used, or in the judgment of the patient offer little reasonable hope of benefit or involve disproportionate burdens. Clearly, experimental procedures are always considered to be extraordinary and disproportionate. Even scientifically established procedures can be considered extraordinary in places where those procedures are not regularly practiced because, ethically speaking, the increased effort to succeed and the risk of failure may constitute a disproportionate burden.

Both ordinary/proportionate and extraordinary/disproportionate means always entail some benefit; otherwise they are futile. The benefits of a procedure are first and foremost the health benefits that the procedure is designed to achieve. Burdens are primarily those to the patient, but burdens to family and caregivers should also be considered. In the final analysis, what constitutes proportionate and disproportionate in a case refers to what the patient judges to be beneficial or burdensome.

Directives 55 to 57 of the *Ethical and Religious Directives for Catholic Health Care Services* deal directly with the application of this principle. They state that patients should receive all the necessary information about their medical condition and options, should receive medical and spiritual support in understanding their condition and evaluating options, and should accept means they judge ordinary and proportionate but may forgo those they judge extraordinary and disproportionate:

> Directive 55. Catholic health care institutions offering care to persons in danger of death from illness, accident, advanced age, or similar condition should provide them with appropriate opportunities to prepare for death. Persons in danger of death should be provided with whatever information is necessary to help them understand their condition and have the opportunity to discuss their condition with their family members and care providers. They should also be offered the appropriate medical information that would make it possible to address the morally legitimate choices available to them. They should be provided the spiritual support as well as the opportunity to receive the sacraments in order to prepare well for death.

> Directive 56. A person has a moral obligation to use ordinary or proportionate means of preserving his or her life. Proportionate means are those that in the judgment of the patient offer a reasonable hope of benefit and do not entail an excessive burden or impose excessive expense on the family or the community.

> Directive 57. A person may forgo extraordinary or disproportionate means of preserving life. Disproportionate means are those that in the patient's judgment do not offer a reasonable hope of benefit or entail an excessive burden, or impose excessive expense on the family or the community.

The difficulty in applying this principle lies in evaluating benefits and burdens and in relating them to each other and to the medical condition of the patient as a whole. The patient needs to make not only objective judgments about how effective a given procedure is likely to be and what burdens it will entail, but also subjective judgments about the benefits and burdens of the procedure in relation to his or her overall condition and relationship to family,

caregivers, and society. While "benefit" refers primarily to the health benefits of the procedure independent of the patient's further goals in pursuing good health, those further goals constitute the personal context in which the judgment is made and are sometimes very important. For example, accepting a burdensome kidney dialysis might be extraordinary but desirable for family reasons, such as a likely reconciliation among family members or one's presence at an important future event. Burdens involve a wide variety of factors, some of which are based on objective (often medical and financial) knowledge and others that are personal to the patient and family.

For many reasons, it is impossible to give a list of procedures that always constitute extraordinary and disproportionate means. The evaluation of benefits and burdens always considers the specifics of the situation, even if there are some procedures, such as physician-assisted suicide and euthanasia, that no situation can justify. The burdens associated with certain procedures can change over time, as in the example above concerning amputation. Moreover, potential benefits and burdens change according to circumstances, including the availability and effectiveness of a procedure, the prognosis, the progression of disease, and the available financial resources.

Nonetheless, it is possible to identify certain types of common burdens:

- *Great effort*: The effort that is required to use certain means is generally considered extraordinary/disproportionate when it becomes too difficult or impossible to use. For example, an asthma sufferer is not expected to move to a different geographical region to improve health.

- *Severe pain*: The pain associated with treatment makes it extraordinary/disproportionate when the pain surpasses what a person can reasonably bear. This burden obviously varies according to a patient's ability to endure pain. Palliative care reduces this burden.

- *Exquisite means and great expense*: Patients are not expected to bankrupt themselves or their families to procure medical treatment. They are not bound to try exotic cures, nor is there an obligation to provide them.

- *Repugnance*: Patients may have a dread of certain treatments, especially those that would constitute mutilation if it were not for the underlying pathology. Moreover, psychological factors can play a large part in one's response to treatment and may reasonably render certain treatments extraordinary/disproportionate.[2]

Assisted Nutrition and Hydration: Points of Clarification and Controversy

The quite legitimate term "proportionate" should not be confused with "proportionalism," a school of ethics that denies the possibility of defining actions, such as euthanasia—which ought never to be done—and that ends up judging all actions in terms of the beneficial and burdensome consequences. The principle of ordinary/proportionate and extraordinary/disproportionate means, however, is used with the principle of double effect, which evaluates the benefits and burdens of actions that are not inherently evil. Moreover, the evaluation of benefits and burdens concerns the benefits and burdens of treatment, not of continued life with the disease from which a patient is suffering. Thus, the question is whether the procedure will bring about the benefit it is designed to accomplish without undue burden under the given circumstances, especially the condition of the patient as a whole. Cardiopulmonary resuscitation, for example, is ordinarily attempted when a patient is likely to be resuscitated and survive a reasonable length of time, but it might not be attempted if its inherent limitations or other medical conditions make resuscitation and survival unlikely. Similarly, if chemotherapy holds reasonable promise of reducing tumors, cancer patients ordinarily continue with it until they judge that the burdens of prolonged treatment or other burdens make it disproportionate to the benefits of reducing the tumors.

Confusion about how to evaluate benefits and burdens is apparent in the recent controversy about the withdrawal of assisted nutrition and hydration (ANH) from patients in a persistent vegetative state (PVS). There seems to be a tendency to compare the benefit of nourishing the body not simply with the burden of treatment, but with the burden of continued life in a PVS. For example, one might argue that ANH should be considered extraordinary and disproportionate when it becomes morally certain that a patient in a PVS will not regain consciousness. This argument suggests that because ANH will not contribute to restoring consciousness in this case, it can be withdrawn.[3] Such reasoning, however, requires ANH to bring about a benefit it is not designed to achieve, and neglects the benefit that it is designed to achieve, namely, nourishing a person's body. Removing ANH from a patient in a PVS who would otherwise be expected to continue living, albeit in a debilitated state, results in death from the lack of food and water rather than death from an underlying pathology. While the physical burden of ANH is typically low compared to the benefit of bodily nourishment, a patient or surrogate might judge that continuation of ANH in certain circumstances constitutes an unreasonable burden for other reasons associated with the treatment, such as lack of access to good medical care in a developing country. In such cases, those burdens could make the means extraordinary and disproportionate for particular patients.

Notes

[1] See also the Congregation for the Doctrine of the Faith, *Declaration on Euthanasia* (May 5, 1980); David F. Kelly, *Contemporary Health Care Ethics* (Washington, D.C.: Georgetown University Press, 2004), 128–131; Benedict M. Ashley, Jean DeBlois, and Kevin D. O'Rourke, *Health Care Ethics: A Catholic Theological Analysis*, 5th ed. (Washington, D.C.: Georgetown University Press, 2006), 185–186.

[2] See also Scott M. Sullivan, "A History of Extraordinary Means," *Ethics & Medics* 31.11 (November 2006): 3–4.

[3] See Ashley, DeBlois, and O'Rourke, *Health Care Ethics*, 194–196. See also William E. May, *Catholic Bioethics and the Gift of Human Life* (Huntington, IN: Our Sunday Visitor, 2000), chapter 7, for a criticism of the view of O'Rourke.

✠

Editorial Summation: Although medical technology has advanced remarkably in recent times, the moral question of what means of treatment are obligatory and what are optional remains unchanged. The patient has a duty to care for and preserve his or her own life, and caregivers have a duty to assist with medical expertise and intervention. These duties, however, are not absolute, and patients, their families, and caregivers may sometimes forgo measures that prolong life. The principle of ordinary/proportionate and extraordinary/disproportionate means guides judgment in this area. Ordinary/proportionate means of medical care are those that have been proved to be successful, are customarily used, and in the judgment of the patient offer reasonable hope of benefit without imposing disproportionate burdens. Accordingly, extraordinary/ disproportionate means of medical care are those that are not proven to be successful, are not customarily used, or in the judgment of the patient offer little reasonable hope of benefit or involve disproportionate burdens. The evaluation of benefits and burdens always considers the specifics of the situation, including the availability and effectiveness of a procedure, the prognosis, the progression of disease, and the available financial resources. These may change over time. Typical categories of extraordinary/disproportionate means include treatments that require great effort, cause severe pain or mental anguish, or are very expensive. These means are not obligatory, though a patient is still free to pursue them.

C. Confidentiality

Kevin J. Murrell, M.D.

Con- (or com-) is a prefix which means "with" (or "thoroughly"). *Fidere*, a Latin verb, means "to trust." *Confidere* or *confidence* implies a relationship of trust, and reliance on another's discretion regarding what belongs to the one who places the trust. It implies a thorough trust in another, that he or she will protect the entrusted information. The application of this meaning of *confidere* is well understood by most medical professionals and is thoroughly considered by physicians and other health care professionals as part of their *fiduciary* (from the Latin *fiduciarius*, "entrusted") responsibility toward their patients. The Hippocratic Oath speaks of this relationship when it says, "What I may see or hear in the course of the treatment or even outside of the treatment in regard to the life of men, which on no account one must spread abroad, I will keep to myself, holding such things shameful to be spoken about."[1] Perhaps not so well understood is the notion of confidence as simple trust in one's fellow men, a trust that both frees and builds relationships. This section of chapter 3 will look at both aspects of *confidere*. The first part will consider the concept of *confidence,* and the second will consider *confidentiality*.

Confidence

A significant aspect of showing love and respect for people is holding them in esteem, that is, regarding them as being of great value. Without such esteem there is something missing in the relationship. One can act as if another is worthy of love and respect while inwardly not really valuing the person as truly worthy. When the relationship is put to a test, this will become evident.

In Christian relationships (in this case, between the Christian physician and his or her patients), mutual esteem is a basis for relationships based on genuine love and respect. It is based on the essential value given each human being by Christ and by the realization that we all share a common humanity. Knowledge of another's faults and weaknesses cannot exhaust this source of esteem. Above the disappointments encountered in our daily contact with each other should live in us a supernatural knowledge of Christ's favor on each person. In his Letter to the Romans, St. Paul tells us, "Love one another with mutual affection; anticipate one another in showing honor" (12:10). According to the Greek text, St. Paul exhorts the Christians not only to deference but to an attitude of esteem. They are encouraged to fight the tendency to place themselves above others because they judge them inferior.

For those in positions of authority, like the physician, the temptation to think more highly of oneself is greater. Therefore, those in positions of authority must practice humility, especially in their hearts, and habitually think of their brethren (their patients in this case) with esteem. This esteem implies an attitude of faith in the grace given to each person. To develop this esteem and make it more concrete, those in authority should make a strong effort to see the personality and good qualities of each person. In looking at those under their care through kindly eyes, physicians should note specific reasons for esteem, appreciating more and more those who are their fellow creatures under God.

In the difficulties and conflicts that arise in the practice of medicine, an attempt to understand rather than judge is necessary. Those in authority must work to grasp the true intentions of those in their care, which may not always be clear in particular situations. Such an attitude of goodwill can enable physicians to receive the confidence of their patients. It is necessary that those for whom we care can say what they wish to express with the certitude of being welcomed and understood. If their confidence in us brings reproach or condemnation, their openheartedness will become impossible.

Esteem implies that physicians not speak of those in their care in depreciative ways. If slander is forbidden to every Christian, it should be more radically excluded from those to whom confidences are entrusted. Physicians should consider as sacred the reputation of those who confide in them. When it is detrimental to their patients, physicians cannot divulge that information which their position has permitted them to observe or be informed of. More will be said of this, including possible exceptions, in our consideration of *confidentiality*.

Physicians should not listen to and favor one person's account or complaints about another. Of course, they must listen to the one who confides in them, but there is an equal duty to protect the reputation of each one entrusted to their care and have the confidence to promote mutual esteem among all. Thus, physicians should habitually speak of others kindly, which should reflect their thinking: appreciating the good will and the efforts of each person.

Love is proved by confidence. If physicians should see those in their care as "sons and daughters of God," they should show the kind of confidence in them merited by this divine affiliation. In the Gospel Jesus shows an amazing confidence in his disciples. He gives them the mission of spreading his testimony throughout the world. He does not withdraw his confidence in St. Peter even after Peter denies him three times. Generally speaking, Jesus did not lose hope in people.

Confidence in others, then, is an inherent disposition of Jesus. Standing in Christ's place, as agents of God's healing, physicians are invited to follow this same kind of confidence, a confidence which does not grow weary. Physicians should remember that they also benefit from Christ's confidence in them and in their leadership and expertise, even with their deficiencies and failings. They should try to transmit this confidence to patients and colleagues, expressing by their actions the confidence that the Lord has in each person.

We physicians appreciate it when patients and colleagues show confidence in what we do; we feel supported in the accomplishment of our duty and have the courage to perform our tasks. We should then provide our patients with like support. In showing our confidence in our patients and colleagues, we encourage them to put all their resources and abilities into the task ahead of them. Where this esteem and confidence are lacking one usually finds mistrust. We then have to work to build confidence. By believing in the good will of our patients and colleagues, we foster their growth and development. It is not the physician's primary task to control and repress, but to promote. Our love for our patients and colleagues will be fruitful to the extent that it expresses our confidence in them.[2]

The Confidentiality of Natural and Professional Secrets

I believe that an understanding of confidence is important to an understanding of confidentiality. Confidentiality comes out of our respect for the dignity and privacy of each person. It is also rooted in the understanding that each person's life is lived in relationships and that such relationships help define the individual as a person. Therefore, each one has the right to determine those who are closest to him and those who are not. Degrees of closeness are usually known by how much about oneself is confided. Those who are closest are entrusted with more knowledge of oneself. Those who are not close are entrusted with less. It is the individual alone who determines where the lines are drawn. Therefore, those who might be privy to certain confidences do not have the right to disclose them to others without the approval of the person whom that knowledge is about. This obligation of confidentiality most surely bears upon physicians who, by their privileged role in a patient's life, have knowledge of such confidences.[3]

In late eighteenth-century England, Dr. Thomas Percival noted that

> secrecy and delicacy, when required by peculiar circumstances, should be strictly observed. And the familiar and confidential intercourse, to which the faculty are admitted in their professional visits, should be used with discretion and with the utmost scrupulous regard to fidelity and honor.[4]

Near the beginning of this section, a portion of the Hippocratic Oath was quoted. Such an understanding of the need to keep confidences, to guard certain secrets, remains consistent throughout history, underscoring the importance of this principle for the good of mankind.

What are some of the obligations one has to keep a secret? It can be said that each person has a natural right to secrecy by the very fact that our intellect and will are inviolable. Under normal circumstances and apart from the use of unjust means, no other human being is physically able to penetrate these faculties. So the knowledge and the thoughts which a person has, and which pertain only to himself, are his own.

A second reason for keeping secrets is based on the natural understanding that human beings live their lives in a society of other human beings. Thus, secrecy is necessary for the public peace and for prosperity. John DeLugo wrote,

We cannot properly inquire about the crimes and secret defects of our neighbor, or broadcast them. For this is very destructive of the public peace and tranquillity. Moreover, that these crimes remain occult and be buried in ignorance and oblivion helps toward avoiding crime and gently correcting faults. Because the conserving of one's good name is a great control and motive for good living; and when that control has been removed and a man's reputation is once lost, human frailty rushes easily and precipitously into desperation, since the hope of preserving a good reputation among men is gone.[5]

Again, on the necessity of proper secrecy for the common good, Robert Regan writes,

To cut men off from the support of their fellow men would tend to disorganize and disrupt society; whereas a properly functioning social life ... is demanded by man's very nature. In certain difficulties men are forced to turn for assistance to others better qualified than themselves. Assurance that they will not be betrayed, and thus find their sorry condition made worse, is a necessary condition for this recourse. For if the needy and unfortunate are persuaded that in their misfortunes they cannot look to others for assistance without the danger of betrayal, which will bring down upon them even greater evils, such as loss of fortune, loss of reputation and honor, great embarrassment, loss of liberty, and even loss of life itself, they will prefer to keep their troubles to themselves. Thus frustration would most certainly engender hopelessness, despondency, and despair, with the fruits of such states of mind and soul, such as recklessness and dereliction of duty. The evils that would befall society if such conditions existed could be enormous.[6]

Two kinds of secrets seem to apply to the physician most directly: the natural secret and the professional secret. The natural secret is one that someone happened to find out, and which the person is unwilling to have disclosed. The obligation to keep the natural secret is due to either charity or justice. If the disclosure of the information would cause displeasure to the person, its disclosure is a violation of charity. If, in addition to the displeasure, the disclosure would cause someone to suffer material loss or bring damage to the reputation of the person, the disclosure is a violation of justice.

The professional secret is a committed secret, binding in justice, by reason of the professional position of the one who receives the secret knowledge. The professional's duty to keep the secret may only be implicit and not explicit, but is morally binding nonetheless. When physicians enter the practice of medicine, they make an implicit contract with all who come to them in their professional capacity. Whatever secrets are imparted to the physician in the doctor–patient relationship will be kept inviolate and will be used only as far as necessary to achieve the purpose for which the patient entered the relationship. Again, the underlying principles on which such confidentiality rests concern the individual's natural right to what resides in his own personal faculties and the common good.[7]

It is commonly understood that parents have a right to know professional information about their children. This certainly applies to children who have not yet reached the age of reason. In the case of older children, the obligation of the physician to reveal professional information to the parents seems less clear. Parents who send their children to a physician for evaluation can regard the physician as their agent in the fulfillment of their duty to protect and safeguard their child and, therefore, expect to be told what is going on. However, information that the child volunteers as a natural secret could be protected by the physician. What is to be revealed and what is to be held secret is often left to the prudential judgment of the physician.

Abuses of confidentiality destroy confidence. They can destroy trust in people and in authority in general. They can destroy the trust of a patient in the physician, with detrimental effects on the care the patient may need. Given the importance of confidentiality and the great duty we have to protect the dignity of each person by protecting the confidences they share with us, it is important to examine instances in which we might be obliged to set aside this important principle.

The Professional Secret and the Common Good

A medical professional is obliged to keep the secrets of his patient as long as the patient retains the right to the secret. This obligation is based on the person's natural right as well as the added obligation of professional secrecy. The professional secret is more specifically founded on the concept of the common good but is still a significant obligation. Given this important understanding, there are circumstances which permit, or even require, the revelation of the professional secret.

An important principle with application to the consideration of revealing a professional secret is that private property, including a secret, becomes commonly held in common necessity. The obligation of professional secrecy comes about because observance of professional secrecy is a necessary means to preserve the common good and the right order of society. If a set of conditions or circumstances is found in which the observance of professional secrecy would be more harmful than helpful for the common good, then the obligation of secrecy ceases and is replaced by the obligation to reveal the secret. For example, if the state considers the reporting of all gunshot wounds to the police as a necessary means of controlling crime, and thus of helping to ensure the common good, then the physician has an obligation to report such wounds to the proper authorities.[8]

The principle that a professional secret may be revealed under certain conditions is also illustrated in the example of the patient who loses his right to secrecy by becoming an unjust aggressor who threatens harm to an innocent third party. This principle was made into law in the 1976 case *Tarasoff v. Regents of the University of California,* in which the California Supreme Court ruled, "When a doctor or psychotherapist, in the exercise of his professional skill and knowledge, determines or should determine, that a warning is essential to avert danger arising from the medical or psychological condition of his patient, he incurs a legal obligation to give that warning."[9] This obligation is most often followed after the physician has tried other methods of preventing the probable harm, such as hospitalizing the patient or obtaining the patient's permission to involve the third party.

This approach is advocated by the code of ethics adopted by the American Medical Association:

> Information disclosed to a physician by a patient should be held in confidence. The patient should feel free to make a full disclosure of information to the physician in order that the physician may most effectively provide needed services. The patient should be able to make this disclosure with the knowledge that the physician will respect the confidential nature of the communication. The physician should not reveal confidential information without the express consent of the patient, subject to certain exceptions which are ethically justified because of overriding considerations.
>
> When a patient threatens to inflict serious physical harm to another person or to him or herself and there is a reasonable probability that the patient may carry out the threat, the physician should take reasonable precautions for the protection of the intended victim, which may include notification of law enforcement authorities.[10]

One area of confidentiality that has posed specific kinds of problems because of to its highly politicized nature concerns HIV-infected patients. To many it follows the reasoning in *Tarasoff.* A particular moral question arises as to a physician's obligation to break confidentiality when the physician is aware that an HIV-positive patient is placing friends, family members, or others at risk because of nondisclosure and high-risk behavior. The American Medical Association takes the following position regarding the duty of the physician to warn endangered third parties:

> If an HIV-positive individual poses a significant threat of infecting an identifiable third party, the physician should: (a) notify the public health authorities, if required by law; (b) attempt to persuade the infected patient to cease endangering the third party; and (c) if permitted by state law, notify the endangered third party without revealing the identity of the source person.[11]

Case law has tended to follow the *Tarasoff* precedent, which limits the duty to warn to cases with identifiable third parties. Included in this category have been the patient's spouse, fiancé(e), lover, and health care workers whose duties place them at risk.

Civil law is another area that may affect professional secrecy. Although there may be differences according to the type of case under consideration, the New York Statute of 1828 has been the model of subsequent statutory law in many other states:

> A person duly authorized to practice physic or surgery, or a professional or registered nurse, shall not be allowed to disclose any information which he acquired in attending a patient in a professional capacity, and which was necessary to enable him to act in that capacity; unless the patient is a child under the age of sixteen, the information so acquired indicates that the patient has been the witness or the subject of a crime, in which case the physicians or nurses may be required to testify fully in relation thereto upon any examination, trial, or other proceeding in which the commission of such crimes is the subject of inquiry.[12]

Mutual Trust and Respect

Confidentiality is a critical relationship principle. It is of significant importance to the physician–patient relationship. In this section I have tried to base the principle of confidentiality on an understanding of its root, *confidere,* "to have confidence." Underlying the duty to protect privileged information is an understanding of the duty we share, not only to protect the dignity of each person by keeping entrusted confidences, but also to inspire confidence—confidence in God, confidence in the physician, and confidence in one's self. When the principle of confidentiality is used well, mutual trust and respect grow, furthering the growth of a community of love and truth. This is fertile ground for good spiritual, emotional, and physical health—the goal of the medical profession.

Notes

[1] Ludwig Edelstein, *The Hippocratic Oath: Text, Translation, and Interpretation* (Baltimore: Johns Hopkins Press, 1943).

[2] J. Galot, *Inspiriter of the Community* (New York: Alba House, 1971).

[3] Robert M. Veatch, *Medical Ethics* (Boston: Jones and Bartlett Publishers, 1989).

[4] Thomas Percival, "Of Professional Conduct," in *Ethics in Medicine*, ed. S. J. Reiser (Cambridge: MIT Press, 1977).

[5] John DeLugo, *De jure et justitia* (Lyons, 1670), disp. 14, sec. 9, n. 143.

[6] Robert Regan, *Professional Secrecy* (Washington, D.C.: Augustinian Press, 1943), 18.

[7] Thomas J. O'Donnell, *Medicine and Christian Morality*, 2nd ed. (New York: Alba House, 1991).

[8] Ibid.

[9] *Tarasoff v. Regents of the University of California*, 118 Cal Rptr 129, 529 P2d 553 (1974).

[10] American Medical Association, *Code of Medical Ethics*, opinion E5.05, Confidentiality (issued December 1983; updated June 2007).

[11] Ibid., opinion E-2.23, HIV Testing (issued March 1992; updated November 2007).

[12] John C. Thomson, ed., *New York Code of Civil Procedure*, 37th ed. (Albany: Matthew Bender, 1912), sec. 834 (amended 1904, 1905).

Editorial Summation: Most health care professionals are well aware of the laws and regulations concerning confidentiality and the disclosure of medical records. Even more important than these, however, is an awareness of confidentiality as a moral principle. Confidentiality is rooted in the trust between professionals and patients that ought to arise from a love—exemplified in Christ—for those who are under our care. The virtues of charity (love), justice, and the principle of the common good provide the moral foundation for the specific obligations regarding confidentiality and disclosure of information in the delivery of health care. Secrets can be natural, when they are discovered by accident, or professional, when they result from medical practice. The first type is universally binding; the second is generally binding but may suffer exception when the common good of society or the particular good of another person is in jeopardy.

D. Double Effect

Edward J. Furton and Rev. Albert S. Moraczewski, O.P.

May one perform an action which is intended to achieve a good effect if it is foreseen that an evil effect will also result? In human affairs, much of what we intend as good in a particular action brings with it undesired consequences. Surgery is done to save the life of a pregnant woman; the cancer is successfully removed but in the process the baby is lost. The gangrenous leg of a diabetic person is amputated at the knee; the patient's life is saved, but the power to walk is greatly impaired. Severe, chronic, and unrelenting pain is markedly reduced by opiates, but the person is rendered partly unconscious. All these examples involve the production of a desired good effect that is intended along with a concomitant evil effect that is not intended.

The principle of double effect governs situations in which one action is followed by two effects, one good (and intended), the other evil (foreseen but not intended). The principle probably arose in the thirteenth century concurrently with the development of moral theology.[1] Its formulation has developed over the subsequent centuries, but even today there are several ways in which the principle is stated and applied—all this, it should be noted, not without some acrimonious debate. For the purposes of this section, a commonly accepted version will be used, and will be followed by commentary and various examples.

Conditions of the Principle

There are four main conditions that govern this principle. A person may licitly perform an action that he foresees will produce good and bad effects provided that these four conditions hold: (1) the action in itself, and considered in its object, is good or at least indifferent (that is, neither good nor bad); (2) the good effect and not the bad effect is intended; (3) the good effect is not produced by means of the bad effect; and (4) there is a proportionately grave reason for permitting the bad effect.[2] To this list some would add a fifth criterion—that the proposed course of action be the least harmful alternative or that the good effect must follow from the action as immediately as does the bad effect—or some other additional requirement. Restricting the present discussion to the four agreed-upon conditions listed above, the proper application of the principle of double effect requires that all be met. If a proposed course of action fails any one of these conditions, it is not permissible.

Before elucidating the criteria in some detail, a word is in order concerning the difference between the facts of a case and their moral evaluation. There are various goods and evil that confront us in medicine, most notably the goods of life and health and the evils of death and disease. These exist prior to our choices. Cervical cancer in a patient, for example, is a tragic condition that occurs in some women. An operation to remove the cancer, if the woman is pregnant, will result in the loss of the child. This too is a fact. We cannot change these facts. We can only make the best possible choices with regard to them through careful inquiry and sound decision making. Moral evaluation concerns the quality of our actions in view of the given facts.

An Action Good in Itself

The first criterion of the principle of double effect is whether a particular action under consideration is itself morally good or evil. This consideration is independent of whatever results follow from the act and is a prerequisite, as it were, for taking any action at all. Simply put, if the contemplated action is itself morally evil, then one should not carry it out even if it produces a good effect. The action must itself be either good or indifferent. Intrinsically immoral actions include the following:

> Whatever is opposed to life itself, such as any type of murder, genocide, abortion, euthanasia, or willful self-destruction; whatever violates the integrity of the human person, such as mutilation, torments afflicted on body or mind, attempts to coerce the will itself; whatever insults human dignity, such as subhuman living conditions, arbitrary imprisonment, deportation, slavery, prostitution, the selling of women and children; as well as disgraceful working conditions, where men are treated as mere tools for profit, rather than as free and responsible persons.[3]

Any freely chosen action that is wrong by its very nature cannot be justified under the principle of double effect.

This is an important point to stress, because it shows that a good intention alone is never sufficient to justify an action. One must not only act for the right reason, but also do what is right by nature. It is possible to do what is right for the wrong reason and it is possible to do what is wrong for the right reason. Neither of these is permissible under the principle of double effect. In philosophical terms, "intention" refers to the mental state of the agent, and "object" refers to what is done by the agent. The first rule of double effect concerns the object. Some actions are objectively wrong and should never be done. For example, the direct killing of the innocent is in principle unjustifiable—regardless of the intention.

The Bad Effect Is Only Foreseen

The second condition is that the intention of the agent be for the morally good effect. This is an easier point to see and agree upon. In a health care setting, the agent of action generally intends to benefit a patient. The physician, the nurse, the lab technician—even the receptionist—intend to do something good for the patient. The intention is the reason why a particular action, surgery, administration of a medication, or some other therapeutic or prophylactic measure is undertaken. Obviously, the intention to kill or cause harm to the patient is intrinsically immoral. This is true not because the thinking alone makes the proposed course of action bad, but because one intends to carry out the very type of intrinsically immoral action that is forbidden under rule number one.

The intention of the agent is often confused with the object, largely because we live in an age where subjective intention is considered the key to moral decision making. That, as we have seen, is only half the story. Just as important is that what is done be good. Merely wanting or intending that our actions be good is not sufficient. We must do what is good in itself or good by its very nature. Thus, curing the patient is good by nature, whether it happens intentionally or by accident. Similarly, the death of the patient is bad regardless of intention. This distinction is recognized in law. No true physician seeks to kill his patients, but if death does happen in spite of the physician's best intentions, there is the possibility of legal action because of the bad result.

Under the principle of double effect, the bad result does not happen by accident, but is judged to be tolerable in view of the good that one hopes to achieve. The bad result is foreseen, but is not intended. Thus, a strong sedative is given to a patient who is in severe pain, even though the sedative may depress breathing and shorten life. Some object to the distinction between intending and foreseeing because they see it as an artificial distinction. How can we not intend what we foresee will happen? But the distinction is fairly obvious if we set aside the principle of double effect, for just a moment, and focus solely on the difference between foreseeing and intending. The CEO of a large hospital knows that a certain number of patients will die each year in his facility because of medical error. He will, of course, want to keep this number to an absolute minimum, but given the human condition, he cannot prevent these errors entirely. Obviously, the CEO does not intend these deaths, even though he foresees very clearly that they will happen.

To return to the principle of double effect, in removing a cancerous uterus from a pregnant woman, the surgeon's aim is to eliminate the disease, not to terminate the life of the child. He knows that an unborn human being is present, and he foresees the certain death of the child as a consequence of his surgery, but he does not desire or intend the death of the child. Indeed, the surgery is necessary if the physician is to save at least one of the two lives. Bear in mind that in this example the first criterion of the principle has already been satisfied. The removal of a cancerous uterus is not immoral, but is an action that is good in itself. The fact that a child is present is tragic, but it does not change the nature of the act. Presuming there is no other less harmful option, the act is good and may be performed, despite the foreseen death of the child.

No Evil Means to a Good End

This leads us to a consideration of the third condition, that the good effect must not be brought about by means of the bad effect. How do we know that this is not happening in the above example? Because the action of the surgeon is directed against the cancerous uterus which must be removed to preserve the life of the mother. The child is not the object of the action. Similarly, in the case of chorioamnionitis, as Peter Cataldo has well argued,[4] it is permissible to evacuate the infected tissues (pla-

cental and chorionic) even though this will result in the death of the child. As before, the object of the surgical action is directed against an infection, not against the child. This also explains why salpingectomy is certainly permissible under Catholic teaching as a remedy for an ectopic pregnancy. Again, the action of the physician is directed against the impacted fallopian tube. The fact that the embryo is lodged within the tube is unfortunate, but the aim of the action is not directed against the embryo. Indeed, a length of the tube is removed.

Other actions, such as craniotomy, in which the surgeon must destroy a child directly by crushing the skull in order to prevent the death of the mother, would not be permissible under the principle of double effect. Here the object of the act, and the intention of the agent, is to destroy the child. The same is true for salpingostomy. In this procedure, there is a direct attack on the embryo. Admittedly, these distinctions may appear very refined to one who is not familiar with the principle, but whenever an action is directed against the life of another innocent human being, it fails the third criteria of double effect. In contrast, whenever the action is directed against the pathological tissues or organs, it fulfills the third criterion. This third rule, in fact, forms part of a general moral principle that is commonly acknowledged by all: we cannot do evil in order that good come of it (see Rom. 3: 8).

Another illustrative case concerns the removal of a healthy uterus from a woman who has a serious heart condition. If a subsequent pregnancy would jeopardize her health or life, is this procedure permissible? In this situation, the good effect, the preservation of the woman's health or life, is secured by means of a bad effect, namely, removal of a healthy uterus. Here there is a mutilation of the body and a loss of reproductive potential. This leads to a difficult result, for it obliges women with this condition to rely either on periodic or total abstinence to avoid the prospective danger of pregnancy. Nonetheless, this result gives us a correct application of the principle.

Yet another illustrative case is the separation of conjoined twins in those cases where the death of one is foreseen. Suppose that the flow of oxygenated blood is currently dispersed between the two in a manner that cannot support both lives. Is the redirecting of the blood flow to one of the twins an action that deprives the other of what is necessary for life? Or is it an act that restores the bodily integrity of the first child to its appropriate condition? If it is the former, then the action is immoral; if it is the latter, then it may be permissible under the principle of double effect. Usually the physiology of the twins will show that the healthier child is supporting the life of the weaker by "sharing" organs, oxygen, or blood. As such, restoring the bodily integrity of the healthier child would not be a direct attack on the weaker child even though the death of the weaker child is foreseen. The surgical operation would instead be a restoration of the flow of blood, direction of the nerve supply, and support of vital organs consistent with the most natural physiological integrity.

A Proportionate Reason

The fourth condition requires that there be due proportion between the good and bad effects. Thus, the bad effect must not exceed the good. What is compared is the good obtained and the good lost by one and the same act. The good which is lost in the case of a hysterectomy is bodily integrity and reproductive potential, and the good which is gained is the health and life of the woman. Sometimes it may be difficult to weigh up goods and evils, especially if the goods are only prospective in nature and are not assured. Nonetheless, life and health are obviously very great goods, and we have a positive duty to preserve them, even at considerable cost, if they can be enjoyed in their fullness for some time.

Consider now the more difficult case of an individual who has cancer of the tongue and surrounding tissue. After careful examination, which requires a biopsy, the surgeon recommends radiation followed by surgical excision of the tongue and possible removal of all or part of the mandible (jawbone). The procedure would also entail removal of one eye and the loss of hearing on the same side. In spite of all those radical procedures, the chances of the individual living at least five years is only 25 percent.

The patient is faced with a difficult and major decision. The disfiguration will be considerable, even with subsequent plastic surgery. Further, the loss of speech and the impaired vision and hearing will make for a difficult life afterward. The surgical procedure is certainly not a moral evil in itself, for the object is the removal of cancerous tissue. The intention of the surgeon is to add a few years to the patient's life. But does this good effect outweigh the many evils, namely, loss of speech, loss of binocular vision, loss of binaural hearing, loss of facial integrity, and normal human physical appearance? Perhaps many would find the postoperative condition to be sufficiently poor to decline the surgery and allow the pathology to take its natural course.

The decision to accept the evil consequences must be proportionate to the good that is gained. In this case, rejecting surgery may be the lesser evil. This last condition of estimating goods and evils is for some the most important, but it is also generally the most difficult to ascertain. The subjective element plays a large role in such a balancing act. Much depends on the values by which one has lived. The principle offers a sure and objective guide, but in the end, as in all moral decisions, a prudential judgment in the application of that guide is required.

Notes

[1] See Joseph T. Mangan, "An Historical Analysis of the Principle of Double Effect," *Theological Studies* 10.1 (March 1949): 41–61.

[2] See ibid., 43.

[3] Vatican Council II, *Gaudium et spes* (December 7, 1965), n. 27.

[4] Peter J. Cataldo, "The Principle of the Double Effect," *Ethics & Medics* 20.3 (March 1995): 1–3.

Editorial Summation: The principle of double effect justifies some good actions that also have bad consequences under certain conditions. The proposed action must be good in itself, must not intend the bad effect, must not use the bad effect to achieve the good, and must present a sufficiently grave reason for tolerating the resulting evil. Some actions are wrong in themselves and can never be justified, no matter how much good might come from them. These are intrinsically immoral. Other actions that are performed by the agent may be good or at least indifferent, but follow from a bad intention. When actions good in themselves follow from a good intention, the evil that is produced cannot result directly, but must only be a foreseen consequence. Moreover, there must be a reasonable proportion between the good that is achieved and the evil that is tolerated. When all of these conditions are met, the action is justifiable under the principle of double effect.

E. Virtue in Bioethics

Rev. David Beauregard, O.M.V.

Since it involves the perfection of the acting agent, virtue is necessary in bioethics as a subjective complement to objective rules, principles, laws, and procedures, which simply define abstractly what should be done, that is, the general rule apart from the concrete historical situation which the acting agent faces. Virtue enables medical personnel to act with greater perception, promptness, facility, responsibility, and pleasure in exercising their talents and applying these general principles, laws, and procedures to particular circumstances. In other words, any given case involves three components: a patient; medical personnel; and principles, laws, and procedures. It further requires the virtuous application—that is, a prudent, compassionate, and just manner of application—of abstract principles and defined procedures to a particular patient in specific circumstances. The virtuous person, through the degree of perfection of his or her dispositions, sensitivity, and perception, will accordingly become a more or less perfect mediating and humanizing link between abstract principles and concrete circumstances, so as to achieve the ultimate goal of the authentic good of the patient and the common good.

The Aim of Bioethics

Both bioethics and medical ethics aim at a certain good, the health of the individual person and the health of society. Since the good of society, or the common good, includes the good of the individuals who compose any given community, the aim and goal of bioethical and medical decisions and actions must be the person as an end, not as a means. Using human beings as a means to an end—in human experimentation, for example—is not consistent with Christian principles. Scientific progress should exist for the sake of the human person, not the human person for the sake of scientific progress. The person is always to be treated as an end in himself.

In order to ensure the common and individual good in health care, especially the inherent dignity and value of the human person, we need laws, rules, and procedures to guide us. St. Thomas Aquinas defines law as "an ordination of reason, directed to the common good, made by one who has care of the community, and pro-

mulgated."[1] Consequently, if we need sound laws, rules, and procedures to guide us toward the common and individual good, we also need virtuous agents to make judgments in applying those laws and to employ skills in using medical procedures during the healing process. Virtue, therefore, is an essential personal component in the management of any health care community directing it toward the realization of its proper good.

The Nature of Virtue

Virtue is defined by Aquinas as "a good quality of mind, by which one lives righteously, of which no one can make bad use, which God works in us, without us."[2] Implicit in this definition is the perfection of the acting agent, whose powers, inclinations, and appetites are directed in a moderate, stable, responsible, motivationally creative, and rightly ordered manner toward the achievement of certain goods. For example, to drink temperately is to enjoy the good taste of wine, a capacity that may increase and grow in time as one learns to perceive the goodness of wine in terms of its color, taste, bouquet, and body. Thus, an appetite for drink is perfected to the point where one's moderation in drinking brings one great physical satisfaction and intellectual enjoyment in, say, considering the superiority of one type of wine over other types. To drink to excess is to destroy this capacity, since excess destroys the ability to discriminate the subtleties of taste and the equilibrium of adequate satisfaction. Not to drink is to deny oneself the goodness that wine can bring. In any case, moderation is usually the key to virtuous behavior, defined as the mean between the extremes of excess and deficiency in relation to any appetite, emotion, or passion.

Law and the Need for a Virtuous Agent

What is paramount here is the human perfection of the acting agent. Action involves both exterior laws and interior dispositions, both an external rule and an acting agent. To simply follow rules and laws is not to be thoroughly moral, but rather to practice legalism, a rather anemic form of morality, a reduction of morality to obedience to law, with too little attention to human inclination and intelligence. A nurse, for example, can follow the rules in *Standards of Clinical Nursing Practice* from the American Nurses Association, but that will make him only an adequate but not a good or excellent nurse, since he will be merely carrying out exterior actions passively without a corresponding interior disposition toward the perfection of nursing, which involves the development of knowledge, talent, sensitivity, patience, and skill actively directed toward the good of the patient. Such activity can become routine, mechanical, and inflexible, in contradistinction to the perceptive creativity, compassionate sensitivity, sense of responsibility, and downright pleasure of acting virtuously. Thus, the perfection of the acting agent, who must carry out the laws, rules, and procedures of good medicine, is essential to the good of the patient.

This is simply to say that the law is an impersonal abstraction and requires an agent to apply it intelligently and dispassionately to given circumstances. Human actions are not isolated events without a context, performed apart from the character and history of the moral agent. Laws, rules, and medical procedures need to be applied in a certain manner, with an intelligent and humane attention to significant circumstances, so as to bring about the end desired, the good of the patient. Again, when there is no law governing a situation, or when there is no time to search out the relevant law, or when circumstances create an intensely pressured situation, a virtuous person is most likely to make a sound practical judgment. Finally, beyond the minimum that the law requires, beyond the merely technical aspects of treatment, there is the dimension of quality care for the patient, a dimension that can be ensured only by virtuous medical personnel interested in the good of the patient and the enjoyable development and exercise of their talents.

Virtues Particular to Bioethics

What, then, are some of the virtues relevant to bioethics and, by extension, the medical profession, that is, to those involved in making bioethical and medical decisions and applying the appropriate rules and procedures?

Faith

It is particularly important to recognize the differences in outlook formed in men and women who have the virtue of faith. Secular society tends to see suffering as pointless, meaningless, and absurd. Moreover, it tends to view life unrealistically as something that ought to be under the imperial control of the individual in every respect, especially in matters affecting birth and death. The aspiration to control and dominate nature by

scientific technology and the body politic by totalitarian governments goes hand in hand with this central secular "value" of imperial control. But in the Christian vision, one must exercise dominion over nature in a more respectful, cooperative, and harmonious way, that is, as a form of stewardship. Thus suffering is seen by the Christian as a part of life that is meaningful in being mysterious, redemptive, and even formative in this "vale of soul-making." One must respect the natural processes of birth, suffering, and death, and act in rational accordance with them, assisting and helping them toward their natural end rather than trying imperiously to control and dominate them.[3]

Charity

This central Christian virtue includes the two minor virtues of *mercy* and *beneficence*. The former is essentially "grief for another's distress," a kind of pity and compassion. The second may be defined as "doing good to someone," and so may be loosely equated with care. Both should be regulated by reason and modified according to due circumstances. This means that beneficence should extend to all persons but must be measured proportionately according to the requirements of time, place, and the matter at hand.

Prudence

As a virtue of the intellect, prudence enables one to make a practical judgment in the present circumstances as to the best possible course of action. It involves being cautious, taking counsel, considering past and present experience, and exercising foresight into what may come about in consequence of the present action.

Justice

Classically defined as "giving every man his due," justice aims at a certain equality, but not an egalitarian equality. What is "due" varies from individual to individual, as, for example, in the matter of organ transplantation. One is not owed an organ, but available organs must be distributed in the manner most fitting to those most in need of them or those who will make the best use of them. The virtue of justice enables one to make the best, most equitable use of medical goods (one's time and medical resources) that is possible under the circumstances.

Patience

To face evils—especially the difficulties of misfortune, suffering, and death—with a certain mental equilibrium and calm for the sake of human good is essential for medical personnel. Without patience, practical judgments about what to do are premature, erratic, distorted, and confused. Clear thinking requires the virtue of patience.

This short list of virtues obviously does not exhaust the topic, but it does give the main outlines of the function of virtues in bioethics.

Notes

[1] Thomas Aquinas, *Summa theologiae* I-II, q. 90, a. 4.

[2] Ibid., q. 55, a. 4.

[3] See especially the introduction to the U.S. Conference of Catholic Bishops' *Ethical and Religious Directives for Catholic Health Care Services*, 4th ed. (Washington, D.C.: USCCB, 2001).

Editorial Summation: Virtue ethics has a long historical pedigree. Indeed, it is the first ethical theory of Western philosophy, inaugurated by Aristotle twenty-four centuries ago. The teaching and the imparting of the virtues should still have a prominent place in medicine today. Unless one is motivated to act by a virtuous character, actions result only from a rote obedience to the rules of morality and the law. This is not genuine virtue, for it does not follow from the interior principles that constitute the rightful disposition of the agent. Neither does it give one the practical ability to resolve more complex, pressing, or novel situations in a virtuous manner. Virtue is generally defined as the rule of reason over one's actions. There are a great variety of virtues at work in the practice of medicine, including the theological virtues of faith and charity, and the natural virtues of prudence, justice, and patience. These enable health care professionals to think accurately about the moral issues that confront them daily in the health care setting.

F. The Common Good

David M. Gallagher

Broadly speaking, a common good is any good which is shared or participated in by many persons. Like the good in general, a common good can take many forms: it may be a good to be produced or achieved like a house built by a construction crew or a victory won by a sports team, or it may be an already existing good, such as natural resources, the beauty of a mountain range, or a work of literature. It can be a means to be used, like a hydroelectric dam, or an end enjoyed in itself, like the beauty of the mountains. It can be a true good, such as health or the common good of a hospital staff, or merely an apparent good, like a bombing in the eyes of a team of terrorists. All these are shared goods, goods pursued or enjoyed by many persons. More specifically, the term "common good" is used to designate the overall good at which society, acting together, aims.

Essential Structure of a Common Good

Why is the notion of the common good essential for ethics? The answer lies in the nature of human fulfillment, the end by which we measure an action's moral goodness. Almost every element of human happiness, whether simple physical health, material well-being, edu-

cation, enjoyment of the arts, or even liturgical worship, can only be achieved by common action, that is, by the organized efforts of many persons. Essential elements of health care would be impossible without hospitals, higher education impossible without universities, hearing a symphony impossible without an orchestra. For this reason, we must work together in communities of all sorts in order to achieve their fulfillment. Thus, the virtuous life and morally good action demand that a person contribute to and share goods held in common in an ordered way. This aspect of the moral life traditionally falls under the virtue of justice, especially *legal justice*, which deals with the obligation of the individual person to contribute to common goods, and *distributive justice*, which is concerned with the fair distribution of common goods to the members of a community.

A common good is relative to a community whose members strive together to achieve that good or share in it. Normally, a single person belongs to many different communities and accordingly is ordered to many common goods. These communities are related to one another according to the goods to which they are directed. This can be seen in an organization like a large firm in which the ends of the lower-level groups are ordered to those of the higher-level groups and all are ultimately ordered to the good of the firm as a whole. Among the communities in the temporal realm, the state has traditionally been considered the highest community, having as its end a common good which includes all the goods of the lower communities. Yet recent Church social teaching has pointed out that it is possible and necessary to think of the entire world as a single community and of the corresponding common good of all peoples. Beyond the temporal sphere, moreover, the community is formed by participation in grace, forming the Church whose common good is the sharing of all men in eternal life. In fact, this constitutes the common good of the whole universe throughout the whole of time.

Within any one community, there is an authority which directs and coordinates the members of the community in achieving the common good. This implies, on the one hand, that the legitimate exercise of authority in any community requires that those who exercise it truly seek the common good. On the other hand, the members of the community, if they wish to promote the common good, should obey the authority. Thus, one's obligation to seek the common good underlies one's moral obligation to obey legitimate authority. So, too, the members of a community should subordinate their particular good to the common good of the community. For example, good parents should choose a vacation spot not merely to satisfy their own particular interests, but rather to do what is best for the family as a whole. This subordination of one's particular good to the common good, however, occurs within the order of that particular community. As a member of the team, the athlete should seek the common good of victory, but as a member of his family, he may not be able to play in an important game because of family obligations. This point takes on special relevance in explaining why the state cannot coerce the conscience of its citizens; the obligations to God and his law transcend the temporal order, and so the state cannot regard the citizen as subject to its authority in all respects.

The Common Good of the Whole of Society

The common good most often discussed is that of a society as a whole, that to which the political community, the state, is directed. It is precisely this meaning of the term that is usually intended when it appears within the Church's social teaching. In this context, the common good is defined as "the sum total of social conditions which allow people, either as groups or as individuals, to reach their fulfillment more fully and more easily."[1] This common good is obviously very complex and contains many elements. Moreover, its concrete form changes as social conditions change through technological, economic, and educational development and by the onset of such conditions as war, economic depressions, and natural disasters.

Among the elements that compose the common good in modern times are the material infrastructure (systems of transportation, information networks, food supply, waste disposal systems, health care systems); a healthy economy—including a stable currency—in which all can productively participate; an educational system that educates the citizens into truth and moral virtue; a morally healthy environment (e.g., clean entertainment); and the administration of justice in all its forms. This last is not limited to the adjudication of disputes between individuals and the punishment of criminals, as advocated in individualistic political philosophies (e.g., those of Hobbes and Locke); justice also includes a fair distribution of the burdens required to bring about the common good (e.g., taxes) as well as a fair distribution to all citizens of society's common goods, such as wealth, property, education, and health care. Such a distribution does not imply absolute equality, but rather, in accord with the principles of distributive justice, will be proportionate to both the needs of individuals as well as their own contribution to the common good. The requirement of justice implies that respect for the dignity and worth of each person is a necessary component of the common good of society.

Within the state, the authority to whom care for the common good is entrusted is the government. Its function is to oversee and coordinate all the various elements of the common good; it carries out this task primarily by making and enforcing laws. This does not mean, however, that the state itself should take over the procurement and distribution of all the common goods. Rather, the state should encourage as much as possible that the components of the common good be achieved by lower communities, especially the family. (This is the principle of subsidiarity.)[2] The government must act to procure those goods which it alone can provide, such as national defense, the currency, the judicial system, and goods which would be unavailable if the government were not to provide them, such as education and health care in some underdeveloped countries. (This is the principle of solidarity.)

It is clear that those in authority, especially political authority, make a special contribution to the common good. Still, every member of society—that is, every citizen—is morally obliged to do so as well, in the first place by obeying the laws made by the competent political authority. Good laws direct citizens to actions which promote the common good, as for example, the observance of traffic laws results in safe and usable roads for all. Second, each person contributes to the common good through his professional work, including homemaking. The division of labor means that each, by his particular expertise, contributes something to the common good of society, giving rise to the obligation to exercise one's professional work primarily as service to the rest of society. A third major contribution lies in the education of the young, particularly that moral and spiritual education which occurs only within the family. Finally, each person contributes to the common good by striving to live a life of virtue. As St. Thomas Aquinas points out, inasmuch as the good of each part is good for the whole, it follows that the virtue of each person contributes to the good of society.[3]

Health Care as a Common Good

Consideration of the common good is relevant for questions involving health care. Health care itself is clearly a common good of society, an essential element of the general common good. It neither is, nor could it be, produced by a single person. In fact, it is the result of the coordinated efforts of a large number of persons, even of many not directly involved in health care. Also, as a common good, it must be distributed to those who use it, which is, in fact, all the members of the society. This implies, in the first place, that the rendering of health care is not just a matter of commutative justice, a simple exchange of goods and services between the provider and the patient. Rather, it must be governed by the principles proper to distributive justice, and implied here is access to health care by all members of society. Second, it falls to the authority within society, ultimately the political authority, to ensure that the distribution of health care takes place and is just and consistent with the overall use of society's resources. Thus, the government's concern in this area is legitimate and necessary. Nevertheless, according to the principle of subsidiarity, the distribution of health care should be entrusted, as much as possible, to the intermediate communities. The government may regulate their activities, ensuring their harmony with the general common good, or may even to some degree take over the distribution itself. But this, according to the principle of subsidiarity, should occur only when it is clear that these lower entities are unable or unwilling to do so themselves.

Notes

[1] *Catechism of the Catholic Church*, n. 1906; Vatican Council II, *Gaudium et spes* (December 7, 1965), n. 26.

[2] See *Catechism*, n. 1883.

[3] Thomas Aquinas, *Summa theologiae* I-II, Q. 58.

Editorial Summation: The common good is a good that is shared or participated in by many persons. Like any good, it is directly connected to the nature of human fulfillment. Securing most human goods requires the assistance of others who have unique skills to contribute to a common effort. The need for coordinated activity among those who pursue a common good gives rise to authority and the political order. The principle of subsidiarity requires that higher authorities permit the smaller communities of which they are composed to secure their own good with minimal interference, unless and until the smaller community fails in its aims. Generally, the government should restrict its action to the securing of the larger human goods, such as national defense, that could not be achieved by any lesser agency. Health care is one of the common goods of society. The benefits of health cannot be secured except through the concerted effort of many individuals. The government has an obligation to ensure that all its citizens have access to health care, but that does not mean that it must take the health care system under its complete direction.

G. Conscience

Rev. Germain Kopaczynski, O.F.M. Conv.

The Christian moral life is a walk of reason in faith. One of the great guides on this journey is conscience, an exercise of the practical reason applying general principles of moral reflection to a particular case in the here and now. Its proper use is one of the glories of the human condition; its possible misuse has occasioned much reflection by Pope John Paul II in *The Splendor of Truth*, the 1993 encyclical on the foundations of Christian morality.

Especially in numbers 54 through 64, we find a reiteration of the central theme of the encyclical: authentic human freedom is allied to the conscientious pursuit of the truth. Since conscience is a function of reason, it must seek the truth of the human condition. The words of Jesus Christ come to mind: "You will know the truth, and the truth will set you free" (John 8:32). A case could be made that *The Splendor of Truth* is a long-running commentary on that one Gospel sentence.

What Is Conscience?

The following definitions ought to help those on ethics committees read the literature with some appreciation for how ecclesiastical documents use terminology regarding conscience:

> *Conscience* may be defined as the intellect itself exercising a special function, the function of judging the rightness or wrongness of our own individual acts according to the set of moral values and principles the person holds with conviction. To put it a bit differently, conscience is a person's reason, making a practical, concrete judgment about the morality of an action that the person is about to perform (or has already performed).
>
> *Certain conscience* is a conscience that judges without doubt or fear that the opposite is true.
>
> *Doubtful conscience* is a conscience that either makes no judgment or judges with fear that the opposite is true.
>
> *Erroneous conscience* is one that judges good as evil or evil as good; in a word, it misreads the objective moral situation.
>
> *Correct conscience* is a conscience that judges good as good, evil as evil; in a word, it accurately gauges the objective moral situation.[1]

Two overarching principles have been formulated to help persons deal with issues of conscience: (1) never act with a doubtful conscience, and (2) always obey a certain conscience.

Conscience and Health Care

Conscience is the subjective guide to morality. Conscience is the source of our great dignity as human beings, the voice of God speaking within us in the core of our being, as the Second Vatican Council stated in *Gaudium et spes* (n. 16). It is extremely important to understand Church teaching on conscience correctly, especially in medical matters involving, as they often do, issues of

life and death. Notice how two of the directives from the 2001 *Ethical and Religious Directives for Catholic Health Care Services* (*ERDs*) employ the notion of conscience in their discussion of important health care decisions:

> Directive 28. Each person or the person's surrogate should have access to medical and moral information and counseling so as to be able to form his or her conscience. The free and informed health care decision of the person or the person's surrogate is to be followed so long as it does not contradict Catholic principles.
>
> Directive 32. While every person is obliged to use ordinary means to preserve his or her health, no person should be obliged to submit to a health care procedure that the person has judged, with a free and informed conscience, not to provide a reasonable hope of benefit without imposing excessive risks and burdens on the patient or excessive expense to family or community.[2]

Much of the discussion swirling around contemporary moral theological reflection deals with conscience and its role in the moral life of each individual human being. To make a long story short, an important element should be kept in mind regarding conscience for the individual on an ethics committee in a Catholic health care facility as well as for the corporate body itself: Conscience is inviolable, yes, but not infallible. It is an exercise of the practical reason and as such shares in the glories and the tribulations of this aspect of who we are as human beings. It is, as the Second Vatican Council says, the voice of God calling from within our depths.[3] It is important that the conscience be seen in this dual aspect: the subjective guide to morality hearing the objective voice speaking to it from within, yet not to be confused with the self.

The National Catholic Bioethics Center and the Catholic Health Association jointly published, in 1984, *Ethics Committees: A Challenge for Catholic Health Care*.[4] One of the topics dealt with conscience and the Catholic health care institution, paying special attention to the role of the "corporate conscience." Such considerations ought to be kept in mind as we examine in this present volume the question of conscience from an individual perspective, that is, the question of the dignity and the formation of the individual conscience.

In developing an appreciation for both the individual and the corporate aspects of conscience, members of ethics committees in Catholic health care facilities will find a most valuable resource in Joseph Cardinal Ratzinger's *On Conscience* (2007), a publication of The National Catholic Bioethics Center. It should find a place on the bookshelves of every Catholic facility interested in pursuing authentic Catholic teaching on this matter. The work contains two seminal essays of Pope Benedict XVI, which are especially illuminating for a treatment of the importance and the seriousness with which the teaching on conscience must be handled.

"The Church has always sought to embody our Savior's concern for the sick." These are the first words to the general introduction of the *ERDs*, and they set the tone by putting Catholic teaching into proper perspective: all Church teaching, including that on conscience, must take its inspiration from Jesus Christ, the divine physician of both body and soul. The general introduction to the 2001 *ERDs* continues, "Jesus' healing mission went further than caring only for physical affliction. He touched people at the deepest level of their existence; he sought their physical, mental, and spiritual healing (John 6: 35 amd 11: 25–27)."

Life and death belong to the Lord, and all decisions about these matters must show that this teaching has pride of place in Catholic health settings: "For the Christian, our encounter with suffering and death can take on a positive and distinctive meaning through the redemptive power of Jesus' suffering and death." Again it is the example of Christ that serves as the touchstone, indeed, Catholic health care comes about in imitation of the divine Master: "In faithful imitation of Jesus Christ, the Church has served the sick, suffering, and dying in various ways throughout history."[5]

Thus, this interest in the sick, with the mind of Christ, is paramount for any authentic directives guiding Catholic institutions: "The Church seeks to ensure that the service offered in the past will be continued into the future." The only way to be assured that this is done is for Catholic health facilities to do everything possible to form their collective judgments regarding health care in the spirit and in the letter of Christ the Healer. In this the bishop serves as a central point of reference. "Catholic health care expresses the healing ministry of Christ in a specific way within the local church. Here the diocesan bishop exercises responsibilities that are rooted in his office as pastor, teacher, and priest." Adherence to the example of Jesus Christ is, then, or ought to be, the touchstone of any authentic Catholic teaching on health-care-related issues. A text of the Second Vatican Council expresses this succinctly:

> The disciple has a grave obligation toward Christ, his Master, to grow daily in his knowledge of the truth he has received from him, to be faithful in announc-

ing it and vigorous in defending it without having recourse to methods which are contrary to the spirit of the Gospel.[6]

Church teaching on medical matters, ultimately binding on the conscience, is formed in an extensive dialogue with the world of science and medicine. Good health care and Catholic moral teaching are never at odds. The American Catholic bishops offer guidance to help in the formation of conscience of the individual as well as of the ethics committee members who will serve on such committees in local facilities:

> In a time of new medical discoveries, rapid technological developments, and social change, what is new can either be an opportunity for genuine advance in human culture, or it can lead to policies and actions that are contrary to the true dignity and vocation of the human person. In consultation with medical professionals, Church leaders review these developments, judge them according to the principles of right reason and the ultimate standard of revealed truth, and offer authoritative teaching and guidance about the moral and pastoral responsibilities entailed by the Christian faith. While the Church cannot furnish a ready answer to every moral dilemma, there are many questions about which she provides normative guidance and direction. In the absence of a determination by the magisterium, but never contrary to Church teaching, the guidance of approved authors can offer appropriate guidance for ethical decision making.[7]

The first mention of conscience in the *ERDs* comes only after the above reflections meant to help conscientious Catholics in fulfilling their responsibilities in health care. A truth of faith and a truth of reason can never contradict each other. Boethius, a fifth-century Roman philosopher, put it very simply: "Join faith and reason if you can."[8] This is the challenge of walking in faith in the health care scene today.

Not all share the Catholic vision. Here, too, their consciences must be respected, yet the *ERDs* are also able to bring home a valuable point on this precise aspect of living in a society with people of varying beliefs:

> Within a pluralistic society, Catholic health care services will encounter requests for medical procedures contrary to the moral teachings of the Church. Catholic health care does not offend the rights of individual conscience by refusing to provide or permit medical procedures that are judged morally wrong by the teaching authority of the Church.[9]

Since conscience is the subjective guide to morality telling us to do or omit doing something here and now, it must be obeyed. But it is most important and indeed crucial to bear in mind that the authentic Catholic view of the matter is that morality has two poles, the subjective and the objective. Many are aware that the Church has always taught that one must always follows one's conscience, but they are perhaps less aware that it is the formation of that conscience according to objective standards that will ensure decisions which are not only certain subjectively but correct objectively. Indeed, the ideal is to have a conscience both certain and correct; anything less is settling for second best, which is never a very sound idea in matters involving who lives and who dies.

Gaudium et spes ties together many of these themes in its reflections on the dignity of the moral conscience:

> By conscience, in a wonderful way, that law is made known which is fulfilled in the love of God and of one's neighbor. Through loyalty to conscience, Christians are joined to other men in the search for truth and for the right solution to so many moral problems which arise both in the life of individuals and from social relationships. Hence, the more a correct conscience prevails, the more do persons and groups turn aside from blind choice and try to be guided by the objective standards of moral conduct.[10]

The question of the formation of conscience may be expressed as follows: How should one forge an alliance of the subjective guide to morality with the objective norms of morality? Regarding the formation of conscience, article 41 of the Canadian bishops' "Statement on the Formation of Conscience" is especially perspicacious:

> For a Catholic, "to follow one's conscience" is not, then, simply to act as his unguided reason dictates. "To follow one's conscience" and to remain a Catholic, one must take into account first and foremost the teaching of the magisterium. When doubt arises due to a conflict of "my" views and those of the magisterium, the presumption of truth lies on the part of the magisterium. "In matters of faith and morals, the bishops speak in the name of Christ and the faithful are to accept their teaching and adhere to it with a religious assent of soul. This religious submission of will and of mind must be shown in a special way to the authentic teaching of the Roman pontiff, even when he is not speaking ex cathedra" [*Lumen gentium*, n. 25]. And this must be carefully distinguished from the teaching of individual theologians or individual priests, however intelligent or persuasive.[11]

If Catholic health care facilities are characterized by a presumption in favor of life, a "bias for bios" as it were, so too ought they be characterized by this presumption of truth spoken of by the Canadian bishops.

Notes

[1] Milton Gonsalves, *Fagothey's Right and Reason: Ethics in Theory and Practice*, 9th ed. (St. Louis: Merrill, 1989), 54.

[2] U.S. Conference of Catholic Bishops, *Ethical and Religious Directives for Catholic Health Care Services*, 4th ed. (Washington, D.C.: USCCB, 2001).

[3] Vatican Council II, *Gaudium et spes* (December 7, 1965), n. 16.

[4] Margaret John Kelly and Donald McCarthy, eds., *Ethics Committees: A Challenge for Catholic Health Care* (St. Louis: Pope John Center and Catholic Health Association, 1984).

[5] USCCB, *Ethical and Religious Directives*, intro.

[6] Vatican Council II, *Dignitatis humanae* (December 7, 1965), n. 14.

[7] USCCB, *Ethical and Religious Directives*, intro.

[8] Boethius, "Whether Father, Son, and Holy Spirit May Be Stustantially Predicated of the Divinity," *De trinitate*.

[9] USCCB, *Ethical and Religious Directives*, part 1, intro.

[10] Vatican Council II, *Gaudium et spes*, n. 16.

[11] Canadian Catholic Conference, "Statement on the Formation of Conscience" (December 12, 1973), http://canada.omsoul.com/Statement_on_the_Formation_of_Conscience.pdf.

✠

Editorial Summation: Conscience is an act of the intellect which guides individual decision making and is naturally suited to formation by objective moral norms. Conscience is a subjective guide in the sense that it operates in concrete situations marked by individual circumstances, but this does not mean that conscience is a purely subjective principle. The subjective side of conscience is the person (the subject) making an intellectual assessment of an individual moral situation in all of its particulars. The objective side of conscience is the subject's act of applying objective moral norms to those same particulars and reaching a conclusion about what to do or not to do. Catholic teaching aims at forming the objective side of conscience by supplying moral norms and principles. The 1993 encyclical of Pope John Paul II, *The Splendor of Truth*, provides an excellent guide to the working of conscience, as do the writings of Pope Benedict XVI on this same subject. The *Ethical and Religious Directives for Catholic Health Care Services* recognize the rightful role of conscience in medical decision making and insist that patients receive all information necessary to form their own conscience. The individual should be free to follow a well-formed conscience, but ultimately, Catholic health care is guided by the teachings of Jesus, who has called us to live in accord with the light of truth. Within a pluralistic society, Catholic health care facilities must be free to form and follow their own corporate conscience based on the teachings of the magisterium.

H. The Natural Moral Law

Edward J. Furton

The Catholic Church remains one of the most consistent defenders of the natural law tradition in the West. The *Ethical and Religious Directives for Catholic Health Care Services* states that the teachings it sets forth for Catholic hospitals and health care workers are derived mainly from a consideration of the natural law: "The moral teachings that we profess here flow principally from the natural law, understood in the light of the revelation Christ has entrusted to his church. From this source the church has derived its understanding of the nature of the human person, of human acts, and of the goals that shape human activity."[1]

Given the centrality of the natural law to Catholic moral teaching in general and to the Church's specific directives in health care, it is important that every member of a Catholic health care ethics committee have at least a general understanding of this moral theory.

The present article will offer a relatively straightforward exposition, suited to one not trained in philosophy. In one sense, everyone who thinks about moral matters in daily life employs natural law reasoning, for this is the method that is universally embraced by all thinking human beings, though most do not articulate their ideas in its technical terms. The situation is similar to the use of logic. Human beings learn to think logically without any formal training in the subject, but it is of course possible to reflect on how logic functions. The same is true in natural law ethics. An individual who is a fair and just person will acquire a set of moral skills without ever receiving any formal training in "ethical theory," but it is also possible to reflect on what it is that we typically do when we use the God-given power of reason to deliberate about how to achieve the good.

Origins and Current Status

The theory of natural law is by far the longest standing and most successful explanation of how we acquire moral knowledge. Natural law reasoning began in the ancient world well before the time of Christ, was embraced by the Church in the Middle Ages, and has been championed by the great defenders of human rights and self-government in modernity. The philosophy of natural law has enjoyed this long history, its adherents would say, because it is the route to moral knowledge that is most natural to the human condition. In this sense, it is the most democratic of all moral systems, being common to the educated and the uneducated alike, and employed by all ranks and divisions of society—even by those who would claim to reject its influence.[2]

Among the ancients, Plato, Aristotle, and the Stoics all qualify as influential defenders of natural law reasoning, with Aristotle clearly the most prominent. Among the Romans, the writings of Marcus Tullius Cicero contain especially insightful defenses of the natural law. When Christendom rediscovered the writings of Aristotle in the Middle Ages, its chief philosophers and theologians embraced the philosophy of natural law as a complement to Christian revelation and as a practical proof that God has given us the power of reason so that we might live an ethical life. The champions of natural law and natural rights among the English and the French political theorists, such as John Locke and the Baron de Montesquieu, held that self-government is the natural duty of free citizens called by God to the pursuit of happiness. John Courtney Murray, S.J., the distinguished defender of religious liberty and influential *peritus* at the Second Vatican Council, argued that the United States is fertile ground for a revival of the natural law tradition that would be compatible with the heritage of the Catholic faith.

General Features of Natural Law

The very features that have made the philosophy of natural law the perennial favorite of Western civilization are the same ones that make it an object of doubt today. A social order committed to moral relativism and the absolute ascendancy of the will is not likely to find natural law theory very appealing, but the resilience of this system is in its practical approach to moral questions. Ultimately, very few people truly believe that all morality is relative, as this would imply that murder, rape, and treason are not wrong in themselves but only from a certain point of view. When a relativist suffers an injustice, all talk about the relativity of morality typically goes out the window. Societies that are wealthy and powerful may be able to prop up broad social illusions—such as moral relativism—for a considerable time, but when a serious crisis arises the validity of natural law reasoning reasserts itself. Thus we were witness to its resurgence at the end of World War II, especially in its use in prosecutions against those who committed crimes against humanity.

All reasoning involves both induction and deduction. Induction derives from observation on experience and arrives at general truths. For example, the fact that every physical action thus far observed has produced an equal and opposite reaction leads to the first rule of Newtonian physics. With this rule in hand, we can deduce that if a new action occurs, it too will produce an equal and opposite reaction. This is simple deductive reasoning on the facts of experience. Natural law reasoning employs the same method, but its objects of concern are not motion and rest, but good and evil. The natural law theorist holds that it is possible to carry out moral inductions (all acts of murder are wrong) and moral deductions (this act is wrong because it is murder). Murder is wrong because reason grasps that it is an injustice committed against the good of innocent human life. Here is a law that is no less objective than those discovered by Newton; indeed, we can safely say that the rules of morality are even more obvious.

The central question facing the defender of natural law morality today is whether the good can properly be called an object of rational comprehension. Can we reasonably say that the existence of the good is no less certain than the existence of motion? Are good and evil objects in nature? This is critical, for if objectivity is not found in ethics at its starting point, it will not be possible to introduce it later. That would give us only a subjective ethics. For ethics to have an objective basis, it must be the case that an action such as murder is wrong prior to any decision on our part and regardless of whether any particular person happens to agree that it is wrong. The truthfulness of morality must exist independently of the human mind and yet at the same time be easily discoverable by it. These two requirements are met only if the natural order is governed by moral laws that stand before the mind as settled and established facts. Thus, the wrongfulness of murder is conceived by natural law theorists to be an objective feature of nature. The goodness of life, and all other such goods, are pre-existing realities that must govern our actions.

Those who deny that morality is objective will say that good and evil are not real features of the world, but constructions of the mind. All moral theories that reduce ethics to a matter of taste or personal opinion, such as relativism, adopt this view. Here again we see why natural law theory does not find favor today. Many have been taught to believe that what is good or evil is arbitrarily decided by the human will. Morality, they say, is a matter of choice, not of fact. Nonetheless, counterexamples are legion. Dirt is not good to eat, nor will it provide sufficient nourishment for me to maintain my health, no matter how much I choose to believe otherwise. We know that food is necessary for health, and that those who do not have food suffer a terrible harm. To pretend that starving people do not need food, but only need to think differently about their circumstances to achieve an abundant supply of nourishment, is hardly worthy of rebuttal. There are many such objective moral facts, and it is irresponsible to deny them.

Of course, we all have different tastes, but the good is not an object of taste or sensation, but of mental apprehension. So too is evil, or the corruption of the good. Thus life is a good and death is an evil, not necessarily in absolute terms, but objectively.[3] Physicians seek to preserve the one and forestall the other. Similarly, health is a good and disease its corruption. Here are the kinds of simple moral facts that serve as the basis for a commonsense ethics that is accessible to all who have reason. Saving a person's life is obviously a good; killing an innocent person is obviously an evil. The self-evident character of such propositions is why natural law ethics is frequently associated with the philosophy of common sense. We all know these truths, and though how we come to know them may be a rather deep subject of theoretical inquiry, no one but the delusional or the wicked would deny what is so obvious.

Choice is an essential part of moral action, but we do not choose the ends of action, but rather the means to the ends. Thus, the physician does not decide whether he will cure patients or not, but decides on the best course of treatment to effect a cure. He is already committed to a life that secures the natural good of human health—and health is a good prior to any of our choices. The same is true of moral action in every profession. The engineer seeks structural stability in buildings, the editor seeks truth in the printed word, the judge seeks justice under law, and so on. The principal ends that are proper to any area of human endeavor are not created by choice, but exist in nature as objects of choice. We do not invent them, but discover them. We live moral lives by directing our actions to the pursuit of these goods, and it is fair to say that those who seek the highest goods and provide the greatest benefits to others have the better and more valuable professions.

The natural law theorist divides ends into primary and secondary. Secondary ends are ordered to those that are higher and primary. If the physician is to secure the health of patients, he must possess a range of knowledge about how the body absorbs nutrients, how the lungs respire, how conception is achieved, and other similar information. But how the stomach contributes to the good of digestion, for example, will not necessarily be evident to the average patient, for this type of knowledge requires experience and education. Unlike the most obvious and self-evident ends, the means that nature has established as the route to the higher and more-encompassing goods such as life and health are typically known only by those who have some degree of training and specialty in a given field. Thus, the good of digestion is a secondary aim that the physician can help the patient to achieve, but it is obvious to all reasoning beings that this good is subordinate to the greater and more-encompassing good of health.

Moral skeptics refuse to acknowledge that there are any objective goods or evils at all. This makes discussion and agreement on questions of ethics very difficult, as it is impossible to find any common starting point. Often skeptics ask us to consider difficult and obscure cases so that they can convince us that objective morality is an impossibility. Thus we are asked, for example, to consider ourselves as the conductor on an unstoppable train that is approaching a division in the tracks; one route will kill an abandoned newborn baby and the other an elderly man who knows the secret to the universe. Such games are entertaining for college sophomores, drinking buddies, and tenured academics, but they have little bearing on real life. For the most part, we are called to live moral lives in which good and evil are relatively easy to see.

The duty to earn a living and care for one's family is not a great moral mystery. Neither is it complicated to understand that you should treat others as you would like to be treated. The broad outlines of morality are not difficult to discern, and the existence of exceptional cases is no proof that objective ethics is a mental fiction.

Nonetheless, there are times when moral problems arise that are not easy to solve. These, in fact, are the common subject matter for ethics committees. Such problems typically occur when two or more goods come into direct conflict, when some good cannot be achieved without also generating a significant evil, or when two evils present themselves as objects of a necessary choice. In these inquiries, the wisdom accumulated by previous thinkers in the natural law tradition is indispensable. The *Ethical and Religious Directives* offers a wide range of guidelines, founded on established moral principles that are crucial in any sound evaluation of cases. Despite their difficulty, the solution of difficult cases is ultimately tied to the simpler truths of ethics that are obvious to everyone. Thus the reason why a particular procedure is forbidden is because it harms a fundamental good. Similarly, the reason why a particular procedure is permitted is because it promotes or preserves a fundamental good or avoids an unnecessary evil. All the subtleties of human reasoning will not bring us any closer to moral truth unless we first acknowledge the objective existence of certain objective goods. Once these are acknowledged, agreement in ethics is at least a theoretical possibility.

Universality of Natural Law

Natural law morality is universal because it is applicable to all rational beings and therefore binding at all times and places. This does not mean that there is no variation in its application to particular cultures or that it does not undergo any development over time. Rather, it means that certain actions, such as the killing of the innocent, have always been wrong and always will be wrong. Similarly, certain other actions, such as kindness to strangers, care of the poor, friendship, and loyalty, have always been right and always will be right. One may be loyal to the wrong cause, love the wrong person, or show a misplaced kindness, but this is not the fault of these good actions; rather it reflects an error in judgment. So, too, when a robber brazenly holds up a bank, his actions are not properly called courageous, for courage, by its very nature, is directed to the good.

Some deny the universality of the natural law by claiming that if morality were truly binding on all, we would all agree on the principles of ethics. This argument confuses the universality of the natural law with the universality of compliance. The fact that some deny or disobey the rules of morality does not prove that the rules are nonexistent. Indeed, it is the very possibility of choosing to live in accord with these universal principles that is the true mark of human freedom. If we were bound to do so, we would not be human, but mere machines. The demand that there be universal agreement on matters of ethics is not realistic. Universal agreement does not exist concerning even the most fundamental truths of science; for example, there still exist those who claim that the earth is flat. Obviously, this is no proof to the contrary. The same is true of the immorality of human sacrifice. There were primitive societies which favored this practice, but the fact that even entire peoples fell into such a grave error is not an argument against the universal character of ethics.

Others suppose that if morality were universal, it could never undergo any change. But change is possible in several ways. First, we can come to better understand the moral law over time. Thus the claim that human sacrifice is morally permissible has rightly been set aside; however, this does not mean that the moral law, objectively considered, has changed, but only that our understanding has improved. New cultural developments can also lead to extensions of the existing principles of natural law. The right to private property is a basic principle of morality, but it took new form with the advent of intellectual property rights. Still other variations are evident as the natural law informs different cultures in unique ways. The moral law that governs a people who live by farming will display different qualities than that which governs those who live by fishing. Thus, the intentional flooding of fields may be a grave injustice to a society that obtains its sustenance from crops but a blessing to those who harvest from the sea. What matters are the general rules governing respect for life, private property, and the satisfaction of human needs. To say that natural law morality is universal is not to say that all of its propositions hold universally. Everyone is bound by the natural law, but not necessarily in the same ways.

There is also a difference between positive and negative precepts. Positive precepts are not always binding; negative precepts are. Thus, it is not necessary to constantly perform acts of charity, even though acts of charity are always worthy of choice, but it is necessary to always avoid acts of adultery, without exception. We are called to pursue the good, but we cannot pursue all possible goods at all possible times. We must choose particular courses of action and limit ourselves to them.

Wrongful actions, in contrast, mandate our complete rejection. But even here we must be careful. When attending to a prohibition in ethics, we must recognize that the general principles of natural law hold only usually and for the most part, thus admitting exceptions. Although it is generally true that killing a fellow human being is wrong, as is done in embryonic stem cell research, the killing of enemy combatants is permissible in war consistent with just war theory, in view of the greater good of the social order. In stating an exceptionless moral norm, we need to specify the subject of the prohibition exactly. Thus murder, properly defined, is always wrong.

Natural Law in Relation to Medicine

Morality and medicine are distinct disciplines, and both make observations and judgments about the order of nature. Morality concerns itself with the ends that are the natural aims of human action, specifically, the good in its various forms, such as health and life, while medicine concerns itself with the means to achieve those ends, sometimes through complicated technological procedures, within a health care setting. As the discipline concerned with ends, morality is in the ruling position, for means must be directed to ends and are therefore subordinate to them. The claim that if we have the technological means to do something we are therefore entitled to do it puts things in reverse order. Mere technological ability is no guarantee that a chosen course of action will be moral. Rather, it is the moral dimension of human decision making that must guide our actions in medicine. This is commonly recognized by all, but nonetheless raises spurious objections among those who wish to be free of all moral constraints.

Given the fact that natural law morality is evident to reason, the guidelines set forth in the *Ethical and Religious Directives* should not be viewed as the doctrinal teachings of the Catholic faith or even as guidelines unique to our religion. They are the commonsense understanding of morality that has been handed down in the West over the course of centuries and developed by many different minds, Catholic and non-Catholic alike. As a result, this moral code within a Catholic health care institution is not in any way an imposition of a particular religious faith on its patients, much less on society at large, but reflects instead the enlivening moral understanding that has long been nurtured at the heart of Western civilization. No one who enters a Catholic health care facility is expected to accept that Jesus Christ is the Second Person of the Trinity, but everyone who enters must understand that the Catholic Church continues to affirm, in keeping with the best moral thinkers of the past, that human life is sacred and cannot be treated as a mere instrument of human use. The same is true of the other moral principles that mark the central ethos of Catholic health care in the United States.

As a philosophical outlook, rather than a body of religious doctrine, society has an obligation to respect the free decision of the Catholic Church to follow this moral understanding in its health care institutions. Those who claim that Catholic health care facilities must provide "services" that are contrary to its understanding of the moral law often fail to see that there is nothing particularly "religious" about the Catholic refusal to do so. We admit to a realm of supernatural truth that makes us unique among the religious believers of the world, but our moral code, in its basic tenets, is not particular to our faith. The philosophy of natural law represents a commonsense approach to ethics that is accessible to all human beings. Reason can know the difference between good and evil, formulate rules for the achievement of the one and suppression of the other, and thus guide us in our moral conduct. No one should deny the right of a Catholic health care facility to follow this moral outlook.

Despite the distinguished history of natural law theory, our own age has grown hostile to it. There are very few natural law theorists outside the Church, and most of them are isolated from the larger moral and cultural views of the intellectual elite. The decline and impending demise of natural law reasoning has been announced many times and in virtually every age, but whenever it appears to be nearest extinction, it returns once again to dominate intellectual and civic discourse.

We live in an age in which natural law reasoning is generally neglected, if not dismissed outright as outdated, but we can safely predict that this is only a sign of a future revival. When the present denial of the objectivity of moral judgment has run its course, when the social order has suffered sufficient decline, when society as a whole once again experiences the need to stand on the terra firma of commonsense reasoning, this outlook will reappear in full flower. While we await its return, we can take comfort in the knowledge that the Catholic Church remains unalterably committed to this timeless approach to moral truth.

Notes

[1] U.S. Conference of Catholic Bishops, *Ethical and Religious Directives for Catholic Health Care Services*, 4th ed. (Washington, D.C.: USCCB, 2001), preamble.

[2] Other moral theories expect individuals to possess fairly remarkable skills of moral analysis. Thus the Kantian asks us to apply the "categorical imperative," a complex theoretical idea for ensuring right action. Similarly, the utilitarian asks us to employ "the principle of utility," another idea known only to the educated. Under these theories, the philosophically trained are best able to achieve the good. As a matter of fact, however, the average person never bothers to formulate such abstract rules but is nonetheless able to choose well in life, often better than the philosophers.

[3] By "absolute" I mean in preference to whatever other goods may be at stake; by "objective" I mean a settled fact of experience. Thus, life is an objective good and will always be so, but when a life is overburdened with a painful and irremediable disease, there is no absolute obligation to preserve it.

✝

Editorial Summation: The Catholic Church remains committed to the timeless moral truths of the natural law. This is a commonsense philosophy of ethics that derives from reasoned reflection on the goods and evils that exist in nature, and from the rules of conduct that issue from a consideration of how to achieve the one and avoid the other. Natural law theorists hold that morality is objective; it exists in nature prior to any choice on our part. Choice is not directed to the ends of action, but to the means by which we might achieve those ends. For example, we do not decide whether health will be the aim of medicine, but how to achieve that good. Primary goods are the most obvious; secondary goods require training to fully appreciate and secure. Thus, everyone knows that health is a good, but the health care professional can best tell us how to achieve this aim through the attainment of intermediate goods. The first principles of natural law do not undergo change, but adapt themselves to different cultures and find new application over the course of time. Natural law morality does not depend on supernatural revelation; therefore, the freedom of Catholic health care to follow this commonsense ethics in its service to the public should be recognized by all.

PART II
ETHICS COMMITTEES

CHAPTER 4

Health Care Ethics Committees: Purpose, Functions, and Structure

Daniel O'Brien

An important premise of Catholic moral teaching is that faith and reason do not necessarily contradict each other.[1] This presupposition is based on the natural law principle that human beings have an innate desire and capacity to know the truth.[2] If faith and human reason are ultimately compatible, since they both proceed from the One Creator, and if the Church is to be both true to itself and an authentic witness to human dignity and the common good, then ongoing dialogue between faith and other scientific disciplines (which all have philosophical presuppositions of their own) must be a constitutive feature of the Church's moral methodology, especially with respect to health care. Following this line of reasoning, ethics committees, sufficiently prepared and grounded, can serve as an important forum and resource for Catholic health care organizations to explore in dialogue the question of whether or not a particular practice, behavior, or development in the health sciences and medicine is, or represents an opportunity for, advancing human dignity and the common good. Such practical reasoning is the substance of ethical inquiry at the organizational level, with implications for all of the organization's decisions, behavior, policies, and practices.

Building on the above presupposition, among others, the *Ethical and Religious Directives for Catholic Health Care Services* identifies several conditions and responsibilities of Catholic health care institutions that illustrate the need for an ethics committee or alternative form of ethics consultation, education, and review service in a Catholic health care institution:

Directive 9. Employees of a Catholic health care institution must respect and uphold the religious mission of the institution and adhere to these Directives. They should maintain professional standards and promote the institution's commitment to human dignity and the common good.

Directive 28. Each person or the person's surrogate should have access to medical and moral information and counseling so as to be able to form his or her conscience. The free and informed health care decision of the person or the person's surrogate is to be followed so long as it does not contradict Catholic principles.

Directive 37. An ethics committee or some alternate form of ethical consultation should be available to assist by advising on particular ethical situations, by offering educational opportunities, and by reviewing and recommending policies. To these ends, there should be appropriate standards for medical ethical consultation within a particular diocese that will respect the diocesan bishop's pastoral responsibility as well as assist members of ethics committees to be familiar with Catholic medical ethics and, in particular, these Directives.[3]

In this chapter, I will briefly explore and review the historical background of health care ethics committees as they developed in the United States. I will then describe the following aspects of an ethics committee: its educational function, its consultation role and decision-making authority, its advisory role, its composition and structure, the various types of ethics committees, and the importance of ethics committee guidelines. I will also discuss the issue of a committee's "expertise." For reasons of organizational integrity, credibility, accreditation, and Catholic identity, I will argue that the ethics committee, or some form of ethics review body, is an essential feature of contemporary Catholic health care organizational life.

Historical Background

Although medical-ethical questions first began to be addressed with some frequency in the sixteenth-century moral manuals, the first set of medical-moral norms for Catholic hospitals in the United States was not published until 1921, by the Archdiocese of Detroit. Many hospitals across the United States and Canada posted these directives or some version of them in their operating rooms. When they proved to be inadequate over time, the more comprehensive *Ethical and Religious Directives for Catholic Hospitals* was developed by a team of American and Canadian theologians led by Gerald Kelly, S.J.; it was published in 1949 and was widely adopted by dioceses across the United States and Canada. After Canada moved to universal health care and the Canadian bishops adopted a new set of directives in 1954, a new, condensed version of the *Ethical and Religious Directives* was developed in the United States; published that same year, it was known as the *Code of Medical Ethics for Catholic Hospitals*, or simply "the U.S. Code." The U.S. Code could easily be hung on operating room walls and in other prominent places in a hospital. In 1956, the Catholic Hospital Association (CHA; now the Catholic Health Association of the United States) revised the 1949 directives in 1956, adding new material on professional secrecy, ghost surgery, psychotherapy, and spiritual care for people of other faiths.[4]

Following the request of the CHA board, the National Conference of Catholic Bishops (now the USCCB) developed the *Ethical and Religious Directives for Catholic Health Facilities* in 1971, which were promulgated by most bishops in the United States, especially following the *Roe v. Wade* decision in 1973. The implementation of these directives, which were revised in 1975, was generally handled directly by hospital administrators, who were usually members of the sponsoring religious congregations. Since that time, Catholic and non-Catholic lay people have assumed most key leadership roles in Catholic health care, along with an increase of physicians not of the Catholic faith and a decrease in nurses graduating from Catholic schools. These changes, as well as rapid advances in medicine and science, stimulated an interest in forming or revitalizing medical-moral committees in Catholic hospitals.[5] Along with new developments and emerging debates in moral theology, the changes also necessitated a reconstitution of the *Directives* which, after several years and numerous drafts, were promulgated in 1994 as the *Ethical and Religious Directives for Catholic Health Care Services,* and revised in 1995 and 2001. In the 1994 edition, ethics committees were officially promoted for Catholic health care institutions for the first time.

Ethics committees are now a common element of Catholic health care institutions across the United States, but this was not always the case. A 1983 annual survey of Catholic hospitals (based on 1982 data) revealed that less than half had ethics committees at that time.[6] The 1983 President's Commission for the Study of Ethical Problems in Medicine and Biomedical and Behavioral Research, in its *Deciding to Forgo Life-Sustaining Treatment: Ethical, Medical, and Legal Issues in Treatment Decisions*, estimated from its research that only about 1 percent of all hospitals in the United States had ethics committees at that time.[7]

There is now a virtual consensus among professional and accreditation bodies in the United States that all health care facilities and organizations should have ethics committees or some alternative form of ethical consultation service available to administrators, professionals, patients, families, and surrogates. In the early 1980s, the American Hospital Association, following the President's Commission, recommended that ethical education, consultation, and review be available to each hospital for difficult decisions in patient care.[8] Since 1995, the Joint Commission on Accreditation of Healthcare Organizations has strongly recommended that each hospital seeking accreditation should have some mechanism available to it for addressing ethical issues and conflicts which arise in the care of patients.[9] The Joint Commission has made similar recommendations for long-term care facilities.

Case law fueled by the rapid changes of medical technology, and even a few criminal law cases generated by challenges to traditional medical practice, created widespread interest in medical-ethical issues.[10] The New Jersey Supreme Court, in its 1976 landmark decision *In the Matter of Karen Ann Quinlan*, was perhaps the most significant catalyst for the establishment of ethics committees in U.S. hospitals. The New Jersey court suggested that the Quinlan case should have gone to an ethics committee for a decision before going to court. This was highly problematic, given that there were then very few ethics committees in U.S. hospitals or long-term care facilities, and none at the institution in question. As a result, great speculation over the proper function of an ethics committee transpired. Although it made the problematic suggestion that an ethics committee should assume a kind of decision-making authority or power to resolve physician-family conflict, the *Quinlan* court provided a great service by generating a profusion of research with a wide variety of opinions on the subject of ethics committees.

The President's Commission identified several potential ethics committee functions: confirming a physician's diagnosis or prognosis, reviewing treatment decisions, making treatment decisions for incompetent patients, providing ethics education programs for staff, formulating policies, and serving as a consultative body for those responsible for making ethical decisions.[11] Only the last three recommendations have proved to be appropriate for an ethics committee, assuming that its members are suitably formed in the necessary competencies. Directive 37 identifies the same three functions. The other three functions identified by the President's Commission involve the exercise of decision-making power. Both the Catholic health care administration which appoints ethics committee members and the committee members themselves must be clear about the inappropriateness of the committee exercising such power. Were a committee to make decisions for an incompetent patient or act as a second opinion, this could both dissuade caregivers from seeking the committee's help and persuade others to seek its help for inappropriate reasons. While it is appropriate for a committee to clarify what certain policies or directives permit or prohibit, it is not the role of the committee to shift responsibility away from those to whom it properly belongs. More will be said about this later.

The Educational Function

Education is arguably the most important function of an ethics committee. One could easily make the case that the other two functions—advisory and consultative—are really only two aspects of the committee's educational role. Committee members are responsible first for educating themselves. Always with the ultimate goal of improving quality of care and organizational processes and behaviors, such education can be accomplished in a variety of ways, such as

- Through shared reading and discussion of the *Ethical and Religious Directives* and expert commentaries;

- Through shared study and discussion of classic cases in the ethical, medical, and legal literature (such as the ones identified in note 10);

- Through role-playing of actual or fictitious cases;

- Through the use of multimedia resources;

- Through the study and development of ethical policies for recommendation to the administration; and

- Through a discussion of actual cases within the institution itself, exercising care to maintain confidentiality.

Care must be taken to avoid making the study of cases an end in itself. While case studies and education are vitally important for committee members to increase their understanding and ability to respond more effectively to cases and crisis situations, there is an increasing recognition that ethics committees must have as a deeper aim the goal of improving quality of care and preventing recurrences of the same ethical problems.[12] Ethical crises in clinical care are often influenced by larger organizational issues that need to be addressed if repeat problems are to be overcome.[13]

In more recent years, the effectiveness of ethics committees has been evaluated not only in terms of how well education is accomplished or individual cases are resolved, but in light of how well the root causes of ethical problems are identified and addressed at the organizational level.[14] As one ethicist observes, it is one thing to resolve *this* conflict over a particular physician order; it is quite another to affect the way orders are sometimes addressed by clinicians in order to avoid conflicts.[15] In other words, ethics committees, if they are to be *truly* effective in impacting and influencing professional behavior and organizational practice, must go beyond case studies and conflict resolution. They must become instruments of organizational change, where the root causes of ethical challenges are addressed within the context of the organization's larger goal of delivering quality care in the moral framework of the healing mission and values of Christ and the Church.

There are a number of things that facilitate a committee's educational function. Meeting regularly, usually once a month, with a well-planned agenda that reflects a variety of topics with obvious application to the everyday work of the committee members, is an important way to maintain interest and ensure that real ethical challenges within the organization are actually being addressed. Rotating presenters as well as discussion facilitators and allowing ample opportunity for everyone to participate and to develop their competencies will also advance a committee's progress. The size of the committee should be neither too small nor too large to impede these goals. I have seen effective committees ranging from a dozen to thirty members. Much depends on the combination of personalities and the skill of the chairperson or discussion facilitators. In addition, professional respect for differences of opinion, mutual respect of persons, supportiveness, sensitivity, compassion, and a commitment to the process of learning and participation are all desirable qualities toward which committee members should aspire.[16]

In one classic study, David Thomasma identified at least five levels of education that should occupy an ethics committee.[17] The first level involves the committee members updating themselves on fundamental theory and "axioms" of medical ethics. The second involves developing clinical ethics skills. The third level is conducting consults. The fourth level is developing practice guidelines. The fifth level is contributing to the institutional conscience and developing a public education program. Thomasma acknowledges that the dominant "four principles" approach to bioethics—the balancing of autonomy, beneficence, nonmaleficence, and justice—has increasingly come into question, but only mentions in passing the vigorous debates which have given rise to alternative ethics theories. Although he cautioned that the committee's self-education should not be directed at members becoming humanities scholars, some of the members should at least be familiar with the recent discussions in the literature. The same holds true today.

One of the more vigorous ongoing theoretical debates, for example, was initiated by the 1982 publication of *In a Different Voice: Psychological Theory and Women's Development*, by Carol Gilligan.[18] Feminist critical theories are not monotypic, but they are pervasive and, in 2008, continue to have a profound impact on all the major professions, including health care professions, which cannot be underestimated. For this reason, it would serve a committee well for at least a few members to familiarize themselves with some feminist theories. I am referring to theories that are not simply critiques of the traditional roles of men and women in society, but a pervasive calling into question the Kantian-based deontological theory that has dominated northern European and American ethics for the last two centuries.[19]

The Consultative Function

Many may be inclined to think automatically of the ethics consultation service as the primary function of an ethics committee. If "consultation" is understood in its broadest sense, this may be true. Ethics committee members often share their insights informally with their coworkers—counseling them, in effect, on important ethical issues of everyday importance in the health care environment. But an ethics consultation service is rarely the most consuming work of an ethics committee. If a committee is initiated with this expectation, the members will quickly become disappointed.

Nevertheless, when the consultation service is accessed, the committee will have an opportunity to foster proper decision-making processes, clarify responsibilities, and promote a heightened awareness and understanding of human dignity, guiding principles, and institutional

policies. The consultation service is principally an educational function meant to facilitate appropriate moral decisions and decision making among patients, surrogates, physicians, nurses, and other caregivers.

Even a request for something that would be inappropriate for an ethics committee to handle—for example, when a family wants it to censure a physician—can be a "teachable moment." Those who screen consultation requests must take care not to miss an opportunity to assist by being too quick to dismiss the case as "a legal problem" for risk management, or "a family communication problem" for pastoral care or social work. Most ethics consultations involve some legal dimensions and communication difficulties.

The ethics consultation service can be a powerful positive force in the institution for improving quality and patient care, for facilitating effective communication among providers and caregivers, and for fostering appropriate respect for human dignity at all levels in the institution. Committee members who are called on to provide an ethics consultation must take great care not to abuse their privileged position by manipulating vulnerable patients and family members (for example, by generalizing or overstepping their authority). They must take care not to allow the consultation session to deteriorate into a "doctor-bashing" tool for disgruntled employees. Consultation protocols can offer a way both to delineate the committee's power and to build appropriate expectations in the participants. Consistent with Thomasma's recommendation, start-up ethics committees should refrain from providing a consultation service for perhaps a year or more—or at least until those members who will actually engage in consultations possess the requisite competencies.

Near the turn of the this century, the American Society for Bioethics and Humanities (ASBH) made a particularly important contribution to this discussion in its comprehensive report, *Core Competencies for Health Care Ethics Consultation*.[20] As the report's name suggests, the professional society set out to identify and make a number of recommendations for developing the core competencies needed for quality improvements in ethics consultations. Consistent with other competency theories, the ASBH identified three components: a knowledge set, a skill set, and character traits. Under core skills needed, it included process and interpersonal skills. It identified nine core knowledge areas that are required for ethics consultation, and several character traits necessary for optimal ethics consultation.

Without repeating the details of the report, a list of the items under each of the three competency areas follows below. Such is the scope of competencies needed. It is important to note that the document also makes specific recommendations concerning how many members of a consultation team or ethics committee ought to have certain skills, possess certain knowledge sets, and at what level of expertise each member should function. Rather than review those details here, it suffices to say that an ethics committee would do well to study this important document and implement its recommendations.

Skills Required for Ethics Consultation

- Skills necessary to identify the nature of the value uncertainty or conflict that underlies the need for ethics consultation
- Skills necessary to analyze the value uncertainty or conflict
- The ability to facilitate formal and informal meetings
- The ability to build moral consensus (not always necessary, but often important)
- The ability to utilize institutional structures and resources to facilitate the implementation of the chosen option
- The ability to document consults and elicit feedback regarding the process of consultation so that the process can be evaluated
- The ability to listen well and to communicate interest, respect, support, and empathy to involved parties
- The ability to educate involved parties regarding the ethical dimensions of the case
- The ability to elicit the moral views of involved parties
- The ability to represent the views of involved parties to others
- The ability to enable the involved parties to communicate effectively and be heard by other parties
- The ability to recognize and attend to various relational barriers to communication

Knowledge Areas Required for Ethics Consultation

- Moral reasoning and ethical theory as it relates to ethics consultation
- Bioethical issues and concepts that typically emerge in ethics consultation
- Health care systems as they relate to ethics consultation

- Clinical context as it relates to ethics consultation
- The health care institution in which the consultants work, as it relates to ethics consultations
- The local health care institution's policies that are relevant to ethics consultation
- Beliefs and perspectives of the patient and staff populations where ethics consultations are done
- The relevant codes of ethics and professional conduct and the guidelines of accrediting organizations as they relate to ethics consultation
- Health law relevant to ethics consultation

With respect to these knowledge sets, in 2003, ethics committee leaders from across Ascension Health reached a consensus that three additional knowledge areas were needed for Catholic-sponsored ethics committees in order for their consultation services to function optimally:

- Catholic moral theory and key ethical principles
- Classic cases beyond health law
- *Ethical and Religious Directives for Catholic Health Care Services*

Character Traits Required for Ethics Consultation

- *Tolerance*, *patience* and *compassion* are traits that enable a consultant to listen well and communicate interest, respect, support, and empathy.
- Honesty, forthrightness and self-knowledge are traits that help prevent the manipulative use of information and help create an atmosphere of trust necessary to facilitate formal and informal meetings.
- *Courage* is sometimes needed to enable various parties, especially the politically less powerful, to communicate effectively and be heard by others.
- *Prudence* and *humility* inform behavior when rash or novel courses of action are being considered, and they enable consultants not to overstep the bounds of their roles in consultation.
- *Integrity* enables consultants to pursue an option or range of options that is ethically required even when it might be convenient to do otherwise.

Finally, with respect to the importance of character, the ASBH report makes a critical observation:

> Good character, and integrity in particular, is not only important for conducting ethics consultation itself, but also for the credibility of those who will be conducting it. Other professionals and layper-

sons understandably expect that good character be exhibited by ethics consultants in their professional roles (and indeed in other quasi-public domains). The perception of a person's character in these other areas will inevitably influence one's effectiveness in doing a consult. For example, a physician who developed a reputation for belittling other members of the health care team or routinely disregarding the wishes of competent patients would face serious credibility problems in performing ethics consultations.[21]

Consultations and Decision Making Authority

In the thirty years following *Quinlan*, most reflections on the proper functions of ethics committees have recommended that decision-making authority rest within the physician-patient or professional-patient relationship, working within the framework of institutional policies and established ethical and legal standards.[22] In the midst of an ongoing discussion in the medical and ethical literature over the tension between patient autonomy and professional integrity (e.g., the futility debates), the *Ethical and Religious Directives* continue to offer a balanced model, in which the professional-patient relationship is understood as a partnership of moral equals who are, however, unequal in power and expertise:

> Neither the health care professional nor the patient acts independently of the other; both participate in the healing process. ... The health care professional has the knowledge and experience to pursue the goals of healing, the maintenance of health, and the compassionate care of the dying, taking into account the patient's convictions and spiritual needs, and the moral responsibilities of all concerned. The person in need of health care depends on the skill of the health care provider to assist in preserving life and promoting health of body, mind, and spirit. The patient, in turn, has a responsibility to use these physical and mental resources in the service of moral and spiritual goals to the best of his or her ability.[23]

A committee must not exercise the moral authority that rightly belongs to the physician and the patient or to those professionals and others who are immediately involved in the patient's care. If decision-making powers were exercised by ethics committees, they could, in effect, distance or remove medical and ethical decisions and moral responsibility from those most accountable for a patient's welfare.[24]

In developing its consultation service, then, the committee members who will participate in this delicate task must thoroughly understand the proper limits of the ethics consultation, and adhere to its primary functions:

- To assist the decision makers by clarifying institutional policy
- To appropriately explain or interpret the *Ethical and Religious Directives* when needed
- To raise questions or alternatives not considered by the decision makers
- To clarify the patient's rights and responsibilities, as well as professional and institutional rights and responsibilities
- To assist surrogates in an appropriate understanding of their role and responsibilities
- To identify and clarify any ethical principles applicable to the particular case
- To foster an appropriate understanding and respect for the human dignity of the patient, the family, and the professional caregivers
- In a word, to educate

Strict consultation protocols and information brochures that discuss the purpose of ethics consultations can diminish the number of inappropriate requests. Occasional articles in the health system or institutional publications and periodic presentations to professional staffs can also help eliminate problematic perceptions and expectations of the committee's responsibilities. Even the perception by others that the committee has the authority to make medical decisions or to reproach physicians and caregivers can be damaging to the committee's credibility and effectiveness. The 1983 opinion of the general counselor for Karen Quinlan's family, Paul W. Armstrong, is still good advice for ethics committees in the early twenty-first century:

> Regularly assigning to ethics committees the task of making decisions on life-sustaining treatment could undermine recognizing the obligations of those who should be principally responsible. The surrogates for an incapacitated person and the health-care professionals should be the primary decision makers who, through the vehicle of the ethics committee, seek the keener insight of an interdisciplinary view in deciding on their course of action.[25]

The Advisory Function

Like the consultative function of an ethics committee, its advisory role is also educational in character. The administration should make liberal use of the committee for reviewing proposed polices on clinical care, on employee relations, and even on managed-care contracts. The experienced committee, under strict obligations of confidentiality, can offer an important perspective to the development of administrative policies and protocols. Ethics committees have long been employed as the principal drafters of treatment-decision and patient-rights policies. But all the organizational aspects of the health care institution have ethical implications that directly or indirectly affect the human dignity of patients and employees alike. It is not the committee's function to implement administrative policies. But their participation in the development of those policies and protocols, whether clinical or business or organizational, would make an invaluable contribution to the mission and ministry of the institution as a whole.

Committee Composition

The progress of a committee's growth is dependent on its composition and reporting structure. In a Catholic-sponsored organization, the committee should be appointed by, and report directly to, the administration, or have a dual-reporting relationship with the administration and board. The committee should have a well-balanced representation from medical and nursing staffs. Representatives from pastoral care, social work, discharge planning, and other areas of direct patient care are also essential for an effective ethics committee. A health-law attorney can be quite effective on a committee, so long as he or she is careful not to put legal concerns above ethical concerns. A person well-trained in the moral methodology and teaching of the Catholic Church can bring an important dimension to the committee's education and discussions, particularly as they pertain to the *Ethical and Religious Directives*. Outside ethicists may also bring an important perspective, but with special caution. They, like anyone else, could undermine the growth and effectiveness of the committee if they openly challenge the mission and identity of the institution or the authority of the *Ethical and Religious Directives,* or if they see the committee as merely an academic exercise. These behaviors and characteristics could be especially damaging on account of an ethicist's recognition as an expert.

A liaison from the administration should be active on every ethics committee. A committee that does not have the full support of the administration is doomed to failure. Indeed, all people serving on the committee must be willing to support the mission of the institution and the standards of the *Ethical and Religious Directives*, even if they personally disagree with certain aspects of either. It is unrealistic to think that everyone serving on the ethics committee will be Catholic. Nor is this even desirable, if the committee is to accomplish one of its principal tasks of self-education. People from diverse religious backgrounds can contribute greatly to a committee's knowledge, skills, and effectiveness in responding to questions raised by employees, professional staff, and patients from other religious backgrounds.

Long-Term Care and System Ethics Committees

Most early studies of ethics committees focused on the hospital. In recent years, however, long-term care facilities, home health and hospice organizations, health systems, and even managed-care organizations have established ethics committees. Long-term care ethics committees will, obviously, be composed largely of nursing personnel, especially nursing supervisors and the director of nursing. But pastoral care personnel, education and activities directors, administrators, physical therapists, speech therapists, and social workers all should play important roles on a long-term care ethics committee. The medical director or a physician directly responsible for the care of several residents should also play an active role on the long-term care ethics committee.

System ethics committees, or ethics coordinating councils, serve a purpose distinct from that of institutional committees. An institutional ethics committee will focus on the various aspects of ethics education, consultation, and policy review or development within a facility or for a particular service (e.g., acute care, skilled care, home health, hospice). Such committees will also sponsor educational opportunities for their immediate communities. A system ethics committee or coordinating council, by contrast, will focus much of its efforts on facilitating the integration of ethical standards and consistency of practice throughout the continuum of care in a system of facilities and services.

Such regional system committees will generally meet only three or four times per year. Members should be selected from the institutional committees, including chairpersons, vice-chairpersons, appropriate delegates, and experts in medicine, nursing, pastoral care, social work, advocacy, administration, legal affairs, mission, and government relations. Meetings of such committees may also be an excellent place for working with sponsors' representatives.

Smaller regional ethics committees may be formed to serve just two or three institutions. These committees, if they take the place of an institutional ethics committee, should meet more regularly, preferably monthly.

In a national or multistate health care system, it may not be feasible to bring representatives of different institutions together as a single-system ethics committee, owing to constraints imposed by local professional commitments, travel, and costs. Use of audiovisual technology may be an option in some systems or, in place of a system-wide committee, a national or multistate system might designate an ethics subcommittee of the board or develop a regular forum for the leadership team to do the following: educate itself, explore and address ethical issues that affect facilities and services across the system, help develop consistent ethical standards and practices, and develop an appropriate understanding and implementation of the *Ethical and Religious Directives*. A system ethicist or theological consultant might facilitate some discussions.

A system ethics committee should not duplicate what the institutional committees do. The principle of subsidiarity applies: the system committee should not secure for itself those actions and responsibilities that can be most effectively accomplished at the local level by institutional committees. However, in these days of system-wide integration, mergers, managed-care contracting, and integrated delivery across a continuum of care, a system-wide forum for ethical inquiry may be needed over and above the institutional ethics committee.

A system ethics committee can provide several benefits to a system as a whole, as well as to local institutional committees within a growing system:

• By sharing ideas and discussing common concerns that cut across institutions and services

• By comparing institutional policies and solutions to similar problems

• By sharing and developing training modules and resources

• By promoting ethical consistency and/or standardization throughout the system and across the continuum of care

• By providing another networking opportunity for people committed to raising ethical awareness in their local institutions

• By promoting a corporate culture informed by catholic social teaching and values throughout the system and across the continuum of care

The list is certainly not exhaustive, but its potential harvest may make such a committee worth planting in the system. The fruits of ethical consistency across facilities and systems should generate several important results: greater confidence and higher expectations of quality among patient and enrollee populations, a deeper clarity and higher level of ethical reasoning and expertise among

the various professional groups who serve within the structures of an integrated system, and greater conviction about the system's distinctive mission and religious identity. Everyone should benefit, but most of all the patients and populations who are served.

Other potential arguments for establishing and developing a system or regional ethics committee include these:

• The work of a system or regional committee cannot be accomplished by a system ethicist. A system ethicist will be helpful for passing on information from one committee to another, for providing theological and philosophical expertise as a consultative resource to governance, administrations, and committees, and for helping to connect members of one committee to another. This provides for some degree of continuity, but the ethics expert cannot substitute for a discourse among members of several committees.

• A system or regional committee, composed as it is of members from several institutional committees, may be the more appropriate forum for developing a system-wide policy. This may be preferable to having policies just handed down "from above," with only cursory input "from below," and may result in greater buy-in and cultural change. Committee members who invest the research, time, and energy in developing and recommending a system-wide policy are more likely to embrace it and defend it in any given situation. It is not simply a matter of pride. It is also a matter of participation, deeper understanding, and ownership.

• A system or regional ethics committee can generate an ethical discourse unmatched by local committees. The system group brings together a broader range of experiences from different institutional and community settings. For example, a system ethics committee can provide the opportunity for one committee delegate to explain to other delegates why a particular policy was developed and the form in which it was developed. They can then bring back to their own committees a greater appreciation for the subtleties and complexities of values, principles, cases, and policy development, and at the same time acquire new skills and language for addressing ethical issues with greater clarity and thoroughness.

• Periodically gathering key people from several committees can be encouraging to fledgling committees, reinvigorating for more established committees, and educational for all.

Finally, consideration ought to be given to the formation of ethics committees to serve boards and administrative teams. Board committees, perhaps in the form of a mission and ethics committee, could serve the educational needs of these bodies by identifying and raising key ethical issues and concerns in the life of the institution, by preparing educational exercises, by recommending certain actions and policies, and by reviewing major transactions as part of a larger mission "due diligence" process. Such committees could enhance the organization's self-understanding and contribute significantly to its sense of Catholic mission and identity. Consideration might even be given to making ethical issues a regular agenda item at quarterly board meetings or monthly at administrative team meetings. A regularly scheduled time for even just a few minutes of reflection can enhance and help develop a board or administrative team's understanding and leadership competencies. Many contemporary Catholic health system boards have mission or mission and ethics subcommittees which serve this function quite effectively.

Ethics Committee Guidelines

The health care administration should establish ethics committee guidelines that clearly articulate the role, purpose, functions, and limited powers of the ethics committee and its services. *Ethics Committees: A Challenge for Catholic Health Care*, by Sr. Margaret Kelly and Rev. Donald McCarthy, offers several models which, for the most part, are still valid today. *Health Care Ethics Committees: The Next Generation*, by Judith Ross and others, and the Fall 1994 issue of *Bioethics Forum* also offer helpful advice for formulating guidelines.[26] Ethics committee guidelines clarify several important things: who is in charge and what the reporting structure is, what is expected of everyone, what the power and function of the committee are, and how long members should serve. Defining the mission, role, purpose, and functions of the ethics committee helps to keep the committee on track and helps guide everyone's expectations both on and off the committee.

Committee Expertise

Many members of ethics committees, if not most, will not have extensive higher education in ethics or moral theology. Nor should this be desirable:

> What is often missing in understanding present ethics committees is that they are not intended to be decision makers or experts in the manner of their ancestor committee. Moreover, the absence of expertise is

not a mistake in the creation of ethics committees; indeed, it is an important part of the reason for coming into being.[29]

The ethical "expertise" of individual committee members will vary and be an ongoing development for each participant. Ethics committee members bring their own professional expertise and perspectives to the committee, backed by an openness and a willingness to contribute, to participate, to study, and to learn. By incorporating gained insights into his or her own thinking and professional practice, each member enriches the institution as a whole, becoming an important resource to other practitioners and decision makers—whether clinician, administrator, manager, patient, or surrogate.

Much of the membership's education and experience will occur in the ethics committee processes—through case studies and retrospective review, topical presentations and discussions, and through policy review and policy development. Ideally, this will be fortified by intensive or informal workshops, conferences, incidental university courses, and independent reading. Many nurses and physicians will have studied ethics during their formal education and training. The rich diversity of professional and community experience and expertise that each member brings to the committee will contribute added insight for every other member. Above all, the work and study of the ethics committee must relate directly to the day-to-day work of the members. The committee will founder if its members see little or no apparent relationship between the work of the committee and their daily work with patients, or if they see little or no impact on the organization's behaviors, policies, and decisions.

Conclusion

An ethics committee's life and sense of purpose rise and fall with the administration's support or indifference. With administrative encouragement, appointment of effective leadership, careful selection of members, appropriate financial support, and welcome participation in the life and heart of the institution, a committee is likely to flourish and contribute significantly to the institution's self-understanding and needed changes in its culture. A healthy, active ethics committee is one convincing sign of an administration that is truly committed to the Catholic mission and identity of the institution or system it serves. Ethics committees can be an invaluable part of the mission and culture of the Catholic health care ministry and a key instrument for deepening our institutional commitment to human dignity and the common good.

Notes

[1] John Paul II, *Fides et ratio* (September 14, 1998).

[2] Thomas Aquinas, *Summa theologiae* I-II, q. 94, a. 2; Servais Pinckaers, "Natural Law and Freedom," in *Morality: The Catholic View* (South Bend, IN: St. Augustine's Press, 2003).

[3] U.S. Conference of Catholic Bishops, *Ethical and Religious Directives for Catholic Health Care Services*, 4th ed. (Washington, D.C.: USCCB, 2001).

[4] Catholic Hospital Association, *Ethical and Religious Directives for Catholic Hospitals* (St. Louis: CHA, 1949); Kevin O'Rourke, Thomas Kopfensteiner, and Ronald Hamel, "A Brief History: A Summary of the Development of the *Ethical and Religious Directives for Catholic Health Care Services*," *Health Progress* 82.6 (November–December 2001): 18–21.

[5] Margaret John Kelly and Donald McCarthy, eds., *Ethics Committees: A Challenge for Catholic Health Care* (St. Louis, MO: Pope John XXIII Center and Catholic Health Association of the United States, 1984), 4–5.

[6] Kelly and McCarthy, *Ethics Committees*, 6.

[7] President's Commission for the Study of Ethical Problems in Medicine and Biomedical and Behavioral Research, *Deciding to Forgo Life-Sustaining Treatment: Ethical, Medical, and Legal Issues in Treatment Decisions* (Washington, D.C.: GPO, 1983), 448.

[8] Kevin D. O'Rourke and Dennis Brodeur, *Medical Ethics: Common Ground for Understanding* (St. Louis: Catholic Health Association, 1987), 45.

[9] Joint Commission for Accreditation of Healthcare Organizations, *2006 Comprehensive Accreditation Manual for Hospitals* (Oakbrook Terrace, IL: JCAHO, 2006).

[10] Such cases are well-known today: *Dax Cowart* (1973), *Roe v. Wade* (1973), *Joseph Saikewicz* (1976), *Baby Doe* (1983), *Claire Conroy* (1983), *Baby Fae* (1984), *Elizabeth Bouvia* (1985), *Sammy Linares* (1988), *Nancy Cruzan* (1990), *Gilgunn v. Massachusetts General Hospital* (1995), *Vacco v. Quill* (1997), *Terri Schiavo* (2003) to name just a few. See Ascension Health ethics resource at http://www.ascensionhealth.org/ethics/public/main.asp. See also Daniel O'Brien, ed., *Ethics in Health Care: Ingredients for Effective Committees* (Ann Arbor, MI: Sisters of St. Joseph Health System), 1995.

[11] President's Commission, *Deciding to Forgo*, 160–161.

[12] Ellen Fox, Mary Beth Foglia, and Robert A. Pearlman, of the National Center for Ethics in Health Care (VHA), "Preventive Ethics: A Quality Improvement Approach to Health Care Ethics," presentation at the 9th annual meeting of the American Society of Bioethics and Humanities, October 18, 2007.

[13] Mary Beth Foglia and Robert A. Pearlman, "Integrating Clinical and Organizational Ethics: A Systems Perspective Can Provide an Antidote to the 'Silo' Problem in Clinical Ethics Consultations," *Health Progress* 87.2 (March–April 2006): 31–35.

[14] See the following articles in *Health Progress* 87.2 (March–April 2006): Francis Bernt et al. "Ethics Committees in Catholic Hospitals," 18–25; Kevin Murphy, "A 'Next Generation' Ethics Committee," 26–30; Foglia and Pearlman, "Integrating Clinical and Organizational Ethics"; John Tuohey, "Ethics Consultation in Portland," 36–41; see also *HEC Forum* 12.1 (January 2000): David C. Blake, "Reinventing the Healthcare Ethics Committee," 8–32; and Janis Rueping and Dan O. Dugan, "A Next Generation Ethics Program in Progress: Lessons from Experience," 49–56.

[15] Ron Hamel, "Ethics Committees: Pursuing Enhanced Effectiveness," *Health Progress* 87.2 (March–April 2006): 17.

[16] Daniel O'Brien, ed., *Ethics in Health Care: Ingredients for Effective Committees* (Ann Arbor, MI: Sisters of St. Joseph Health System, 1995); American Society for Bioethics and Humanities, *Core Competencies for Health Care Ethics Consultation* (Glenview, IL: ASBH, 1998).

[17] David C. Thomasma, "Education of Ethics Committees," *Bioethics Forum* 10.4 (Fall 1994): 12–18.

[18] Carol Gilligan, *In a Different Voice: Psychological Theory and Women's Development* (Cambridge, MA: Harvard University Press, 1982); Mary Jeanne Larrabee, ed., *An Ethic of Care: Feminist and Interdisciplinary Perspectives* (New York: Routledge, 1993).

[19] See, for example, Marilyn Friedman, "Beyond Caring: The De-Moralization of Gender," in *An Ethic of Care: Feminist and Interdisciplinary Perspective*, ed. Mary Jeanne Larrabee (New York: Routledge, 1993), 258–273; and Joan C. Tronto, "Beyond Gender Difference to a Theory of Care," in *An Ethic of Care: Feminist and Interdisciplinary Perspectives*, 240–257. Catholic moral theory can bring much to the debate; see John E. Tropman, *The Catholic Ethic in American Society: An Exploration of Values* (San Francisco: Jossey-Bass, 1995); and Sidney Callahan, "A Feminist Case Against Euthanasia," *Health Progress* 77.6 (November–December 1996): 21–29. In particular, Catholic moral theory counters the claim that there are only two basic ethics—an ethics of justice and rights, and an ethics of care and response; see Gilligan, *In a Different Voice*. Recognizing the value of these feminist theories as critiques of Kantian-based ethics should not be construed as an agreement with any position the authors may take that is contrary to Catholic teaching.

[20] American Society for Bioethics and Humanities, *Core Competencies for Health Care Ethics Consultation* (Glenview, IL: ASBH, 1998). The actual preparation of the report was completed by the Society for Health and Human Values and the Society for Bioethics Consultation, with the participation of the president of the American Association of Bioethics. The report was reviewed and adopted by the American Society for Bioethics and Humanities, the successor to these three organizations, on May 8, 1998. The development of the report is described on pages 1 and 2 of the document.

[21] ASBH, *Core Competencies*, 23.

[22] Judith Wilson Ross et al., *Health Care Ethics Committees: The Next Generation* (Chicago: American Hospital Publishing, 1993), 91–107.

[23] USCCB, *Ethical and Religious Directives* (2001), part 3, introduction.

[24] O'Rourke and Brodeur, *Medical Ethics*, 45–48.

[25] P. Armstrong, "Legal and Judicial Issues of Ethics Committees," in *Ethics Committees*, ed. Kelly and McCarthy, 51.

[26] See Kelly and McCarthy, eds., *Ethics Committees*, 113–144. See also Ross et al., *Health Care Ethics Committees*; and *Bioethics Forum* 10.4 (Fall 1994). This issue of *Bioethics Forum* is devoted entirely to ethics committees.

[29] Ross et al., *Health Care Ethics Committees*, 3.

Editorial Summation: This chapter shows that the educational function of a health care ethics committee is central to all its other functions, especially its consultative and policy development and review functions. The educational function is critical because decision makers in health care, and not just ethics committees, must have the internal resources that will enable them to reason and make good moral judgments about the care of patients and about organizational systems and processes that affect that care. The ethical dimension of providing health care cannot be extrinsic to the health care provider. In the delivery of health care, there is no substitute for moral judgments that arise from, and are embraced by, the individuals who provide the care. The ethics committee must always be at the task of educating itself and others. This is directly accomplished through specific programs, but it happens no less through consultations on specific cases, and through the review and development of policy. The need for ethics committees will always be present. Nevertheless, the greater the transfer of the bases for moral decision making to the people directly responsible for patient care, the better that care will be.

CHAPTER 5

The Dynamics of Ethics Committee Operation

A. Health Care Ethics Committee Meetings

Sheila O'Friel, D.C.

In many cases, the effectiveness of a health care ethics committee reflects the meetings of the members. For that reason, the meetings must have specific measurable goals and a clear agenda which reflects efforts to attain these goals. Good minutes should report the goals, agenda, and outcomes.

Meeting Minutes

Meeting minutes are an important record. Minutes should accurately report a committee's agenda items, whether they be on policy writing, education and case reviews, or ethical dilemmas. The minutes should state the options available to the committee, the actions taken, and, when appropriate, the reasons that the committee has chosen a specific course. Minutes need not and should not be excessively detailed, but they should make clear the issues the committee considered, the conclusions they reached, the reasons for conclusions, and the possible effects that decision-making outcomes may have on patient, family, and provider. If a committee develops good meeting agendas and adheres to them, allotting a planned time for each topic, the minutes should flow easily from the agenda items. The minutes are an account of the progress on the agenda items. The minutes should also provide those who are unable to attend a meeting with an adequate account of what transpired.

Some committees may want to include summaries of case reviews in the minutes or may prefer to develop separate case review records, noting in the minutes only that a case review was conducted. However, confidentiality is respected and the records should not include patient names. Code names or numbers may be used for identification.

The goals, agenda, and minutes of health care ethics committee meetings will depend on the type of meeting being conducted. Some of the most common types of meetings are

- Regularly scheduled, periodic meetings of the committee

- Emergency meetings, for consultation on cases

- Educational meetings, for updating members and for other purposes

- Orientation meetings for new members

- Subcommittee meetings for possible subgroups:

  - Steering, to formulate agenda, for example

  - Policy, to develop or review policies

  - Corporate, to consider challenges in business ethics

  - Education, to address educational needs

The formats for meetings may also vary. For instance, an interdisciplinary, large-group meeting may be used for strictly educational ethics programs for the ethics committee members as well as for other interested persons, but also for discussion of problems and recommendations. In meetings of the ethics committee only, smaller groups will discuss issues and make decisions. In other meetings, an invited guest may speak on an issue of concern. In all cases, the goal of the meeting will determine the size, format, and agenda that will be most effective for the purpose outlined.

Planning and Agendas

Regardless of goal, size, format, or agenda, one necessary element common to all meetings is *planning*. Satisfying, productive meetings do not just happen. They must be thought out and organized ahead of time. One way to focus on planning is to establish a definite time, place, and responsible parties for the implementation of planning. A steering committee could consist of the chairperson and several other members, such as the secretary and chairpersons of all standing subcommittees, or a group of long-term members. The steering committee's responsibility is the planning and evaluation of meetings. The work of the steering committee should result in more energetic and imaginative planning. Even a chairperson gifted in planning and running meetings alone will benefit from the support of a team. In addition, a team effort demonstrates the multidisciplinary commitment of the group.

An effective chairperson or steering committee will create both short-term and long-term agendas for the health care ethics committee. The chairperson or steering committee may plan for the short term by first examining the past meeting. The committee may want to meet for fifteen minutes at the end of the regular meeting or schedule a longer meeting within a few days. A retrospective look at the last meeting asks: Is there anything we learned from the last meeting that can help next time? Did the meeting accomplish its goals? What worked well? What caused a problem? Did unresolved matters remain, which can be included in the agenda of the next meeting? Some committees have their members spend the last few minutes of each meeting filling out a brief evaluation of the meeting. The steering committee then takes these evaluations seriously, giving committee members feedback on how they plan to respond to the evaluations. If people are asked to express their concerns, either their concerns should be addressed by the committee or a committee leader should explain why they cannot be addressed.

After the last meeting has been evaluated by the steering committee, an agenda may then be established for the next meeting. Not only subject matter, but also process issues that different topics require must be addressed.

Agendas may differ greatly in their substantive and process complexity. It is not just that they include different subject matters; it is also that the reality behind the agenda items differs in many significant ways. In case presentations, for example, which are a common agenda item, every case is unique, and family wishes and patient's illnesses vary—significant differences that may not be revealed by a typical agenda.

A sample agenda may read as follows:

1. Review the minutes of the last meeting
2. Old business: Reports on tabled topics
3. Case presentation: Patients' right to refuse CPR
4. Education: Use of advance directives

It is important to plan the format, or process, of the meeting to fit its particular content and the human realities underlying it.

More sophisticated methods for dealing with the various agenda items can be developed by committees. For example, work on a specific subject might best be developed by means of a worksheet or short questionnaire. Group process techniques such as role-playing and brainstorming can be planned. Developing ways to help address affective dimensions of issues or stretch the customary boundaries of topics may be time-consuming, but often is effective. Primary focus is on patient-care issues.

Long-term planning also deserves attention by the whole committee in order to appreciate how the individual meetings are part of a larger plan. Generally, it is useful to develop a year's plan for committee efforts, including educational projects, policy reviews, surveys to be conducted, documents to be drafted, and similar projects. Some committees during their initial meeting of the year develop a general plan for the year or present a plan that has been developed by the steering committee. Other committees formulate the plan at the end of the year. When the plan is accepted, each member should be urged or required to assume some responsibility for a part of the plan during the year. A sample ethics committee plan for a year could include goals like these:

- Design and conduct a survey on utilization of ethics committee consultation service by physicians and staff.

- Develop a system by which committee members keep abreast of new technological developments and their moral and ethical implications for patients and staff.

- Formulate educational programs in ethics for new members, the committee members, and the community in general. Include focus on ethics of dilemmas and patient rights.

It is essential to committee success that members have a sense of participation and responsibility and not be merely passive attendants at a series of presentations or experiences formulated by others.

Managing Meetings

In order for the meetings of the health care ethics committee to be productive and effective, it is essential that they be managed well. For this reason, the meeting leader must consider three major concerns: getting the meeting started on time, keeping it moving, and generating action.

Integral to the success of a meeting is the leader's defining its purpose, creating the agenda, and letting all the participants know why the meeting is to be held. Defining the purpose and desired outcome is a crucial initial step. The group leader should determine why the meeting is being held (purpose) and what it is to accomplish or achieve (objectives). At times this is more difficult to determine for a routinely scheduled meeting, but it can be combined with creating the agenda.

Creating the Meeting Agenda

The agenda, an important tool for a well-managed meeting, is a map to keep the meeting on track and on time. The following questions will help with the formulation of the agenda: What are the topics for consideration? For each topic, what should be accomplished? Who is responsible for each topic? What are committee members expected to do: contribute information, make recommendations, make a commitment, give feedback, approve? How much time should be allotted to each topic? Which topics have priority?

Communicating Purpose and Desired Outcome

Mailing the agenda a week in advance along with all the documents that need to be read ahead of time is an excellent means of communicating the purpose and plan of the anticipated meeting. In addition, this serves as a reminder to the committee members of the meeting time and place.

Managing the Meeting in Motion

A good meeting needs a good leader who knows how to attend to both content and process. Certain steps may help to achieve this goal: reviewing the meeting agenda, defining or reviewing the ground rules for the meeting, focusing the discussion on the purpose and desired outcome, setting the pace, and articulating the conclusions:

- Reviewing the meeting agenda is an important first item of business since it focuses the group on the task at hand. This is a good time to ask for any changes or additions to the agenda as well as for a reallocation of time for topics that may need it.

- Defining or reviewing the ground rules for a meeting may only be needed for newly established groups. Typically, ground rules pertain to the kind of participation expected, nonnegotiable matters, confidentiality, and role assignments.

- Focusing the discussion on the purpose and the desired outcome makes the meeting more effective. The leader needs skills to keep the discussion

moving from point to point of the agenda. When redirecting the discussion, the leader should ask questions and make statements that will lead the discussion back to the objectives of the specific agenda topics or to the general purpose of the meeting.

- Setting the pace is another skill needed by the meeting's leader. Even when focused on the objective, the discussion may move too quickly or slowly for appropriate consideration of contributions.

- Articulating conclusions should take place throughout the meeting, for instance, after each major topic or item is considered, after all relevant information has been presented, after all sides of an issue have been expressed, and when the group decides it is ready to make a decision.

The third responsibility of the leader in managing committee meetings well is that of generating action. It is common for people to comment that, "when all is said and done, a lot more is said than done." To avoid this, it is important that the leader help the group formulate an action plan after each conclusion is reached. Then members will leave the meeting with a sense of accomplishment and will expect follow-through. In order to formulate an action plan, it is helpful to:

- Specify what action needs to be taken.

- Make specific assignments for specific people with completion dates.

- Agree on how to monitor progress and/or evaluate outcomes and who will do the monitoring.

A format for committee minutes may appear in block form, as shown on the following page.

Three related points may be helpful in planning successful health care ethics meetings. Many other points could be considered as well, but the important ones relate to the leadership skills of the meeting leader, time management skills (beginning and ending the meeting on time), and the distribution of materials for committee members.

Leadership Skills. In addition to being able to organize and manage the process of a meeting, a leader also needs to have personal leadership skills which focus on handling behavior central to group interaction. The leader needs to give special attention to encouraging participation, handling disruptive behavior if necessary, and managing diversity.

Group participation is influenced by the leader's behavior. An effective leader will specify the type of participation that is desired, create a participatory cli-

	DISCUSSION	
Issue	Progress	Action
Discussion of DNR orders in surgery	Committee unwilling to make recommendations without input from surgery	Smith will discuss with chairman of surgery

mate, skillfully draw out contributions from specific individuals, protect persons with a minority view, as well as acknowledge and reinforce constructive participation from all the members.

Disruptive behavior is usually unintentional. Examples include bringing unrelated subjects into the discussion, discouraging group action by saying things like "This will never work" or "There is no solution to this problem," dominating the discussion and preventing others from contributing, interrupting others, and disagreeing with everyone. Since most persons are unaware of this behavior and how it blocks group progress, the leader might try using a paradigm to analyze an ethical dilemma or answering these questions: What is the problem? Whose problem is it? What are the patient's wishes? What is the diagnosis and prognosis? What is the dilemma? What ethical principles are in operation here? The leader's goal should be to preserve everyone's self-esteem while, at the same time, stopping the disruptive behavior. A private talk with the person is preferable to a confrontation at the meeting.

Managing diversity is an art to be acquired. For the enrichment of the group, diversity is a primary value of ethics committees. An effective leader needs to be able to encourage the creative flow of ideas from those with different experiences while maintaining positive results. Focusing on agreement puts things into perspective, for the areas of disagreement are usually small in comparison to the areas of agreement.

Having the trust and respect of members and being able to stimulate productivity from them are the marks of a skilled meeting leader. The better the leadership, the more efficiently and effectively a group works. The leader must take responsibility for guiding the process, but all committee members should be aware of their own responsibilities and should work to become productive members of the group and to effectively contribute to the group process.

Time Management. Not beginning and ending meetings on time can be costly. Starting late reinforces tardy behavior, and it devalues the substance of the committee's

work as well as the time of those who made the effort to arrive punctually. Time management is equally important at the end of the meeting. Permitting a meeting to drag on while members look at their watches and endeavor to escape at intervals is demoralizing for all. Meetings that consistently begin and end as scheduled reinforce the work of both the participants and the issues.

Related to this management of time is the allotting of time limits for the agenda items by those planning the work of the meeting. If the time allotments are insufficient, the time can be extended if the chairperson, with the committee's concurrence, judges it appropriate. In this way, the allocation of time is explicitly handled by both those planning the meeting and all members in attendance. An alternative is to place the topic on the agenda for the next meeting.

Distribution of Materials

Minutes, policies, patient information, and other such documents, as well as educational materials, all require that members have some time for review outside committee meetings. If necessary, changes in policies or other textual materials should be highlighted as to what is critical and useful and what is for information only.

Educational materials relevant to discussion require particular attention. Good use of them results from consistently taking time for discussion of articles which were sent by the leader, setting a time and keeping to the limit for discussion, as well as providing an outline to focus reading and guide discussion. An outline could include the following questions:

• What do you consider the three main points of the author?

• Were the opinions of the author persuasive?

• Can you identify other articles on this topic that have a different perspective?

• Would you recommend this article as helpful to someone interested in health care ethics? Why or why not?

It has been helpful in some committees to assign one or two members to lead the discussion of an article or ask for volunteers. Other committees ask the members who lead a discussion to choose the articles and formulate discussion questions.

Key Questions

In order to gauge the success of health care ethics committee meetings, a few simple general questions can be asked. Do members attend? Do they come on time? Are discussions lively? Are there moments of humor as well as moments of seriousness? Do people continue to talk about issues discussed in the meeting after it is over? Are people eager to belong to the committee? More specific questions may afford more definitive evaluation. For instance:

- What were the results of the consultation evaluations?

- Was the group a "patient advocate"?

- Did the ethics committee promote help and assistance to those who initiated consultation?

- Do people feel free to consult the ethics committee?

- Were educational endeavors successful?

- Were policies developed, reviewed, or revised?

- Were decisions effective and valued?

- Did the outcome produce customer satisfaction?

All health care ethics committees may benefit from greater attention to the conduct of their meetings. Each committee might develop a means for periodic evaluation of its meeting activity. The key is for each committee to give enough thought and imagination to its own expectations of meetings to tailor its own instrument of review and self-renewal.

Editorial Summation: This nuts-and-bolts chapter outlines the elements necessary for successful health care ethics committee meetings. When ethics committee meetings are run with professionalism, are organized, have a clear agenda and purpose, and are held to strict time limits, the committee and its work can become an integral part of the health care system. When these tasks not carried out well, the committee may seem to be adrift, morale suffers, and members come to think that their talents are not being utilized correctly. The two keys to successful meetings are (1) adequate preparation and (2) time management.

B. The Evaluation of Ethics Committees

Rev. Dennis A. Brodeur

When evaluating ethics committees in Catholic health care facilities, one can raise several questions: (1) What are the weaknesses and strengths of *existing* committees? (2) What are the weaknesses and strengths of the ethics committee *concept*? (3) What are the weaknesses and strengths of a Catholic ethics committee in a *pluralistic society in a time of health care reform*? These questions will be addressed in light of this author's experience.

Assumptions

To begin, let me state some assumptions. My first assumption is that ethics committees are not equally good. Some ethics committees work very well, and some ethics committees are not doing a very good job

for their institutions. If we want to do something positive for the future of ethics committees, we need to identify the problem areas.

A second assumption is that an ethics committee is not an isolated group. One problem is to try to understand in a systemic manner the way in which ethics committees are connected to a variety of other activities, some of which may be part of our substantive Catholic identity.

People and health care facilities are parts of communities and states. Community health status must be measured, and risk and responsibility assumed for the improvement of that health status in a new, reformed model of health care. Many committees also deal with a variety of state issues applicable to Medicaid or particular state laws. These include everything from the standards of evidence necessary to know that one has a valid living will or durable power of attorney to knowing how to override legally a parent's insistence on withholding lifesaving treatment for an ill child.

Many Catholic hospitals are parts of systems. System membership has an impact on the way things are addressed by committees. The impact may be from the system's overarching policy—a mandate to establish an ethics committee—or the requirement to develop a resuscitation policy, with the clinical details left to the hospital. Membership and ownership concerns are sometimes a vital part of policy. Regional networks will have an impact on local institutions regarding a variety of issues—employment issues, insurance issues, access issues, all of which can bring to the surface fundamental ethical concerns.

Some issues have notable regional and local (and diocesan) differences. An important issue for a hospital in Michigan, Washington state, Oregon, or California will be physician-assisted suicide, which is not so pressing an issue in Kansas, Oklahoma, or South Carolina.

Regulations are also a concern. Ethics committees will have to respond to the kinds of regulations that are promulgated by the joint commission, other outside monitors, or those suggested by payers. Ethical issues related to access, patient care, confidentiality, or other clinical concerns are then raised.

A third assumption is the purposeful identification of the mission and purpose of the committee. What is the mission of the committee? What are our expectations? Is it to deal only with clinical matters? Or are there other areas of concern, such as access to care, public policy, and organizational ethics? Does the agenda of the ethics committee reach beyond the walls of the health care facility? For example, are home health care agencies, home hospice programs, or durable medical equipment programs subject matter for ethics committee evaluation? A clearly articulated mission helps establish a meaningful agenda.

The education and qualifications of the personnel serving on ethics committees affect committee performance. My assumption is that what a committee needs, how it responds, and perhaps even how it assesses its strengths and weaknesses is dependent on both its composition and whether it is a board committee, a committee of the medical staff, or a committee of the administration. Evaluation questions follow from this identification. Who are appointed as members? Do the members represent the power structures of the institution? If the persons with real power are not represented on the committee, do the members feel free to make decisions and are they

then supported in their decisions and activities? Also, is the effectiveness of the committee meetings evident in follow through activities? This varies greatly.

Finally, the strength or weakness of an ethics committee is proportional to the rest of the institution's ethics commitments. If the ethics committee is the sole locus of systematic thinking on ethical matters, it probably is going to be weak. On the other hand, if the institution is strong in assessing ethical issues that arise in nonclinical areas, such as human resources and labor relations, in internal business matters, and in its relationship to the community, then the work of the committee in clinical ethical matters is likely to be stronger and taken more seriously. It is unlikely that ethical clinical matters will receive a great deal of attention if other ethical issues are not also systematically addressed.

Strengths

One strength of Roman Catholic ethics committees is Catholic anthropology. The anthropological considerations that underlie Roman Catholic theological thinking, and moral theology in particular, are outlined fairly clearly. This anthropology establishes a starting point for considerations concerning the nature of the human person and specifically the purpose of human life. These considerations are not necessarily shared by people who do not share a particular religious framework. Sometimes this makes conversation more difficult. Other philosophical or contemporary principle-based medical-ethical approaches (known as "principlism") do not always reflect the Catholic anthropological underpinnings and moral principles. This results in an approach that reduces bioethics to one set of principles. Principles like autonomy, for example, can then become the sole focus of ethical debate.

There are scriptural roots to the moral enterprise that are an attempt to understand how God interacts with humankind. Our moral analysis is not an application of a moral code fully revealed in Scripture. Rather, we struggle with the ethical concerns of modern medicine from a theological and anthropological backdrop that provides structure, nuance, and direction to our ethical concerns. Granted, there are parts of the moral system which are debated. But there *is* a moral system, and that is a strength in doing ethical reflection in a Catholic institution.

A second strength is that most of our Catholic institutions seem to have the service of trained moral theologians. Although not everywhere present, they add a dimension to the ethics committee's work. Where these theologians immerse themselves in the clinical and organizational realities of health care, they bring an added dimension to the discussion.

A third strength is an articulated sense of mission in Catholic health care facilities. We may not have complete agreement on what the mission of Catholic health care is today, but we have a general sense of mission as being "sent." We may question whether this or that aspect of hospital practice is Christian or is specifically Catholic. How do we articulate the healing ministry of Jesus Christ today? What do we mean by it? We can raise these questions, but the very fact that we raise them makes our mission very different from, for example, that of the VA system, where the mission of care is focused on a set of people who do not have care and rely on their veteran's status for services.

Basic to our mission, of course, is a fundamental commitment to the dignity of the patient as a person. We may not always be faithful to that principle, but there remains a fundamental awareness that the sacredness and dignity of the human person are not to be violated. We care for patients as ends in themselves and not merely as means to organizational goals. In the Catholic tradition we have a fundamental commitment to the human person from the moment of conception to the moment of natural death. We have a long tradition of moral concern which provides a priceless guide. For over four hundred years the Catholic Church has been at the forefront of discussing these issues.

Fourth, there are dedicated research groups, such as the Catholic Health Association of the United States (CHA), the National Catholic Bioethics Center (NCBC), and many diocesan groups, with dedicated people who are focused on identifying, clarifying, and solving health care issues. How do we best address old and new issues and what assistance might we have? Whom do we call to find suitable help? There is an already established sense that even if there is disagreement—and there is, from time to time—at least a common understanding of the basic values exists. There is also a commitment to a list of concerns, for patients and families as well as for staff, through pastoral care, through social services, and through general education centers in our institutions. Such educational commitments are supportive of the activities that go beyond the ethics committee meeting.

On this set of strengths we should build. Members of ethics committees need to have some understanding and appreciation of these strengths if they are going to be effective agents in the development and strengthening the Catholic identity of our health care institutions.

Weaknesses

A first potential weakness is a loss of focus on the ethics committee's true agenda. Despite our clear moral tradition, our developed anthropology, and our theological convictions, ethics committees often get embroiled in heated discussions about the application of principles, moral methods, and the tension between religious and secular approaches to problems. The methods used to assess issues and do ethical evaluations are not easily made into agenda items for an ethics committee meeting. Instead, they should be the substance of the personal education of ethics committee members.

These methodological discussions will continue as part of a self-education process. Some issues, such as the meaning and purpose of sexuality, are the subjects of substantive debate. For example, it is asked how one should properly understand Catholic moral teaching on the procreative and unitive dimensions of the conjugal act in relation to other assessments of sexuality in our culture. In particular, what are the implications of the differences between Catholic teaching and broader cultural views on human sexuality in the matter of contraception and surgical sterilization?

Second, weaknesses sometimes arise in areas of moral authority. The committee may be too dependent on the moral authority of a single member, particularly the bishop's delegate, a theologian, a professional ethicist, or a physician. Similarly, a sister or a priest or someone in pastoral care may, because of their position, be considered an ethics expert. Often he or she is not, for these ,e,bers do not always have the necessary specialized training to act in this role. Some members also may have the naive belief that the magisterium has answers for every question which can be raised.

A third notable weakness is an overemphasis on the obstetric/gynecologic and death-and-dying questions. Obstetrical and death-and-dying questions are fundamental concerns in our tradition and in our hospitals. I was once asked to review ethics committee minutes of a hospital for a bishop, and I requested ethics committee minutes for the previous five years so that I could get a sense of what the ethics committee had done. I was somewhat dismayed. What arose during that period were tertiary care obstetrical issues, sterilization issues, contraception issues, death-and-dying issues, and nothing else. These are a staple of Catholic hospital ethics committees, but they are not all the issues. Those who establish an ethics committee agenda should be alert to additional ethical matters which do arise and require careful analysis and discussion.

Another weakness, alluded to above, is that committee members do not always have a sufficient education about moral systems or about the application of moral principles. How does one apply the principle of double effect to a particular case? When does it work? When does it not? What about the principle of totality, or the principle of cooperation, or other traditional principles are used in ethical analysis? The need is not for uninformed belief, but for cognitive appreciation of the intellectual dimension and appropriate application of Catholic moral and theological principles.

Another difficulty is that many of our Catholic institutions are connected solely to a network of other Catholic institutions. Discussions centered on Catholic values and principles can be very difficult to understand in larger, pluralistic settings. Catholic institutions will benefit from dialogue and interactions with non-Catholics. The challenge is to find common points of understanding as we move forward in dialogue. This problem is clearly seen as ethics committees engage ethical discussion in health care delivery settings such as hospitals that are jointly owned or managed by non-Catholic partners and work with other community groups.

There is also confusion about the consultative role of ethics committees. When an ethics committee goes into the consultative process, is it really consulting? Is the committee merely giving nice opinions? Is it hand-holding? Is it comforting? When the ethics committee makes a recommendation, is it mandatory? Is it optional? Is the consultation intellectually stimulating? Ambiguity about the role of consultation leaves people confused, and if this occurs often, they become uninterested in this service.

Finally, it is not clear that ethics committees are oriented to the future. The already changing world of health care will change even more rapidly tomorrow. Ethics committee agendas, from around the country, do not have many items that anticipate future concerns. For example, what are the ethical issues for an integrated network with capitation, or managed care, and other possible finance mechanisms? It is not clear that the ethics committees of today appreciate what it means to deal with a "capitated life," or what it means to be a hospital that will take a "per diem." "Risk" is a huge financial issue and, by implication, a huge ethical issue. How do we address such issues or at least prepare for those issues before they occur?

Outcome Measures

The final issue is the lack of quality outcome indicators for ethics committees. The absence of outcome indicators is the biggest weakness. There is very little in the literature which offers the outcome measures expected for successful ethics committees. What might these be? One measure might be clarity of terms and meanings. For example, a good outcome should be that when a meeting occurs and terms like "brain death" are used in a medically and legally correct manner. When committee members talk about an issue of informed consent, they should all have a sense of what that presupposes: knowledge of what is wrong with the patient; knowledge about options, patient alternatives, and the risks and consequences of proposed procedures; and the use of clear language. There should also be an expectation of clarity concerning any moral principles used. Thus, if the principle of totality is referenced, it can be assumed that the committee members have a basic sense of what this principle means. Without a commonly understood language, discussion is futile. This is an outcome measure internal to the committee.

External outcome measures are different. These are measures of institutional ethics goals which the ethics committee can set for the institution. There ought to be measures that show that an institution has become increasingly sensitive to ethical issues. Do ethical issues regularly surface at department meetings, service-area meetings, and meetings about patient care? Has the ethics committee developed mechanisms and avenues by which its agendas are built from clinical practice? Or is it only an individual (e.g., the chairperson or the ethics expert) who decides the particular issues that the ethics committee needs to address? The use of outcome measures can impose a difficult discipline on those in the humanities—theology, sociology, and philosophy. However, ethics committees should state the specific outcomes they expect to occur in the institution, which could include outcomes regarding the organization's stewardship responsibilities and the allocation of resources. The institutional use of ethics committees is a relatively young movement, but it is time to identify solid external outcome measures so that ethics committees may be fully utilized.

Finally, there are questions that we can raise about the "blueprint" of possibilities for ethics committees in the future. Are there ways to share information and processes that allow replication of best practices across institutions? Is there a possibility for cross-institutional learning, involving multiple Catholic institutions, as well as networks of shared information? Is there any way to cross-educate ourselves, to benchmark successful programmatic activities, and to transmit what is learned throughout the delivery system? This will require a sharing of measures, open communication, a sharing of failures and successes, and a willingness to change.

✠

Editorial Summation: The strengths of an ethics committee in a Catholic health care facility are several: (1) The Church has an established anthropology which is used as one source for ethical considerations concerning patients. (2) The Catholic hospital usually has available the services of trained moral theologians or ethicists. (3) The sense of mission has been well articulated by the Church and the Catholic health care facilities which serve it. (4) There are a variety of ethics research groups within the Church available for consultation, such as the Catholic Health Association, in St. Louis, Missouri, and The National Catholic Bioethics Center, in Philadelphia, Pennsylvania. The weaknesses are also evident: (1) There are conflicting moral approaches, which can divide the attention and energy of the ethics committee. (2) There is often too great a dependency of the committee on the moral authority of one person. (3) A tendency exists to focus on issues in only two areas, namely, ostetrics/gynecology and death and dying. (4) Catholic hospitals are often tied in with non-Catholic institutions which have different values. (5) Insufficient use has been made of modern communication systems. (6) There are no adequate outcome indicators for ethics committees. It would be helpful for Catholic health care delivery facilities to share information about the experiences of their ethics committees. This would facilitate the development of stronger and more effective ethics committees, resulting in an overall improvement in health care delivery.

C. Diocesan Health Care Ethics Committees

Rev. Thomas Knoblach

The relationship between a diocese and the health care organizations serving in that diocese is one of collaboration in the healing mission of Christ. However, the mechanics of that relationship cannot be captured in a single model. Since dioceses can be involved in Catholic health care in a diversity of ways—some immediate, others more peripheral—no universal template for diocesan health care committees exists.

Indeed, not every diocese has such a structure. At times, when the diocese itself is not directly involved in providing health care services, an individual is designated, more or less formally, as a liaison for the bishop with health care providers. Often this person may have multiple roles—sometimes as part of a social concerns office, as vicar general or chancellor, or in another existing role. In other situations, a diocese may be directly involved in the provision of health care through hospitals, long-term care facilities, clinics, and other entities. In such a case, the role of a diocesan health care committee will obviously be far more extensive. In any case, whatever form it takes, the two key points of reference are the direction given by the bishop for this committee, and the *Ethical and Religious Directives for Catholic Health Care Services.*[1]

Given this range of possible structures, this chapter will be somewhat general in discussing the purpose, role, functions, and operation of a diocesan health care committee. Yet even such a necessarily rough sketch may help dioceses and health care organizations reflect on and be more intentional about their own particular relationships, and may help them brainstorm ways to enhance their mutual efforts to embody the healing mission of Jesus for those in need.

The Diocesan Bishop and Health Care Organizations

Over time, in response to the Gospel, the healing mission of Christ has developed concrete structures and institutions to make accessible and effective this care for the sick and vulnerable in the name of Jesus. Hospitals, nursing homes, clinics, and other organizations embody the love of God that ministers to the whole person, body and soul. Much of the history of Catholic health care in the United States is grounded in the courageous and generous witness of religious communities of women and men who responded to the unmet needs of the people in the communities they served. Sometimes this outreach even predated the establishment of dioceses.

The diocese is, at the same time, central to the structured organization of the universal Church. The diocese is a specific portion of God's people (usually in a specific geographical territory) in which the mystery of the Church is truly present and active. For that reason, the general introduction to the *Ethical and Religious Directives for Catholic Health Care Services* describes the relationship of the local church to Catholic health care through the role of the diocesan bishop as pastor, teacher, and priest. It states,

> As the center of unity in the diocese and coordinator of ministries in the local church, the diocesan bishop fosters the mission of Catholic health care in a way that promotes collaboration among health care leaders, providers, medical professionals, theologians, and other specialists. As pastor, the diocesan bishop is in a unique position to encourage the faithful to greater responsibility in the healing ministry of the Church. As teacher, the diocesan bishop ensures the moral and religious identity of the health care ministry in whatever setting it is carried out in the diocese. As priest, the diocesan bishop oversees the sacramental care of the sick. These responsibilities will require that Catholic health care providers and the diocesan bishop engage in ongoing communication on ethical and pastoral matters that require his attention.

This broad description of the role of the bishop is made more specific in a handful of directives. Directive 8 speaks of the ecclesial nature of Catholic health care institutions and the need to observe the relevant requirements of canon law. Directives 21 and 22 relate to appointments of Catholic and non-Catholic clergy to pastoral care staffs. Directive 37 calls for each diocese to have "appropriate standards for medical ethical consultation" so that such consultation, whether through an ethics committee or some other mechanism, is informed by Catholic moral teaching and particularly the ERDs.

Expanding on directive 8, part 6 of the ERDs describes in more detail the complexities of partnerships between Catholic and non-Catholic providers. Consultation with the diocesan bishop (directly or through his delegate) is counseled when decisions may have a significant impact on the identity or mission of Catholic health care services (directives 67 and 68). Any such partnerships with this potential impact on Catholic identity must have the approval of the diocesan bishop if they are subject to his governance, or his nihil obstat for partnerships sponsored by religious institutes of pontifical right (directive 68). The responsibility for assessing and addressing the potential for scandal in such partnerships rests ultimately with the diocesan bishop (directive 71).

However, these specific provisions of the *ERDs* do not exhaust—and ought not overshadow—the relationship between the local church and the health care organizations serving in the diocese. The diocese does not stand primarily in a position of oversight and monitoring, but aims to coordinate the larger collaboration in the mission of the Church to live out the Gospel. Thus, directive 3 is a significant point of reference for this shared responsibility:

> In accord with its mission, Catholic health care should distinguish itself by service to and advocacy for those people whose social condition puts them at the margins of our society and makes them particularly vulnerable to discrimination: the poor; the uninsured and the underinsured; children and the unborn; single parents; the elderly; those with incurable diseases and chemical dependencies; racial minorities; immigrants and refugees. In particular, the person with mental or physical disabilities, regardless of the cause or severity, must be treated as a unique person of incomparable worth, with the same right to life and to adequate health care as all other persons.

This directive outlines both the distinctive actions and the underlying attitudes that are to mark all aspects of the Church's ministry in the world, and the values that inform the joint effort by bishops and health care organizations who both seek to serve the mission of the Gospel.

Role and Membership

Given the range and scope of his responsibilities, the bishop cannot personally attend to every aspect of the mission of the local church. Yet he needs to be kept informed and effectively involved when appropriate or necessary. The role of a diocesan health care committee, then—whatever form it takes in a particular diocese—is to assist the bishop in shaping the response to the Gospel vision sketched in directive 3 and made more explicit throughout the *ERDs*, in collaboration with health care organizations serving in that territory.

Ideally, a diocesan health care committee is interdisciplinary, representing the key areas of concern and expertise in providing Catholic health care. It is best if members appointed by the bishop include persons with knowledge of Catholic moral theology and the *ERDs*, as well as those versed in canon and civil law; administrators of Catholic health care organizations working in the diocese or their representatives; and representative physicians, nurses, social workers, members of spiritual care departments, and perhaps community members.

At the same time, the group must not become so large that it cannot function effectively or meet regularly; perhaps eight to ten persons is a workable size. While this will vary with the particular group, some rotation of members every few years is often helpful to enhance the group's objectivity and bring fresh perspectives.

The bishop or his designated health care coordinator chairs the group, which works collaboratively to maintain good lines of communication and address issues related to Catholic identity and mission in whatever ways the bishop directs. Meetings need to have a clear purpose and agenda, with a reporting relationship to the bishop if he is not present. Outlining these details in written form in a mission statement and a set of procedures is helpful to ensure continuity and clarity in purpose and function.

Unless the committee is established to have legitimate oversight responsibilities for health care providers directly under diocesan control (hospitals, clinics, long-term care facilities, etc.), it generally has only a consultative voice and functions as a resource for the bishop to facilitate mutual awareness, education, and coordination of this aspect of the larger mission of the Church in the diocese.

Whatever form the committee takes, the *Ethical and Religious Directives* and the broader Catholic moral vision that informs them are the central and common point of reference for all parties. Understanding of and commitment to the *ERDs* is at the heart of the role, function, and operation of any diocesan health care committee.

Qualities Required

Effective interaction between the local Church and health care organizations has several key qualities. Among them are a genuine spirit of respectful collaboration, a shared commitment to the principle of subsidiarity and to the vision and norms outlined in the *ERDs*, open lines of communication, and mutual trust.

Collaboration

Because the Gospel mandate to care for the sick is a responsibility of the whole Church, the provision of Catholic health care must be a shared and collaborative effort. The need for collaboration is, of course, generally evident in health care itself. Good working relationships among physicians, nurses, administrators, and other health care professionals are essential to effective care for patients and families.

For Catholic health care, this "internal" collaboration extends also to the relationship with the local Church, so that there is a sense of mutual effort toward a common goal. Among all those involved—the bishop, health care administrators and boards, professional providers and volunteers, and community leaders—each has a particular role in caring for the health of the community. Awareness of these various roles and respect for the good faith, diligent work, and sincerity of those who work at all levels create a healthy climate.

At the same time, true collaboration also implies the commitment to identify and resolve conflicts in a constructive way for the sake of the larger mission. Without this ability, unhealthy trends develop: "turfdom," wasteful parallel efforts, mistrust, divisiveness, resentments, and avoidance of others to the detriment of those who are to be served. The interdisciplinary nature of a diocesan health care committee can both model and at times help toward resolution of conflict through respectful and honest dialogue.

Subsidiarity

The principle of subsidiarity fosters good order by normally reserving authority and decision making to the most immediate level. Those who are involved at that immediate level are presumed to have the best knowledge of the particularities of persons, situations, policies, and procedures in play, and are capable of making prudential judgments in accord with the mission and goals of the organization. Higher levels of authority and oversight are engaged only when there is some conflict or obstacle that cannot be effectively resolved at the more immediate level.

Beyond the question of authority, subsidiarity fosters respect and trust for those who are engaged in the day-to-day work of providing health care. Relative to diocesan health care committees, subsidiarity is important so that the committee does not become distracted with the temptation to micromanage, second-guess, or interfere with the operation of organizations. Rather, its purpose is to coordinate, encourage, and provide a resource to keep in focus the broader overall mission and values of Catholic health care that all Catholic organizations hold in common, regardless of the particularities of each institution.

Commitment to the
Ethical and Religious Directives

The *ERDs* provide a snapshot of the broader Catholic moral tradition as applied to specific (and evolving) questions in the ethical provision of health care. Those who serve on a diocesan health care committee need familiarity with both the *ERDs* themselves and with this larger moral tradition that informs their interpretation in accord with the mind of the Church. Regular study of the *ERDs*, perhaps in sections, and case studies discussed in light of the *ERDs* can help educate and update members in this area.

One hospital with which I consult has taken the *ERDs*, one by one, and laid out how each directive is adhered to in the hospital: what departments and initiatives meet that directive, what policies govern its implementation, and who is ultimately responsible for its fulfillment. The list is reviewed annually and updated as needed. While this is a considerable undertaking, it is a concrete demonstration of institutional commitment to the *ERDs* and a resource for board, committees, staff, and the public.

In addition to this self-education regarding the *ERDs*, the committee must also strive to stay abreast of the larger context of the field of health care. Study and presentations on the various social, political, scientific, and economic trends that affect health care in general, and challenge the mission of Catholic health care in particular, are essential.

Communication and Trust

Communication and relationships of respect and trust are essential to the effective work of a diocesan health care committee. Developing these relationships takes time and regular contact, both formally through scheduled meetings and informally through casual contacts and genuine interest in how each organization is contributing to the mission.

Understanding the dedication, commitment, experience, and expertise that each brings to the committee, and to the leadership of health care organizations at work in the diocese, requires attention to communication. Reporting on events and initiatives, sharing satisfactions and challenges in realizing the mission, and seeking consultation can only enhance the function of the committee. It will also make the more difficult moments that may arise more manageable through collaborative effort.

It is to be expected that some of the questions a committee will address will be controversial, generating strong feelings and touching on staunchly held opinions. This is often true, not only in society as a whole, but also among committed Catholics. Skills of respectful dialogue, consensus, appropriate confidentiality, collaboration, and appreciation of the unique contributions of Catholic health care to the larger society will make for an effective and supportive committee, always guided by the authentic moral tradition and mission of the Church.

Some Common Concerns

Because of the variety of forms this committee might take, as well as the rapidly changing field of health care and the new challenges to organizational and biomedical ethics such change creates, it is not possible even to sketch all the issues that might come before a diocesan health care committee. However, by way of illustration, several common concerns are predictable: (1) the formation of new partnerships and collaborative initiatives with both Catholic and non-Catholic providers; (2) issues in reproductive health, particularly sterilization, contraception, abortion, and related issues; (3) issues in end-of-life care, particularly withholding and withdrawing of life-sustaining treatments, pain management, palliative care, and advance directives; (4) organizational ethics issues—expansion and collaborative efforts in a given service area, personnel and specialty area shortages, just compensation, "mission vs. margin" concerns; (5) collaboration in community wellness education and initiatives; and (6) responses to legislative initiatives and regulatory requirements as they affect Catholic health care.

Depending on its membership, expertise, and the direction of the bishop, the committee may address these concerns in various ways. It may do research and make recommendations to the bishop. It may provide education and consultation on relevant issues for Catholic providers and the general public. It may draft or review diocesan policies regarding Catholic health care when appropriate.

Support, Affirm, Guide, and Challenge

The role of a diocesan health care committee is not to oversee and scrutinize Catholic health care providers in the diocese, but to support, affirm, guide, and when necessary challenge them to serve the common good as a ministry of the Church. In collaboration with other works of the local Church under the direction of the bishop, such a committee—whatever form it is given by the local bishop—seeks to ensure that the work of all parties conforms to the *Ethical and Religious Directives* and the larger Catholic moral tradition they enshrine, and functions as a true ministry of the Church to carry out the healing mission of Jesus in the world for the sake of the Gospel.

Notes

[1] U.S. Conference of Catholic Bishops, *Ethical and Religious Directives for Catholic Health Care Services*, 4th ed. (Washington D.C.: USCCB, 2001).

✠

Editorial Summation: Not every diocese has a diocesan health care ethics committee, nor is there one model for all. Such committees seek to advance the love of God that ministers to the whole person, body and soul, through the various organizations that comprise the Catholic health care mission. The diocese is central to the structural organization of the universal Church, and the *Ethical and Religious Directives for Catholic Health Care Services* describe the general role of the bishop in the delivery of this Christian care. The diocese does not stand primarily in a position of oversight and monitoring, but aims to coordinate the larger collaboration that marks the mission of the Church to live out the Gospel in its concern for others. While the bishop cannot attend to every aspect of the mission of the local church, he needs to be kept informed and effectively involved when appropriate or necessary. Ideally, a diocesan health care committee will be interdisciplinary, representing the key areas of concern and expertise in providing Catholic health care. Some of the qualities necessary for membership are the ability to collaborate, an appreciation for the principle of subsidiarity, a commitment to the *ERDs*, and a willingness to communicate and trust.

D. The Ethics Committee in Long-Term Care Facilities

Rev. James A. O'Donohoe

Historical Development of the Long-Term Care Facility

A long-term care facility can be generally described as an institution which provides assistance for people who are not able to take proper care of their own health at home and no longer require or cannot afford formal hospitalization.[1]

In health care circles, long-term care facilities have become practically synonymous with what have been called "nursing homes." There are many different types: (1) residential care homes in which residents are able to provide most of their own care; (2) nursing facilities in which immediate care is provided; (3) skilled nursing facilities in which skilled care is provided by licensed health-care professionals; (4) subacute care facilities in which residents require complex care but are medically stable; and (5) retirement communities in which care ranges from independent living to total dependence.[2]

The origins of present-day long-term care facilities can probably be found in the almshouses provided for the handicapped, indigent, and homeless in earlier times. In the 1930s, legislation for the creation of a social security system contributed toward the growth of public care for the sick and elderly. Most nursing-home-type facilities as we know them today date from that period. In 1965,

Titles XVIII and XIX of the Social Security Act (Medicare and Medicaid) contributed to the growth of government-subsidized homes for the sick, the elderly, and the indigent. The nursing home industry was considerably stimulated and, despite several periods of difficulty, continues to this day. Inasmuch as these services help large sections of the population, they are strictly governed by civil legislation and must provide frequent reports on the care they offer.

Ethical Issues in the Long-Term Care Facility

One area for which reports are requested is the "ethical performance" of these facilities. The law addresses such matters and for good reason, as the points made below should demonstrate.

The word *ethics* is frequently used in contemporary society but there is a good deal of misunderstanding about its meaning. Put simply, the fundamental purpose of ethics is the determination of what constitutes "the good which humanizes," that which contributes to human flourishing. Philosophical ethics attempts to determine this through the use of human reason, while theological ethics tries to discover it through reason enlightened by a religious faith. The ultimate good for the former is justice, that is, giving to the other what is due; the ultimate good for the latter is "love which brings about justice." As a discipline, ethics can be best defined as "an attempt to articulate the behavioral implications of human flourishing." Since the civil law is concerned with the ethical practices of the institutions which the government aids economically, long-term care facilities are required to report in detail on how they contribute to the human growth of their residents as well as how they handle situations which might detract from the residents' overall good both physically and spiritually.

It can well be imagined that those who are in charge of such facilities are not infrequently faced with a good number of ethical dilemmas occasioned by the day-to-day care for their residents. An example is the situation in which a decision has to be made about continuing a treatment that appears to be simply prolonging a patient's dying process and that offers no reasonable hope of benefit to the patient.

It is for that reason that the U.S. Conference of Catholic Bishops suggests the following in the *Ethical and Religious Directives for Catholic Health Care Services*: "An ethics committee or some alternate form of ethical consultation should be available to assist by advising on particular ethical situations, by offering educational opportunities, and by reviewing and recommending policies."[3]

The number of ethical dilemmas which can arise in a long-term care facility over a period of time can be large. These are some of the most common:

First are instances which can affect the well-being of an individual resident: (1) personal assault (i.e., threatening bodily harm to force a resident to do something against his or her will); (2) battery (i.e., hitting or even touching a resident's body without a sufficient reason; (3) invasions of privacy (i.e., improperly exposing a resident's body or going through his or her personal belongings); (4) failure to respect confidentiality (i.e., discussing the case of a resident with others who are not entitled to such information); and (5) staff negligence in giving a resident care.

In addition to all the situations mentioned above, one might also cite incidents which do violence to a proper understanding and interpretation of the resident's advance directive; situations in which do-not-resuscitate orders are not properly observed; occasions in which there has been little attention given to the determination of proper and adequate pain medication.

Of special help in determining other ethical issues is the so-called residents' bill of rights, which lists most of these issues and also calls attention to certain other ethical problems which can easily be forgotten: a resident's

rights to civil and religious liberties, to file complaints without fear, to inspect his or her records, to be free from verbal abuse, to refuse treatment which is offered, to be informed of his or her medical condition, and to take part in the planning of treatment.[4]

Primary Functions of the Long-Term Care Ethics Committee

In determining the proper functioning of an ethics committee, one must not give the impression that this group must be consulted every time situations similar to those described above occur. Many incidents can be simply and adequately handled by the customary triad of patient, physician, and family. Other issues may be sufficiently taken care of by appropriate consultation with the administration and the staff. However, when an ethical issue has serious implications for the good of a resident or even of the facility, the services of the ethics committee should be sought through the proper channels.

At this point, it is important to point out that it is not the function of the ethics committee to make decisions. Decisions are ultimately and ideally made by the resident or the resident's proxy and, if the resident is no longer competent, the primary physician and the family. The role of the ethics committee must always be advisory only.

Even though the committee is not a decision-making body, it can and does serve the health-care facility in many other capacities: to educate the staff and the administration on the complexity and ambiguity of many contemporary health-care dilemmas; to recognize the need for open and honest dialogue among those concerned in the welfare of the patient; to be conscious of the fact that many things which are legal are not, in fact, moral; to understand that ethical responsibility does not lie merely in a simplistic response to the rules of a static code but in a deep penetration of the moral values which the law intends to communicate and defend.

It must be understood that the formation of an ethics committee in any health care institution can be either auspicious or inauspicious. Where it is poorly prepared for and inadequately formed, it can become a source of increased tension, confusion, and conflict. However, where it has been carefully planned, is open to genuine dialogue and the pursuit of the truth, and enjoys the support—as well as the encouragement—of the administration, it can have a tremendously renewing and invigorating effect on the individual members of the staff, the residents, and their families.

A few concluding remarks may be in order. First, it is important that the members of the committee establish definite goals and make the committee's purposes clear to all concerned. Again, before the committee goes into full operation, it should devote several meetings to the education of its own members. (A working familiarity with the ERDs is basic to such an endeavor.) Finally, the members of the committee must always remember that ethics is much broader than medical and legal issues, and they must always remain conscious of the need to be seen as a group that is not *sui iuris* in the facility but is always responsible to and at the service of the institution's board of governance.

Notes

[1] Peggy A. Grubbs and Barbara A. Blasband, *The Long-Term Care Nursing Assistant*, 2nd ed. (Upper Saddle River, NJ: Prentice Hall Health, 2000).

[2] Donna D. Ignatavicius, *Introduction to Long Term Care Nursing: Principles and Practice* (Philadelphia: F. A. Davis, 1998).

[3] *Ethical and Religious Directives for Catholic Health Care Services,* 4th ed. (Washington D.C.: USCCB, 2001), n. 37.

[4] Grubbs and Blasband, *Long-Term Care Nursing Assistant*, 25.

Editorial Summation: Any long-term care facility which provides nursing care should have an ethics committee. There certainly are enough ethical dilemmas and questions in the long-term care facility to warrant one. The facility routinely faces issues of informed consent, confidentiality, privacy, patient abuse, advance directives, DNR orders, and a variety of end-of-life ethical issues. Ethics is best understood as an inquiry into what constitutes human flourishing. Ethics committees are not called upon to resolve all moral issues, but should be ancillary to the triad of patient, physician, and family. These parties, ideally, should be the decision-makers. The committee does need to emphasize the importance of the moral dimension in all medical decision-making at the facility and should devote a significant amount of time to education, both of its own members and of the staff at large. Moral decision-making is not simply a matter of applying rules to given cases, but is directed toward understanding the deeper moral import of the law that is embodied in those directives. The committee needs to bear in mind at all times that it is in service to the institution as a whole.

PART III

BEGINNING-OF-LIFE ISSUES

CHAPTER 6

The Fetus and Human Embryo

A. Abortion

Rev. Albert S. Moraczewski, O.P.

Abortion means "the directly intended termination of a pregnancy before viability or the directly intended destruction of a viable fetus ... which, in its moral context, includes [also] the interval between conception and implantation of the embryo."[1] In the moral order, an abortion can never be justified. There exists no condition which objectively can justify an abortion as defined above.

The basic reason for the Church's consistent and vigorous opposition to abortion is that it is the unjust killing of a human person. Historically, the Church has been vigorous in defending the dignity of the human individual from the beginning of life in the womb of the mother. The Church has also been cautious as to precisely when human personhood begins, because there has not been a consensus among scientists and theologians as to the moment when infusion of a spiritual soul is accomplished. Even if this is delayed, the human being who has been conceived is already on its way to being a human person, and one should not risk killing a human person. The Church teaches in the *Declaration on Procured Abortion*,

> This declaration expressly leaves aside the question of the moment when the spiritual soul is infused. There is not a unanimous tradition on this point, and authors are as yet in disagreement. For some it dates from the first instant; for others it could not at least precede nidation [implantation]. It is not within the competence of science to decide between these views because the existence of an immortal soul is not a question in its field. It is a philosophical problem from which our moral affirmation remains independent for two reasons: 1) supposing a belated animation, there is still nothing less than a *human* life, preparing for and calling for a soul in which the nature received from

parents is completed; 2) on the other hand, it suffices that this presence of the soul be probable (and one can never prove the contrary) in order that the taking of life involve accepting the risk of killing a man, not only waiting for, but already in possession of his soul.[2]

This text should be considered in the light of another document from the Congregation for the Doctrine of the Faith written thirteen years later, *Donum vitae* (Instruction on Respect for Human Life in Its Origin and on the Dignity of Procreation):

> Certainly no experimental datum can be in itself sufficient to bring us to the recognition of a spiritual soul; nevertheless, the conclusions of science regarding the human embryo provide a valuable indication for discerning by the use of reason a personal presence at the moment of this first appearance of a human life: how could a human individual not be a human person? ... The human being is to be respected and treated as a person from the moment of conception; and therefore from that same moment his rights as a person must be recognized, among which in the first place is the inviolable right of every innocent human being to life.[3]

The Church's prohibition against abortion was most emphatically stated by Pope John Paul II in his encyclical *Evangelium vitae* (The Gospel of Life):

> Therefore, by the authority which Christ conferred upon Peter and his successors, in communion with the bishops ... *I declare that direct abortion, that is, abortion willed as an end or as a means, always constitutes a grave moral disorder*, since it is the deliberate killing of an innocent human being. This

doctrine is based upon the natural law and upon the written Word of God, is transmitted by the Church's Tradition, and taught by the ordinary and universal magisterium.[4]

Modern biological data regarding the earliest stages of human embryological development, properly interpreted, support the position that there is present a being who is the proper subject of moral rights, namely, a human person, from the moment of conception. This moment is the completion of fertilization when the zygote is formed, that is, the new human organism.[5]

While the Bible does not supply proof-texts which specifically treat dilemmas related to embryological questions, it does provide a profound teaching on the origin of every human person. Throughout the Old Testament there is a growing emphasis on the I–Thou relationship established by the Creator with each of his human creatures from the outset of his or her existence. At the same time a similar relationship is constituted among all members of the human community. In the New Testament, the incarnation of the Divine Son in Jesus Christ provides the archetype by which Christians understand their own personal relationship with the Father. This is a relationship celebrated in baptism, and initiated in grace by the divine call which brought them into existence as human beings.

Since the first century the Church has affirmed the moral evil of every procured abortion. In the patristic period, the time of the Church Fathers from the late first century to the middle of the eighth century, abortion was generally rejected as a form of infanticide. Medieval theologians, occupied with the classification of sins and influenced by ancient Greek philosophy and biology, took the view that abortion was not technically homicide, although it was a grave sin against nature even when it took place during the earliest period of fetal life. In the Renaissance and Reformation periods, moral theologians, with the tolerance of Church authorities, permitted some forms of therapeutic abortion. However, with the rise of modern embryology and a greater concern for consistency in Church discipline, the Holy See took a strict anti-abortion position, reaffirmed by Vatican II.[6] As the *Catechism of the Catholic Church* likewise makes clear, direct abortion—that is, abortion willed either as an end or as a means—is gravely contrary to the moral law (nn. 2270 and 2271).

Human life must be respected and protected absolutely from the moment of conception. From the first moment of existence, a human being must be recognized as having the rights of a person—among which is the inviolable right of every innocent human being to life. This means that there can be no situation, no combination of circumstances, which would morally permit a *direct* abortion. It can be granted that there may arise some rare situation where it would seem that the life of both mother and child are at stake. Certainly one may not take the life of the child to save the mother, nor can the life of the mother be directly taken to save the child. Two examples may help to clarify the problem and the correct application of the principles.

Case 1: *A woman with a heart condition unintentionally becomes pregnant. Her physician tells her that to attempt to carry the child to term will increasingly and seriously threaten her life and that of her child. Better, the doctor tells her, to abort the child promptly. She is reluctant to do so and consults a pro-life obstetrician who advises her that with careful management and the use of modern medical knowledge and technology it is possible to bring the child beyond the point of viability, so that if the child must be delivered early he or she will have a good chance of survival.* In any event, even in the worst-case scenario, it is not morally acceptable directly to abort the child. One may not intend or use any chemical or physical means of directly bringing about the expulsion of a living human fetus before it is able to survive with or without technological life support, for any reason whatever.

Case 2: *A pregnant woman is diagnosed with uterine cancer. Her physician advises her that she needs to have surgery promptly and have the cancer removed which also would entail removal of her uterus. Since the surgery is to take place before the child in her womb reaches viability, the death of the child is inevitable. Is this morally permissible?* Yes, because there are significant medical and moral differences between this case and Case 1. In this second case, the surgery itself is directed toward removing the cancer. Moreover, the surgeon (and the patient) directly intend and act to remove the cancer, even though the process also requires the removal of the uterus. Although the inevitable death of the child in the womb is foreseen, it is not intended. The will of the surgeon is directed to the removal of the cancer in this case, while in the first the direct and immediate intention of the surgeon is to destroy the child, even if he also further intends to preserve the life of the mother.

In sum, one may never directly take the life of an unborn child even if one does so in order to preserve the health and life of the mother (Case 1). One may not use an evil means to achieve a good end.[7] However, one may undertake a procedure whose immediate effect is to remove some lethal pathology, even if in so doing the death of the unborn child is foreseen but not intended (Case 2).

While there is no doubt with regard to the Church's absolute prohibition of direct abortion, there can be, and indeed there are, situations where it is not at all clear whether direct abortion is involved. In such cases, wide consultation among physicians, ethicists, and hospital personnel will be necessary in order to ensure a correct course of action.

Abortifacients

Abortifacients are substances, chemical or otherwise, whose actions include the prevention of implantation by a fertilized oocyte, that is, an embryo. Since, the human embryo is already a human being (i.e., a human person), as already noted, such an abortifacient action is morally equivalent to abortion. The use of a chemical substance that includes effects such as interfering with tubal transport or modifying the state of the endometrium (the lining of the uterus) so that it is not able to receive the developing embryo for normal implantation is equivalent, morally, to abortion. The deliberate use of such substances is a grave moral evil. No desired objective or intention, no matter how noteworthy and noble, can morally justify the knowing and deliberate use of abortifacients.[8]

The French company Roussel Uclaf manufactures and markets the most widely known abortifacient, RU-486 (mifepristone). This drug is also increasingly used in smaller doses for "emergency contraception." It consists of a synthetic steroid compound that blocks progesterone, a hormone needed to continue a pregnancy. The rate of success when it is used alone is around 60 percent, so a second drug, a prostaglandin, is given forty-eight hours later to increase effectiveness. The drug can produce significant complications for women, including death. Since mifepristone received FDA approval in 2000, eight women in the United States, two women in the United Kingdom, one woman in Sweden, and one in Canada have died following its use. These deaths should be added to those of the unknown number of unborn children who have been aborted using this method.

Although the concept of an abortifacient is clear, it is not easy to determine whether a particular chemical agent, such as an oral contraceptive, includes an abortifacient effect among the several effects that may be associated with it. An agent may well act as a contraceptive in the strict and correct sense of the word; that is, it prevents ovulation. But these substances usually have multiple effects that differ depending on the specific combination of estrogen and progestin as well as the dosage level of each. The scientific and medical literature on particular agents, such as Ovral (norgestrel and ethinyl estradiol) and Plan B (levonorgestrel), is not very helpful for determining the mode of action of these substances. One possible reason for this situation is that the secular medical interest in this area is the prevention of pregnancy (understood as established at the time of implantation), not simply of conception. As a consequence, one finds in some of the medical literature that the medically traditional definition of conception is now applied to the time after implantation. From that perspective, the prevention of implantation would be called a contraceptive rather than abortifacient effect. Yet some reports bring out the multiple effects that an anovulant may have—namely, preventing ovulation, modifying the viscosity of the cervical mucus, modifying tubal motility, and rendering the uterine lining hostile to implantation—and consider all these simply as contraceptive actions.[9]

Hence, in considering the oral contraceptives from a moral point of view, it is not sufficient to consider only the adverse side effects associated with them (which are often related to the dose level), such as the potential for causing thrombi. It is also necessary to consider the possibility that a contraceptive may also bring about an abortion, that is, prevent the implantation of the fertilized oocyte (i.e., the embryo), which is already the beginning of a human life, a human person with a right to life.

It is theoretically possible that one could use, for its anti-ovulatory action, a contraceptive that also includes an abortifacient effect. For example, in a case of rape, a contraceptive with an abortifacient effect could be used to prevent conception *if* (and that is a large *if*) one could be morally certain that fertilization had not already taken place, that there was no embryo on its way to implantation. One needs moral certitude that a human life would not be destroyed as a result of administering the contraceptive drug. In practice, however, it is generally difficult to obtain the kind of information one needs from or about a patient to determine that no fertilization has taken place or is about to take place. There are tests which have been developed that can help make this determination.[10] Eventually, a drug may be discovered that has only a contraceptive effect with no abortifacient action.[11] Morally, abortifacient drugs or procedures are considered equivalent to abortion and must be so treated.

Partial-Birth Abortion

The term "partial-birth abortion" has been described as covering "all methods that involve the vaginal delivery of most of the baby's body before the baby is killed, generally by stabbing the baby at the base of the skull with surgical scissors. The baby's brain is then removed by suctioning to collapse and complete the delivery."[12] In the Partial Birth Abortion Ban Act of 1997 (H.R. 1122), partial-birth abortion was defined as "an abortion in which the person performing the abortion partially vaginally delivers a living fetus before killing the fetus and completing the delivery."[13]

The Partial Birth Abortion Ban was enacted in 2003 to prohibit this barbaric practice, and its constitutionality was affirmed by the U.S. Supreme Court in *Gonzalez v. Carhart* in 2007.[14] The law states that "any physician who, in or affecting interstate or foreign commerce, knowingly performs a partial-birth abortion and thereby kills a human fetus shall be fined under this title or imprisoned not more than 2 years, or both." The statute also states that partial birth abortion "is a gruesome and inhumane procedure that is never medically necessary" and notes that "twenty-seven states [have] banned the procedure as did the United States Congress which voted to ban the procedure during the 104th, 105th, and 106th Congresses." This bill represents a significant victory for pro-life voices. It was preceded by the passage, in 2002, of the Born Alive Infants Protection Act (Public Law 107-207), signed into law by President George W. Bush on August 5 of that year.[15]

The 1997 effort to enact the Partial Birth Abortion Ban had ended with a veto of the bill by President Bill Clinton. He stated his reason as follows:

> Unfortunately, H.R. 1122 does not contain an exception to the measure's ban that will adequately protect the lives and health of a small group of women in tragic circumstances who need an abortion performed at a late stage of pregnancy to avert death or serious injury.[16]

This contradicted the best medical evidence, as later indicated in the Congressional record. The effect of this veto was to keep this gruesome and inhumane procedure before the public mind for many years, energizing the pro-life community and causing shudders among the general voting population. To kill a child during the process of birth is infanticide.

After the 1997 veto, there was a growing and realistic fear that the next step for public policy would be the legal sanctioning of death for born children who have gross or not so gross abnormalities. Instead, public law went the other way with passage of the Born Alive Infants Protection Act in 2002. This legislation ensures that any child who survives an attempted abortion and is born alive will receive proper care and treatment.

A Catholic physician, whether practicing in a Catholic health care facility or not, may not perform a direct abortion or a partial-birth abortion. Similarly, nurses and other medical personnel may not cooperate with physicians doing such procedures. Both procedures involve the direct and intentional killing of an unborn innocent human person. There is no valid exception to this principle.

Notes

[1] U.S. Conference of Catholic Bishops, *Ethical and Religious Directives for Catholic Health Care Services* (*ERDs*), 4th ed. (Washington, D.C.: USCCB, 2001), n. 45.

[2] Congregation for the Doctrine of the Faith, *Declaration on Procured Abortion* (November 18, 1974), n. 19.

[3] Congregation for the Doctrine of the Faith, *Donum vitae* (February 22, 1987), I, 1.

[4] John Paul II, *Evangelium vitae* (March 25, 1995), n. 62 (original emphasis).

[5] See Benedict Ashley and Albert S. Moraczewski, "Is the Biological Subject of Human Rights Present from Conception?" in *The Fetal Tissue Issue: Medical and Ethical Aspects* eds. Peter Cataldo and Albert S. Moraczewski (Braintree, MA: Pope John Center, 1994), 33–59.

[6] See Donald G. McCarthy and Albert S. Moraczewski, eds., *An Ethical Evaluation of Fetal Experimentation: An Interdisciplinary Study* (St. Louis, MO: Pope John Center, 1976), 62–63.

[7] See Romans 3:8.

[8] See *ERDs*, n. 45.

[9] See Joseph W. Goldzieher, *Hormonal Contraception: Pills, Injections and Implants* (Dallas, TX: Essential Medical Information Systems, 1989), 34–36, 82.

[10] See Joseph J. Piccione, "Rape and the Peoria Protocol," *Ethics & Medics* 22.9 (September 1997): 1–2.

[11] See, for example, Ralph Miech, "A Proposed Novel Treatment for Rape Victims," *National Catholic Bioethics Quarterly* 5.4 (Winter 2005): 687–695; and Robert L. Barbieri, "Gonadotropin Releasing Hormone Analogues for Contraception," in *Fertility Control*, 2nd ed., eds. Stephen L. Corson, Richard J. Derman, and Louise B. Tyrer (Pearl River, NY: Parthenon, 1994).

[12] National Conference for Catholic Bishops, Secretariat for Pro-Life Activities, *Life Insight* 6.5 (June–July 1995), 3.

[13] *Partial Birth Abortion Ban Act of 1997* (H.R. 1122), 105th Cong., 1st sess. (March 19, 1997), 2.

[14] *Partial Birth Abortion Ban Act of 2003*, Public Law 108-

105, *U.S. Statutes at Large* 74 (2003): 1201–1208. *Gonzales v. Carhart*, 550 U.S. 124 (2007).

[15] *Born Alive Infants Protection Act of 2002*, Public Law 107-207, *U.S. Statutes at Large* 116 (2002): 926.

[16] William J. Clinton, Letter to the U.S. House of Representatives on H.R. 1122, October 10, 1997, http://clinton6.nara.gov/1997/10/1997-10-10-president-letter-to-the-house-on-the-veto-of-hr.html.

✠

Editor's Summation: Abortion is the unjust killing of an unborn human being. This includes the act of destroying an embryo in the period of time between conception and implantation. Although the Catholic Church has never expressly stated that human life begins at conception, and although it denies that this question can be answered in purely scientific terms, it has consistently condemned the destruction of innocent human life at any stage of existence. This teaching has been reaffirmed many times in various magisterial documents. The early Church condemned abortion as a form of infanticide. Debate in the Middle Ages and the Renaissance focused on whether abortion was solely a sin against nature or also homicide. With the advent of modern science and increased biological knowledge, the Church affirmed with even greater vigor that abortion is an intrinsic evil. Some cases of indirect abortion are permissible on moral grounds. These occur when the direct effect of a medical action is genuinely therapeutic and the death of the child is an unavoidable, indirect, foreseen, and unintended consequence. Abortifacient drugs, such as RU-486, are likewise intrinsically immoral. Abortion can also occur with the use of some contraceptives, though the likelihood of such an effect is difficult to determine, given the state of the medical evidence. In such matters, it is necessary to err on the side of caution, for a human life may be at stake. Recent legislative history in the United States has been moving in the direction of increased protection for unborn human life, although progress is minimal considering the magnitude of the problem. The brutal practice of partial-birth abortion has been banned, and some protection is now afforded children who are born alive after an attempted abortion. Catholic health care workers and Catholic health care facilities must not carry out or cooperate with abortion in any way.

B. Human Cloning

John B. Shea, M.D.

The human being typically comes into existence as soon as the sperm penetrates the oocyte, but human cloning uses genetic engineering techniques that involve asexual or a combination of asexual and sexual means to produce a human organism. These techniques include somatic cell nuclear transfer, pro-nuclear transfer, mitochondrial transfer, germ cell nuclear transfer, recombinant gene transfer, artificial recombinant gene transfer, parthenogenesis, and embryo splitting (fission). All of these techniques involve the in vitro production of, or the attempt to produce, a human being.

In somatic cell nuclear transfer, a woman's oocyte (human egg cell) is stripped of its DNA nucleus and the nucleus of a somatic (body) cell is put in its place. The new human being is almost an identical twin of the one who provided the somatic cell. The twin is not actually identical, because the clone contains foreign DNA from the mitochondria present in the cytoplasm of the oocyte.[1]

Thus far, there has been no successful instance of human cloning, although many scientists and researchers have tried. The reasons for embryo splitting include assisted human reproduction and also research. The other techniques are used for various reasons, including the prevention or cure of disease or congenital abnormality, eugenic human enhancement, basic research into disease mechanisms, and pharmacological research. Typically, reproductive and therapeutic cloning are distinguished, although they are accomplished by an identical technique. In reproductive cloning, the cloned human being is implanted in a woman's uterus with the aim of bringing it to birth. In therapeutic cloning, the human being is destroyed for its embryonic stem cells.

Catholic Teaching

The Church teaches that there is an "inseparable connection, willed by God and unable to be broken by man on his own initiative, between the two meanings of the conjugal act: the unitive meaning and the procreative meaning."[2] The Congregation for the Doctrine of the Faith states in *Donum vitae* that

> The transmission of human life is entrusted by nature to a personal and conscious act and as such is subject to the all-holy laws of God. ... Advances in technology have now made it possible to procreate apart from sexual relations through the meeting *in vitro* of the germ cells previously taken from the man and the woman. But what is technically possible is not for that very reason morally permissible. ... No one can, in any circumstance, claim for himself the right directly to destroy an innocent human being. ... *Attempts or hypotheses for obtaining a human body without any connection with sexuality through "twin fission," cloning or parthenogenesis are to be considered contrary to the moral law.*[3]

Pope John Paul II said that, to the list of the world's injustices, "we must add irresponsible practices of genetic engineering, such as the cloning and use of human embryos for research."[4] In addition, "human embryonic cloning also poses great threats to the rule of law by enabling those responsible for cloning to select and propagate certain human characteristics based on gender, race, etc. and eliminate others."[5]

Ethical Problems with Human Cloning

Genetic engineering, the controlled modification of the human genome, has two main objectives: eugenics, or the enhancement of human abilities, and the cure or prevention of disease. Human cloning is deeply connected to the eugenics movement initiated by Sir Francis Galton as early as 1865. Segregation and sterilization of "defectives" was recommended by early eugenicists, but today genetic engineering that involves human cloning is promoted. Scientists also see human cloning as a means of producing embryonic stem cells that can be used in medical therapies. Cloning that involves the reproduction of a human being by somatic cell nuclear transfer has not yet had any eugenic effect or cured any disease. The reasons are that embryonic stem cells are associated with immune response tissue rejection and tumor formation, and their production would involve the use of far more oocytes than are available.

The basic difference between Catholic doctrine and that of modern eugenics is that the former teaches that the final end of man is eternal life, while the latter places it in civic worth. For the Church, bodily and mental cultures must submit to morality. Eugenics makes morality subservient to the bodily and mental cultures of the day.[6]

Medical Problems with Human Cloning

According to Harold Varmus and other advocates, cells derived from somatic cell nuclear transfer have the potential to cure many diseases, such as diabetes, heart disease, and cancer. This opinion was given in evidence before the House Committee on Commerce, Subcommittee on Health and Environment, on February 12, 1998. This potential is purely speculative. No successful clinical trial of embryonic stem cell therapy has yet been done. Embryonic stem cells have a known tendency to form tumors and to cause tissue rejection. Tissue rejection can occur even with tissues derived by somatic cell nuclear transfer from the patient's own somatic cells because the DNA in the mitochondria of the oocyte's cytoplasm is foreign to the patient. Tissue rejection requires treatment with drugs that may have to be taken for a lifetime, carry a high risk of causing infections, and are associated with a 5 percent increase in the incidence of cancer after a few years. The Rand Corporation has shown that only 2.8 percent of the approximately four-hundred thousand frozen in vitro embryos in the United States have been designated for research, and that only 275 stem cell lines could be developed from those embryos.[7]

Those who support human cloning claim to have good motives such as curing or preventing disease. However, one should not do evil in order to achieve a good. Furthermore, as Pope John Paul II has stated, "Science itself points to other forms of *therapeutic intervention* which would not involve cloning or the use of embryonic cells, but rather would make use of stem cells taken from adults. This is the direction that research must follow if it wishes to respect the dignity of each and every human being, even at the embryonic stage."[8]

The Do No Harm Coalition of Americans for Research Ethics keeps a running tally of current successes involving adult stem cell research, along with additional information about the field.[9] David Prentice, senior fellow for life sciences of the Family Research Council, has stated that adult stem cells are already being used clinically to treat many diseases in human patients:

> These include reparative treatments with various cancers, autoimmune diseases such as multiple sclerosis, lupus, and arthritis, anemias including sickle cell anemia, and immunodeficiencies. ... [Adult stem cells

have also been used] in growing new corneas to restore sight to blind patients, treatments for stroke, … [and] to repair damage after heart attacks. In most cases, the patient's own stem cells can be used for the treatment, circumventing the problems of immune rejection, and without tumor formation.[10]

The United Nations and the Church

On March 23, 2005, the United Nations called on all member states to "prohibit all forms of human cloning inasmuch as they are incompatible with human dignity and the protection of human life."[11] Since it is obvious that cloning is totally incompatible with human dignity and the protection of human life, the UN declaration was intended to ban "all forms" of human cloning, including both its reproductive and therapeutic forms. Supporters of human cloning hold that the phrase "inasmuch as" means "to the extent that." However, the phrase is commonly used to mean "because." They use this ambiguity to argue that some human cloning is allowed. Even though the declaration is nonbinding, it is of great importance.

John Paul II has said that "faith and reason are like two wings on which the human spirit rises to the contemplation of truth; and God has placed in the human heart a desire to know the truth."[12] Pope Benedict XVI has stated, "The real problem of our historical moment lies in the imbalance between the incredibly fast growth of our technical power and that of our moral capacity, which has not grown in proportion." He also added, "Catholicism is not a collection of prohibitions: it is a positive option."[13]

The Church teaches God's truth to the world. It does not seek to manipulate or dominate. The Church's teaching on human cloning is a truth that sets man free to live a morally good, healthy, and beautiful life and spares him from sin and moral, psychological, and pathological disease and degradation. The present moment is one that calls for "solidarity between science, the good of the person and of society."[14] This moment also calls for what Pope John Paul II has named a

> contemplative outlook … the outlook of those who see life in its deeper meaning, who grasp its utter gratuitousness, its beauty and its invitation to freedom and responsibility. It is the outlook of those who do not presume to take possession of reality but instead accept it as a gift, discovering in all things the reflection of the Creator and seeing in every person his living image.[15]

Catholic caregivers and health care facilities are presented today with a great opportunity to fulfill their lay apostolic duty to bring the truth of Christ to our complex world by providing an example in the way they perform their duties, and by informing the world about Catholic teaching in the realm of bioethics "with gentleness and reverence" (1 Peter 3: 15).

Notes

[1] It is of interest that the creation of hybrid clones is now allowed in Great Britain. A human somatic cell nucleus is inserted into the oocyte of a rabbit or cow from which the nucleus has been removed. This technique avoids the need to ask women to donate eggs for nuclear transfer, a process that involves hormonal stimulation of the ovaries that can be hazardous to women's health. Hybrid cloning is intended to create banks of cells that are useful for more effective pre-clinical research into drug toxicity, and pharmacological research aimed at the provision of more effective drug treatment of specific diseases. The direct use of stem cells derived from clones, however, may cause tissue rejection due to the presence of foreign protein in the mitochondrial DNA.

[2] Paul VI, *Humanae vitae* (July 25, 1968), n. 12.

[3] Congregation for the Doctrine of the Faith, *Donum vitae* (February 22, 1987), intro., 4, 6; I, 6 (original emphasis).

[4] John Paul II, Message for the Celebration of the World Day of Peace (January 1, 2001), n. 4.

[5] Intervention by the Holy See Delegation at the Special Committee of the 57th General Assembly of the United Nations on Human Embryonic Cloning (September 23, 2002), http://www.vatican.va/roman_curia/secretariat_state/documents/rc_seg-st_doc_20020923_martino-cloning_en.html.

[6] *The Catholic Encyclopedia*, s.v. "The Church and Eugenics," by Thomas J. Gerrard (New York: Encyclopedia Press, 1914), www.newadvent.org/cathen/16038b.htm.

[7] Rand Institute for Civil Justice and Rand Health, "How Many Frozen Embryos Are Available for Research?" Law and Health Research Brief RB-9038 (2003) summarizing D. I. Hoffman et al., "Cryopreserved Embryos in the United States and Their Availability for Research," *Fertility and Sterility* 79.5 (May 2003): 1063–1069.

[8] John Paul II, Address to the 18th International Congress of the Transplantation Society (August 29, 2000), n. 8.

[9] Do No Harm: The Coalition of Americans for Research Ethics, "Adult Versus Embryonic Stem Cells: Treatment," http://www.stemcellresearch.org/.

[10] David Prentice, "Adult vs. Embryonic Stem Cells," testimony against House Bill 1183 (*Maryland Stem Cell Research Act of 2005*) before the Maryland House, Health and Government Operations Committee and House Appropriations Committee, March 2, 2005.

[11] UN General Assembly, Fifty-ninth Session, Sixth Committee, "United Nations Declaration on Human Cloning" (A/RES/59/280), March 23, 2005, 2.

[12]John Paul II, *Fides et ratio* (September 14, 1998), opening statement.

[13]Pope Benedict XVI, Interview in Preparation for the Upcoming Journey to Bavaria (August 5, 2006).

[14]Pontifical Academy for Life, "Reflections on Cloning" (1997).

[15]John Paul II, *Evangelium vitae* (March 25, 1995), n. 83.

Editor's Summation: Human cloning generally involves the insertion of the nucleus of an ordinary body cell into a woman's ovum (egg cell), whose own nucleus has already been stripped away. The fusion of the new nucleus with the empty ovum results in a complete human being. This human being will be the genetic twin of the one from whom the original body cell was taken. Two types of cloning are commonly mentioned in the political arena. Reproductive cloning produces a human being in vitro who is then placed into the uterus and brought to term. Therapeutic cloning produces a human being who is then destroyed through the extraction of embryonic stem cells. Scientifically, the cloning procedure is exactly the same in both methods. New human life should arise through sexual union in marriage, not through laboratory techniques. Cloning is part of the larger eugenic project that has been made possible by reproduction in vitro. The effort to fashion new medicines and therapies from embryonic stem cells—held out as the promise of cloning—faces significant obstacles, including tissue rejection, tumor formation, and the need for a vast number of donated ova. Adult stem cells have already proved to be far more successful in the cure and amelioration of disease. The United Nations has condemned all forms of human cloning, as has the Catholic Church. The progress of science should stand in harmony with the highest regard for the dignity of human life in its origins.

C. Stem Cell Research

E. Christian Brugger

A stem cell is an undifferentiated cell that possesses two broad capacities: first, for *proliferation and self-renewal* over months, even years, into identical daughter copies of itself; and second, for *differentiation* into specialized cell types within the organism, e.g., liver cells, neural cells, and blood cells.

The "potency" of a cell refers to its capacity for differentiation and development. If a cell possesses the ability to differentiate and develop into the entire organism, including extraembyonic tissues, placenta and umbilical cord, the cell is called *totipotent* (e.g., a zygote, or single cell human embryo); if it is able to differentiate and develop into many if not all the cell types of the human body, but not the entire organism as a living integrated entity, the cell is called *pluripotent* (e.g., embryonic stem cells); if it can differentiate only into cell types of a related family of cells (e.g., blood cells), it is called *multipotent*; and if it can differentiate into only a single cell type, it is called *unipotent*.

Embryonic stem (ES) cells are undifferentiated, self-renewing cells taken from early human embryos, at or before the blastocyst stage. They are obtained from the inner part of the embryos, called the inner cell mass. This extraction of the cells is lethal to the embryo.

Adult, or somatic, stem (AS) cells are undifferentiated, self-renewing cells found in differentiated human tissue. They are called "adult" not because they are found only in adults, but because they are found in mature (i.e., differentiated) tissue. Because they ordinarily have the capacity to differentiate only into the types of cells found in the tissues or organs from which they derive, most adult stem cells are multipotent.

Adult and Embryonic Stem Cell Research: Hope for Cures

Human stem cell research, part of the larger field of regenerative medicine, is still in its early years. (The first embryonic stem cell line was not derived until 1998, by researchers at the University of Wisconsin-Madison.) Responding to pressure from opponents of embryo-destructive experimentation, President Bill Clinton signed a law in 1995 making it illegal for federal funds to be used for embryo-destructive stem cell research. Advocates for the controversial research began an active campaign against the new legislation. The political heat increased steadily until President George W. Bush, in August 2001, implemented an executive policy which he believed struck a balance between the needs of science and the demands of morality. He permitted, for the first time, the federal funding of human embryonic stem cell research, but only on sixty stem cell lines created before that day, August 9, in which cases "the life and death decision [had] already been made."[1] Since then pro-embryonic-stem-cell activism has grown remarkably, utilizing the mainstream media to advance a permissive message toward embryo destruction—"they're only tiny clumps of cells"—and hyperbolic publicity on their clinical promise. In July 2006, both houses of Congress passed a law to fund embryonic stem cell research that would encourage the destruction of so-called spare embryos stored at IVF clinics to derive new stem cell lines. President Bush vetoed this legislation—the first veto of his presidency.

Until that time, claims were repeated in scientific and journalistic literature for the vastly superior potential of embryonic stem cells over adult stem cells. Cures for conditions like Parkinson's disease, Alzheimer's disease, diabetes, heart disease, strokes, spinal cord injuries, and burns were touted, if only more money could be invested in this promising research. In 2004, the state of California passed Proposition 71, which earmarked three billion dollars of taxpayer-funded grants for embryonic stem cell research. Non-federally-funded research institutes were set up at Harvard and Stanford, underwritten with hundreds of millions of dollars of privately solicited funds. Despite the projections and massive fundraising efforts, as of October 2007, embryonic stem cell research had produced *no* useful therapies, nor had there been any FDA clinical trials.[2] This is not to say there never will be. embryonic stem cell research is a young science and scientists are learning from it rapidly. It may be naive, and certainly premature, to argue that adult stem cells will have equal or superior clinical utility to embryonic stem cells, but the moral arguments do not change. The *foundational* arguments against embryo-destructive experimentation must be made on ethical grounds, and not on scientific predictions that may be falsified.

Nevertheless, at present, adult stem cells have shown greater clinical benefit. Research using adult stem cells derived from bone marrow, umbilical cord blood, nasal mucosa, and other sources have already begun to be used in treating diseases such as lupus erythematosus, multiple sclerosis, leukemia, coronary heart disease, ovarian cancer,

brain tumors, Parkinson's disease, and spinal cord injuries. Further, numerous studies demonstrate that some adult stem cells have a differentiation potential similar to that of embryonic stem cells.[3] In August 2006, for example, researchers at the University of Florida reported finding adult stem cells from the human brain expressing the same potential as embryonic stem cells.[4] Also in August 2006, researchers at the University of Kyoto, Japan, demonstrated that mouse fibroblasts (connective tissue cells) could be induced in vitro to a state of pluripotency; they named the cells iPS (induced pluripotent stem) cells.[5,*] And German scientists in April 2006 demonstrated that adult stem cells from mouse testis expressed embryonic-stem-cell-like properties, and, they said, there is good evidence that these type of cells can be isolated in adult humans.[6] These claims have yet to be fully explored, and even if adult sources of pluripotent stem cells are established, the cells may have somewhat different properties than embryonic stem cells. Still, the findings are very significant. Interestingly, almost immediately after the Bush veto in July 2006, scientists who had hyped the potential therapeutic benefit of embryonic stem cell research began to moderate their projections.[7]

Stem Cell Research: Ethical Reflection

In assessing the morality of any type of deliberate human behavior, one needs to assess the goodness of both an act's *end(s)* (i.e., that for the sake of which the action is chosen, sometimes called the "intention"), and the proximate *means* by which the end is pursued (sometimes called the moral "object"). Since both bear in a determinate way upon goods fundamental to human flourishing, and since "the morality of acts is defined by the relationship of man's freedom with the authentic good,"[8] both an act's end *and* means need to be good for the act to be good.

In the case of both adult stem cell and embryonic stem cell research, the ends sought are good and praiseworthy, namely, the advancement of scientific knowledge and the development of viable clinical therapies for improving health and diminishing suffering. An upright end, however, is not enough to allow us to conclude that an act is unqualifiedly good. With respect to chosen means, adult stem cell and embryonic stem cell research are—morally speaking—radically different kinds of acts.

---

* Further developments on this front are described below under *Adult Cell Reprogramming*—ED.

Embryonic Stem Cell Research

The two chief ethical problems with embryonic stem cell research concern the manner in which embryos are derived and the destructive means to which they are subject. As noted, securing embryonic stem cells requires the isolation of the inner cell mass from the living body of an embryo, which kills the embryo. The Pontifical Academy for Life, in its document on human embryonic stem cell research, teaches that this lethal surgical procedure "is a *gravely immoral* act and consequently is *gravely illicit*."[9] This judgment is derived from the prior ethical judgment affirmed in the Congregation for the Doctrine of the Faith (CDF) instruction *Donum vitae* and again in the papal encyclical *Evangelium vitae*, which asserts that "the human being is to be respected and treated as a person from the moment of conception; and therefore from that same moment his rights as a person must be recognized, among which in the first place is the inviolable right of every innocent human being to life."[10]

The instruction should not be misunderstood. It does not say with certitude that the human embryo is a human person, but "is to be respected and treated as a person." Since in Christian anthropology personhood is predicated of ensouled human beings, and the moment of ensoulment is neither taught in sacred scripture nor subject to empirical verification, no one can say with certitude that the embryo from its first moments of existence possesses full personhood, although there are good reasons to conclude that it does.[11] This leaves the doubt unresolved. Consequently, to lethally experiment upon embryos, knowing they might be innocent human persons, means one is willing to kill innocent human persons, which is gravely immoral. Despite the admittedly good intentions with which embryo-destructive experimentation is usually chosen, the adopted means are gravely evil. To choose evil means even with a good intent is to render one's act and oneself morally evil: "no evil done with a good intention can be excused."[12] The only type of experimentation upon embryos that is licit are procedures "which respect the life and integrity of the embryo and do not involve disproportionate risks for it, but rather are directed to its healing, the improvement of its condition of health, or its individual survival."[13]

The second ethical problem concerns the way embryos are derived. Although the long-term aim of many scientists is to create embryos through somatic cell nuclear transfer ("therapeutic cloning"), human cloning technology, as illustrated by the Woo Suk Hwang scandal,[14] has not yet achieved this stage of sophistication. Consequently, stem cell researchers presently rely on in vitro fertilization. Because IVF instrumentalizes the bringing about of new human life by replacing the marital act with the fertilization of gametes through a calculated laboratory procedure, it *always* violates the dignity of the human embryos brought into existence. By violating "the right of every person to be conceived and to be born within marriage and from marriage," IVF is a grave injustice against the embryos it creates and therefore is always gravely immoral to choose.[15]

Some argue that given the approximately four hundred thousand "spare" embryos presently frozen and stored at IVF clinics in the United States,[16] and given that their likely fate will be death, great good could be achieved if they were earmarked for destructive embryonic stem cell experimentation; it is therefore morally legitimate to use them for embryonic stem cell research. The argument presupposes the false premise that it is sometimes licit to do evil in order to achieve good. The constant and ancient teaching of the Catholic Church, however, reasserted by Pope Paul VI in *Humanae vitae* (n. 14) and Pope John Paul II in *Veritatis splendor* (n. 80), is that although sometimes "it is lawful to tolerate a lesser moral evil in order to avoid a greater evil or in order to promote a greater good, it is never lawful, even for the gravest reasons, to do evil that good may come of it."

The question as to what people of good will can do on behalf of the thousands of frozen embryos is a difficult one. Some Catholic moral theologians faithful to the magisterium have proposed "embryo adoption" (or "embryo rescue") as a life-saving alternative, i.e., the choice of able adult women to gestate abandoned embryos. It should be said, however, that the Catholic Church has not yet provided a moral judgment on the procedure, and some moral theologians think it is illicit.[17]

Adult Stem Cell Research

Because adult stem cell research involves neither the creation of embryos through IVF nor their killing through destructive research, it does not violate the two norms discussed above. Its legitimacy therefore is subject to the same norms that govern all scientific and clinical research, specifically, truth-telling with respect to all threatened burdens and promised benefits, informed consent in all dealings with subjects of experimental and tested therapies, honesty in reporting research and data, refrainment from all unwarranted promises of benefit, and professionalism in all doctor–client relations. It should be noted that the Vatican and the USCCB have repeatedly endorsed ethically legitimate research on stem cells that does not exploit or destroy human embryos.[18]

Adult Cell Reprogramming

An extraordinary breakthrough in stem cell research was published in November 2007. Two teams of researchers, one from the University of Wisconsin-Madison,[19] and the other from Kyoto University in Japan,[20] announced contemporaneously that they had successfully transformed human fibroblast cells into pluripotent stem cells (called induced pluripotent stem, or iPS, cells). By injecting four genes into adult skin cells, the teams were able to induce (or "reprogram") the cells to a state of pluripotency believed by the researchers to be functionally identical in key respects to that of embryonic stem cells. One of the researchers on the Wisconsin team, Dr. James Thomson (who is sometimes referred to as the founder of embryonic stem cell research, since he was the first to isolate embryonic stem cells through embryo-destructive means in 1998), stated,"The induced cells do all the things embryonic stem cells do. It's going to completely change the field."[21] Since iPSCs can be derived from a patient's own cells, patient-specific stem cells can be produced avoiding problems with tissue rejection.

The breakthrough provides the scientific community with an alternative means for deriving pluripotent stem cells without needing to use human embryos. Dr. Thomson admitted to struggling with the ethical implications of his original research: "If human embryonic stem cell research does not make you at least a little bit uncomfortable, you have not thought about it enough."[22] He stated frankly that this breakthrough marks "the beginning of the end of the controversy" over embryonic stem cell research.[23] "A decade from now this will be just a funny historical footnote."[24] Dr. Shinya Yamanaka, leader of the Japanese team, also expressed misgivings over destroying embryos: "We can't keep destroying embryos for our research," he said. "There must be another way."[25] After examining the work of Yamanaka and his colleagues, Professor Ian Wilmut, the pioneer cloning researcher who created Dolly the sheep, decided to abandon therapeutic cloning in favor of the new reprogramming technology. The research, he said, was "extremely exciting and astonishing" and represents, he believes, the future for stem cell research.[26]

Catholic Hospitals, Universities, and Research Institutions

An important question to address is whether it is licit for Catholic institutions to undertake research or utilize cures derived from embryo-destructive experimentation. In Catholic tradition this is a question of the permissibility of cooperating with the wrongdoing of others.

With respect to embryo-destructive experimentation and the illicit production of embryos through IVF, not only the persons who carry out the acts, but anyone who "commands, directs, advises, encourages, prescribes, approves or actively defends" the acts does wrong.[27] Such persons are said to *formally cooperate* in the wrongdoer's evil action. In choosing to instigate another's wrongdoing, the cooperator includes in his choice the evil object chosen by the wrongdoer. *Formal cooperation in destructive embryo experimentation and the production of embryos through IVF is always gravely wrong, and therefore it is never licit for Catholic institutions to formally cooperate in such acts.*[28]

The more difficult question pertains to situations where formal cooperation is excluded—that is, where there is no instigation of evil—but where one's actions contribute in some way to the success of the wrongdoing. This is called *material cooperation*. Because in the case of material cooperation one does not include in one's own choice the evil chosen by another, material cooperation can sometimes be licit. At the same time, one willingly does something that contributes to the success of wrongdoing. If by refraining from acting, or actively opposing the wrongdoing, one has a reasonable chance of preventing the evil or minimizing its harm, then such cooperation, even though free from instigating evil, can be morally wrong. The former (legitimate) type of cooperation is called *remote material cooperation*, and the latter (illicit) type is called *proximate material cooperation*.

Presuming formal cooperation by a Catholic institution is excluded, the legitimacy of three types of material cooperation needs to be assessed: (1) utilizing previously isolated undifferentiated embryonic stem cells and cultured stem cell lines derived from embryo-destructive experimentation, (2) utilizing differentiated cells obtained from previously isolated embryonic stem cells, and (3) utilizing therapies and medicines derived from embryonic stem cell research.

To determine when and how it is morally permissible to utilize and benefit from research that relies in part on what has been unjustly obtained, one needs to assess the relevant facts and prevailing circumstances of the contemplated alternatives, especially their likely consequences. *The central moral consideration must be fairness to those unjustly harmed by the research.* A more permissive view poses the risk of giving an example that could be exploited to strengthen the argument of advocates of immoral research—that the promise of new biomedical breakthroughs demands more and more destructive research. To obviate this hazard, Catholic institutions should resist the first and second type of cooperation stated above, that is, resist any use of embryonic stem cells, stem cell lines, or differentiated cells obtained from embryonic stem cells, even if acquired from other researchers or secured by commercial means. This includes participating in therapeutic trials, constructing disease models, and testing pharmaceutical products using embryonic stem cells. Successes (or claims of success) in these areas would only be used to bring pressure for more embryo killing. The use of embryonic stem cells or the differentiated lines derived from them would be permissible only where there is no likelihood or substantial possibility that it would have this effect.[29]

As for using tested and approved therapies or pharmaceuticals derived from research involving embryo killing, Catholic institutions (and clinicians and patients) should resist this form of material cooperation *if there is a reasonably accessible morally legitimate alternative.* If such an alternative is available by reasonable effort, one has a serious duty to utilize it. In addition, if one has reason to believe that publicizing one's conscientious objection could assist in minimizing harm to victims, one should make public one's objections.

If, however, a therapy presents itself for which there is no reasonably accessible alternative, if the therapy promises a reasonable probability of success, and if the consequences of not undergoing the therapy would be grave, then undergoing the therapy would not necessarily constitute illicit participation. In order to avoid scandal, however, one would have a moral duty to make known to all parties to whom scandal could be given of one's firm opposition to the two injustices (at least) that were done to make the therapy possible, specifically, the creation of embryos through IVF and embryo killing.

Notes

General information on stem cells is available at http://stem-cells.nih.gov/, http://www.umdnj.edu/gsbsnweb/stemcell/, and http://www.news.wisc.edu/packages/stemcells/.

[1] White House, "President discusses stem cell research," press release, August 9, 2001.

[2] The National Institutes of Health confirms this on its Web site (accessed 12/12/2008); see Healthcare Question 2 under "Frequently Asked Questions," at http://stemcells.nih.gov/info/faqs.asp.

[3] For a list of journal references for more than seventy different conditions treated with adult stem cells, see the Family Research Council's Center for Human Life and Bioethics under Resources, http://www.frc.org/life--bioethics#stem_cells. See also Do No Harm, "Benefits of Stem Cells to Human Patients" (April 11, 2007), http://www.stemcellresearch.org/facts/treatments.htm.

[4] John Pastor, "Healing potential discovered in everyday human brain cells," University of Florida, *Health Science Center News*, August 16, 2006, http://news.health.ufl.edu/story.aspx?ID=4180.

[5] K. Takahashi, and S. Yamanaka, "Induction of Pluripotent Stem Cells from Mouse Embryonic and Adult Fibroblast Cultures by Defined Factors," *Cell* 126.4 (August 25, 2006): 1–14. For an essay demonstrating that "pluripotency" genes are expressed in lung AS cells, see T. Ling, "Identification of Pulmonary Oct-4+ Stem/Progenitor Cells and Demonstration of their Susceptibility to SARS Coronavirus (SARS-CoV) Infection In Vitro," *Proceedings of the National Academy of Sciences of the United States of America* 103.25 (June 20, 2006): 9530–9535.

[6] K. Guan et al., "Pluripotency of Spermatogonial Stem Cells from Adult Mouse Testis," *Nature* 440.7088 (April 27, 2006): 1199–1203; see also M. Kanatsu-Shinohara and T. Shinohara, "The Germ of Pluripotency," *Nature Biotechnology* 24 (June 2006): 663–664. Also, researchers at Kansas State University have shown that stem cells isolated from the umbilical cord of swine possessed "properties of primitive pluripotent stem cells." R. Carlin et al., "Expression of Early Transcription Factors Oct-4, Sox-2 and Nanog by Porcine Umbilical Cord Matrix Cells," *Reproductive Biology and Endocrinology* 4.1 (February 6, 2006): 8.

[7] Nicholas Wade, "Some Scientists See Shift in Stem Cell Hopes," *New York Times*, August 14, 2006. See also M. Enserink, "Selling the Stem Cell Dream," *Science* 313.5784 (July 14, 2006): 160–163.

[8] John Paul II, *Veritatis splendor* (August 6, 1993), n. 72.

[9] Pontifical Academy for Life, *Declaration on the Production and the Scientific and Therapeutic Use of Human Embryonic Stem Cells* (August 25, 2000). See also John Paul II, *Evangelium vitae* (March 25, 1995), n. 63; and Holy See, *Charter of the Rights of the Family* (October 22, 1983).

[10] Congregation for the Doctrine of the Faith, *Donum vitae* (February 22, 1987), I, 1; and *Evangelium vitae*, n. 60.

[11] See *Evangelium vitae*, n. 60; and Germain Grisez, "When Do People Begin?" *Proceedings of the American Catholic Philosophical Association* 63 (1989): 27–47.

[12] *Veritatis splendor*, n. 78. See Romans 3:8.

[13] *Evangelium vitae*, n. 63. See *Donum vitae*, I, 3.

[14] See Kevin Shapiro, "Lessons of the Cloning Scandal," *Commentary* (April 2006): 61–64; and W. S. Hwang et al., "Evidence of a Pluripotent Human Embryonic Stem Cell Line Derived from a Cloned Blastocyst," *Science* 303.5664 (March 12, 2004): 1669–1674. *Science* subsequently retracted this essay.

[15] See *Donum vitae*, I, 6, also note 32.

[16] See D. I. Hoffman et al. for the Society for Assisted Reproduction (SART) and RAND, "Cryopreserved Embryos in the United States and Their Availability for Research," *Fertility and Sterility* 79.5 (May 2003): 1063–1069.

[17] See, for example, Thomas V. Berg and Edward J. Furton, *Human Embryo Adoption: Biotechnology, Marriage, and the Right to Life* (Philadelphia and Thornwood, NY: National Catholic Bioethics Center and Westchester Institute for Ethics & the Human Person, 2006).

[18] Pontifical Academy for Life, *Declaration on Human Embryonic Stem Cells*, 2000; U.S. Conference of Catholic Bishops, "Catholic Support for Ethically Acceptable Stem Cell Research," Office of Pro-Life Activities, n.d., http://www.usccb.org/prolife/issues/bioethic/stemcell/stemcath.shtml; and Catholic Online, "American Bishops Reaffirm Church Support for Adult Stem-Cell Research," *Catholic.org*, June 26, 2006, www.catholic.org/national/national_story.php?id=20275.

[19] J. Yu et al., "Induced Pluripotent Stem Cell Lines Derived from Human Somatic Cells," *Science* 318.5858 (December 21, 2007): 1917–1920.

[20] K. Takahashi et al., "Induction of Pluripotent Stem Cells from Adult Human Fibroblasts by Defined Factors," *Cell* 131.5 (November 30, 2007): 861–872.

[21] Catharine Paddock, "Reprogrammed Skin Cells Could Replace Embryonic Stem Cells, *Medical News Today*, November 26, 2007, http://www.medicalnewstoday.com/printerfriendlynews.php?newsid=89799.

[22] Gina Kolata, "Man Who Helped Start Stem Cell War May End It," *New York Times*, November 22, 2007. Thomson is quoted similarly in Colin Nickerson, "Breakthrough on Stem Cells: Reprogramming of Human Skin May Circumvent Ethics Controversy," *Boston Globe*, November 21, 2007.

[23] Marie McCullough, "Stem Cells Without the Fuss? Possibly," *Detroit Free Press*, November 21, 2007.

[24] Kolata, "Man Who Helped Start Stem Cell War."

[25] Martin Fackler, "Risk Taking Is in His Genes," *New York Times*, December 11, 2007.

[26] Roger Highfield, "Dolly Creator Prof. Ian Wilmut Shuns Cloning," *London Telegraph*, November 16, 2007.

[27] Germain Grisez. *The Way of the Lord Jesus*, vol. 1, *Christian Moral Principles* (Chicago: Franciscan Herald Press, 1983), 300.

[28] See *Evangelium vitae*, n. 74.

[29] With regard to alternative sources, Robert George notes: "One possible example is the use of ES cells as epigenetic reprogramming agents in somatic cell dedifferentiation strategies for producing pluripotent stem cells. This use could very well render embryo-destructive research entirely obsolete without a single embryo being killed. It should be said clearly though that if it involved killing even a single embryo, it should be opposed. But unlike other possible uses, success in this speculative area of research would not indicate the "need" for additional stem cell lines and more embryo killing. In fact, the opposite would be true. Of course, if it is possible to reprogram somatic cells to the pluripotent state without using existing cell lines, that is even better." Robert P. George, personal communication, 2006. See also the President's Council on Bioethics, "Alternative Sources of Human Pluripotent Stem Cells" (May 2005), www.bioethics.gov/reports/white_paper/alternative_sources_white_paper.pdf. NOTE: Not all the procedures discussed in this white paper are compatible with the principles set forth in the present essay.

✠

Editorial Summation: A stem cell is an undifferentiated cell that can produce identical daughter copies of itself. These cells can be differentiated into specialized cells for use in medical therapies and cures. Embryonic stem cells are extracted from embryos in a procedure that kills them. Adult stem cells are undifferentiated cells found within an organism's mature tissues. The prospects of new cures and therapies via embryonic stem cells have been trumpeted by its advocates for many years, although there is little evidence of success thus far. Success may indeed come in the future, but at present, adult stem cells have proved far more useful in combating a variety of serious diseases. Although the aim of finding cures is laudable, the destruction of human embryos is gravely immoral. We can never choose an evil means to a good end. The production of embryos in vitro is itself an injustice. The use of adult stem cells, in contrast, poses no significant moral difficulties and has been consistently encouraged by the Catholic Church. The recent discovery of induced pluripotent stem cells opens a door to all the potential benefits of embryonic stem cell research without the moral difficulties. Adult stem cell reprogramming can provide researchers with an abundant supply of embryonic-like stem cells without the destruction of human embryos. Catholic hospitals and research facilities face the question of whether they may use embryonic stem cell lines that were created by others. This is a question of cooperation. Generally, Catholic institutions should resist using any embryonic stem cells, cell lines, or differentiated cells obtained from these lines, even though the destruction of embryonic life and the culturing of the cells were done by others. An argument can be made that the use of a particular therapy that has its origins in embryonic stem cell research may be permissible for a Catholic patient if there is no alternative available and the patient suffers from a serious disease.

CHAPTER 7

Chemical, Barrier, and Surgical Contraception

John M. Haas

There are two directives in the *Ethical and Religious Directives for Catholic Health Care Services* which deal with contraception. Directive 52 reads, "Catholic health institutions may not promote or condone contraceptive practices but should provide, for married couples and the medical staff who counsel them, instruction both about the Church's teaching on responsible parenthood and in methods of natural family planning." Directive 53 reads, "Direct sterilization of either men or women, whether permanent or temporary, is not permitted in a Catholic health care institution. Procedures that induce sterility are permitted when their direct effect is the cure or alleviation of a present and serious pathology and a simpler treatment is not available."[1] The second sentence in directive 53 refers to indirect sterilization.

There is undoubtedly no area of Catholic teaching which is more controversial—or, frankly, less understood—in contemporary American society than that which deals with the moral regulation of births. Because many means of birth regulation have entered into the realm of medical practice, Catholic health care services must have a clear understanding of Church teaching in this area. For purposes of easy reference and for the sake of clarity, the application of the teaching of the Catholic Church will be presented first in this chapter before there is any attempt to explain the philosophical and theological foundations of the teaching.

Direct and Indirect Contraceptive Sterilization

Contraceptive sterilization can be understood in both a medical and a moral sense. In a medical sense, it includes any medical, surgical, or other intervention which renders the persons engaging in intercourse sterile either permanently or temporarily. In a moral sense, it is direct sterilization if the purpose of the intervention is precisely to render the person sterile or infertile for whatever reason. However, if there is a surgical, medical, or other intervention directed at some present pathology and the purpose of the intervention is specifically therapeutic, even though it is foreseen that the intervention may unintentionally render the patient sterile or infertile, the action is referred to as indirect sterilization. Indirect sterilization can be considered morally licit in Catholic teaching if it is done for a proportionately grave reason and if no other, simpler therapy is available. Because indirect sterilization results from a legitimate, moral medical procedure directly correcting a pathology of some sort, it is not considered immoral. What is considered immoral is an action which directly renders a person sterile so that intercourse freely chosen in the future would be deprived of its inherent, fertile end.

The central governing and teaching agency of the Catholic Church, the Vatican, has been quite clear on the matter of direct sterilizations in Catholic health care institutions. In 1975, the Congregation for the Doctrine of the Faith, which maintains the integrity of Catholic teaching and practice, made an unequivocal statement with respect to the involvement of Catholic hospitals with direct sterilization. It is known as a *responsum*, since it was issued in response to a question posed to the congregation by the U.S. bishops. It is also known by the first Latin word of the document, *Quaecumque*.

> Any sterilization which of itself, that is, of its own nature and condition, has the sole immediate effect of rendering the generative faculty incapable of pro-

creation is to be considered direct sterilization. ... Therefore, notwithstanding any subjectively right intention of those whose actions are prompted by the care or prevention of physical or mental illness which is foreseen or feared as a result of pregnancy, such sterilization remains absolutely forbidden according to the doctrine of the Church. And indeed the sterilization of the faculty itself is forbidden for an even graver reason than the sterilization of individual acts, since it induces a state of sterility in the person which is almost always irreversible.[2]

The teaching of the Congregation is also clear about the cooperation of a Catholic health care facility with a contraceptive act. Once again, there is an undeniable clarity to the Church's position, even if one should disagree with it:

> Any cooperation institutionally approved or tolerated in actions which are themselves, that is, by their nature and condition, directed to a contraceptive end, namely, that the natural effects of sexual actions deliberately performed by the sterilized subject be impeded, is absolutely forbidden. For the official approbation of direct sterilization and, *a fortiori*, its management and execution in accord with hospital regulations, is a matter which, in the objective order, is by its very nature (or intrinsically) evil. The Catholic hospital cannot cooperate with this for any reason. Any cooperation so supplied is totally unbecoming the mission entrusted to this type of institution and would be contrary to the necessary proclamation and defense of the moral order.[3]

This is a strong judgment passed by the Vatican on Catholic facilities cooperating in the provision of direct sterilizations. In 1977, the administrative committee of the National Conference of Catholic Bishops approved a commentary on the Vatican *responsum*.[4] It reiterated the statement of the Congregation for the Doctrine of the Faith quoted above and added guidelines for hospital policy. The Vatican later required that the commentary no longer be used, because it lacked a certain clarity in some areas. However, there was no lack of clarity in the greater specificity the U.S. bishops provided with respect to the kinds of conditions to which appeal could *not* be made to justify the direct sterilization of individuals:[5]

> As it was stated in the Roman document, the Catholic hospital can in no way approve the performance of any sterilization procedure that is directly contraceptive. Such contraceptive procedures include

sterilizations performed as a means of preventing future pregnancy that one fears might aggravate a serious cardiac, renal, circulatory, or other disorder. Freely approving direct sterilization constitutes formal cooperation in evil and would be "totally unbecoming the mission" of the hospital as well as "contrary to the necessary proclamation and defense of the moral order."[6]

It has sometimes been maintained that sterilizations for the sorts of conditions identified by the bishops (e.g., a uterus that has undergone several cesarean sections, diabetes mellitus, cardiovascular disease, kidney disease, or serious psychiatric illness) are "medically indicated" and therefore moral if a future pregnancy would constitute a health risk to the wife. In the commentary on the Vatican document, the U.S. bishops made it very clear that such an appeal could not be legitimately made:

> If the hospital cooperates because of the reason for the sterilization, e.g., because it is done for medical reasons, the cooperation can hardly be considered material. In other words, the hospital can hardly maintain under these circumstances that it does not approve sterilizations done for medical reasons, and this would make cooperation formal.[7]

Despite this clear teaching there have been representatives of Catholic health care who have tried to make the case for direct sterilization for "medical reasons." But as one obstetrician and one maternal-fetal specialist have put it, they know of no medical condition which is alleviated, cured, or ameliorated by cutting or tying the fallopian tubes. Any Catholic hospital which permits tubal ligations or vasectomies because they are supposedly medically indicated would be formally cooperating in direct sterilization and betraying the ethical mission of Catholic health care.

Despite these clear teachings of the Church, the pervasiveness of sterilizing procedures in health care institutions in the United States and the dominant social attitude with respect to contraception led the bishops to issue *another* statement on the matter on July 3, 1980. It sought to reassure Catholic health care institutions that they were legally protected in the United States from having to violate their religious and ethical mission by cooperating in contraceptive sterilizations. "Catholic health care facilities in the United States complying with the *Ethical and Religious Directives* are protected by the First Amendment from pressures intended to require material cooperation in contraceptive sterilization."[8]

"Uterine Isolation" and Further Specification of Direct and Indirect Sterilization

A surgical approach was developed in some Catholic health care institutions which claimed to be indirectly sterilizing and, therefore, permitted. It is known as uterine isolation. As seen above, it was already well-established Catholic medical moral teaching that it would be morally permissible to remedy a present pathology, even though it was anticipated that the treatment for the pathology would result in sterility. A well-known Catholic moral theologian, Rev. Gerald Kelly, S.J., argued in his 1958 book *Medico-Moral Problems* that there were cases in which a "weak uterus" could be considered to be in a pathological condition and could be removed. He wrote, "When competent physicians judge that, by reason of repeated cesareans (or some similar cause) a uterus is so badly damaged that it will very likely not function safely in another pregnancy, they may, with the consent of the patient, remove the uterus as a seriously pathological organ."[9]

Another moral theologian carried the argument further. Rev. Thomas J. O'Donnell, S.J., argued that if the pathological condition of the "weakened uterus" was such that it could legitimately be removed, then it ought to be legitimate to isolate the "weakened uterus" by cutting the fallopian tubes. This could only be done in those cases in which it would be legitimate to remove the uterus.[10] A number of Catholic hospitals and health care systems came to accept this argument and developed policies of "uterine isolation."

The Congregation for the Doctrine of the Faith was asked to assess the morality of this practice and responded in 1993. Three cases had been presented to the CDF. The first dealt with a hysterectomy for an actual, pathological uterus, that is, a uterus with "a hemorrhage which cannot be stopped by other means," the second dealt with a hysterectomy for a uterus that might not be able to carry a future pregnancy without medical risk, and the third dealt with a tubal ligation for the same reason. The CDF responded,

> In the first case, the hysterectomy is licit because it has a directly therapeutic character, even though it may be foreseen that permanent sterility will result. In fact, it is the pathological condition of the uterus ... which makes its removal medically indicated. The removal of the organ has as its aim, therefore, the curtailing of a serious present danger to the woman independent of a possible future pregnancy. ... From the moral point of view, the cases of hysterectomy and

"uterine isolation" in the circumstances described in numbers 2 and 3 are different. These fall into the moral category of direct sterilization. ... In point of fact, the uterus as described in number 2 does not constitute in and of itself any present danger to the woman. Indeed the proposal to substitute "uterine isolation" for hysterectomy under the same conditions shows precisely that the uterus in and of itself does not pose a pathological problem for the woman. Therefore, the described procedures do not have a properly therapeutic character but are aimed in themselves at rendering sterile future sexual acts freely chosen. The end of avoiding risks to the mother, deriving from a possible pregnancy, is thus pursued by means of a direct sterilization, in itself always morally illicit, while other ways, which are morally licit, remain open to free choice [e.g., complete or periodic abstinence]. The contrary opinion which considers the interventions described in numbers 2 and 3 as indirect sterilizations, licit under certain conditions, cannot be regarded as valid and may not be followed in Catholic hospitals.[11]

Even this clear teaching was misunderstood by some. It was suggested in a memorandum from a Catholic hospital association to its members that the Congregation for the Doctrine of the Faith considered the uterus described in numbers 2 and 3 as being in a pathological state which would be aggravated in the future by a pregnancy. However, the CDF clearly taught that the uterus cannot be considered pathological in its current condition such that its removal would be medically indicated, as was the situation in the first case. Also, there are studies which would call into question whether multiple cesarean sections rendered a uterus so weakened that it could be considered pathological and could be legitimately removed or "isolated."[12] The intent in such cases, however, is clearly contraceptive and therefore cannot be allowed in Catholic health care institutions.

Explanation of the Church's Teaching on the Moral Regulation of Births

If there is a grave reason for avoiding a child at a given point in a marriage, such as the mother's poor physical or emotional health or economic hardships, the Church holds that the couple may quite legitimately avoid another child. What is morally relevant is the method of birth regulation which the couple uses, not birth regulation as such. The avoidance of a child in marriage could be accomplished either through complete abstinence or by simply abstaining from marital intercourse during the wife's fertile period. This is known as natural family planning (NFP), and instruction in this method should be made available through Catholic health care services. More will be said on this later.

We often do not think of it, but there are many ways for married couples to regulate conception which have nothing to do with the practice of medicine as such. Abstaining from or engaging in marital intercourse during the wife's fertile period has nothing to do with medicine. Neither does the use of a condom to avoid a pregnancy. Obviously, the prescription of drugs or the performance of surgical sterilizations do require the involvement of health care professionals; yet in most cases of birth regulation there is no need for a health care professional to be involved. However, today, a married couple seems to consider consultation with a physician to be necessary if they are going to plan their families.

The situation has been complicated further by the fact that many would also list abortion as one means of regulating births. Yet the termination of a pregnancy was, until very recently, considered to be vastly different from the prevention of a pregnancy and would never have been considered a means of birth control. In fact, in a brochure titled *Plan Your Child for Health and Happiness*, published by Planned Parenthood in 1968, the facts were more clearly stated than is usually done today. In response to the question "Is birth control an abortion?" the Planned Parenthood brochure stated, "Definitely not. An abortion kills the life of a baby after it has begun. ... Birth control merely postpones the beginning of life." However, a generation later, Planned Parenthood had become the largest perpetrator of abortion in the country.

General Cultural Rejection of Contraception

One will still find considerable social agreement with the Catholic position on abortion, so that the exclusion of direct abortion from Catholic health care facilities usually does not engender great controversy. However, Catholic teaching on contraception leaves most in contemporary American society thoroughly perplexed. Because contraception has come to be seen as a medical matter and as part of the "full range of women's reproductive health services," it has become a matter of incredulity to many Americans that Catholic health care services will not "provide it." Catholic institutions and agencies, and the bishops who guarantee the authenticity and integrity of their health care ministry, must face this harsh cultural reality.

It is often forgotten that the moral aversion to contraception used to be far more widely felt in American society than is the case today. Many states had laws against the sale and distribution of contraceptives as late as the 1960s, and these laws had not been passed by legislatures dominated by Catholics. In many states, for example, condoms could not be sold as contraceptives but had to be sold as prophylactics, that is, devices to prevent or diminish the spread of disease. Yet, while social attitudes have changed radically in the last fifty years, the Church continues to uphold an ethic which has survived much longer.

Until relatively recently, contraception was considered more a "lifestyle" choice rather than a medical choice, much like a decision whether to have cosmetic plastic surgery. After all, condoms or IUDs or even birth control pills do not constitute medical interventions to overcome a pathology and restore health. In fact, the couples making use of them usually enjoy healthy reproductive systems; that is why the contraceptives are being used. Furthermore, these contraceptives themselves do nothing to enhance the health of the individuals using them. They may help avert a pregnancy that could possibly aggravate a pathological condition in the future, but there is no present pathology which these contraceptives are addressing, nor is a future pregnancy itself a pathology. However, as stated, contraception has now come to be so generally perceived as "health care" that we have reached the point that some state legislatures have required that any health plan which provides prescription drugs must also provide oral contraceptives. Such laws not only violate the consciences of many Catholic health care workers, they also violate notions of sound medical practice.

A brief chapter in a manual for health care ethics committees can hardly provide a major defense of the Catholic moral tradition on contraception. However, a few words on the reasons for the teaching may well be in order since ethics committees will on occasion be required to make moral assessments of cases brought before them which deal in some way with contraception.

The Role of Bishops

Before looking at some of the reasons for Catholic teaching on contraception, we should remind ourselves that the leaders of the Catholic Church, the bishops, have the responsibility to ensure the integrity of the various ministries of their church, in this case, health care ministry. This does not mean that Catholics believe that the bishops have answers for every moral difficulty that can arise. Indeed, the bishops themselves state in the general introduction to the *Ethical and Religious Directives for Catholic Health Care Services*, "The

Church cannot furnish a ready answer to every moral dilemma." However, the bishops go on to say that there are many questions about which the Church does provide "normative guidance and direction." Among the moral norms which the Church through its bishops has taught with consistency throughout its history is the one which states that direct sterilization of either the husband or the wife, whether temporary or permanent, is immoral; it is simply not appropriate human conduct. It is certainly not sound medical care, notwithstanding how it is viewed by the medical community in general and the public at large. And the bishops are certainly not presuming to be making *medical* judgments but rather moral ones.

The health care professionals associated with a Catholic facility are highly trained in their respective disciplines and deeply committed to providing the best care possible to those who come to them for help. Indeed, they are the ones who actually carry out this particular ministry of the Church under the direction of the bishops. Catholic health care facilities and those associated with them are aware of the fact that professional competency is not enough, however. There must be a concern always to be engaged in promoting the good of the human person and to avoid anything which would violate human dignity. Indeed, those are the ends toward which their professional competencies are ordered.

It goes without saying that in our pluralistic society there are different visions of what constitutes a fulfilled human life and what constitute true human goods. It is to be expected that Catholic institutions will bring their vision of the human person to the health care which is provided under their auspices and will expect those sharing in their ministry to respect their particular commitment to what constitutes human goods. The Church can hardly be viewed as trying to impose its understanding of what constitutes good health care if it has made clear what it understands such health care to be. Furthermore, health care professionals freely choose to associate themselves with this particular ministry of the Church.

Another point should be made at the beginning of this discussion with respect to the use of terminology. "Birth control" could be used to cover even methods considered morally licit by the Catholic Church, but since it refers almost exclusively to contraceptive or sterilizing procedures, the term will not be used in this chapter. Therefore, no distinction will be made between artificial and natural birth control, for example, as though there were a significant moral difference between the two. Nor will a distinction be made between artificial and natural contraception. It is contraception which is considered immoral, not whether it is done in an "artificial" or "natural" manner. "Contraception" will refer to any intervention on the part of a married couple which is directly and specifically intended to deprive the freely chosen marital act of one of its inherent, natural ends, in this case, a child.

The Natural Moral Law and Contraception

The Catholic Church believes that its ethical teachings can be *understood* by anyone even if they do not necessarily agree with them. In this particular case, it believes that its teachings on the moral regulation of births are not uniquely Catholic, any more than its teachings against theft or lying are uniquely Catholic. If one reads through the *Ethical and Religious Directives for Catholic Health Care Services,* there are very few directives which would be considered controversial in any sense. Who, for example, would find exception with directive 26 which requires the informed consent of patients before they be subjected to a treatment? "The free and informed consent of the person or the person's surrogate is required for medical treatments and procedures, except in an emergency situation when consent cannot be obtained and there is no indication that the patient would refuse consent to the treatment."

Just as the ethical correctness of such directives as number 26 appears self-evident, the Church believes that its teaching on euthanasia, contraception, and abortion should be self-evident as well. After all, even the pagan Hippocratic Oath required a physician to swear that "I will give no deadly medicine to anyone if asked, nor suggest any such counsel, and in like manner I will not give to a woman a pessary to induce an abortion."

The Catholic tradition believes that there are common, universal, societal norms against killing the innocent and lying or stealing because these are commonly seen to be actions contrary to human nature and to the good of society in which all human beings must live. This general awareness of what conduct conforms to and enhances human nature, and what is contrary to it, is known by an expression which is older than the Catholic Church itself: the natural moral law. Although opposition to contraception is now seen as a uniquely Catholic position, the fact is that until relatively recently most religious and even secular moralists found contraception to be inappropriate human behavior since it allowed men and women, even unmarried ones, to seek actions for the sake of pleasure without fully embracing the full consequences of those actions and without being open to the fundamental *social* good of marriage, the bearing and raising of future responsible citizens. For example, one reads in Sigmund Freud's *Introductory Lectures on Psycho-Analysis*, "It is a characteristic common to all the [sexual] perversions that in them reproduction as an aim is put aside. This is actually the criterion by which we judge whether a sexual activity is perverse—if it departs from reproduction in its aims and pursues the attainment of gratification independently."[13] Charles Darwin worried that contraceptive technology would "spread to unmarried women and would destroy chastity on which the family bond depends; and the weakening of this bond would be the greatest of all possible evils to mankind."[14]

The fact that social consensus has been lost on the immorality of contraception does not mean that it might not be regained, nor does it mean that if contraception is not ethical, it can be made ethical by popular opinion.

General Christian Teaching on Contraception

The Christian Church from its beginnings had considered contraception and abortion to be immoral, as had the Jewish tradition before it. In the first book of the Bible there is the famous account of *coitus interruptus* and the "spilling of the seed" by Onan, which incurred God's displeasure (Gen. 38:6–11). Barrenness was invariably seen as a great curse in the Old Testament. And one can read in the Talmud such passages as the following: "A man who does not concern himself with procreation should be considered to be shedding human blood" (Talmudic Tractae Yebamoth, fol. 63b).

From the beginnings of Christianity, the Church has taught that contraception is immoral. There are Bible scholars who argue that the Greek word *pharmakeia* in Paul's letter to the Galatians, which used to be translated as "witchcraft" or "sorcery," ought to be understood as referring to the use of sterilizing potions or "pharmaceuticals." Such a translation would actually seem to make more sense in the context: "Now the works of the flesh are obvious: immorality, impurity, licentiousness, idolatry, '*pharmakeia*,' hatreds, rivalry, jealousy, outbursts of fury, acts of selfishness, dissensions, factions, occasions of envy, drinking bouts, orgies, and the like" (Gal. 5:19–21).

St. Justin Martyr wrote in the second century: "We Christians either marry ... to have children or, if we refuse to marry, are completely continent" (*First Apology for Christians*, 29). St. Clement of Alexandria wrote in the third century, "A man who marries for the sake of begetting children must practice continence so that it is not lust he feels for his wife, whom he ought to love, so that he may beget children with a chaste and controlled

will" (*Stromata*, bk. 3, 7.58). Indeed, our popes are teaching what was already taught in the early fifth century by St. Augustine, the bishop of Hippo in North Africa, who succinctly condemned both abortion and contraception by speaking of those married couples who "sometimes go to such lengths as to procure sterilizing poisons, and if these are unavailing, in some way to stifle within the womb and eject the fetus that has been conceived. They want their offspring to die before it comes to life or, if it is already living in the womb, to perish before it is born" (*On Marriage and Concupiscence*, ch. 17). Such was the common teaching of Christians until contemporary times. Admittedly, however, it has been increasingly and even fiercely challenged in our own day.

In 1968, Pope Paul VI continued the presentation of this teaching when he issued an encyclical, or "circular letter," on the moral regulation of births, titled *Humanae vitae*. He was fully aware that he was merely reiterating what the Church had always taught, that is, "a coherent teaching concerning both the nature of marriage and the correct use of conjugal rights and duties of husband and wife."[15] However, the document engendered considerable controversy which has not yet subsided.

In *Humanae vitae*, the Pope addressed the kinds of acts which the moral person ought to avoid. To be excluded, he said, "is direct sterilization, whether perpetual or temporary, whether of the man or of the woman. Similarly to be excluded is every action which, either in anticipation of the conjugal act, or in its accomplishment, or in the development of its natural consequences, proposes, whether as an end or as a means, to render procreation impossible"[16]

Here Paul VI was reiterating what Pope Pius XI had taught in his encyclical on chaste marriage, *Casti connubii*, issued in 1930: "Any use whatsoever of matrimony exercised in such a way that the act is deliberately frustrated in its natural power to generate life is an offence against the law of God and of nature."[17] But again, what has been taught by our modern popes is what has been taught consistently by the Church throughout its history.

The Catholic Church Is Not Opposed to Birth Regulation

Despite some popular thinking, the Catholic Church has never taught that married couples, even Catholic married couples, should have as many children as they are physically capable of engendering. The Church has taught that couples should act reasonably in determining how many children they are morally, physically, emotionally, and economically capable of bearing and raising. In fact, *Humanae vitae* mentions specific factors which may morally lead a couple to decide to delay or avoid a pregnancy, such as poor health or financial difficulties.[18]

What has always been morally decisive for the Catholic Church, however, has been the manner in which couples regulate the births of their children. In the Church's estimation, some methods of birth regulation correspond to the dignity of the human person as a free and reasonable individual, and some approaches simply violate human dignity by denying the person's nature as a free moral agent. There also used to be general social consensus for this understanding of responsible sexual conduct.

Pregnancy results from actions in which a man and a woman freely choose to engage.[19] With some of the language used today, one would almost think that pregnancy is a contagious disease unwittingly contracted by a woman against her will. If a couple does not want to conceive a child, they can simply refrain from sexual intercourse. There is no inevitability to pregnancy. All the Catholic Church is saying is that a couple is able to regulate the births of their children by freely choosing to engage in, or by choosing to refrain from, conjugal intercourse. They should be able to control and direct their sexual urges and act like free, reasonable persons, fully cognizant of the consequences of their sexual activity.

It should be pointed out that we have always without hesitation sterilized pets or farm animals if we did not want them to conceive because the lower animals are driven by instinct. Human beings have the same biological urges as lower mammals; however, human beings are not driven solely by instinct and can choose their actions using their intellect and exercising their free will. They understand the nature of their biological urges and the consequences of acting on them and therefore make their choices accordingly. This indeed reflects the dignity of human beings. This is why the Catholic Church considers it beneath human dignity surgically to sterilize a man or a woman as though they were animals—or for human beings to render themselves permanently, or even temporarily, sterile using other methods.

The position of the Catholic Church would seem to be perfectly understandable, since marriage is defined as the lifelong union of one man and one woman for the establishment of a family through the engendering and raising of children. The Catholic Church has taught this clearly in the documents of its last great ecumenical council:

> For God himself is the author of marriage and has endowed it with various benefits and various ends in view: all of these have a very important bearing on the continuation of the human race, on the personal development and eternal destiny of every member of the

family, on the dignity, stability, peace, and prosperity of the family and of the whole human race. By its very nature the institution of marriage and married love is ordered to the procreation and education of offspring, and it is in them that it finds its crowning glory.[20]

If a man and woman entered into a personal relationship rejecting or denying any of those purposes of marriage, they simply would not be entering into a marital union but into some other form of union. To act against the engendering of children by the use of contraception would mean acting against the very meaning of marriage. It would be an unreasonable act. As Paul VI taught in *Humanae vitae*, "To use this divine gift [i.e., conjugal union] destroying, even if only partially, its meaning and its purpose is to contradict the nature both of man and of woman and of their most intimate relationship."[21]

But again, the Church has never taught that a couple has to have as many children as physically possible. It has taught that if a couple were to avoid having a child it must be done in a reasonable fashion. Since it is the marital act which gives rise to a new life, if a couple for grave reason should avoid having children at a given time, they simply restrain from the marital act. With our enhanced knowledge of a woman's physiology, it is now known that the couple need only restrain from the marital act for rather brief periods of time, perhaps eight days a month.

It was not until 1930 that medical science discovered that a woman ovulates (and hence is fertile) in the middle of her monthly cycle. In the years since, it has been learned how long the ova live after ovulation (thirty-six to forty-eight hours) and how long the sperm will likely live after intercourse (as many as five days). By observing signs in her body, such as the consistency of her cervical mucous, the wife can now determine the time of her fertility with remarkable accuracy, and couples can ascertain when to avoid or when to engage in conjugal intercourse depending on whether they hope to conceive a child or not. This approach is commonly known as natural family planning (NFP) and is considered to be morally licit by the Catholic Church if it is used with proper motives.[22] Natural family planning simply refers to the use of periodic abstinence to avoid pregnancy, or the planned use of fertile periods of the woman's cycle to achieve pregnancy, using the physiological criteria mentioned which facilitate the determination of the time of fertility. This is to be done with an upright and moral intention.

The same year that it was discovered that a woman was not fertile during most of her cycle, Pope Pius XI issued his encyclical on chaste marriage, *Casti connubii*, mentioned above, in which he taught that it would be morally licit if the couple restricted conjugal relations to the infertile period if they needed to avoid having a child at a particular time in their marriage. Such a conjugal act would *not* be immoral, the Pope taught, "though on account of *natural* reasons *either of time* or of certain defects, new life cannot be brought forth."[23]

If a couple chooses not to have children, then they should simply avoid marital relations at the time when the wife is fertile. This seems a very reasonable (and healthy) approach to the regulation of births. Husband and wife are looked on as free, rational beings who ascertain the time of their fertility and then simply control their actions by choosing to engage in or to forgo conjugal relations. One would think this approach would have a certain appeal in our day, since such a manner of regulating births is "natural"; it does not require the ingestion of chemicals with adverse side effects, or the use of spermicidal foams, or surgical procedures with their risks, or latex condoms which can give rise to allergic reactions and which have a significant failure rate, or diaphragms which must be fitted by a physician and assisted by spermicidal agents. The NFP approach to birth regulation means making informed choices about when to have conjugal relations and not allowing oneself to be driven by passions without regard to consequences.

There are many married Catholics who joyfully live their lives in accord with the Church's teaching on marital intimacy. However, it must be admitted, in today's culture that the Church's insistence on the immorality of contraception has frankly led to the alienation of many Catholics, the ignoring of the teaching by many other Catholics, and the derision of the Church by many who are not Catholics. Yet the bishops of the United States in their *Ethical and Religious Directives for Catholic Health Care Services* make it quite clear that Catholic institutions may not permit or promote contraceptive practices (directives 52 and 53) in Catholic health care services because (1) they ought not properly to be considered health care, and (2) they violate the dignity of persons by treating them as though they were not free moral agents able to make responsible choices about their sexual behavior.

What Procedures Are Not Permitted in Catholic Health Care Services

Abortion is not contraception and is not covered by directives 52 and 53. It is a different kind or species of act and is addressed directly or indirectly in directives 36, 39, 45 to 48, 50, 54, and 66. Abortion and contraception are both intrinsically evil, or objectively disordered, actions,

according to Catholic teaching and, as has been argued, do violence to human dignity. Direct abortion, that is, an abortion knowingly, willfully and directly chosen, is far more grave than contraception, since it is the destruction of an innocent life, whereas contraception is the prevention of the beginning of a new life, as pointed out in the 1968 Planned Parenthood brochure quoted earlier. Nonetheless, the Catholic Church still considers the direct permanent or temporary sterilization of men or women as constituting a grave violation of their moral, physical, and spiritual integrity, even when they request it. And obviously physicians have a right, indeed an obligation, not to do anything to violate a patient even when the patient requests it of them. As we have seen, in the Hippocratic Oath, the physician promises never to give a sick patient a deadly medicine even when requested.

The following example may not be useful because it may appear too outrageous, but it might help explain by analogy the aversion of many people to contraception. If an individual suffering from kleptomania came to a physician and asked to have his right hand amputated because it would make it more difficult for him to steal, the physician would of course refuse such a request. He would counsel the man simply to stop stealing or to seek psychological help in gaining control over this compulsive urge. The physician would rightly refuse to remove a perfectly healthy and functioning hand to help a man avoid a problem in the future. Likewise, there are physicians who would see it as senseless, and not at all a question of the practice of medicine, to render a person's perfectly healthy reproductive system surgically (or chemically) inoperative because the individual feared he or she would not be able to make sound choices with respect to his or her sexual activity in the future. In the absence of a current pathology being worsened by the continued production of the sexual hormones, for example, it simply is not good medicine to disable one of the body's principal physiological systems which is perfectly healthy.

Other Ways to Explain the Immorality of Contraception

There are many different ways in which the immorality of contraception might be explained. The wrongness of contraception has been explained by saying that the marital act is both "unitive" and "procreative" by its very nature. It unites husband and wife to one another and leads to the living expression of their love, a child. To act against either the unitive or the procreative meanings of the conjugal act is to deprive it of its full significance and to turn it into some act other than the marital act. To deprive it of an essential part of its meaning is to deprive it of its full meaning; it is to make the act more or less "meaning-less." It is perhaps instructive to note that contraception always involves an act other than the marriage act (such as the use of a condom, a diaphragm, a pill, a patch, a tubal ligation, a spermicidal foam), and this act has no other purpose than to prevent the procreative good (the child), which is inherent in the act, from materializing.

It could also be said that contraception is a sort of lie. The marital act of its nature is ordered to the generation of new life. This is one of the social tasks which a man and woman take on when they marry. To deny the very meaning of what they are doing in and through the marital act by depriving the act of its natural end, one of the purposes for which the act even exists, is to turn the act into a kind of a lie. However, no lie is involved if the couple avoids the marital act when there is a serious reason why they should not have a child at a given time, or if they engage in the marital act at a time when the woman cannot conceive in any event. The act is naturally, quite apart from the will of the couple, infertile at that time.

Kinds of Contraception

There are new methods of contraception being developed all the time, and so it would be pointless to try to list them all. However, they can be categorized. There are hormonal or *chemical contraceptives,* such as the "birth control pill" and oral contraceptives as well as implants (like Norplant) and patches which release the effective sterilizing agents over an extended period of time. Others are *barrier methods*, such as condoms and diaphragms, which usually also require a spermicidal or chemical agent to enhance their effectiveness. And finally there are *surgical interventions,* such as tubal ligations, vasectomies, and even hysterectomies. If any of these is used specifically and directly for the purpose of rendering a person temporarily or permanently sterile, it is considered immoral and is not permitted in a Catholic health care facility or service.

It is clearly conceivable that an individual could take a medication for an illness which would secondarily or indirectly render him or her sterile, and it is possible that the individual could undergo surgery for a pathology which would have the same indirect effect. This could be considered moral according to Catholic teaching and could be allowed in a Catholic health care institution (see chapter 3D): "Procedures that induce sterility are permitted when their direct effect is the cure or alleviation of a present and serious pathology and a simpler treatment is not available."[24]

The Individual Physician, Institutional Witness, and Contraception

There are, of course, Catholic physicians and physicians of other faiths who will not prescribe contraceptives or surgically sterilize patients. They give witness to their consciences, to their concern for the good of the patient, and to their professional competencies. However, the social reality today is such that most physicians in practice in the United States write prescriptions for contraceptives, fit for diaphragms, dispense condoms, and perform tubal ligations and vasectomies. Many of these physicians are Catholics perpetrating these acts on other Catholics. It must be admitted that there have been theologians and priests who have not faithfully taught or represented the Church's teaching on this matter, so it may well be that these individual Catholics are confused about what the Church actually teaches and what is morally required of them. If they know what the Church teaches and if they profess to be practicing Catholics, then they clearly should not engage in these activities. If they are confused, they have an obligation to learn what the Church actually teaches. Whether they perform their professional work in accord with the moral teachings of the Church is a matter between them, God, and their confessor or spiritual director.

However, because individual Catholic physicians normally do not practice medicine as a public Catholic ministry, they are not held to the same kind of standards as institutions or health care services which identify themselves as Catholic. These institutions are publicly identified as carrying out the healing ministry or apostolate of the Catholic Church and must take particular care to see that their ministry is indeed consonant with Catholic teaching.

Catholic institutions must be held to higher standards of conduct than an individual Catholic physician because they constantly make public witness to the Catholic Faith. Individual physicians do not act in a public, official capacity *as Catholics*. Indeed, their patients may not even know that they are Catholic. Catholic hospitals, medical centers, and clinics, on the other hand, make a public witness to the Faith and carry out their work specifically as an expression of the Church's public ministry. Consequently, the local bishop cannot allow a hospital which ministers in the name of the Church, which is actually in the name of Jesus Christ, to do anything that would violate the dignity of the human person. The bishop, who Catholics believe has been charged by God with protecting and preserving the moral teachings and practices of the Church, must make certain that people are not led into confusion about what is morally right or wrong by what a given Catholic health care institution may do or allow.

Quite apart from Catholic physicians who do not live in accord with the teachings of their religion, there are, of course, many physicians associated with Catholic health care services who are not Catholic and who do not accept Catholic moral teaching. This creates tension between the Catholic institution and those who are not Catholic but who work there or perhaps receive care there. Non-Catholic physicians in Catholic health care institutions must be respectful of Catholic teaching in this regard and should not involve the Catholic institution in the promotion of contraception if they prescribe or recommend it in their own practices. Physicians associated with a Catholic health care institution should respect the consciences of the Catholics with whom they work as well as the conscience of the Catholic institution by not involving them in any way in contraception.

A Catholic hospital or other facility which grants privileges to a physician does not of course take over or control that physician's practice. The physician establishes a professional relationship with a patient and works with the patient in providing care and treatment in conformity with the wishes of the patient, so long as the physician does not consider the patient's wishes to be bad medicine or contrary to his moral beliefs. As stated in the introduction to Part 3 of the *Ethical and Religious Directives for Catholic Health Care Services*, "When the health care professional and the patient use institutional Catholic health care, they also accept its public commitment to the Church's understanding of and witness to the dignity of the human person." This can lead to very complicated situations, since the Catholic health care institution would hold that contraception violates the dignity of the human person, whereas the physician who has privileges at a Catholic hospital and the patient who comes to the physician simply may not share that view.

However, under no circumstances should a physician associated with a Catholic facility do anything which would implicate it in the practice of contraception. Consequently, prescriptions for contraceptives should not be written on prescription pads of the hospital, nor can the physicians expect prescriptions for contraception to be filled at the pharmacy of the Catholic institution. Furthermore, it would be preferable if such practices did not take place in the medical arts or professional building of a Catholic hospital. However, arrangements are sometimes made so that the medical arts building does not belong to the Catholic institution and is independent of it, even though it might be close or even contiguous to the Catholic institution. Also, although not ideal, allowances are made for physicians renting space in a medical arts building owned by a Catholic institution to dispense contraceptives in their private practice, using their own prescription pads and making clear that the promotion or distribution of contraception is contrary to the Catholic institution itself. Following this chapter are guidelines which might be useful in helping physicians who regrettably are unable to see or understand the moral law on this matter and yet nonetheless rent space in a Catholic facility. This tolerance and level of cooperation cannot be extended to any procedure, device, or medication which is promoted as contraceptive but which is in reality abortifacient.

Contraception and Collaboration between Catholic and Non-Catholic Institutions

The teaching on contraception has admittedly led to great difficulties in collaborative ventures between Catholic and non-Catholic health care institutions. Bishops sometimes have to reject proposed collaborative arrangements because of this issue. If the Catholic institution has not worked closely with the bishop and has not received his permission for a collaborative venture, his rejection of it can lead to considerable public embarrassment and sometimes considerable financial loss for the parties involved. The ethical question of cooperation is covered in this volume; I merely point out here that it is often the question of contraception which leads to difficulties between collaborating Catholic and non-Catholic institutions.

It must be said that the moral dilemmas between cooperating Catholic and non-Catholic institutions arise almost exclusively today in terms of contraceptive tubal ligations, since the facilities and surgical license of a hospital or ambulatory surgical center are needed for that procedure. Even though the Church considers vasectomies to be as immoral as tubal ligations, vasectomies seldom come into conflict with the policy of a Catholic hospital since they can be done on an outpatient basis in a physician's office. Similarly, the prescribing of oral contraceptives and diaphragms seldom causes problems because it is done in a physician's office and under the physician's auspices, not those of the Catholic medical center or hospital. It is undoubtedly true that most obstetrician-gynecologists who have privileges at Catholic institutions are prescribing contraceptives. As deplorable as that may be, it is not the Catholic institutions themselves that are sponsoring, promoting, or prescribing it.

If a physician's practice is owned and managed by a Catholic institution, the administrators must take steps to ensure that contraception and abortion are not promoted or provided in the practice. Physicians who have privileges at a Catholic hospital might do such things in their private practices, but they should never be seen as doing them under the auspices of the Catholic institution.

The administrators in Catholic institutions should do their utmost to see that all physicians who have privileges understand the Church's position in this matter, and should make it clear that the institution itself will never be involved in or promote contraception or abortion. And if the institution provides services touching on human procreation, administrators should positively take steps to see that natural family planning is taught and promoted under the auspices of the hospital or Catholic health care services.

When it comes to collaborative ventures with other hospitals and medical centers, the Catholic institutions should not be involved in any way in these activities and should find contractual means to avoid involvement. Catholic institutions should consider involvement with medical centers engaged in these violations of human dignity only if such involvement is seen to be necessary to achieve some other important good and to avoid other, more grave evils. In such cases, the principle of cooperation should be seen as allowing but limiting the involvement with such other entities. Catholic institutions should avoid being party to legal documents which have the effect of ensuring that these immoral practices continue after the institutional collaboration has been established.

In Summary

• Catholic hospitals may not promote or permit on their premises contraceptive sterilizations, whether temporary or permanent.

• Catholic hospitals may mediately materially cooperate with other health care institutions which engage in such activity for a grave reason and with the permission of the local bishop. (See Chapter 25, on cooperation, for the meaning of the terminology.)

• Catholic hospitals may permit procedures aimed at correcting a present pathology which may indirectly render the patient infertile if there is no other procedure reasonably available. For example, a male cancer patient may undergo radiation treatment which may render him sterile, or a female cancer patient could have a diseased uterus removed, thus rendering her infertile. Indeed, healthy testes in a male may be removed if their secretion of hormones accelerates or aggravates the growth of a cancer.

• Catholic hospitals and pharmacies may not promote or provide for contraceptive practices, nor may their personnel be engaged in such activities in the Catholic-owned facilities. Physicians who rent space in a medical arts or professional building owned by a Catholic entity may provide contraceptives, but only in their capacities as private physicians, never as members of a Catholic-owned practice, while at the same time making it clear that such practices are contrary to the beliefs of the Catholic Church and are being provided in a private capacity. The guidelines on pages 91 to 93 may help clarify this point.

Notes

[1] U. S. Conference of Catholic Bishops, *Ethical and Religious Directives for Catholic Health Care Services*, 4th ed. (Washington, D.C.: USCCB, 2001).

[2] Congregation for the Doctrine of the Faith (CDF), *Quaecumque sterilizatio* (March 13, 1975), n. 1.

[3] Ibid., n. 3a.

[4] National Conference of Catholic Bishops (NCCB), *Commentary on the Reply of the Sacred Congregation for the Doctrine of the Faith on Sterilization in Catholic Hospitals*, September 15, 1977 (Washington D.C.: United States Catholic Conference, 1983).

[5] See Lawrence J. Welch, "An Excessive Claim: Sterilization and Immediate Material Cooperation," *Linacre Quarterly* 66.4 (November 1999): 4–25.

[6] NCCB, *Commentary*.

[7] Ibid.

[8] NCCB, *Statement on Tubal Ligation* (Washington, D.C.: United States Catholic Conference, 1980.)

[9] Gerald Kelly, *Medico-Moral Problems* (St. Louis, MO: Catholic Hospital Association of the United States and Canada, 1958), 214.

[10] Thomas J. O'Donnell, *Medicine and Christian Morality*, 2nd ed. (New York: Alba House, 1991), 138–144.

[11] CDF, *Responses to Questions Proposed concerning "Uterine Isolation" and Related Matters* (July 31, 1993), q. 3, explanation.

[12] See R. M. Farmer et al., "Uterine Rupture during Trial of Labor after Previous Cesarean Section," *American Journal of Obstetrics and Gynecology* 165.4 (October 1991): 996–1001; A. S. Leung, E. K. Leung, and R. H. Paul, "Uterine Rupture after Previous Cesarean Delivery: Maternal and Fetal Consequences," *American Journal of Obstetrics and Gynecology* 169.4 (October 1993): 945–950; and T. M. Goodwin, "'Medicalizing' Moral Decisions in Reproductive Medicine," in *Faith and Challenges to the Family*, ed. Russell E. Smith (Braintree, MA: Pope John Center, 1994), 79–99.

[13] Sigmund Freud, *A General Introduction to Psycho-*

Analysis, trans. Joan Riviere (New York: Liverwright, 1935), 277.

[14] Charles Darwin, letter to Charles Bradlaugh, June 6, 1877, in Janet Browne, *Charles Darwin: The Power of Place* (New York: Alfred A. Knopf, 2002), 468.

[15] Paul VI, *Humanae vitae* (July 25, 1968), n. 4.

[16] Ibid., n. 14.

[17] Pius XI, *Casti connubii* (December 31, 1930), n. 56.

[18] *Humanae vitae,* nn. 10 and 16.

[19] We are here excluding from consideration those very rare instances in which conception may occur from rape.

[20] Vatican Council II, *Gaudium et spes* (December 7, 1965), n. 48.

[21] *Humanae vitae,* n. 13.

[22] See Benedict Guevin, "A Theological Caution on NFP," *Ethics & Medics* 25.9 (September 2000): 2–4.

[23] Pius XI, *Casti connubii,* n. 59 (emphasis added).

[24] USCCB, *Ethical and Religious Directives,* n. 53.

Editorial Summation: The moral regulation of births is one of the most controversial issues in contemporary American society. In a *medical* sense, contraceptive sterilization includes any medical, surgical, or other intervention which would render the act of sexual intercourse temporarily or permanently sterile. In a *moral* sense, it is direct sterilization if the purpose of the intervention is to render the person sterile or infertile for whatever reason. If, however, the procedure is directed at some present pathology, and the ensuing sterility is foreseen but not intended, it is considered to be indirect sterilization. If there is no other suitable conservative means and there is a proportionate reason for the surgical intervention, indirect sterilization may be considered morally licit. This is the Catholic Church's teaching. The Vatican is the central teaching agency of the Church and has issued a number of authoritative documents on the topic of contraceptive sterilization. "Uterine isolation" was suggested and promoted by some as means of pregnancy prevention in the presence of a concern for a future pathology, but the Vatican ruled that this was not morally acceptable because in such cases there is no present danger. The bases for this teaching on the regulation of births are to be found in the Sacred Scriptures, the Church's moral tradition, and the natural law. The Church is not opposed to the regulation of births. As Pope Paul VI's encyclical *Humanae vitae* recognized, there are times when a couple could seek to avoid the conception of another child. However, the means employed to achieve this end are morally important. An acceptable means, granted that there are proportionate reasons for limiting conception, is natural family planning. This procedure utilizes the natural fertility/infertility cycle of the wife and limits conjugal intercourse to those times when the wife is naturally infertile. Catholic health care facilities may not engage in those contraceptive and birth-regulating procedures which are judged to be morally unacceptable, including and especially abortion. A particularly vexing issue is that of collaboration with non-Catholic institutions which perform direct sterilizations.

Model Clinical Practice Ethics Guidelines for Affiliated Health Care Professionals with Respect to Prescription of Contraceptives

The health care professionals affiliated with [Name of Hospital] are critical to its mission. The mission of [Name of Hospital] is to provide, within the Catholic vision of health care, health, healing, and hope to all. [Name of Hospital] and its sponsor, the [Name of Sponsor], fully appreciate the fact that the health care professionals affiliated with [Name of Hospital] are highly competent experts in their respective health care specialties. The health care professionals of [Name of Hospital] seek to provide dedicated, quality health care to those whom they serve.

[Name of Hospital], the [Name of Sponsor], and the health care professionals affiliated with [Name of Hospital] all recognize that the provision of health care is as much about serving the human good and dignity of the patient as it is about exercising professional competency and expertise. In fact, everything that is done in the name of good medicine is done because it is regarded by the health care provider as ultimately comporting with the human dignity of the patient. No one would provide health care if it were known to be contrary to the human good of the patient.

The Catholic identity of [Name of Hospital] is founded upon a vision of the human good and dignity of the person. This vision permeates all that [Name of Hospital] does and is the ultimate measure by which [Name of Hospital] provides health care. Consistent with a health care provider's vision of human dignity, certain procedures and activities will be either allowed or disallowed. Therefore, the particular configuration of health care provided by [Name of Hospital] does not represent an interference by the Catholic Church in the practice of medicine. Rather, it represents the provision of health care consistent with a vision of human dignity that can be different from other views in some respects.

The *Ethical and Religious Directives for Catholic Health Care Services* (ERDs) represents the model of Catholic health care to which [Name of Hospital] adheres. All services provided by [Name of Hospital] and its subsidiaries must comply with the ERDs. The ERDs are promulgated by the bishop of [Name of Diocese] in fulfillment of his responsibility for the Catholic identity of Catholic health care organizations and services in the diocese.

Given the obligations of [Name of Hospital] and the [Name of Sponsor] to preserve the Catholic identity of [Name of Hospital], and to ensure that [Name of Hospital] acts according to its vision of the human dignity of the patients it serves, the guidelines below are established for physicians, nurse practitioners, and physician assistants affiliated with [Name of Hospital] who prescribe contraceptives.

1   Owned Physician and Independent Nurse-Practitioner Practices

1.1   Any physicians or independent nurse practitioners whose practices are owned by [Name of Hospital] and who do not have a limited private-practice capacity may not prescribe contraceptives.

—continued—

These guidelines were developed by the NCBC ethicists and are recommended by the NCBC for use by Catholic health care organizations and dioceses.

1.2   Any physicians or independent nurse practitioners whose practices are owned by [Name of Hospital] and who prescribe contraceptives do so in a limited private-practice capacity contrary to any intention on the part of [Name of Hospital] or the [Name of Sponsor].

1.3   No prescription pad printed with the names of [Name of Hospital], any of its subsidiaries, or any associated logos may be used for the prescription of a contraceptive.

1.4   Any physician, nurse-practitioner, or physician-assistant salary paid by [Name of Hospital] does not cover work associated with the prescription of contraceptives by the health care professional in his or her limited private-practice capacity.

1.5   [Name of Hospital] will not process bills or collect revenue for work exclusively identified with the prescription of contraceptives by a physician, nurse practitioner, or physician assistant in his or her limited private-practice capacity.

1.6   [Name of Hospital] will not provide liability insurance for work associated with the prescription of contraceptives by the physician, nurse practitioner, or physician assistant in his or her limited private-practice capacity. The health care professional will need to supply his or her own supplemental liability insurance for such work.

1.7   All activities associated with the prescription of contraceptives can only be performed by the physician, nurse practitioner, or physician assistant, who must make it clear to patients and office staff that he or she is providing the prescription in a limited private-practice capacity.

1.8   Any physician, nurse practitioner, or physician assistant offering obstetrical or gynecological services must provide natural family planning literature and be able to make referrals for NFP instruction.

1.9   Signage must be provided which explains that prescriptions for contraceptives are provided by the health care professional in his or her limited private-practice capacity.

1.10   Physicians, nurse practitioners, and physician assistants cannot provide or prescribe any medication or device which acts primarily as an abortifacient.

1.11   Physicians, nurse practitioners, and physician assistants cannot provide counseling or referrals for abortion.

2   Physician and Independent Nurse-Practitioner Tenants

2.1   Any physician or independent nurse-practitioner tenants who prescribe contraceptives on the premises of [Name of Hospital] or its subsidiaries do so in a limited private-practice capacity contrary to any intention on the part of [Name of Hospital] or the [Name of Sponsor].

2.2   No prescription pad printed with the names of [Name of Hospital], any of its subsidiaries, or any associated logos may be used for the prescription of a contraceptive.

2.3   [Name of Hospital] will not process bills or collect revenue for work exclusively identified with the prescription of contraceptives by a physician, nurse practitioner, or physician assistant in his or her limited private-practice capacity.

2.4 [Name of Hospital] will not provide liability insurance for work associated with the prescription of contraceptives by the physician, nurse practitioner, or physician assistant in his or her limited private-practice capacity. The health care professional will need to supply his or her own supplemental liability insurance for such work.

2.5 Any physician, nurse practitioner, or physician assistant offering obstetrical or gynecological services must provide natural family planning literature and be able to make referrals for NFP instruction.

2.6 Signage must be provided which explains that prescriptions for contraceptives are provided by the health care professional in his or her limited private-practice capacity.

2.7 Physicians, nurse practitioners, and physician assistants cannot provide or prescribe on [Name of Hospital] premises any medication or device which acts primarily as an abortifacient.

2.8 Physicians, nurse practitioners, and physician assistants cannot provide on [Name of Hospital] premises counseling or referrals for abortion.

3   Physicians with Privileges

3.1 The use of medical or surgical privileges at [Name of Hospital] or any of its subsidiaries must comply with the ERDs.

3.2 No physician will receive privileges at [Name of Hospital] or any of its subsidiaries, or be leased space by [Name of Hospital] or any of its subsidiaries, if that physician performs abortion or prescribes abortifacient medications as defined in the *ERDs*.

CHAPTER 8

Reproductive Technologies

Peter J. Cataldo

The *Merck Manual of Diagnosis and Therapy* reports that up to 10 percent of couples in the United States experience infertility.[1] One in six couples are estimated to be infertile worldwide.[2] Infertility is usually regarded as the inability to conceive after at least one year of unimpeded sexual intercourse. There can be many causes of infertility, ranging from low sperm count and blocked fallopian tubes to causes which are not demonstrable. It is important that a Catholic health care ethics committee which is considering a case or issue regarding reproductive technologies grasps the basic moral principles and criteria that should be used in the evaluation process. This chapter will focus on a review of these principles and criteria in order to provide ethics committee members with a starting point from which to make a moral evaluation of the many reproductive technologies that exist and continue to be introduced. Some of the major technologies are examined as examples of how Catholic teaching may be applied.

Fundamental Principles

Chapter 1 of this manual shows how human life is a gift from God, who has sole dominion over his creation. Human life is therefore entrusted to each person, who is called to act as a steward of the gift and not treat the gift of life as an object of manipulation. Simply because we are free to use available technology to overcome infertility does not mean that we ought to do so, or that there is a moral right to do so.[3] This gift must not be abused or destroyed, precisely because it is a gift. Some have argued that if life were truly a gift from God, He would not retain a claim over the gift and that the recipients of the gift should be able to do what they wish with it. Thus, it is concluded that if it is wrong to destroy human life—for example, in the case of suicide—it is not because life is a gift.

To answer this objection it is important to understand the way in which the term "gift" is used in Catholic teaching on the subject of the gift of life. There are several qualities of human life that are inextricably bound up with the fact that life is a gift from God: (1) God shares something of himself in giving life to man, (2) God is the Lord of life, (3) life is sacred and inviolable, (4) the gift of life is a commandment, and (5) life is not a mere object of manipulation.

How each of these qualities is related to life as a gift is masterfully articulated in the teaching of *Evangelium vitae*, by Pope John Paul II. As to the first quality, the Pope explains that the gift of life should be understood as an act of sharing on the part of God. God's gift of life to man is at once also an act of sharing, not an act of surrender. Moreover, it is a sharing of something that the recipient completely lacks apart from God, and upon which the creature utterly depends. God creates man from nothing and in doing so gives man being and life. Because God is the cause of man's being, man shares in God's being analogously. In other words, man exists and has being because of God but does not exist in the same way that God exists. "The life which God offers to man," John Paul II states, "is a gift by which God shares something of himself with his creature."[4] "Man's life comes from God; it is his gift, his image and imprint, a sharing in his breath of life."[5]

Second, because the gift of life results from God sharing with his creature, God does not relinquish control over the gift. The Pope states that "God therefore is the sole Lord of this life: man cannot do with it as he wills."[6]

Life "does not belong to [man], because it is the property and gift of God the Creator and Father."[7]

Third, human life is also both sacred and inviolable because the gift of life is a sharing in God's image and likeness:

> Human life is sacred because from its beginning it involves "the creative action of God," and it remains forever in a special relationship with the Creator, who is its sole end. God alone is the Lord of life from its beginning until its end. ... God proclaims that He is absolute Lord of the life of man, who is formed in his image and likeness (cf. Gen. 1:26–28). Human life is thus given a sacred and inviolable character, which reflects the inviolability of the Creator himself.[8]

Fourth, the gift of life is entrusted to man—it is an obligation of stewardship. The gift of life comes with demands that are ultimately for the good of the receiver. Life is not simply a gift of a specific sort, but it is also an obligation that bears upon our moral agency. As John Paul II explains,

> The *Gospel of life* is both a great gift of God and an exacting task for humanity. It gives rise to amazement and gratitude in the person graced with freedom, and it asks to be welcomed, preserved, and esteemed, with a deep sense of responsibility. In giving life to man, God *demands* that he love, respect, and promote life. *The gift* thus *becomes a commandment, and the commandment is itself a gift.*[9]

The gift of life in the sense described by the Pope can be regarded as an embodied obligation; that is, our obligations toward life are an inherent part of life itself. The other side of the coin is that the responsibilities inherent in the gift of life in turn allow for human flourishing.

Fifth, because life is something shared from God and is entrusted to man as an obligation, life ought not be subject to the domination of man and become an object of manipulation. Rather, man's responsibility inherent to the gift is to respect the specific nature of the gift of life: "Life is indelibly marked by *a truth of its own*. By accepting God's gift, man is obliged to *maintain life in this truth* which is essential to it."[10] If life is not regarded as God's shared gift that has a nature containing specific ends which constitute human good, then, as John Paul II points out, "life itself becomes a mere 'thing,' which man claims as his exclusive property, completely subject to his control and manipulation."[11]

The second through fifth qualities of the gift of life follow from the first, namely, that man analogously shares in God's being. Given what these qualities are, it

is entirely correct to hold that life may not be treated as an object of manipulation either at its beginning or end precisely because life is a gift. Simply having life as a gift does not by that mere fact allow the recipient to use the gift in any way whatsoever. To use the gift of life properly is to respect its God-given nature.

Chapter 1 also explains that the human person is not simply and only a physical body with physical functions, but is a composite unity of body and soul. Thus, bodily functions, though in themselves physical (including reproductive functions), take on a spiritual and moral significance because they are ordered toward purposes and ends other than simply their physical function.[12] Physical functions are each an integral part of a whole who is the unified person—both body and soul. Therefore, as stewards of this body–soul unity, we have an obligation to respect the moral ends of the reproductive powers which God has inscribed in the very natures of man and of woman.

Because the procreative aspect of the reproductive powers is ordered toward a complete unity between the man and the woman, the procreation of children should only take place within marriage, and must respect the inseparability between the procreative and unitive meanings of the conjugal act in marriage (see chapter 8). Vatican II addressed this critical point:

> By their very nature, the institution of matrimony itself and conjugal love are ordained for the procreation and education of children, and find in them their ultimate crown. Thus a man and a woman, who by their compact of conjugal love "are no longer two, but one flesh" (Matt. 19:6), render mutual help and service to each other through an intimate union of their persons and of their actions. Through this union they experience the meaning of their oneness and attain to it with growing perfection day by day. As a mutual gift of two persons, this intimate union and the good of the children impose total fidelity on the spouses and argue for an unbreakable oneness between them.[13]

The *procreative meaning* of the conjugal act is fulfilled in and through the unitive meaning insofar as the complete, reciprocal gift of the spouses to each other necessarily includes the mutual gift of their procreative capacity; and the *unitive meaning* of the conjugal act is fulfilled in and through the procreative meaning insofar as the conjoining of the spouses' generative powers makes for a complete interpersonal union.

Given the inseparability of the procreative and unitive meanings of the conjugal act, any technology that separates the two meanings from each other corrupts both. The actions of the spouses who engender a child in this way are neither procreative nor unitive. They are not truly procreative because the child has been engendered apart from the conjugal act of husband and wife; and their actions are not truly unitive because they have acted independent of each other in the engendering of the child. The procreative meaning of the conjugal act cannot be reduced to fertilization because this meaning encompasses all aspects of the procreative capacity. The unitive meaning cannot be reduced to the contribution of gametes because this meaning of the conjugal act is inclusive of a full and complete interpersonal union.

Ethical Criteria for Evaluating Reproductive Technologies

Catholic teaching on marriage and conjugal love is brought to bear on the issue of reproductive technologies precisely at the point concerning the role of the conjugal act in these technologies. Reproductive technologies must respect two essential goods: (1) the conjugal love between spouses expressed in and through specific conjugal acts, and (2) the dignity of the child, which requires that he or she be the fruit of the conjugal union between mother and father. This teaching results in a critical distinction for determining the moral acceptability of reproductive technologies: it is the distinction between procedures which "*assist* the conjugal act either in order to facilitate its performance or in order to enable it to achieve its objective once it has been normally performed" and those that *substitute for or replace* the act.[14] Those procedures that assist or facilitate the conjugal act in the ways mentioned can be morally permissible; those that replace the conjugal act are not. This distinction will be called the moral norm of *Donum vitae*. A number of technologies will be evaluated below in the light of this distinction.

It is commonly but erroneously assumed that marriage gives the spouses a right to a child. It is thought that the spouses' love for each other and for children gives them sufficient warrant to have a child by whatever means available. However, marriage only enables the spouses to engage in those conjugal acts which may lead to procreation of new life, which is a moral option quite different from a right to another human being. *Donum vitae* makes this very important distinction:

> On the part of the spouses, the desire for a child is natural: it expresses the vocation to fatherhood and motherhood inscribed in conjugal love. This desire can be even stronger if the couple is affected by sterility which appears incurable. Nevertheless, marriage does not confer upon the spouses the right to have a child, but only the right to perform those natural acts which

are *per se* ordered to procreation. A true and proper right to a child would be contrary to the child's dignity and nature. The child is not an object to which one has a right, nor can he be considered as an object of ownership: rather, a child is a gift, "the supreme gift" and the most gratuitous gift of marriage, and is a living testimony of the mutual giving of his parents. For this reason, the child has the right, as already mentioned, to be the fruit of the specific act of the conjugal love of his parents; and he also has the right to be respected as a person from the moment of his conception.[15]

Donum vitae also teaches against "surrogate" motherhood. According to *Donum vitae*, a "surrogate mother" is a woman who carries an embryo obtained through the union of sperm and egg from two separate donors, or a woman who carries an embryo obtained by the insemination of her own ovum by the sperm of a man other than her husband. In both cases the surrogate pledges to surrender the baby to the party who contracted the agreement. Surrogate motherhood is morally illicit for two primary reasons, as *Donum vitae* states: "it is contrary to the unity of marriage and to the dignity of the procreation of the human person."[16]

Ethical Assessment of Specific Reproductive Technologies

In Vitro Fertilization (IVF)

IVF is known as an assisted reproductive technology (ART). ART is defined by the Centers for Disease Prevention and Control as "all treatments or procedures that involve surgically removing eggs from a woman's ovaries and combining the eggs with sperm to help a woman become pregnant."[17] An ART cycle encompasses actions from ovarian hyperstimulation to the transfer of human embryos. IVF usually begins with ovarian hyperstimulation in order to generate multiple mature eggs or oocytes. The oocytes are then "retrieved by direct needle puncture of the follicle, usually transvaginally with ultrasound guidance or less commonly with laparoscopy."[18] Sperm is collected by masturbation, then "washed" (a process to collect the most motile sperm) and used to fertilize the oocytes in vitro. The resulting embryos are then cultured for about forty hours, at which time two to five embryos can be transferred into the uterine cavity depending on the prognosis.[19] A process known as "assisted hatching" is sometimes used prior to embryo transfer to dissolve a portion of the zona pellucida surrounding the embryo in an attempt to assist implantation of the embryo. To reduce the risk of multi-fetal pregnancy, some countries by law restrict to three the maximum number of embryos transferred. Currently, the United States does not have legal restrictions. ART cycles of IVF and other techniques may use non-donor eggs and sperm, or embryos that are either "fresh" (nonfrozen), or previously frozen and then thawed for the procedure. Success rates for IVF and other reproductive technologies vary depending on the different ART cycle segments measured and on the country from which data are taken. For example, in 2003, the rate for newborn deliveries per transfer of embryos after IVF ranged from 7.5 percent to 31.6 percent among twenty-eight European countries,[20] and in the United States the rate for live births per retrieval of eggs was 32.9 percent in 2004.[21] *Donum vitae* teaches the following about IVF:

> Homologous IVF [between married spouses using non-donor eggs and sperm] and ET [embryo transfer] ... is brought about outside the bodies of the couple through actions of third parties whose competence and technical activity determine the success of the procedure. Such fertilization entrusts the life and identity of the embryo into the power of doctors and biologists and establishes the domination of technology over the origin and destiny of the human person. Such a relationship of domination is in itself contrary to the dignity and equality that must be common to parents and children. Conception in vitro is the result of the technical action which presides over fertilization.[22]

In vitro fertilization actually replaces the conjugal act between wife and husband and therefore is contrary to the moral norm of *Donum vitae* for morally acceptable technologies. This is true whether or not the semen is collected in a morally acceptable manner. The same moral evaluation holds true for any other procedure that is associated with or relies upon IVF (see below).

There are a number of other immoral aspects of IVF. The domination of technology over the human embryo in IVF entails its destruction and exposes the embryo to death. These factors are also present in other procedures that rely upon IVF. The Church considers such acts morally equivalent to induced abortion and condemns them in the same manner.[23] In vitro fertilization often involves the donation of gametes (reproductive cells) from a donor other than the spouses. This is contrary to the unity of marriage (as would be any other reproductive technology in which gametes from someone other than the spouses are used). The bond of marriage requires that the use of the spouses' procreative powers to engender human life be exclusively reserved for each other so that they become a mother and a father only through each other. Moreover, given the procreative purpose of the conjugal act, the Church also teaches that it is a natural right of

each person to have life as a result of a conjugal act of the spouses in cooperation with God.[24] This right is an integral component of the human dignity of the child.

Zygote Intrafallopian Tube Transfer

The zygote intrafallopian tube transfer (ZIFT) procedure retrieves and fertilizes oocytes in vitro in the same way as IVF. Then, within twenty-four hours after fertilization, the single-cell zygote is transferred into the fallopian tube by laparoscope. In 2004, the success rate in the United States for live births per retrieval of eggs using ZIFT was 30 percent, but the procedure represented only 0.3 percent of the total ART procedures performed.[25]

Intrauterine Insemination

In intrauterine insemination (IUI), sperm is directly transferred into the uterine cavity. Sperm is deposited "in the uterine cavity by means of a catheter that has been passed through the cervical canal. In this way, an increased number of sperm cells can be brought instantaneously to the proximity of the fertilization site, while the cervical barrier has been bypassed."[26] The procedure is also performed intravaginally, intracervically, or pericervically. A recent study has shown that controlled ovarian stimulation in IUI cycles using GnRH antagonists resulted in a pregnancy rate of 53.8 percent.[27]

Intracytoplasmic Sperm Injection

Intracytoplasmic sperm injection (ICSI) is a microsurgical procedure in which sperm is collected, treated, and directly injected into oocytes by means of a microinjection needle. After fertilization occurs in vitro, embryos are cultured and transferred into the uterus. ICSI is used after other methods have failed or are unlikely to succeed or to bypass severe sperm disorders.[28] IVF in combination with ICSI represented 57.5 percent of ART procedures in the United States in 2004. The overall rate of live births per retrieval of eggs using IVF with ICSI was 30.9 percent, and for women under thirty-five the rate was 41 percent.[29] Related procedures to alleviate anomalies of human gamete interaction are known as partial zona dissection (PZD) and subzonal sperm insertion (SZI).[30]

Gamete Intrafallopian Transfer

In gamete intrafallopian transfer (GIFT), oocytes are retrieved in the same manner as in IVF. The sperm are washed and transferred together with the oocytes by laparoscopy into the distal fallopian tubes (point nearest the ovaries) for fertilization to take place. In 2004, GIFT made up only 0.1 percent of the total ART procedures performed in the United States. The success rate for live births per retrieval of eggs was 23.3 percent.[31] This procedure may be morally permissible under certain conditions (see below).

Infertility Drugs

The treatment of infertility using ovarian stimulation with timed intercourse (or with IUI) can meet the norm of *Donum vitae* for moral acceptability if the stimulation is controlled and mild, and if all other steps are taken for avoiding the risk of multi-fetal pregnancy.[32] The stimulation protocol cannot be used in conjunction with IVF, and abortion cannot be an option in the event of a multi-fetal pregnancy. Moreover, the couple must be able and willing to accept a possible multi-fetal pregnancy.

Natural Procreative (NaPro) Technology

This technology includes a method for directly treating infertility due to female factors as well as a natural family planning method. NaProTechnology was developed by Thomas Hilgers, M.D., director of the Pope Paul VI Institute for the Study of Human Reproduction and director of the Institute's National Center for the Treatment of Reproductive Disorders. Dr. Hilgers has described NaProTechnology as "the use of one's medical, surgical, and allied-health energies in a way that is cooperative with the natural procreative systems."[33] There are two premises on which the use of NaProTechnology for the treatment of infertility is based and because of which this method is distinguished from most other approaches to infertility. The first premise is that "infertility is only a symptom of underlying organic and hormonal dysfunction or diseases," and the second is that success in the treatment of infertile couples can be found by treating the underlying disease process. By treating the underlying disease causing female subfertility, NaProTechnology does not directly affect the conjugal act and is therefore consistent with the moral norm of *Donum vitae.*

Conditional GIFT and IUI

Some Catholic moral theologians and ethicists have argued that the GIFT procedure might have the potential to satisfy Church teaching, but only if it is performed under certain conditions.[33] Conditions that must be fulfilled in order for GIFT to be morally acceptable are as follows: (1) the procedure can only be performed for married couples using only the gametes of the wife and husband; (2) the husband's semen cannot be collected by means of masturbation; (3) the semen must be collected as part of a conjugal act in which a perforated Silastic sheath is used;

(4) the ovum should be collected on the same day as the conjugal act; (5) the husband's sperm must be used within seventy-two hours of its collection so that it is not used after its natural viability for fertilization; and (6) an air bubble must separate the gametes as they are transferred through the catheter, so that if fertilization occurs, it will occur at the natural site in the fallopian tube.

Under these conditions, GIFT can be morally acceptable because, as explained above, it assists or facilitates the conjugal act of the spouses to achieve its objective and does not substitute for or replace the act. Performed under all the conditions given, GIFT assists the conjugal act by eliminating physiological hindrances to fertility, which allows the causal power of the conjugal act to reach the objective of fertilization as it naturally occurs. Moreover, although conditional GIFT includes discrete actions that can diminish the personal intimacy of the marital act, this fact is not sufficient to eliminate the unitive meaning of the spouses' act because the unitive aspect of the conjugal act is more than and not reducible to personal intimacy.

IUI also has the potential to fulfill Catholic teaching, but only if it is performed under the same five conditions as GIFT (adjusted for the absence of an ovum in the procedure) and without superovulation. In answer to the question "How is homologous artificial insemination to be evaluated from the moral point of view?" *Donum vitae* states, "Homologous artificial insemination within marriage cannot be admitted except for those cases in which the technical means is not a substitute for the conjugal act but serves to facilitate and to help so that the act attains its natural purpose."[35]

Homologous artificial insemination is defined as "the technique used to obtain a human conception through the transfer into the genital tracts of a married woman of the sperm previously collected from her husband."[36] This definition is consistent with the clinical description of IUI above. Therefore, if IUI can be performed under conditions that would prevent it from being a substitute for the conjugal act, it would be an instance of the morally acceptable exception to the prohibition against homologous artificial insemination found in the teaching of *Donum vitae* quoted above. At the present time, the teaching office of the Church has not voiced any objections against GIFT or IUI in the forms described here.

It must be recognized that other moral theologians and ethicists hold that the conditional GIFT procedure in fact replaces the conjugal act.[37] They argue that even if the spouses' act of sexual intercourse could be considered genuinely conjugal, it is still radically disassociated from the technical method by which a child might be engendered. The act of intercourse, according to this interpretation of GIFT, amounts to a non-masturbatory way of obtaining the husband's sperm for the purpose of using it in a procedure, which substitutes for the couple's conjugal act. The technical acts performed in the procedure are outside the reality of the conjugal act and, in fact, destroy and replace the causal power of the spouses' conjugal act to procreate.

Thus, on the issue of conditional GIFT, there are two opposing bodies of strong, probable arguments by theologians and ethicists faithful to the magisterium on a subject for which there has been an absence of specific Church teaching. Given this situation, and until the Church teaches otherwise, individual Catholics may, according to a rightly informed conscience, choose to act according to either moral evaluation of the conditional GIFT or IUI procedures. Catholic health care institutions have a similar option of providing or denying conditional GIFT or IUI for the same reasons.

Notes

[1] See Mark H. Beers, ed., *Merck Manual of Diagnosis and Therapy*, 18th ed. (Whitehouse Station, NJ: Merck, 2006), 2138.

[2] European Society of Human Reproduction & Embryology, "World Report on ART (Assisted Reproductive Technology) Fact Sheet" (June 21, 2006), http://www.eshre.com/emc.asp?pageId=807.

[3] Congregation for the Doctrine of the Faith (CDF), *Donum vitae* (February 22, 1987), Introduction, 2.

[4] John Paul II. *Evangelium vitae* (March 25, 1995), n. 34.

[5] Ibid., n. 39.

[6] Ibid.

[7] Ibid., n. 40.

[8] Ibid., n. 53, quoting *Donum vitae*, Introduction, 5.

[9] Ibid., n. 52 (original emphasis).

[10] Ibid., n. 48 (original emphasis).

[11] Ibid., n. 22.

[12] See *Donum vitae*, Introduction, 3; and II (B), 4b.

[13] Vatican Council II, *Gaudium et spes* (December 7, 1965), n. 48.

[14] *Donum vitae*, II (B), 6 (emphasis added); see also n. 7. Also, U.S. Conference of Catholic Bishops, *Ethical and Religious Directives for Catholic Health Care Services*, 4th ed. (Washington, D.C.: USCCB, 2001), nn. 38–41.

[15] *Donum vitae*, II (B), 8.

[16] Ibid., II (A), 3.

[17] See U. S. Department of Health and Human Services (DHHS), Centers for Disease Control and Prevention, *2004 Assisted Reproductive Technology Success Rates: National Summary and Fertility Clinic Reports* (Atlanta, GA: DHHS, December 2006), 503.

[18] See Beers, *Merck Manual*, 2142.

[19] See American Society for Reproductive Medicine, *Guidelines on Number of Embryos Transferred* (Birmingham, AL: American Society for Reproductive Medicine, November 1999); and DHHS, *2004 Assisted Reproductive Technology Success Rates*, 41.

[20] See A. N. Andersen et al., "Assisted Reproductive Technology in Europe, 2003," *Human Reproduction* 22.6 (June 2007): 1518.

[21] All U.S. statistics for ART procedures reported here are for techniques that use non-donor unfrozen eggs or embryos. See DHHS, *2004 Assisted Reproductive Technology Success Rates*, 37.

[22] *Donum vitae*, II (B), 5.

[23] Ibid., I, 5 and 6.

[24] Ibid., II (B), 5.

[25] See DHHS, *2004 Assisted Reproductive Technology Success Rates*, 36–37.

[26] A.R. Martinez et al., "Basic Questions on Intrauterine Insemination," *Obstetrical and Gynecological Survey* 48.12 (December 1993): 818.

[27] See A. Allegra et al., "GnRH Antagonist-Induced Inhibition of the Premature LH Surge Increases Pregnancy Rates in IUI-stimulated Cycles: A Prospective Randomized Trial," *Human Reproduction* 22.1 (January 2007): 101–108.

[28] See Beers, *Merck Manual*, 2142.

[29] See DHHS, *2004 Assisted Reproductive Technology Success Rates*, 36–37, 39.

[30] M. Alikani, "Micromanipulation of Human Gametes for Assisted Fertilization," *Current Opinion in Obstetrics and Gynecology* 5.5 (October 1993): 594–599.

[31] See DHHS, *2004 Assisted Reproductive Technology Success Rates*, 36–37.

[32] See B.J. Cohlen et al., "Controlled Ovarian Hyperstimulation and Intrauterine Insemination for Treating Male Subfertility: A Controlled Study," *Human Reproduction* 13.6 (June 1998): 1553–1558.

[33] Thomas W. Hilgers, "Answers for Infertility," *Celebrate Life* (May–June 1995): 34.

[34] See Peter Cataldo: "Reproductive Technologies," *Ethics & Medics* 21.1 (January 1996): 1–3; "The Newest Reproductive Technologies: Applying Catholic Teaching," in *The Gospel of Life and the Vision of Health Care*, ed. Russell E. Smith (Braintree, MA: Pope John Center, 1996), 61–94; and "GIFT as Assistance," *Ethics & Medics* 22.12 (December 1997): 3–4. See also Donald G. McCarthy, "GIFT? Yes!" *Ethics & Medics* 18.9 (September 1993): 3–4; Thomas J. O'Donnell, *Medicine and Christian Morality*, 2nd ed. (New York: Alba House, 1991), 239–240; Donald G. McCarthy, Response to Donald T. DeMarco, "Catholic Moral Teaching and TOT/ GIFT," in *Reproductive Technologies, Marriage and the Church,* ed. Donald G. McCarthy (Pope John Center, 1988), 140–145, 174–182; James J. Mulligan, *Choose Life* (Pope John

Center, 1991), 226–240; and Orville Griese, *Catholic Identity in Health Care: Principles and Practice* (Pope John Center, 1987), 47–48.

[35] *Donum vitae*, II (B), 6.

[36] *Donum vitae*, II, note b.

[37] See Benedict M. Ashley, Jean DeBlois, and Kevin D. O'Rourke, *Health Care Ethics: A Catholic Theological Analysis.* 5th ed. (Washington, D.C.: Georgetown University Press, 2006), 87; John M. Haas and William E. May, "Pastoral Concerns: Procreation and the Marital Act," in *Reproductive Technologies, Marriage and the Church*, ed. McCarthy, 166 (Haas), 166 and 167 (May), and 178–179 (Haas); and "GIFT? No!" *Ethics & Medics* 18.9 (September 1993): 2–3; William E. May, "Catholic Teaching on the Laboratory Generation of Human Life," in *The Gift of Life*, eds. Thomas Hilgers and Marilyn Wallace (Omaha, NB: Pope Paul VI Institute Press, 1990), 88; Donald DeMarco, *Biotechnology and the Assault on Parenthood* (San Francisco: Ignatius Press, 1991), 225–238, and "GIFT as Replacement," *Ethics & Medics* 22.11 (November 1997): 3–4; Nicholas Tonti-Filippini, "*Donum vitae* and Gamete Intra-Fallopian Tube Transfer," *Linacre Quarterly* 57.2 (May 1990): 74–75; John F. Doerfler, "Technology and Human Reproduction." *Ethics & Medics* 24.8 (August 1999): 3–4.

✣

Editorial Summation: Up to 10 percent of couples in the United States experiences infertility. In recent years a number of reproductive technologies have been introduced to manage infertility; therefore, it is important to know and correctly apply the pertinent moral principles contained in the Church's moral tradition. The basic operative principle is that human life is a gift from God, the Creator of the Universe and all its parts. With that life comes the responsibility to preserve and promote it in oneself and in others. This stewardship applies not only to human life but also to the means by which humans procreate. In accordance with God's revealed truth, humans are to be begotten by consensual sexual intercourse between a man and a woman who are married to each other. This conjugal act has two meanings, procreative and unitive, which must not be deliberately separated. Hence, each of the reproductive technologies briefly described in this chapter is to be morally evaluated in light of these principles. The use of a particular reproductive technology must not result in the death of a human being and it must not replace or substitute for the conjugal act. Nor should one or the other of the conjugal act's two meanings be excluded from even a single act of conjugal intercourse. The technology may assist this act by facilitating its performance or by enabling it to achieve its inherent objective once it has been properly performed.

CHAPTER 9

Early Induction of Labor

Peter J. Cataldo and T. Murphy Goodwin, M.D.

Induction of labor refers to the process by which uterine contractions and dilatation of the uterine cervix are provoked pharmacologically or mechanically with the goal of evacuating the pregnant uterus to address certain types of complications. Induction of labor is one way of treating conditions with the result of ending pregnancy; other means include cesarean section (usually only after the gestational age at which the newborn is expected to survive) and instrumental evacuation of the uterus, so-called dilatation and curettage (before about fourteen weeks' gestation), and dilatation and evacuation (after about fourteen weeks' gestation). Early induction of labor refers to induction prior to the time in pregnancy at which the fetus is presumed to be mature—normally thirty-seven weeks' gestation (269 days from the first day of the last menstrual period, with 280 days being the normal length of gestation). Because of the error inherent in estimating gestational age, fetal maturity is presumed in practice to have occurred by thirty-eight to thirty-nine weeks' gestation. In any discussion of induction of labor, the first decision is whether the pregnancy should continue in view of existent or pending complications; if the only way to treat the fetal or maternal problems is by doing something that results in the end of the pregnancy, the second decision is whether this should be unintentionally allowed by induction of labor or should occur by one of the other techniques mentioned above.

Induction of labor is commonly employed in obstetrics. While many decisions about induction of labor are straightforward, some decisions about when and if to induce labor can be among the most complex medically and ethically. The complexity is due in part to the fact that there are two patients involved in each decision, the mother and the child in utero; the interests of the mother and the fetus often conflict to some degree. For both the mother and the fetus, the burden of continuing the pregnancy must be weighed against the benefit of treating problems with the result of ending the pregnancy. Another layer of complexity is introduced by the fact that the estimation of the burden and benefit changes with gestational age. The same clinical factors in the same patient can allow a fundamentally different assessment when reconsidered a few weeks later.

When induction of labor is considered at a gestational age when the fetus is presumed to be mature, there is seldom controversy from the point of view of fetal well-being, since delivery poses no added risk to the child. If a disease of the mother or the fetus poses a risk to either or both after thirty-seven weeks' gestation, the only reason not to induce labor is if the burden of induction on the mother (such as increased risk of cesarean birth, rare complications of induction, or the expense of the induction process) is greater than the benefit of avoiding the risks to maternal and fetal health. When early induction of labor is considered, the burden of newborn prematurity, which is greater with younger gestational age, must also be considered.

Having described what induction and the early induction of labor are and the general parameters of their benefits and risks, this essay will now review several categories of clinical settings in which there are medical indications for inducing labor, even though induction would result in the certain death of the fetus or neonate or significantly shorten its life. Cases involving early induction of labor may be categorized by whether the indication for induction arises from disease of the fetus or disease of the mother and whether induction poses risks to the fetus alone or to both the mother and fetus.

Risk to the Fetus Alone

In some cases, a fetal disease process poses a significant risk to the fetus itself while there is no appreciable risk to the mother of continuing the pregnancy. In fetal hemolytic disease, for example, incompatibility between maternal and fetal blood causes destruction of fetal red blood cells, which can lead to death or disability. This can be treated by blood transfusion to the fetus, but if the transfusion is unsuccessful or if gestational age is advanced to the point where the risks of the transfusion are greater than the risks of preterm birth, induction of labor is offered.

Risk to Both the Mother and Fetus

Two of the most common indications for considering early induction of labor are preeclampsia (high blood pressure of pregnancy), and preterm premature rupture of membranes (PPROM), in which the bag of water that surrounds the fetus ruptures before labor and before the fetus is mature. These may serve as useful examples of ethical decision making for early induction of labor.

The pregnant mother who develops severe preeclampsia is at increased risk for seizures and other complications, such as hemorrhage and stroke. Generally, these risks increase as the pregnancy progresses. The fetus is at increased risk of death or injury related to adverse effects of the maternal hypertension on placental function. The benefit of induction of labor, therefore, is to reduce both maternal and fetal morbidity.

The principle risk of induction to the mother is relatively discrete—an increased rate of cesarean birth compared to women who enter spontaneous labor, and rare, direct adverse effects from the medications used for induction. The risk of induction to the fetus, on the other hand, depends on the gestational age. Earlier in gestation the risk to the fetus is greater because of the complications of premature birth. In a mother who develops severe preeclampsia at twenty-five weeks' gestation, for example, induction of labor with subsequent delivery carries for the child an approximately 40 percent risk of death and, if the child survives, a 40 percent risk of cerebral palsy or other major disability. In such cases, delaying induction of labor in the face of a significant risk of maternal morbidity constitutes an aggressive treatment strategy for fetal well-being in which the mother accepts risks, allowing a delay in delivery to improve outcomes for the fetus. Nevertheless, this strategy usually runs its course in a matter of days, when the mother's deteriorating condition necessitates delivery of the extremely premature infant.

A second common indication for early induction of labor is preterm premature rupture of membranes. The main risk to mother and fetus in PPROM is the development of infection within the uterus, since the amniotic sac no longer serves as a barrier against infection. The burden on the mother and the fetus is the risk of infection, but depending on how early in pregnancy the rupture occurs, the risk of prematurity may be more significant for the fetus.

The decision-making process, balancing maternal and fetal benefits and burdens, changes categorically at the limit of newborn viability. There is substantial ethical controversy about induction of labor in these cases. In most economically developed countries, viability begins at around twenty-three weeks' gestation (161 days from the first day of the last menstrual period). Survival of children born right at twenty-three weeks' gestation is approximately 10 percent, and most survivors have major handicaps (cerebral palsy, blindness, deafness, or mental retardation); at twenty-four weeks, by comparison, the survival rate is around 50 percent.

Preeclampsia diagnosed prior to twenty-three weeks' gestation is often severe, with the risk of maternal complications increasing with the passage of time. There are also substantial risks to the fetus, including a high likelihood of death in utero. Induction of labor removes the risk to the mother, since preeclampsia in its various forms is caused by hormonal products of the placenta acting on the maternal circulation. For the fetus, however, induction of labor prior to twenty-three weeks' gestation means that death is likely.

When the continuation of the pregnancy itself poses continued and usually increasing risk to the mother, the source of the pathologic process is often traceable to the placenta. The disease process in preeclampsia, for example, is understood to be the failure of the trophoblast cells of the placenta to take over the maternal blood vessels in the uterine wall in the normal way in the first few weeks of gestation, resulting in chronic underperfusion of the placenta by the maternal blood vessels. A hormonal signal (not yet fully characterized) is elaborated by the placenta; this signal seeks greater perfusion of the placenta, to which the mother responds with increasing blood pressure.

When rupture of membranes occurs before twenty-three weeks' gestation, especially when it occurs several weeks before this time, induction of labor is often advocated as a means of preventing infection from developing within the mother. There is ample published evidence, however, that when no clinical or laboratory evidence of infection is present, expectant management and use of antibiotics is an acceptable course that can result in fetal survival and acceptable maternal morbidity. If evidence of intrauterine infection develops, however, progressive, severe infection of the mother and the fetus can be expected within hours, a life-threatening situation for both. In this setting, induction of labor for maternal benefit is commonly recommended in practice, even though the fetus cannot be expected to survive.

Can induction of labor before twenty-three weeks' gestation ever be justified ethically? In Catholic moral teaching and tradition, all cases of induction of labor may be evaluated by the principle of the double effect.[1] This moral principle has been developed over centuries as a guide to evaluate whether an act that has foreseeable good and bad effects is morally justified. There are four conditions of the principle, each of which must be fulfilled for such an act to be justified: (1) the act performed is in itself morally good or at least indifferent; (2) the good effect is directly intended, and the bad effect is foreseen but unintended; (3) the good effect is not achieved by means of the bad effect; (4) the good effect is proportionate to the bad effect. The principle can be helpfully applied, for example, in cases of preeclampsia and PPROM.

Induction of labor is not an intrinsically evil act (first condition). The evil of the newborn death is reasonably foreseen but not intended (second condition). In the case of preeclampsia prior to twenty-three weeks' gestation, the intention of the physician inducing labor is to remove the diseased organ (the placenta), thus curing the preeclampsia. In the case of PPROM with evidence of infection in the uterus, the intention of the physician inducing labor is to cure the infection by removing the infected placenta and membranes of the gestational sac. The good effects of curing the mother of preeclampsia and PPROM are not caused by the death of the baby (third condition). In both settings, the removal of the offending organ, the placenta and membranes, allows survival of the mother, which would otherwise be in doubt (fourth condition).[2]

Abortion to treat the conditions considered here is never morally justified. Pope John Paul II reaffirmed Catholic teaching on abortion in *Evangelium vitae*: "Abortion willed as an end or as a means always constitutes a grave moral disorder, since it is the deliberate killing of an innocent human being. This doctrine is based on the natural law and on the written Word of God, is transmitted by the Church's Tradition and taught by the ordinary and universal Magisterium."[3]

On the basis of Catholic teaching and tradition, the U.S. bishops define abortion in this way:

Abortion (that is, the directly intended termination of pregnancy before viability or the directly intended destruction of a viable fetus) is never permitted. Every procedure whose sole immediate effect is the termination of pregnancy before viability is an abortion, which, in its moral context, includes the interval between conception and implantation of the embryo.[4]

Early induction of labor guided by the principle of the double effect is not abortion, because adherence to the principle ensures that the act in itself and the intention of the one acting do not have the sole immediate effect of killing the innocent child. Directive 47 of the ERDs, which permits early induction of labor, does so on the basis of the principle of the double effect: "Operations, treatments, and medications that have as their direct purpose the cure of a proportionately serious pathological condition of a pregnant woman are permitted when they cannot be safely postponed until the unborn child is viable, even if they will result in the death of the unborn child."

In other indications for early induction of labor that involve maternal illness, the normal function of the placenta changes the maternal body in such a way as to increase the risk of maternal death or disability. For example, a fundamental change mediated by placental hormones in pregnancy is an increase in blood volume, which is commonly experienced as the natural swelling of pregnancy. A woman with severe heart disease, however, may be unable to tolerate this added stress on the heart, which places her at risk of dying. Whether the principle of double effect can be applied when the normal homeostatic changes of pregnancy induced by the placenta place a mother's life at risk is worthy of further discussion.

Of note, the alternative means of terminating a pregnancy by dilatation and extraction does not fulfill the terms of the principle of double effect (specifically, the first condition), because this procedure involves directly killing the fetus prior to its extraction or the extraction of the placenta.

Early Induction of Labor for Fetal Anomaly

Apart from the risk of death or serious morbidity to the mother (as in early preeclampsia), the other broad category cited as an indication for early induction of labor is fetal anomaly. The majority of major congenital anomalies can now be identified by ultrasound alone or in combination with tests of amniotic fluid or fetal blood. With rare exceptions, the health of the mother is not affected in cases of fetal anomaly. There is no physical benefit to the mother or fetus in early induction of labor or termination of pregnancy by any means (abortion). Some have identified psychological benefits to the mother in that the emotional burden of carrying a child with a major anomaly is alleviated. This will be discussed below.

Cases of fetal anomaly may be broadly classified into several groups for ethical decision making: (1) lethal anomalies of the fetus, where in almost all cases the fetus will die in utero or shortly after birth; (2) nonlethal anomalies with grave disability, and (3) nonlethal anomalies with serious disability that is generally not life-threatening. Let us consider early induction of labor in each of these categories.

Lethal Fetal Anomalies

Some lethal anomalies of the fetus are anencephaly, renal agenesis, trisomy 13, trisomy 18 with severe cardiac defects, other rare trisomies, triploidy (a complete set of extra chromosomes), and skeletal dysplasias with failure of thoracic development. In trisomy 13, for example, the in the most common scenario the mother is found by ultrasound to have a fetus with defects in several major organs. Examination of fetal cells from amniocentesis confirms a diagnosis of trisomy 13. The extra chromosome causes a syndrome characterized by abnormal formation of the brain, heart, face, and other organs. Almost all fetuses with this condition die in utero or within hours of birth. Early induction of labor or early termination of pregnancy by other means (abortion) provides no physical benefit to the mother under normal circumstances; for the fetus, it inevitably shortens life.

If the mother carrying a child with trisomy 13 encounters no health risks beyond those of a normal pregnancy, is early induction of labor justified? The benefit of continuing the pregnancy is the prolongation of the life of the child for the remaining weeks of the pregnancy, which under these circumstances is a moral right that the child arguably has. This is a good which may be weighed against the proposed benefits of induction of labor. In the absence of a physical malady in the mother, some have contended that the emotional burden of continuing the pregnancy when the child will ultimately die at birth should be weighed against the benefit of continuation of fetal life, and that this could justify early induction of labor in some cases. However, this proposed psychological benefit of early induction of labor has not been demonstrated scientifically. Its use in considerations of early induction of labor is speculative and has been specifically proscribed.[5] The use of emotional distress or trauma has been prohibited as a proportionate reason under these circumstances because the early induction is not directed at some serious maternal pathology but at removal of the child as a means of alleviating the emotional burden.

In assessing the emotional burden of a pregnancy with a fetal anomaly such as trisomy 13, the expected grief response must be distinguished from the much less common clinical depression. The latter can represent a substantive risk to the mother. In the absence of this, however, it can be argued that the only reason to induce is to hasten the death of the child for the purpose of ending the parents' grief. But to hasten the death of the child, either as an end or a means, is never permissible. It is crucial to the parents' understanding to remind them continually that the dignity of the child demands careful application of the principles proper to every member of the human family. To induce labor in order to shorten their emotional suffering is to declare that this child is less than fully human. Sadly, the longed-for resolution of the emotional suffering may actually be put off by the failure to acknowledge and accept the child fully despite its defects.

If a mother carrying a child with trisomy 13 encounters health risks related to a pathologic condition of pregnancy, the benefit of early induction compared to continuation of the pregnancy is weighed in the same way that it is for any pregnancy. This means that the moral considerations are different if, for example, this mother develops mild preeclampsia (a condition which poses some risk but which can often be managed for some time without induction of labor early in pregnancy) compared to what they were when she had only normal health risks. The benefit of early induction of labor to the mother is that the preeclampsia is not allowed to progress to a more severe state. The effect of the early induction on the fetus is to shorten the life of the fetus by the weeks or months that would normally be remaining in pregnancy. Continuation of the pregnancy when there is any risk or physical burden to the mother is, in a sense, an aggressive treatment on behalf of the fetus. When the fetus no longer benefits substantially, prompt induction of labor for maternal benefit is recommended. Thus, labor is commonly induced for even mild preeclampsia, since the benefit to the fetus of delaying delivery is no longer proportionate to the risk the mother and the fetus face should the mother's condition deteriorate rapidly.

In the case of a lethal anomaly, the mother with preeclampsia may accept the physical risks of the disease as well as the burden of the expense of hospitalization and physical limitations of bed rest, in exchange for the benefit of prolonging her child's life for those weeks or months at the end of pregnancy. This good for the fetus may be evaluated in light of when an adult has cancer, for example, late in life. In some cases, life can be prolonged by further chemotherapy, but only as the result of treatment that has become ethically disproportionate because it offers no reasonable hope of benefit or is excessively burdensome. In this instance there is no obligation for the patient to accept another round of chemotherapy, which is not the same thing as hastening the patient's death. Similarly, when a mother is carrying a fetus who is in the process of dying, the additional burden she should be expected to accept is limited in comparison to the burden normally accepted when the benefit to a child is not so constrained. As with the cancer patient, under no circumstances may actions be taken for the purpose of hastening the child's death, as is argued above concerning the moral status of emotional distress. This approach to decision making when a fetus has a lethal anomaly is the same throughout the pregnancy, both before and after the limit of newborn viability at twenty-three weeks' gestation.

Nonlethal Anomalies with Grave Disability

Nonlethal anomalies with grave disability include less common chromosomal defects in which fetal imaging shows multiple anomalies, massive hydrocephalus, and hydrancephaly. In these "intermediate" cases, there is some uncertainty about how long the child may live after birth and some variability in the prognoses overall. In general, the life expectancy of the child is very short, and the suffering and disability are great; in most cases there is profound retardation, and the child lacks an awareness of surroundings and the ability to respond to cognitive stimuli.

Early induction of labor is sometimes considered when the burden of risk for the mother is more than that of a usual pregnancy. This should not be confused with the use of a subjective quality-of-life standard to reach a moral judgment about obligations. Certain physical functions may be lacking in quality, but human life itself is not subject to a quality-of-life standard. The human person may never be reduced "to the value of his qualities."[6] In these cases, a child will most often live only weeks or months after birth, although in some cases children have been reported to live for years. Importantly, because of the range of prognoses, these cases require very careful assessment of the fetus to inform the ethical decision making.

Nonlethal Anomalies with Serious Disability
That Is Not Generally Life-Threatening

More common than cases in which the mother is carrying a fetus with a lethal anomaly or a nonlethal anomaly with grave disability are cases in which the fetus has an anomaly that is serious but nonlethal. The

best example is trisomy 21 (Down syndrome). For the fetus, early induction because of Down syndrome offers no benefit, and continuation of the pregnancy offers the same substantial benefits as in any pregnancy—less risk of mortality due to very early induction and less risk of prematurity-related morbidity due to later (but still early) induction. For the mother, the burden of continuing the pregnancy under usual circumstances is the same whether the child has Down syndrome or not—that is, the need to manage the usual physiologic changes and discomforts of pregnancy. In cases of fetal anomalies that are associated with significant but manageable disability and are consistent with long life, making decisions about early induction of labor is substantially the same as in cases where the fetus is healthy.

Anomalies with serious disability that is not generally life-threatening include, in addition to trisomy 21, omphalocele, neural tube defect, and hydrocephalus. In many cases in which fetal anomaly is taken as an indication for early termination of pregnancy before viability (up to and in some cases even beyond twenty-three weeks' gestation), dilatation and evacuation is used. This technique always involves primary destruction of the fetus and is an abortion.

In each of these scenarios, whether early induction is undertaken because of maternal or fetal indication, the exact nature of the disease state must be known before an informed ethical decision can be made. Although this is a commonplace consideration in medical ethics, there is no other area of medicine where the need for precise characterization of the condition in mother and fetus is more crucial.

Mother–Child Dialogue in Ethical Decision Making

For the moral evaluation of inducing labor under the circumstances described above, we start from the premise that it is appropriate to the dignity of all human beings to live to the natural terminus of life. The importance of emphasizing this point to the couple who have just learned of their child's grave condition is often underestimated. The child, no matter how gravely malformed, is to be shown respect and acknowledged as a member of the human family; one way we do this is by applying the same ethical principles we apply when dealing with all other persons. Often the clinical setting, where the initial diagnosis and discussion of prognosis occurs, in a sense strips the child of its attributes—intelligence, physical beauty, the ability to interact, all the expectations for the future. But the child is still a human being, made in the image and likeness of God. And by applying the ethical principles common to all human beings, we are not heartless, but compassionate.

The process of deliberation on the ethical aspects of such cases can ennoble the family and restore to them their child as someone for whom they are providing the best care they can in this decision. By contrast, the alternative of abortion says to the mother, in effect, "Your child is not part of the family of humans who are treated equally, but is somehow less, a kind of thing that can be set aside without the full acknowledgment that all humans require." Abortion, especially for the family that would not have otherwise considered it, often fails to bring the prompt resolution of the suffering that the abruptness and finality of the procedure itself seem to promise. Much the same may be said of routine early induction after viability.

In order to apply common ethical principles to decisions about early induction, we must understand the unique and complex nature of the maternal–fetal interaction. This interaction model, in which mother and child speak to the moral values at stake, may be helpfully used to evaluate the various conditions described in the previous parts of this essay. First, as was pointed out earlier, while decisions about therapy based on the benefit and burden to the mother change only with the course of the disease, such decisions for the fetus change constantly with advancing gestational age. All decisions about induction of labor must take into account that the fetal "benefit and burden" considerations are constantly changing, from the point of viability up to term.

Second, neither the fetus nor the mother should be treated as being entirely independent of the other. In addition to the usual posing of risk versus benefit, the mother must ask, "Are the risks to my baby proportionate to the benefits I receive?" At the same time, the fetus must ask, "Are the risks to my mother proportionate to the benefits I receive?" The child cannot ask for its own annihilation. It can decline, as it were, treatment intended to prolong its life if the benefit of the prolonged life is outweighed by the burden on itself or on its mother. Just how natural and "taken for granted" this mutual consideration is can be seen in the exceptional cases where a mother or, more rarely, a fetal advocate decides about therapy without regard to the other.

In cases where continuation of a pregnancy poses any substantive risk to the mother, prompt induction of labor (or delivery by cesarean section, as appropriate) is usually the best way to preserve maternal health, as shown earlier. When delivery is delayed in spite of a sub-stantive maternal risk, this delay of delivery becomes an active medical intervention on behalf of the fetus. This is readily perceived in obstetric practice where strategies for delaying delivery for fetal benefit (as in the case of preeclampsia early in gestation) are described as "aggressive." Delaying delivery for fetal benefit in the face of maternal risk is a specific fetal treatment strategy.

Through a surrogate, the child in utero may evaluate this "treatment strategy" as to whether it offers a reasonable hope of benefit or poses excessive burden on itself or on its mother. For patients who face these difficult decisions, the image of this continual dialogue between the child and the mother is not only comforting but serves as a firm touchstone for the ethical decision-making process.

Such reasoning could be said to allow for the possibility of abortion, since the child in utero with a lethal anomaly could be said to benefit little from simply remaining alive in utero for the next four to five months. This benefit could be considered so small as to allow for the possibility that any burden on the mother would outweigh it, leading to a decision to end the pregnancy. To understand why this cannot be so, we must understand the meaning of the term "viability."

This viability is a true dichotomy at the lower end. Below this point, there is no possibility of neonatal survival. From an ethical point of view, viability is the threshold at which proportional benefits and risk can be considered. This is so in practice for all conditions, even those for which the gestational age of viability is nearly theoretical. An example of the latter is diaphragmatic hernia, in which the particular malformation reduces survival after very early preterm birth to almost zero. Even though a child with a serious anomaly may not make use of all the tools available at birth or not use them for long, these are available. This is seen in the way that, in most tertiary perinatal centers, the neonatal resuscitation team attends all deliveries to see how the baby responds to efforts in the first few moments of life. The postnatal decision as to what measures will be used is independent of the anomaly—guided in the main by principles of "reasonable hope of recovery" and "excessive burden."

Anencephaly is one type of fetal anomaly for which some have recommended early induction of labor. In this condition, the covering skull bones (calvarium) are missing and the underlying brain is largely absent. In such cases there is, for all intents and purposes, no chance of survival beyond the neonatal period and no chance of higher brain function. Most physicians advocate abortion if the diagnosis is made early in pregnancy. If the diagnosis is made later in gestation, early induction of labor is often advocated. As mentioned above, even in Catholic institutions, early induction has been proposed as a humane option.

In justification of early induction, one rationale that has been offered is that there is no benefit to the fetus to continue to term, since he or she will almost certainly die shortly after birth and, in any case, will never have any awareness of its family or surroundings. But as we have set out above, the dialogue about early induction of a viable fetus must always begin with the mother's condition. If there is no substantive risk to the mother's health, then it is appropriate to the child in utero, no matter how malformed, to continue to the natural terminus of its existence. If some tangible risk from continuing the pregnancy does develop for the mother, the anencephalic fetus, through its surrogate, could evaluate the treatment strategy of delaying delivery much as an end-stage terminal cancer patient might evaluate further chemotherapy, as was noted above. The aggressive treatment strategy of delaying delivery could be refused, since the proportionate benefit to the fetus of living a few more weeks is outweighed by almost any substantive burden on the mother and the family.

Case Study

A thirty-five-year-old mother in her sixth pregnancy was found to have increased amniotic fluid volume (polyhydramnios) and a fetus with clenched hands at twenty-two weeks' gestation. This suggested trisomy 18, a diagnosis confirmed by amniocentesis. The mother was presented with the option of pregnancy termination, and the genetic counselor told her, "We will respect whatever decision you arrive at, but we have never had anyone who did not opt for abortion in recent years." Nevertheless, the mother refused abortion.

Subsequent counseling was directed toward a thorough understanding of the natural history of trisomy 18 and the postnatal prognosis. This involved detailing exactly which organs were involved and to what extent. An important finding was that the heart was unaffected, since complex heart defects usually result in death early in the neonatal period unless surgery is undertaken. The stomach "bubble" was absent in the child, a condition that suggests esophageal atresia. This was significant, since a gastrostomy tube for feeding the infant and some sort of palliative procedure to prevent aspiration of oral contents would be necessary to prevent death from starvation or lung infection.

The couple learned that in the best-case scenario, 5 to 10 percent of children with trisomy 18 could live for

one year, and 1 to 3 percent could live for five years, but this figure is much lower for boys (their baby was a boy). Also, these figures do not apply to babies with the specific defect of esophageal atresia, which their child was thought to have. The parents wondered if placing a gastrostomy tube after birth to feed their baby would be excessively burdensome. What about surgery to bypass the possible esophageal obstruction?

As the pregnancy progressed, emotional and physical burdens increased. The continued accumulation of excess amniotic fluid resulted in a uterine size twice that of a normal pregnancy at the same gestational age. It was difficult for the mother to perform household duties, and the mother's frequent emotional letdowns affected the entire family.

By thirty-two weeks' gestation, the mother experienced intermittent difficulty breathing because of the size of the uterus, and she felt "at her wits' end." The decision-making process was framed in terms of the benefit to the baby versus the burden of the baby on the family. What is the proportional benefit to the baby of simply living at least another five weeks in utero? To what extent should the emotional burden on the mother be factored into this decision? To what extent should the psychological burden on the rest of the family be factored in? How important is the burden on the family of the mother's being unable to fulfill her role around the house?

The framework for approaching these questions was similar to that applied in all early induction decisions: with each passing day, the benefit to the baby of delaying delivery was less and, therefore, correspondingly smaller burdens on the mother and family might be considered sufficient to justify early induction of labor. In this specific circumstance, it was felt that inducing labor at thirty-two weeks reduced the child's chance of surviving longer than a few months without burdensome intervention to less than 1 percent, as compared to 5 percent for a child delivered after thirty-seven weeks' gestation. This was especially so if intubation and mechanical ventilation were viewed as burdensome intervention. There did not appear to be any tangible medical risks at the time. The principal burden at the time was the distress of the parents. This was not considered sufficient to justify delivery.

On the basis of these considerations, labor was not induced. One week later, however, when the mother developed significant respiratory difficulty, a decision was made to induce delivery. This was justifiable, given the goal of preserving the lives of mother and child to the extent possible under the circumstances. Consideration was given to amniocentesis or other approaches to reduce the amniotic fluid volume, but it was felt that the risk to the mother was not justified by the slight benefit to the child. As Paul Ramsey has pointed out, weighing all the factors that pertain in such a complex decision requires, above all, a pure heart.

Notes

[1] See Peter J. Cataldo, "The Principle of the Double Effect," *Ethics & Medics* 20.3 (March 1995): 1–3.

[2] It can be argued that the placenta is a fetal organ, not a maternal organ, since it is a product of the fetal genome. On the other hand, its intimate relationship with maternal tissues and its direct effect on maternal health argue for its consideration as a maternal organ in some senses. Moreover, the placenta is not part of the body by which the individual is identified; therefore, to take actions to remove it when it is diseased is not an attack on the person.

[3] John Paul II (March 25, 1995), n. 62.

[4] U.S. Conference of Catholic Bishops, *Ethical and Religious Directives for Catholic Health Care Services* (Washington, D.C.: USCCB, 2001), n. 45.

[5] National Conference of Catholic Bishops, "Moral Principles concerning Infants with Anencephaly" (September 19, 1996), http://www.nccbuscc.org/dpp/anencephaly.htm.

[6] Pope John Paul II, Message to those attending an international congress sponsored by the Pontifical Council for the Family, the Bioethics Institute of the Catholic University of the Sacred Heart, and the Pontifical Athenaeum Regina Apostolorum, for the anniversary of the encyclical *Evangelium vitae* (April 23, 1996).

Editorial Summation: Abnormal pregnancies can set the interests of mother and child in conflict. These are among the most difficult cases. In severe preeclampsia, the risks increase for the mother the longer she maintains the pregnancy, but the risks increase for the child the earlier labor is induced. In preterm premature rupture of membranes, there is a risk of infection for both mother and child. If none has appeared, expectant management and the use of antibiotics can be a sound course of action. The principle of double effect permits induction of labor to remove a diseased placenta even though the death of the child is foreseen. Here the object of action is the removal of diseased tissue. Direct abortion is never permissible. There is no evidence that early induction of a child with fetal anomalies provides psychological benefits to the mother. The use of early induction to eliminate fetuses with anomalies (e.g., Down syndrome) is immoral. Every consideration of an abnormal pregnancy should start with the premise that all human beings should live to the natural terminus of life. The mother and child should never be treated as if they existed independently of each other, but should be considered as if in active dialogue over their shared predicament.

CHAPTER 10

Ectopic Pregnancy

This two-part chapter offers opposing moral assessments of how to treat ectopic pregnancy, in which an embryo begins to develop outside the uterine cavity. Salpingectomy is generally recognized as moral, but salpingostomy and the use of methotrexate remain controversial. The opposite opinions presented here reflect the current unsettled status of the question among experts whose work is in accord with the magisterium of the Church.—Ed.

A. Arguments Against Salpingostomy and Methotrexate

William E. May

The relevant directive regarding ectopic pregnancies in the 2001 *Ethical and Religious Directives for Catholic Health Care Services* is by no means as explicit as that expressed in the earlier directives of 1971. The more recent version says simply, "In case of extrauterine pregnancy, no intervention is morally licit which constitutes a direct abortion."[1] But what "constitutes" a "direct abortion?" This is a legitimate question, and different answers are given by theologians.

The earlier directive from the National Conference of Catholic Bishops' *Ethical and Religious Directives for Catholic Health Care Facilities* stated:

> In extrauterine pregnancy the affected part of the mother (e.g., cervix, ovary, or fallopian tube) may be removed, even though fetal death is foreseen, provided that: a) the affected part is presumed already to be so damaged and dangerously affected as to warrant its removal, and that b) the operation is not just a separation of the embryo or fetus from its site within the part (*which would be a direct abortion from a uterine appendage*) and that c) the operation cannot be postponed without notably increasing the danger to the mother.[2]

This directive, as the added emphasis makes clear, excludes as immoral and as constituting direct abortion the management of a tubal pregnancy by means of a salpingostomy. In this procedure an incision of the affected fallopian tube is made, and "the products of gestation [the

unborn baby] are gently expressed from the lumen [the cavity of the tube]. Because a certain amount of separation of the trophoblast has usually occurred, the conceptus can generally be easily removed from the lumen."[3]

The Use of Methotrexate

This directive would also seem to exclude as immoral and as an instance of direct abortion the management of tubal pregnancies by removing the unborn child from its site by means of methotrexate. Methotrexate (MTX) is a highly toxic drug that interferes with the synthesis of DNA (deoxyribonucleic acid) and cell multiplication in the trophoblastic tissue, that is, the outer layer of cells produced by the growing baby and connecting it with its mother.

The trophoblast is a vital organ of the unborn baby during gestation. Although it is discarded later on, it must be regarded as an integral part of the body of the unborn child. The trophoblast, as L. Cannon and H. Jesionowska say, is "exquisitely sensitive" to the destructive effect of MTX. Indeed, it is precisely for this reason that MTX is recommended for ectopic pregnancies.[4] In short, MTX manages tubal pregnancies by destroying the trophoblast and thereby killing the baby, whose dead body is then flushed from its site.

The View of Albert Moraczewski, O.P.

Albert Moraczewski, O.P., founding president of the National Catholic Bioethics Center, has argued that it is morally licit and does not constitute direct abortion to manage tubal pregnancies by salpingostomy and the use of methotrexate.[5] Moraczewski first emphasizes that in a tubal pregnancy, implantation of the embryo has not been successful, that the unborn child is doomed to death no matter what one does, and that tubal implantation is "life-threatening not only for the child, but also for the mother." This, of course, is true. Yet it is crucially important to recognize that an inevitably dying person is still a person, whose life is to be respected and whose death, even if inevitable, is not to be hastened for the benefit of any other person (as debates over the use of organs from freshly dead individuals make clear).

In defense of salpingostomy, Moraczewski claims that "the specific focus of the surgical action is the removal of the damaged *tubal tissue* and damaging trophoblastic tissue, not the destruction or death of the embryo" (emphasis added). However, Thomas Hilgers, M.D., and John Bruchalski, M.D., with whom I have corresponded, challenge this claim. Hilgers says that the focus of a salpingostomy is to enucleate (that is, remove) the ectopic pregnancy (the unborn child) from the fallopian tube and is not, as Moraczewski claims, to remove "damaged tubal tissue." Hilgers sees "no difference between … a salpingostomy and D&C entering through the cervix to remove the embryo and placental tissue." Bruchalski—a convert to the pro-life cause, who at one time performed salpingostomies and other operations that he now deems immoral—testifies that "the focus of the surgical action when I did the procedure was the removal of the ectopic," and as a result, he deems the procedure a direct abortion.

Is Death the Object Chosen?

With respect to the use of methotrexate, Moraczewski says that it "inhibits or stops further activity of the trophoblastic part of the embryo because that activity is injurious to the mother and ultimately to the embryo itself." His claim is that the moral object chosen in the use of methotrexate is not the death of the unborn child but "stopping the destructive action of the trophoblastic cells." While one foresees that the unborn child, who is inevitably dying anyway, will die as a result of being removed from its site, this death is not the means chosen to secure the good effect, nor is its death the end for whose sake the procedure is chosen.

Moraczewski apparently thinks that the unborn child who tragically happens to become implanted in the fallopian tube is the agent causing its own mother's death simply by growing, and that it is morally licit to stop it from growing in order to stop this lethal effect on the mother, even though one realizes that as a result the unborn child will die. But, as Bruchalski comments on

Moraczewski's essay, "the preborn child did not ask or will to be implanted in the tube. It is still innocent whether it is implanted in the uterus or in the tube." Moreover, one chooses to use MTX precisely because one knows that it will destroy the trophoblast, that is, a vital organ of the unborn child. Its "therapeutic" effect is achieved only by means of its lethal effect on the unborn child. Moreover, the "therapeutic effect" does not benefit the unborn child but the mother, and does so only because its nontherapeutic effect destroys the trophoblast of the unborn child, thus causing its death.

"Removal" versus "Killing"

Moraczewski's basic argument is that salpingostomy and the use of MTX can be regarded merely as the "removal" of the unborn child from its site within the mother. This "removal," so the reasoning seems to go, has a bad effect, the death of the unborn child, and a good one, the preservation not only of the mother's life (which also could be protected by a salpingectomy) but also, allegedly, of the fertility of one of her fallopian tubes. The bad effect, according to this line of reasoning, is foreseen but not intended, and can therefore, under conditions in which the mother's life is imperiled, be accepted as a side effect of an action otherwise not immoral. Moraczewski seems to distinguish between abortion as a "removal" of the unborn from its site with its death, a foreseen but not intended result, and abortion as a "killing" of the unborn child. Only the latter constitutes an intrinsically immoral act. (The former would be immoral were there no morally justifying reasons to accept or tolerate the evil effect.)

His argument is basically the same as that first advanced by Germain Grisez, an argument expanded and defended by Joseph Boyle and, more recently, Patrick Lee.[6]

A Contrary Point of View

In a previous essay, "The Management of Ectopic Pregnancies: A Moral Analysis,"[7] I concluded that both salpingostomy and the use of MTX to cope with tubal pregnancies amount to direct abortion. In reaching this conclusion, I found very helpful an article by Kevin Flannery, S.J.[8] Flannery underscored the logical difference between a hysterectomy (or salpingectomy) whose removal led to the death of an unborn child within it, and the "removal" of an unborn child by a craniotomy (and, similarly, so it seems to me, by salpingostomy and MTX), which also lead to the child's death.

In the first instance, the hysterectomy (and, similarly, the salpingectomy in a tubal pregnancy), the medical intervention is performed on the mother, whereas in the "removals" of the unborn child by craniotomy, salpingostomy, and MTX, the interventions are performed on the unborn child. Moreover, they are undertaken, not for the benefit of the unborn child, who is killed as a result of their use, but for the benefit of another, that is, the mother. These procedures are not necessary to protect the mother's life, which can be protected by salpingectomy, but are undertaken because, allegedly, they will help preserve the fertility of the affected fallopian tube.

Hilgers and Bruchalski inform me that the alleged medical benefits to the mother of using MTX or performing a salpingostomy can be seriously questioned, and both judge MTX and salpingostomy to be direct attacks on the life of the unborn, not mere "removals." Moreover, Bernard Nathanson, M.D., in an address to the Natural Law Study Center of Virginia (January 19, 1998), stressed that in coming years the drive to use chemical means, preeminently MTX, to perform abortions will become intense, because this will enable "respectable" doctors to offer the "service" of abortion in their private offices. Nathanson holds that use of MTX to manage tubal pregnancies can only be regarded as a direct abortion and an attack on the life of the unborn.

Immoral Methods

Moraczewski's attempt to justify salpingostomy and the use of MTX to cope with tubal pregnancies ultimately rests, I think, on the claim that we can validly distinguish between abortion as merely the "removal" of the unborn child from its site within the mother and abortion as "killing" the unborn child. This distinction, introduced by Germain Grisez, defended by Joseph Boyle and Patrick Lee, and now operative in Moraczewski, perhaps has a certain plausibility. I think it amounts to a euphemistic description of what is actually going on: all that is chosen and done, so it is said, is the "removal" of the nonviable unborn child from a site where it cannot survive and where its presence and continued growth is threatening the mother's life.

But this description ignores the important issue: how is the unborn child removed? It is removed by an interven-

tion on its own body-person, an intervention known to be lethal and undertaken not for the unborn child's benefit but for the benefit of another person. Even if its death is not precisely the means chosen, one cannot exclude from the means chosen the intentional violation of the bodily integrity of the unborn child and the causing of its death, and the doing so, not for its benefit, but for the benefit of another. I thus conclude that these methods of managing ectopic pregnancies are immoral and must be regarded as direct abortion.

Notes

This article originally appeared in *Ethics & Medics* 23.3 (March 1998). It has been lightly edited for this edition.
[1] U.S. Conference of Catholic Bishops, 4th ed. (Washington, D.C), n. 48.
[2] National Conference of Catholic Bishops, *Ethical and Religious Directives for Catholic Health Care Facilities* (Washington, D.C., NCCB, 1971), n. 16 (emphasis added).
[3] John A. Rock, "Ectopic Pregnancy," in *TeLinde's Operative Gynecology*, eds. John D. Thompson and John A. Rock (Philadelphia: J.P. Lippincott Co., 1992), 422–423.
[4] L. Cannon and H. Jesionowska, "Methotrexate Treatment of Tubal Pregnancy," *Fertility and Sterility* 55.6 (June 1991): 1034.
[5] Albert S. Moraczewski, O.P., "Managing Tubal Pregnancies," part 1, *Ethics & Medics* 21.6 (June 1996): 3–4; and part 2, *Ethics & Medics* 21.8 (August 1996): 3–4.
[6] Germain Grisez, *Abortion: The Myths, the Realities, and the Arguments* (Cleveland/New York: Corpus Books, 1970), 340–341; Joseph M. Boyle, Jr., "Double Effect and a Certain Kind of Craniotomy," *Irish Theological Quarterly* 44 (1977): 303–318; and Patrick Lee, *Abortion & Unborn Human Life* (Washington, D.C.: Catholic University of America Press, 1996), 110–120.
[7] William E. May, "The Management of Ectopic Pregnancies: A Moral Analysis," in *The Fetal Tissue Issue,* eds. Peter J. Cataldo and Albert S. Moraczewski (Braintree, MA: Pope John Center, 1994), 121–148.
[8] Kevin Flannery, "What Is Included in a Means to an End?" *Gregorianum* 74.3 (1993): 499–513.

B. Arguments in Favor of Salpingostomy and Methotrexate

Rev. Albert S. Moraczewski, O.P.

Extrauterine pregnancies continue to rise. The proper management of these potentially lethal events remains both a medical and an ethical issue. The principal current procedures for the management of tubal pregnancies are:

• *Expectant management*—nothing is done besides closely monitoring the situation. Estimates are that about half of tubal pregnancies spontaneously resolve.

- *Salpingectomy—full*: the entire fallopian tube containing the ectopic pregnancy is surgically removed; *partial*: only the segment of the tube containing the ectopic pregnancy is removed, and the cut ends of the tube are brought together and sutured.
- *Salpingostomy*—generally the tube is sliced longitudinally and the portion of the tube containing the damaged tissue and the ectopic pregnancy is extracted with forceps or scooped out with an appropriate instrument.
- *Methotrexate treatment*—the drug, administered systemically or injected at the site, inhibits DNA synthesis so that the otherwise normal implantation enzymatic activity ceases.

The Moral Issue

At stake here is what procedures, if any, are morally acceptable in light of the clear Church teaching against direct abortion. Expectant management is morally acceptable because even though the embryo is permitted to die, death results without human intervention. Salpingectomy is acceptable because the surgical action is on the tube, a portion of which is pathological and poses a significant threat to the health and life of the mother. This is an indirect abortion because there is no intention to destroy the child; rather, the intention is to preserve the health and life of the mother. The surgical action is the removal of the pathological tissue which, unfortunately, concurrently and necessarily involves the removal of the embryo. The child's death is foreseen but not intended. Salpingostomy poses a significant moral problem, for it seems like an instance of direct abortion; many moralists view it that way. Methotrexate treatment poses a similar moral problem, and many moralists judge it to be morally unacceptable.

An Alternative Viewpoint

As in my previous articles on this subject,[1] the following moral analysis depends critically on what the physician or surgeon is doing from a moral perspective. What matters is the moral dimension of the doctor's action and not just his medical or surgical procedure. This requires analysis of what constitutes the moral quality of a human act. Traditionally in Catholic moral teaching, there are three components of a human act that determine its morality: the intention (why the person performs this action), the moral object of the act itself (what is the precise good freely willed in this act), and the circumstances (such as persons, place, time, and condition of the persons involved). For a human act to be deemed morally good, all three components must be good.

Of these three, the intention is the focus of most people when they try to assess the morality of an action. One may foresee death without willing it, but one may never directly intend the death of an innocent. But having a good intention is not sufficient, and it will not render the moral object or the circumstances good if they are not good in themselves. The really critical element, and perhaps the most difficult to grasp, is the moral object: the precise, proximate objective perceived as good that is freely willed in this action. What is the moral object of a salpingostomy? Clearly, it is not the salpingostomy by itself that has a moral object; it is the surgeon who wills that action.

Let us say that the surgeon's intention is good: to preserve the health and life of the mother. He slits the tube carefully and with a pair of forceps he removes the damaged portion of the tube. (This description of the procedure is based in part on information provided by T. Murphy Goodwin, M.D., UCLA School of Medicine.) The specific objective and good of that act is the removal of the damaged tissue and the stopping of the enzymatic activity of the trophoblast. That enzymatic action would be normal and proper in the uterus, but it causes severe damage in an abnormal site, the tubal lining. The embryo, of course, is necessarily also removed in the process. One can consider this an indirect abortion. This conclusion is not based on the distinction between removing the embryo from the site and destroying it in situ. It is based on stopping the destructive activity of the trophoblast by removing the invasive trophoblastic cells along with the damaged tubal tissue.

The Case of Methotrexate

Analysis on the use of methotrexate (MTX) for managing a tubal pregnancy proceeds along a similar line of reasoning except that the action is biochemical rather than surgical. The trophoblast is a special group of cells which very early in development are separated from the embryo proper. Normally, once the blastocyst (the embryo proper and the trophoblast) arrives at the uterus and sheds the zona pellucida (the outside protective covering), it begins to burrow into the lining of the uterus. This occurs through the release of certain substances that enable the blastocyst eventually to establish contact with the maternal circulation. The trophoblast, which is the layer of cells external to the embryo proper (at this point only two or three cells), together with maternal components, will then form the placenta. However, when this normal process takes place in an abnormal site, such as the fallopian tube, the trophoblast causes damage that eventually leads to severe hemorrhaging and possibly death for the mother and the child.

Methotrexate acts to inhibit DNA synthesis. Because the trophoblastic cells are rapidly dividing, they are affected more quickly and fully than cells of the embryo proper. These are relatively quiescent until an adequate supply of nourishment is available to them. Once the synthesis of proteolytic enzymes stops (as a result of MTX), the trophoblastic activity ceases and further damage is prevented. The embryo proper also dies eventually; this is foreseen but not willed as an end or as a means.

In summary, let us assume that the intention of the doctor is good: to save the health and life of the woman. The immediate objective and good which the physician wills in the use of MTX is the curative inhibition of DNA synthesis in order to stop the destructive enzymatic activity of the trophoblast. He can will this specific activity of MTX as the desired good of his action without intending the death of the child; it is foreseen but not willed either as an end or as a means. The unfortunate death of the child is not the precise reason for the termination of the destructive activity of the trophoblast.

The line of argument I have briefly outlined here is offered for discussion and is subject ultimately to the judgment of the Holy See. The argument depends on a clear understanding of the three components which determine the moral quality of a human act as understood in the moral tradition of the Church. The critical point, I believe, is to assess properly the moral object of each medical procedure as carried out by an informed surgeon or physician of good will. This having been said, I believe a case can be made for the moral goodness of the procedures when carried out in the manner described.

Notes

This article originally appeared in *Ethics & Medics* 23.3 (March 1998).

[1] See "Managing Tubal Pregnancies," part 1, *Ethics & Medics* 21.6 (June 1996): 3–4; and part 2, 21.8 (August 1996): 3–4.

✠

Editorial Summation: Currently there is disagreement among Catholic ethicists about the use of salpingostomy and methotrexate in cases of ectopic pregnancy. Those who are opposed to their use argue that both procedures involve a direct attack on nascent human life and therefore cannot be justified under the principle of double effect. Salpingostomy has as its object the removal of the embryo from the fallopian tube, while methotrexate attacks the trophoblast, which must be seen as an essential part of the embryo's body. Those who justify the use of salpingostomy and methotrexate argue that the object of both actions is the removal of the enzymatic action of the trophoblast and the damaged tissue. Thus, the act of the physicians is directed to the pathology, and the death of the embryo is foreseen but not intended. Resolution of this debate will depend on further specification of the exact nature of these medical procedures and further refinement of the arguments about the moral object of each act. Generally, if there are two compelling but contrary bodies of theological opinion about a moral issue, each held by experts whose work is in accordance with the magisterium of the Church, and if there is no specific magisterial teaching on the issue that would resolve the matter, then the decision makers may licitly act on either opinion until such time that the magisterium has resolved the question. Salpingectomy is recognized as morally licit by all, while salpingostomy has found only a few defenders. Its claim to morality is therefore suspect. Opinion about methotrexate appears to be more evenly divided and therefore is more appropriately subject to the rule given above.

CHAPTER 11

Pregnancy Prevention after Sexual Assault

The debate over the appropriate treatment of victims of sexual assault has been a subject of Catholic medical–moral discussions for several decades. In an effort to reflect the full range of that debate, this chapter presents various responses to the central problem raised in this discussion, namely, whether it is necessary to test for ovulation in the victim of sexual assault prior to the decision of whether or not to administer an anovulatory drug to prevent conception by the rapist.

There are complex questions of medical fact present here, especially those concerning the possible abortifacient effect of levonorgestrel, the active ingredient in the widely used commercial product Plan B. Hence, some sections are followed by brief rebuttals from those who hold the opposite view. Gerald McShane, M.D., provides a review of the past and present medical data, examin-

ing the known effects of Plan B (levonorgestrel) and the earlier Ovral (a combination of ethinyl estradiol and norgestrel). Peter Cataldo argues that testing for ovulation is unnecessary before administering levonorgestrel because the probability of an abortifacient effect is so small. Patrick Yeung Jr., M.D., Erica Laethem, and Rev. Joseph Tham, L.C., M.D., take the opposite view, arguing that the likelihood of an abortifacient effect is sufficiently high to forbid any use of levonorgestrel whatsoever. They conclude, like Cataldo, that ovulation testing is unnecessary. Finally, Marie Hilliard, R.N., argues in favor of ovulation testing on the grounds that levonorgestrel may have an abortifacient effect, depending on the timing of the victim's ovulatory cycle. Of these views, the latter has been and remains the position of The National Catholic Bioethics Center.

A. Postcoital Anovulatory Hormonal Treatment: An Overview of the Medical Data

Gerald J. McShane, M.D.

The purpose of hormonal intervention in a woman who has been sexually assaulted is the inhibition of ovulation to prevent a pregnancy resulting from the assault. Three central questions need to be resolved before such intervention can be considered morally permissible in a Catholic health care setting: (1) whether the female survivor of the sexual assault is an appropriate candidate for hormonal treatment to inhibit ovulation, (2) how effective such treatment is, and (3) whether the treatment has any post-fertilization effect.

Candidates and Effectiveness

A woman is not an appropriate candidate for postcoital anovulatory hormonal treatment if she is already pregnant,

if she has had a prior hysterectomy, if she is postmenopausal, or if she is currently taking oral contraceptives. These are obvious exclusions.

Whether postcoital anovulatory hormonal treatment is appropriate in other women depends on precise dating of ovulation in each woman. This medical judgment requires greater medical inquiry than mere historical dating based on the dates of the woman's last menstrual period. Laboratory tests that help determine whether ovulation has occurred or is about to occur include the serum progesterone test and the urine test for luteinizing hormone (LH).

A woman's progesterone level begins to rise at the time of ovulation, continues to rise for six to ten days, and then falls again if fertilization does not occur. Lutein-

Table 1. The Pharmacological Effects of Postcoital Anovulatory Hormonal Agents

Day in cycle:[1]	6	7	8	9	10	11	12	13	14	15	16	17	18	19	20	21	22	23	24	25	26	27	28
Phase:	Follicular phase							Ovulation		Luteal phase													
Day pre- or post-ovulation:		-7	-6	-5	-4	-3	-2	-1	0	+1	+2	+3	+4	+5	+6	+7	Zero						
Probability of pregnancy:[2]	Nearly zero			10%	16%	14%	27%	31%	33%	Nearly zero	Zero												
	Pre-ovulatory							LH surge Ovulation		Post-ovulatory													
										Early Post-ovulatory			Late Post-ovulatory										
										Menses expected in >7 days							Menses expected in <7 days						
Cervical mucus property:[3]	Thick							Strong Ferning		Thick													
Urine luteinizing hormone:[4]	-	-	-	-	-	-	-	+	+	-	-	-	-	-	-	-	-	-	-	-	-	-	-
Serum progesterone level:[4]	<1.5 ng/ml							≥ 1.5 and ≤5.9 ng/ml			≥6 ng/ml						<6 ng/ml						
Pharmacological effect:[5]	Anovulatory effect							Potential Abortifacient Effect									Psychological benefit						

This graphic adaptation of the Saint Francis Medical Center protocol, by Ralph P. Miech, M.D., Ph.D., is intended to help the clinician evaluate the potential pharmacological effect of a postcoital anovulatory hormonal agent in a rape victim. NOTES: (1) The numbers of the days are based on a twenty-eight-day cycle. Days 1 through 5, which are not shown, represent the menses. (2) See Wilcox, Weinberg, and Baird, "Timing of Sexual Intercourse in Relation to Ovulation: Effects on the Probability of Conception, Survival of the Pregnancy, and Sex of the Baby," *New England Journal of Medicine* 333.23 (December 7, 1995): 1517–1521. (3) See T.W. Hilgers, G.E. Abraham, and D. Cavanagh, "Natural Family Planning: The Peak Symptom and Estimated Time of Ovulation," *Obstetrics and Gynecology* 52.5 (November 1978): 575–582. (4) See Saint Francis Medical Center, "Interim Protocol for Sexual Assault: Anovulatory Hormonal Treatment Component," October 1995, which appears here on pp. 125 to 127. (5) The particular pharmacological effect of a postcoital anovulatory hormonal agent depends on three factors: Where in the menstrual cycle did the rape occur? Where in the menstrual cycle did or will ovulation occur? How long after the rape will the postcoital anovulatory hormonal agent be administered?

izing hormone surges briefly and dramatically just before ovulation. If results of serum progesterone and urine LH tests show that ovulation has not yet occurred, postcoital anovulatory hormonal treatment may be appropriate. The use of serum progesterone and urine LH tests in identifying women who are candidates for treatment that inhibits ovulation and those who are not is described in some detail in the Saint Francis Medical Center ("Peoria") protocol for the treatment of victims of sexual assault, reprinted here on pp. 131 to 133.

The second question relevant to Catholic health care focuses on the effectiveness of hormonal treatment in sexual assault. A number of possible hormonal combinations have been tried in the emergency setting, more commonly as postcoital treatment for cases of consensual sexual intercourse. The standard hormonal drug used today in hospital emergency departments is levonorgestrel (Plan B). Before the year 2000, a combination of ethinyl estradiol and norgestrel (Ovral) was the standard treatment. A rather large study in 1998 compared the effectiveness of levonorgestrel and Ovral and showed that levonorgestrel has a higher efficacy for the prevention of pregnancy with a lower incidence of side effects than the standard Ovral method.[1]

The medical literature does not contain a sufficient number of scientific studies relevant to sexual assault. A valid scientific design for studying sexual assault would be extraordinarily difficult to set up. Extrapolation from reported postcoital data for pregnancy prevention in cases of consensual sexual intercourse (i.e., reports on the use of the so-called morning-after pill) may be somewhat helpful for understanding the effectiveness of hormonal treatment. However, rape can cause an altered ovulatory physiology in the survivor, which skews conclusions inferred from postcoital pregnancy-prevention data in non-sexual assault cases. Studies of the medical effectiveness of hormonal treatment—the degree to which it inhibits ovulation—after sexual assault center on interpretations of related scientific data, not data specific to rape situations. In the pre-2000 era, assertions about the mechanism of action of postcoital hormones were speculative. Since then, more objective data, both human and animal, have provided a better understanding of how postcoital contraception works.

Ovulation occurs during a narrow window of time in a woman's menstrual cycle (Table 1). The signal for ovulation is the release of LH from the pituitary gland in the brain. Once the LH surge begins, ovulation will occur over the next twenty-four to forty-eight hours. A large study of the LH surge in women showed that by twenty-four hours after the surge, 35 percent of the women had ovulated, and

by forty-eight hours the other 65 percent had ovulated.[2] Ovulation thus follows predictably from the LH surge, and the main mechanism of action of the typical oral contraceptive pill is the inhibition of LH release.[3] Whether the acute administration of levonorgestrel is effective in inhibiting the LH surge needs to be determined.

A Summary of Post-2000 Data: Postcoital and Post-fertilization Studies of Levonorgestrel

In an article published 2004, H. B. Croxatto et al. assessed the extent to which levonorgestrel affected the ovulatory process when given to fifty-eight women in the pre-ovulatory phase.[13] They found that levonorgestrel disrupted the process in 93 percent of cycles treated. More recently, N. Novikova et al. determined the effectiveness of levonorgestrel administered before or after ovulation in ninety-nine women in a postcoital emergency-contraception study, in which subjects were assessed for ovulatory status at entry.[14] Three women became pregnant. These three women were among the seventeen who received levonorgestrel after ovulation (two days after ovulation, on average). Statistically three to four pregnancies were predicted, and three were observed. Among the thirty-four women who had intercourse just before ovulation (during the fertile period), four pregnancies were predicted; none were observed. The authors conclude that levonorgestrel has few or no post-ovulatory effects and that it is highly effective when given before ovulation. This study suggests no post-fertilization effects, but statistically the study is limited by the small number of subjects.

Animal studies using both rats and the new-world monkey *Cebus apella* have attempted to determine the effects of levonorgestrel on post-fertilization events.[15] In each study levonorgestrel had no effect on fertilization. Pregnancy rates and implantation with levonorgestrel were identical to placebo findings in each study.

P. G. Lalitkumar et al. performed studies on human blastocysts to determine whether levonorgestrel or mifepristone (RU-486) inhibited blastocysts in an in vitro endometrial cell culture model.[16] Their findings using receptors confirmed blastocyst attachment when the blastocysts were cultured with levonorgestrel. Blastocysts cultured with mifepristone failed to attach to the endometrial construct.

Another study, which examined endometrial and serum patterns of glycodelin-A, a potent inhibitor of sperm–oocyte binding, showed different levels when levonorgestrel was given before or after the LH surge.[17]

Although complex, the glycodelin-A level increases sooner than in controls when levonorgestrel was given in the pre-ovulatory state. The inference is that the presence of glycodelin-A in the serum can affect sperm–oocyte binding and subsequent fertilization. In the same group (those who received levonorgestrel in the pre-ovulatory phase), however, this glycoprotein was less present in the endometrium. The authors speculate that this effect in the endometrium would serve to interfere with implantation. Others speculate that these effects are purely the result of the LH-surge inhibition and not an effect of levonorgestrel or reduced progesterone levels (the effect of not ovulating). Clearly, the clinical effects are speculative.

One other study looked at the effects of levonorgestrel on human spermatozoa.[18] K. Brito et al. evaluated the effects of levonorgestrel on the acrosome reaction of capacitated and noncapacitated sperm. Their study failed to show any effects of levonorgestrel on the sperm acrosome reaction. Other, older studies have looked at the effects of levonorgestrel on sperm migration in the three- to nine-hour postcoital time frame. It is considered proved that levonorgestrel, soon after intercourse, will substantially reduce the number of sperm found in the uterine cavity. Overall, the effect on sperm motility is not thought to be a significant mechanism of emergency contraception.

Another study looked at whether the probability of fertilization is associated with levels of LH, follicular stimulating hormone (FSH), and steroids in preovulatory follicular fluid. Using in vitro fertilization techniques, Willem Verpoest and colleagues hypothesized that these levels are associated with the probability of fertilization.[19] Their findings show that eggs from women whose follicular fluid was low in LH were unlikely to be fertilized.

An inference can be drawn that when levonorgestrel is given before ovulation, the LH surge is completely stopped in a majority of cases. There are times when a limited LH surge occurs, enough to cause the egg to erupt from the ovary. It is speculated that these eggs are resistant to fertilization.

Pre-2000 Data:
Three Postcoital Studies of Ovral

This section summarizes the data showing the response of women who have not been sexually assaulted to acutely administered Ovral intervention. The end point of these studies is the determination of the effect of the intervention on the LH surge. It must be emphasized that the volunteers in these studies were women who were not sexually assaulted.

In 1979, W. Y. Ling et al. published "Mode of Action of dl-Norgestrel and Ethinylestradiol Combination in Postcoital Contraception."[4] In 1996, M. L. Swahn et al. published "Effect of Post-Coital Contraceptive Methods on the Endometrium and the Menstrual Cycle."[5] Both studies provide information about the effectiveness of hormonal intervention. The goal of each study was to determine the frequency with which Ovral delayed or totally inhibited the LH surge and consequent ovulation. A better end point would have been the degree to which ovulation was inhibited as verified on sonographic examination. However, studies with that design are not available.

Ling et al. estimated the cycle date and ovulation date, and hence the day to give Ovral, by using the woman's cycle from the prior month as a control.[6] This method of assigning the exact day in the cycle in reference to the LH surge is imprecise. Swahn et al. used both the prior month's cycle and urine LH testing to better determine the woman's particular menstrual-cycle phase during the time of hormonal intervention.[7]

In the study by Ling et al., day 0 is considered to be the day of the LH surge; day -1 is one day before the LH surge; day -2 is two days before the LH surge, and so forth.[8] The following is a summary of the findings:

- *Group 1*: In three women given Ovral on days 0, -1, and -3, the LH surge was completely inhibited.
- *Group 2*: In one woman given Ovral on day -1, the LH surge was delayed by thirteen days.
- *Group 3*: In two women given Ovral on days -1 and -2, LH peak levels were substantially reduced but not totally inhibited.
- *Group 4*: In two women given Ovral on day 0, LH levels were suppressed significantly but not totally.[9]
- *Group 5*: Ovral given to one woman on day -4 had no effect on the LH surge.

Ovral appears to have reliably inhibited the LH surge in groups 1 and 2. In group 3, Ovral did not suppress the LH surge or ovulation in one woman. In group 4, there would not have been an expectation of LH surge inhibition. Underlying these results is the inexactness of the dating methodology used in the study. The last woman was given on Ovral on day -4 with no effect on the LH surge.

An issue facing clinicians is whether ovulation needs to be delayed in the instance described by group 5—that is, in a woman who was assaulted on day -4. The lifespan of sperm (about ninety-six hours) is an important factor, because ovulation takes place twenty-four to forty-eight hours after the LH peak. Consequently, sperm are not likely to remain viable over the five- to six-day period from day -4 to ovulation.

Using the findings from Ling et al., and assuming that a woman is in a preovulatory state (and more specifically a pre-LH surge state), I would estimate that there is a 70 to 80 percent chance that Ovral would inhibit LH. The chances of inhibiting LH actually could statistically be higher if women in the LH-positive preovulatory state were excluded from the study.

The study by Swahn et al. looked at eight volunteers with control months before and after the administration of Ovral (by groups):[10]

- *Group 1*: In three women, the LH surge was undetectable after the administration of Ovral.
- *Group 2*: In two women, the LH surge was delayed twenty-six and twenty-seven days, respectively.
- *Group 3*: In three women, the LH surge was noted on cycle day 13 for two women and cycle day 22 for another.

In group 1, LH was totally suppressed. In group 2, ovulation was postponed for more than three weeks. In group 3, there was no postponement of ovulation in two women, and an eight- to ten-day postponement of the LH surge in one. In conclusion, rather substantial suppression or delay of ovulation occurred in approximately 75 percent of women in this small study. Hence, Ovral administered in the preovulatory state is approximately 75 to 80 percent effective in inhibiting ovulation. In the preovulatory state,

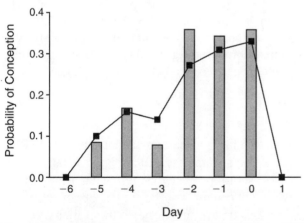

Figure 1. Probability of conception on specific days near the day of ovulation, from Wilcox, Weinberg, and Baird (1995). The bars show probabilities calculated from data on menstrual cycles in which sexual intercourse was recorded as having occurred on only a single day during the six-day interval ending on the day of ovulation (day 0). The solid line shows probabilities based on all cycles for which the dates of ovulation could be estimated. © 1995 Massachusetts Medical Society. Used with permission.

Ovral's principal effect is ovulation inhibition. In the early postovulatory state, the principal effect has to be other than ovulation inhibition.

A clinical study by A. J. Wilcox, C. R. Weinberg, and D. D. Baird estimated the probability of conception on specific days near the day of ovulation.[11] Figure 1 shows the probabilities. In this study, day 0 is considered ovulation. The LH peak day shown in Figure 1 is actually day -2, two days before ovulation, and the probability of conception on day 0 and day -1 are nearly equal. (Ovulation actually takes place, on average, over a one- to two-day period, not just on one day.) The probability of conception on the fourth day prior to the LH peak is essentially zero.

The efficacy of Ovral in postcoital intervention for the prevention of pregnancy was also demonstrated in an international study where in nine hundred treatment episodes it reduced the expected pregnancy rate from 76 to 31 for women with a variety of cycle dates.[12] This is a reduction of approximately 57 percent in the number of pregnancies. Compared to the pregnancy rate reduction of 70 to 80 percent for women in the preovulatory state, the reduction in this group of nine hundred women is less than would be expected from strict anti-ovulatory treatment. Although the data from this study are limited, one could speculate that they support the anovulatory effects of Ovral.

From the data in Wilcox et al., it could be argued that on the day following ovulation the chances of pregnancy are about zero, and hence a sexual assault occurring one to two days after ovulation poses no risk of pregnancy. The key factors for the use of Ovral as a postcoital anovulant intervention are that the timing of ovulation must be precisely determined by identifying the LH signal, that this timing is critical, and that prior to the LH surge the use of Ovral has a significant anovulatory effect.

Whether Ovral also affects implantation is unclear. Although it has varying cytological effects, alteration of implantation would be exceedingly difficult to prove by any large clinical trial. Interestingly, if Ovral truly does affect implantation, it does so rather poorly. Pregnancy rates are reduced by only slightly greater than half of what is expected. What can be said with some greater certainty is that Ovral used prior to the LH surge reduces pregnancy by an anovulatory mechanism in the vast majority of the cases.

Before the year 2000, Ovral was the drug most commonly used to inhibit ovulation in women who had been sexually assaulted. Today, levonorgestrel is most commonly used. In summary, the science behind the mechanism of levonorgestrel supports the anovulatory effect when levonorgestrel is given during a woman's preovulatory phase. Animal data on levonorgestrel show an absence of post-fertilization and implantation effects; one experimental laboratory study shows no interference with implantation; and one human study shows anovulatory effects of levonorgestrel and a lack of post-fertilization events, although the number of participants in that study was small.

Notes

[1] Task Force on Postovulatory Methods of Fertility Regulation, "Randomised Controlled Trial of Levonorgestrel versus the Yuzpe Regimen of Combined Oral Contraceptives for Emergency Contraception," *Lancet* 352.9126 (August 8, 1998): 428–433.

[2] A. C. Pearlstone and E. S. Surrey, "The Temporal Relation Between the Urine LH Surge and Sonographic Evidence of Ovulation: Determinants and Clinical Significance," *Obstetrics and Gynecology* 83.2 (February 1994): 184–188.

[3] W. L. Larimore and J. B. Stanford, "Postfertilization Effects of Oral Contraceptives and Their Relationship to Informed Consent," *Archives of Family Medicine* 9.2 (February 2000): 126–133.

[4] W. Y. Ling et al., "Mode of Action of dl-Norgestrel and Ethinylestradiol Combination in Postcoital Contraception," *Fertility and Sterility* 32.3 (September 1979): 297–302.

[5] M. L. Swahn et al., "Effect of Postcoital Contraceptive Methods on the Endometrium and the Menstrual Cycle," *Acta Obstetricia et Gynecologica Scandinavica* 75.8 (September 1996): 738–744.

[6] Ling et al., "Mode of Action of dl-Norgestrel."

[7] Swahn et al., "Effect of Postcoital Contraceptive Methods."

[8] Ling et al., "Mode of Action of dl-Norgestrel."

[9] Of course, one would not expect LH suppression on day 0 if the LH surge had already fired. This to me shows the inherent flaw in this study. Ling and his colleagues really needed to know whether the subjects were truly preovulatory and in the pre-LH surge. A. J. Wilcox, C. R. Weinberg, and D. D. Baird, "Timing of Sexual Intercourse in Relation to Ovulation: Effects on the Probability of Conception, Survival of the Pregnancy, and Sex of the Baby," *New England Journal of Medicine* 333.23 (December 7, 1995): 1517–1521, attempts to answer that question by performing the LH detection to help identify the circumstances of the individual women in their study.

[10] Swahn et al., "Effect of Postcoital Contraceptive Methods."

[11] Wilcox et al., "Timing of Sexual Intercourse."

[12] Task Force on Postovulatory Methods, "Randomised Controlled Trial of Levonorgestrel."

[13] H. B. Croxatto et al., "Pituitary-Ovarian Function Following the Standard Levonorgestrel Emergency Contraceptive Dose or a Single 0.75 mg Dose Given on the Days Preceding Ovulation," *Contraception* 70.6 (December 2004): 442–450.

[14] N. Novikova et al., "Effectiveness of Levonorgestrel Emergency Contraception Given Before or After Ovulation: A Pilot Study," *Contraception* 75.2 (February 2007): 112–118.

[15] M. E. Ortiz et al., "Postcoital Administration of Levonorgestrel Does Not Interfere with Post-Fertilization Events in the New-World Monkey *Cebus paella*," *Human Reproduction* 19.6 (June 2004): 1352–1356; A. L. Muller et al., "Postcoital Treatment with Levonorgestrel Does Not Disrupt Post-Fertilization Events in the Rat," *Contraception* 67.5 (May 2003): 415–419.

[16] P. G. Lalitkumar et al., "Mifepristone, But Not Levonorgestrel, Inhibits Human Blastocyst Attachment to an In Vitro Endometrial Three-Dimensional Cell Culture Model," *Human Reproduction* 22.11 (November 2007): 3031–3037.

[17] M. Durand et al., "Late Follicular Phase Administration of Levonorgestrel as an Emergency Contraceptive Changes the Secretory Pattern of Glycodelin in Serum and Endometrium during the Luteal Phase of the Menstrual Cycle," *Contraception* 71.6 (June 2005): 451–457.

[18] K. Brito et al., "The In Vitro Effect of Emergency Contraception Doses of Levonorgestrel on the Acrosome Reaction of Human Sperm," *Contraception* 72.3 (September 2005): 225–228.

[19] W. M. Verpoest et al., "Relationship between Midcycle Luteinizing Hormone Surge Quality and Oocyte Fertilization," *Fertility and Sterility* 73.1 (January 2000): 75–77.

Editorial Summation: There are laboratory tests that assist in determining whether ovulation has occurred or is about to occur, thus identifying whether a female survivor of sexual assault is an appropriate candidate for hormonal treatment to inhibit ovulation. These tests include a serum progesterone test and a urine test for detection of luteinizing hormone. The medical literature does not contain a sufficient number of scientific studies relevant to sexual assault to determine how effective such treatment may be. Extrapolation from literature reporting postcoital data for pregnancy prevention after consensual sexual intercourse (i.e., studies of the morning-after pill) is somewhat helpful; however, the circumstances of rape can cause an altered ovulatory physiology in the survivor. In consensual sexual intercourse, the efficacy of Ovral administered in the preovulatory phase is approximately 75 to 80 percent. Levonorgestrel (Plan B) is the drug most commonly used in sexual assault cases now. Studies indicate that levonorgestrel is highly effective for inhibiting ovulation when given in the preovulatory phase. Most studies also indicate that levonorgestrel has no post-fertilization or implantation effects, although the number of studies and their sample sizes have been small.

Protocol for Sexual Assault:
Anovulatory Hormonal Treatment Component

Saint Francis Medical Center

This protocol is intended for use at Saint Francis Medical Center, Peoria. It supplements the existing general protocol for treatment of sexual assault. As additional clinical data are developed, this protocol will be reviewed.

Part I: Introduction

This protocol provides guidelines for a contraceptive intervention in those cases in which there is a clinical indication that the effect of the intervention will be truly contraceptive, and not abortifacient. Such clinical determination will be based on (1) a menstrual history provided by the survivor, (2) hormonal levels evidenced by a blood test that would help better categorize the timing of her own ovulatory cycle (this test is to be utilized only when the results can be provided in a timely manner), and (3) the results of the OvuKIT urine test, which is a reliable guide to the prediction of ovulation. If the urine test is negative, it could be an indication that the LH surge has not been initiated, and a contraceptive intervention would be appropriate. If the test is positive, it would signify that the hormonal shift that leads to ovulation has begun, and could not be blunted or halted by the contraceptive formulation. An effect of a contraceptive intervention could be abortifacient, and is thus excluded, even though there is no evidence that conception has occurred.

Throughout their years of health care ministry, the Sisters of the Third Order of St. Francis have cared for women who have been the survivors of rape. The sisters believe, in the words of the *Ethical and Religious Directives for Catholic Health Care Services* (*ERD*), that "compassionate and understanding care should be given to a person who is the survivor of sexual assault" (directive 36), and that, in Catholic health care services, this must be given in a manner consistent with Catholic moral insights and teachings.

Explanation of the Protocol

"A female who has been raped should be able to defend herself against a potential conception from the sexual assault. If, after appropriate testing, there is no evidence that conception has occurred already, she may be treated with medications that would prevent ovulation, sperm capacitation, or fertilization. It is not permissible, however, to initiate or to recommend treat-

—continued—

The Saint Francis Medical Center *Protocol for Sexual Assault: Contraceptive Treatment Component*, also known as the Peoria protocol, is reprinted here with permission. References cited in the protocol are to R.B. Everett and G.K. Jimerson, "The Rape Victim: A Review of 117 Consecutive Cases," *Obstetrics and Gynecology* 50.1 (July 1977): 88–90; and Sandra Mahkorn, "Pregnancy and Sexual Assault," *The Psychological Aspects of Abortion*, ed. D. Mall and W.F. Watts (Washington, D.C.: University Publications of America, 1979), 55–69.

ments that have as their purpose or direct effect the removal, destruction, or interference with the implantation of a fertilized ovum" (*ERD*, n. 36).

Rape is an act of aggression, and as an individual is justified in repelling an act of such aggression, she is also justified in thwarting the continuing effect of the aggression, namely, the progress of sperm before conception could occur. Fortunately, conception rarely (0 to 4 percent; Everett and Jimerson 1977, Mahkorn 1979) results from the violence of rape. In those cases in which conception is a potential, then, the *ERD* would permit an intervention that would be truly contraceptive in its effect, but not one that would be abortifacient; that is, "the removal, destruction, or interference with the implantation of a fertilized ovum."

If a female survivor of sexual assault shows a negative result for pregnancy on the blood test, and negative with respect on the urine dip-stick test, and her history corresponds to this, she will be offered a contraceptive intervention of Plan B (levonorgestrel). If she accepts this treatment, the dose will be provided to her in the emergency department to achieve the contraceptive effect. (If the survivor is merely given a prescription and delays filling it, ovulation could occur in the meantime, and a possibly abortifacient effect follow.)

If the survivor presents a positive result on the tests she will be counseled that the emergency department will not offer her the formulation. If the blood test result is positive for pregnancy, she will be counseled that this is a pregnancy that is not of immediate or recent origin. If the urine test is positive and relates to her history, it indicates that the LH surge is under way or that the woman is ovulating, and that a contraceptive formulation would not be effective in preventing ovulation. Consequently, this information indicates a risk that should not be taken by a Catholic hospital.

All survivors will be referred to an obstetrician-gynecologist for a suggested follow-up visit. If an individual who is not offered a contraceptive formulation in the emergency department requests this formulation at such a visit, a number of area obstetrician-gynecologists would probably provide such. Physicians employed by the Catholic health care sponsor, OSF Healthcare System, will appropriately participate in the emergency department protocol; however, physicians employed by a Catholic entity should not provide a contraceptive intervention outside the guidelines of this protocol.

In addition to the benefit of a sound protocol for treating survivors of sexual assault, this protocol and the test it suggests will be of benefit to those women who have been reluctant to accept a contraceptive intervention due to their concern of an abortifacient result. This should provide sound information and peace of mind to survivors and the professionals caring for them.

Part II: Clinical Application

I. If a woman is determined to be in the preovulatory phase of her cycle, then Plan B (levonorgestrel) will be immediately available for the most effective contraceptive intervention as a single dose of 1.5 mg.

   1. History: compatible with preovulatory phase

   2. Physical examination: compatible with preovulatory phase

3. LH urine: negative. Progesterone level: less than 1.5 ng/ml

II. If a woman is determined to be in her (1) midcycle LH surge phase or (2) early postovulatory phase, Plan B (levonorgestrel) is not to be given by the emergency medicine department physician:

1. LH urine: positive. Progesterone level: unnecessary to perform

2. LH urine: negative. Progesterone level: greater than or equal to 1.5 or less than or equal to 5.9 ng/ml. Menstrual history: compatible with midcycle and early postovulatory phase (menses expected in more than seven days).

III. If the woman is determined to be past the early postovulatory phase (LH urine negative; progesterone greater than or equal to 6 ng/ml), because the timing of the sexual assault could not have coincided with the presence of an ovum, it is not unethical to prescribe Plan B (levonorgestrel) for the psychological benefit of the woman who requests it.

IV. If the woman is determined to be in the late postovulatory phase, because the timing of the sexual assault could not have coincided with the presence of an ovum, it is not unethical to prescribe Plan B (levonorgestrel) for the benefit of the woman who requests it:

1. Progesterone level: less than 6 ng/ml (Testing for progesterone level will be given only when results can be provided in a timely manner.)

2. LH urine: negative

3. Menstrual history: anticipation of menses in less than seven days (usually three to five days).

V. Dr. Gerald McShane will act as a consultant to the emergency department for the implementation of this protocol.

VI. As part of follow-up for all alleged sexual-assault patients (including referral to Peoria City Health Department for six-week follow-up VDRL [for venereal disease], and material on VD medication, state compensation act, and sexual assault), the patient will be referred to her private physician or obstetrician-gynecologist. Emergency medicine department physician will be available to discuss this patient's case with the private physician.

VII. The treatment provided under this protocol is intended to prevent ovulation, sperm capacitation, or fertilization. Excluded from this protocol are treatments that would have as their purpose or direct effect the removal, destruction, or interference with the implantation of a fertilized ovum.

VIII. State law does not require religious-sponsored hospitals to engage in activities unconscionable to them and provides: "Information which describes fertility status, available types of prevention of unwanted pregnancy and side effects, contraindications, complications, etc. If a hospital does not provide such counseling because of religious preferences, this requirement may be met by listing various sexual assault counseling centers available in the area" (77 Illinois Admin. Code, Ch. I, sec. 545. APP.A, subchapter f, 5[e]). Ethical and Religious Directive 36 calls on Catholic providers to, inter alia, "cooperate with law enforcement officials, offer the person psychological and spiritual support, and accurate medical information."

June 2009

B. Argument in Favor of the Use of Levonorgestrel in Cases of Sexual Assault

Peter J. Cataldo

The Significance of the Role of Freedom for the Moral Analysis

A woman who is sexually assaulted has the right to defend herself against this unjust aggression before, during, and after the assault. Any semen that might have been deposited in the reproductive tract of the survivor by the attacker is one of the lingering effects of the assault and can be considered part of the aggression. The woman has the right to defend herself against this effect and the possibility that it will lead to fertilization. It has been long recognized in the Catholic moral tradition that if it is morally justifiable for a woman to take measures to prevent a sexual attack, then it is justifiable for her to prevent any continuation of the same attack.[1] Every aspect of the act (including the attacker's semen and the risk of fertilization) is forced upon her, and is against her free choice of the will and consent. As an act of self-defense, the woman may take measures to prevent fertilization. She may stop the lingering effect of the attack by not allowing her fertility to be integrated with that of her attacker.[2]

A question arises. How can the Catholic moral tradition consistently hold that the deliberate suppression of fertility is morally unacceptable in some cases but not in others? The morally decisive difference between deliberately suppressing fertility as a defensive measure against unjust aggression and deliberately suppressing fertility only for the sake of preventing fertilization (e.g., direct contraception) rests on these facts: (1) the suppression of fertility in the case of rape is in response to an involuntary act of assault that includes the unjust use of the aggressor's reproductive powers, and (2) the suppression of fertility in the case of contraception is part of a voluntary sexual act. Thus, the presence or absence of voluntariness (i.e., free consent to the act of intercourse) is an essential condition that determines a moral difference between what may otherwise be similar in some physical aspects, namely, taking hormonal medication to suppress ovulation in the context of freely chosen intercourse on the one hand and, on the other, taking the same medication after a sexual assault.

The Church's prohibition against contraception and direct sterilization is, among other things, premised on the fact that those for whom the prohibition applies freely engage in sexual intercourse.[3] If an act of sexual intercourse is voluntary, then neither contraception nor direct sterilization may be used. If one is free to choose regarding the use of the reproductive powers, then one is under the moral obligation to act in accordance with the inherent good of those powers and avoid what is evil in fulfillment of that freedom. The voluntary use of the reproductive powers must therefore be reserved for genuine conjugal acts in marriage. Pope Pius XII explicitly states the link between the voluntary use of the reproductive powers and their inherent goal: "The Creator himself, for the good of the human race, has indissolubly bound up the voluntary use of those natural energies [of sexuality] with their intrinsic purpose."[4] It follows from this statement that the Church's prohibition against contraception also rests on the same foundation of freedom of action.

This point is made in the following two texts from the Congregation for the Doctrine of the Faith:

> Sterility intended in itself is not oriented to the integral good of the person as rightly pursued, "the proper order of goods being preserved," inasmuch as it damages the ethical good of the person, which is the highest good, since it deliberately deprives *foreseen and freely chosen sexual activity* of an essential element.[5]

In its *Declaration on Certain Questions concerning Sexual Ethics*, the CDF again indicates the role of freedom in the Church's prohibition against use of the reproductive powers outside conjugal relations in marriage:

> The deliberate use of the sexual faculty outside normal conjugal relations essentially contradicts the finality of the faculty. For it lacks the sexual relationship called for by the moral order, namely, the relationship which realizes "the full sense of mutual self-giving and human procreation in the context of true love." *All deliberate exercise of sexuality must be reserved to this regular relationship.*[6]

Free use of the reproductive powers carries the obligation to use them only for their inherent ends, namely, their procreative and unitive meanings. If a sexual act is forced upon a woman and is not freely engaged in by her, then the prohibition against deliberately suppressing the procreative dimension of the act does not apply. From a moral point of view, the act of preventing fertilization in this situation is different in kind from an act of contraception. The absence of the essential condition of freedom in a sexual assault makes the prevention of fertilization after the assault an act of self-defense rather than a contraceptive act (in the moral sense). Given that it is morally justifiable to suppress ovulation and to prevent the meeting of gametes as an act of self-defense against sexual assault, is it morally acceptable to achieve this by hormonal intervention?

The Moral Status of Postcoital Anovulatory Hormonal Drugs for the Treatment of Sexual Assault Survivors

The disagreement already mentioned among physicians, theologians, and ethicists who are in accord with the magisterium of the Church is specifically over whether the use of drugs such as levonorgestrel (Plan B) in the treatment of the survivor of sexual assault constitutes a morally legitimate act of self-defense, or whether use of the drug under certain circumstances constitutes the moral equivalence of abortion primarily by preventing implantation. This debate in turn has engendered a debate over testing for the ovulation phase of the survivor of sexual assault. Thus, there is disagreement as to whether compliance with all parts of directive 36 of the *Ethical and Religious Directives for Catholic Health Care Services* is morally possible at the present time. The directive states:

> Compassionate and understanding care should be given to a person who is the victim of sexual assault. Health-care providers should cooperate with law enforcement officials and offer the person psychological and spiritual support as well as accurate medical information. A female who has been raped should be able to defend herself against a potential conception from the sexual assault. If, after appropriate testing, there is no evidence that conception has occurred already, she may be treated with medications that would prevent ovulation, sperm capacitation, or fertilization. It is not permissible, however, to initiate or to recommend treatments that have as their purpose or direct effect the removal, destruction, or interference with the implantation of a fertilized ovum.[7]

The directive allows for medications that would "prevent ovulation." This point, together with the proscription against preventing implantation in the last sentence of the directive, implies that the health care provider must have a prudential or moral certitude (based on current medical and pharmacological knowledge) that the medication will more likely prevent ovulation than act primarily as an abortifacient in any case in which such the drug is administered. Therefore, the debates over directive 36 have generated two crucial questions for the moral evaluation of medications administered to prevent ovulation in rape protocols: (1) what is the evidence for and against an abortifacient effect of postcoital hormonal drugs (such as levonorgestrel) used in the treatment of sexual assault survivors; and (2) in light of this evidence, is it morally required for Catholic hospitals to test for the ovulation phase of the survivor, and administer the drug on the basis of such testing, in order to have greater certitude that the drug will not result in an abortifacient effect when it is administered.

Outline of an Argument Against the Use of Postcoital Hormonal Drugs

The argument against the use of postcoital hormonal drugs for their anovulatory effect may be summarized in this way:

> The use of postcoital hormonal drugs administered only for their anovulatory effect to treat the survivor of sexual assault is not morally permissible, because
>
> A. The evidence indicates that these drugs can also prevent implantation of the embryo, which is morally equivalent to abortion, and
>
> B. The principle of double effect does not validly apply, if attempted.

It is argued that the inability to know whether hormonal drugs will only "prevent ovulation, sperm capacitation or fertilization" (and not the implantation of an embryo) makes their use morally impermissible. As long as there is a possibility that the drug can have the post-fertilization effect of preventing implantation, the drug can cause the death of a newly conceived human being, which would be morally unacceptable. If it is not known that conception has occurred in any given case, even the risk of causing the death of a human being is not morally justified, especially in light of the fact that the life of the woman is not at stake. To employ such hormonal treatment when it is foreseen that there is a possibility that the drug could have an abortifacient effect is to be morally responsible for causing the death of the human being should this effect occur. Moreover, to risk the possibility of an abortifacient action is itself a morally reprehensible act even if no human being is killed.

Therefore, the argument continues, because the possible abortifacient effect of these drugs is known and accepted by many in the medical community, Catholic health care institutions may not use these drugs in the treatment of sexual assault survivors. Moreover, one cannot appeal to the principle of double effect, because it does not validly apply in the case. There are not two concurrent effects (one good and the other bad) caused by the act of administering the drug. Rather, in each particular case, only one of two possible effects occurs—either suppression of ovulation or prevention of implantation.[8]

Outline of an Argument in Favor of the Use of Postcoital Hormonal Drugs

An argument in favor of using postcoital hormonal drugs for their anovulatory effect may be summarized in this way:

> The use of postcoital hormonal drugs administered only for their anovulatory effect to treat the survivor of sexual assault is morally permissible, because
>
> A. The evidence indicates that it is unlikely that these drugs act as an abortifacient, and
>
> B. The remote possibility of a secondary mechanism occurring which might prevent implantation is morally justifiable under the proper circumstances and conditions of moral certitude using a three-moral-fonts approach.

This argument applies the traditional three fonts or sources of the moral act to the question, rather than the principle of double effect. The question is not one that can be judged by the principle of double effect in the first place, but for reasons other than what have been mentioned earlier in the argument against the use of postcoital hormonal drugs. Understanding why the principle does not apply is instructive for the argument in favor of hormonal intervention.

The principle of double effect requires that one can reasonably foresee that two effects of an act (one effect good and the other evil) will occur as a result of the act. This prerequisite condition for applying the principle does not obtain in the question of anovulatory hormonal treatment of a survivor of sexual assault. The improbable evil effect of preventing the implantation of a fertilized ovum as a result of using anovulatory hormonal drugs cannot be reasonably foreseen given what the scientific evidence currently indicates and because at the time of treatment there is no evidence of a human being present (presuming a negative pregnancy-test result).[9]

If one of two possible effects is improbable, then that effect does not bear the sort of causal relation to the act that would warrant an evaluation through an application of the principle of double effect.[10] But the fact that a particular effect is highly probable indicates a stronger causal connection to the particular act, which in turn has a corresponding influence on the moral status of the act and makes the effect morally significant. The inability to foresee reasonably that an abortifacient effect will occur as a result of receiving an anovulatory hormonal medication disqualifies this possibility as a trigger for the application of the principle of double effect. There is no morally significant evil effect which could be factored into a double-effect analysis because there is no convincing evidence that an abortifacient effect will occur, and because evidence to the contrary is inconclusive. Therefore, a different sort of moral evaluation is needed, namely, one that applies the traditional three fonts or sources of a moral act: the object, intention, and circumstances of an act.

The sexual assault survivor commits an act containing both physical and moral components which occur during her consented and voluntary treatment.[11] Physically and biologically there is an external act of receiving an anovulatory drug, which morally is an act of self-defense. This external act, as an act of self-defense, is a morally good kind of act. The *moral object* of the act may be identified as self-defense against the consequences of the unjust sexual aggression of the attacker. However, the fact that the moral object of the act is good does not by itself justify the act. The intention and circumstances of the act must also be morally right.

The intention of the survivor must be to suppress ovulation in order to prevent the unjust circumstance of the gametes meeting, and not to cause the death of a newly conceived human being if fertilization has occurred. The good moral object notwithstanding, *if* the intention of the survivor also includes intending the possible abortifacient effect of the drug, then the act is morally defective, or immoral, because the survivor is intending the killing of an innocent human being. This sort of intention must be distinguished from knowing the possibility that the drug might prevent implantation, however improbable that may be. The fact that an improbable abortifacient effect may be known is not part of the survivor's intention. Knowing and intending are acts of two related but different human powers. To know the possibility of something is an act of the intellect, and to intend something is to perform an act of the will. Thus, to know that an abortifacient effect is possible but improbable is not necessarily to will (intend) it.

The moral object of the act might be good, and the intention of the survivor might be right; but if the circumstances surrounding the act are not in due proportion, that is, if they are morally defective, then the act is immoral. Traditionally, the circumstances of a human act comprising this third moral font include who, what, by what means, where, why (the intention just discussed), how, and when. Here is an example illustrating all seven circumstances and their traditional terms as they pertain to a typical case of a nurse administering pain medication:

Quis (who): a registered nurse

Circa quid (about what) or simply *quid* (what):

1. "by reason of quantity," a therapeutic dose of a medication

2. "by reason of quality," morphine

3. "by reason of the effect," direct alleviation of pain

Quibus auxiliis (by what means): an intravenous line

Ubi (where): a health care facility

Cur (why): to provide palliative care to a dying person

Quomodo (how): competently and with compassion

Quando (when): at the time when pain is experienced, or in anticipation of the pain

These same types of circumstances may be applied to anovulatory hormonal intervention for the treatment of a survivor of sexual assault:

Who: the survivor and the attending health care professionals

What: receiving a drug, for example, levonorgestrel for its anovulatory action

By what means: oral ingestion of the medication

Where: emergency department of a Catholic hospital

Why: to prevent fertilization resulting from an unjust act

How: with a pregnancy test; possibly (but not necessarily) with tests to determine serum progesterone or luteinizing hormone (LH) levels; with knowledge of the survivor's ovulation history; delivered in acute doses

When: after negative results on a pregnancy test and possibly (but not necessarily) also on a serum progesterone or LH test

For the anovulatory hormonal intervention to be justified, these circumstances must be in due proportion to the possibility that the drug might prevent implantation. This means that the circumstances of the act must be such that they produce a moral certitude that the hormonal intervention will not prevent the implantation of a fertilized ovum. The relevant facts that coalesce to provide this certitude are (*a*) the primary mechanism of the drug is the inhibition of ovulation;[12] (*b*) there is no definitive evidence that levonorgestrel will prevent implantation in any given case; (*c*) the evidence purporting an abortifacient effect can be convincingly countered; (d) there is increasing evidence, which has not been successfully opposed, that levonorgestrel most likely does not cause an abortifacient effect; (*e*) assuming a negative pregnancy test, there is no evidence of the presence of an embryo at the time of treatment (either implanted or unimplanted); and (*f*) a possible abortifacient or post-fertilization effect cannot be reasonably foreseen given points *a* through *e*.

Thus, even if there is a remote chance that a drug like levonorgestrel can have an abortifacient effect, the three fonts or sources of a good moral act are nevertheless fulfilled, and the morally certain judgment may be reached that the administration of the drug is justified.[13] What this alignment of object, intention, and circumstances entails for the question regarding ovulation-phase testing is that a drug such as levonorgestrel may be administered either with or without serum progesterone or LH testing, but after a negative pregnancy-test result, which would show that there was no pre-existing pregnancy prior to the rape. The moral certitude that a postcoital anovulatory hormonal agent such as levonorgestrel will not directly interfere with implantation precludes any moral obligation to test first for the ovulation phase of the survivor following a negative pregnancy test. However, this fact does not preempt protocols that in the interests of informed consent and the assuagement of individual conscience provide for both an explanation of the improbable abortifacient effect and an offer of ovulation testing to the survivor. She should be free to consent to an ovulation test or refuse consent, yet in either case still be free to consent to treatment with an anovulatory hormonal agent such as levonorgestrel.

Moral Certitude in Hormonal Intervention

The Catholic moral tradition has long recognized that certitude in a judgment about human action is not the same as what is sometimes required in the physical sciences or in mathematics. The reason for the difference is that certitude is proportionate to the nature of the subject matter known. This principle was first articulated by Aristotle in his *Nicomachean Ethics*, was adopted by St. Thomas Aquinas, and has guided the Catholic moral tradition ever since. Referring to the nature of ethics, Aristotle explains that "our discussion will be adequate if it has as much clearness as the subject matter admits of, for precision is not to be sought for alike in all discussions." He states that we should "look for precision in each class of things just so far as the nature of the subject admits." [14] Because moral judgment concerns the practical realm of acting, it must proceed on the basis of things that are often unclear, changeable, and variable (though not completely). In contrast, a scientific conclusion or one in mathematics is based on things that are largely (though not completely) predictable, universal, and uniform. This difference in subject matter has been traditionally characterized as a difference resulting in what is known as *moral certitude* for practical judgments and *scientific or mathematical certitude* for scientific judgments.

The certitude of a moral judgment about human action need not be, and indeed cannot be, absolute. A morally certain judgment is one that does not include any prudent fear of erring, but does include reasons that might militate against the truth of what is judged. However, these reasons are indecisive and are eclipsed by evidence to the contrary. This fact about moral certitude does not preclude strict certainty about assents to relevant moral principles that a person makes leading up to a particular moral judgment, for example, assenting with strict certainty to the truth of the moral principle that innocent human life ought never be directly taken. However, assent to the judgment that this action, under these circumstances, does not directly take innocent human life and is morally acceptable may contain inconclusive evidence to the contrary. Such a judgment is made with moral certitude. The certitude of this moral judgment is not the same as that with which we assent, for example, to the truths of mathematics, such as the Pythagorean theorem, which states that for a two-dimensional surface, the square of the hypotenuse of a right triangle equals the sum of the squares of the other two sides. However, the certitude of the moral judgment in question is sufficient for the nature of the subject matter that is judged.

A judgment that is made with moral certitude has the trait of being what the Catholic moral tradition calls a "solid probability." [15] A threefold test may be applied to determine if a moral judgment is solidly probable: (1) the argument in its favor would be considered significant by a recognized authority; (2) there can be no decisive argument from authority or reason against the judgment; and (3) the arguments in favor of the judgment are not all satisfactorily refuted by the arguments for the contrary judgment. [16] The moral acceptability of receiving an anovulatory hormonal drug such as levonorgestrel appears to meet the criteria for solidly probable moral certitude. First, arguments like the one proposed here in favor of hormonal intervention have been considered significant by notable theologians who are in accord with the magisterium. [17] Second, there is no decisive evidence from authority or reason against the claim that in any given case the hormonal drug is likely not to act as an abortifacient and may be licitly used in those circumstances. [18] Finally, the arguments against the moral permissibility of hormonal intervention do not pose alternative explanations that are more satisfactory. In fact, there is significant evidence both about the anovulatory effectiveness of the drug and its lack of an abortifacient effect. [19]

It may be objected that the Catholic moral tradition has always recognized an obligation to follow the safer course of action when there is doubt about a matter of great value which would be put at risk, such as the loss of an innocent human life. According to the tradition, one must pursue the safer course rather than expose oneself or another to great harm. There were two classic examples of this obligation to take the safer course: (1) the case of a person suspecting that a drink he or she wishes to have is poisonous, and (2) the case of a hunter's doubt about whether an object that he or she is set to shoot is a human being. The person in these cases is obliged to take the safer option of refraining from acting. From this perspective it has been argued that any doubt about the possibility of an abortifacient effect from anovulatory hormonal intervention is analogous to the classic cases of the rule always to follow the safer course. The risk to innocent human life from the hormonal intervention is analogous to the risk in the classical cases and, therefore, warrants the safer course of not providing the intervention.

On the contrary, the objection is not applicable for two reasons. First, the case of anovulatory hormonal treatment is essentially different from the classic cases. In the classic cases the fact that an object (i.e., the drink, the animal) exists is not in question. The doubt does not concern *that* there is an object, but *what* the object is. The poisonous-drink case poses doubt about what type of drink is in the glass, not whether there is a beverage for drinking. The hunter case poses doubt about what sort of animal or object is in sight, not whether there is a target for shooting. The doubt in these cases is generated in the first place because it is strictly certain that an object exists. It is this particular certainty that gives rise to a doubt about what the nature of that object, or entity, might be. By contrast, in the case of anovulatory hormonal treatment the doubt concerns whether there is an object, namely, a newly conceived being in the woman's reproductive tract. If there is an object, its nature is not in doubt—it is a human being. The question in the case of anovulatory hormonal treatment is not whether a physical object that exists is a human being, but rather whether any human being exists at all (relative to the person's act).

In the case of the hunter, the fact that a target exists (which might be human) is by itself an added reason for taking the safer option where there is doubt as to the nature of the object in sight. However, in the case of anovulatory hormonal intervention there is significantly less reason to believe that a human being will be harmed than in the classic cases, because the doubt in the anovulatory hormonal intervention case is about whether there is any entity at all which might be affected by the action. The evidence indicates that it is likely that there is no individual human being who could be harmed by the intervention, because the intervention effectively prevents conception. Moreover, if ovulation is not suppressed, there is no evidence of a human being present, but if one is present the preponderance of evidence suggests that its implantation will not be prevented.[20]

This fact about what the evidence indicates is related to the second reason why the traditional rule to take the safer course does not apply to the case of anovulatory hormonal treatment. The safer-course rule was often applied in cases of "negative doubt." A person's conscience was considered to be in negative doubt if there were no reasons of any significance on either side of two opposing possible actions. A conscience in this state would be resolved by a governing obligation if fulfilling that obligation were the safer course. However, in the case of anovulatory hormonal intervention there is not an equal lack of significant reasons for acting or not acting. Given the state of the scientific evidence regarding levonorgestrel, there are significant reasons to believe that if a pre-implanted human being is present (even though this cannot be known at the time of treatment), it will probably not be harmed by the hormonal intervention. This fact indicates that the case of anovulatory hormonal intervention is not an instance of traditional negative doubt, which might otherwise be settled by an obligation not to act because this would be the safer course. Therefore, because of the improbability of harming an innocent human being and the absence of negative doubt, the traditional rule always to follow the safer course does not apply.

In conclusion, the acts of administering and taking an anovulatory hormonal drug such as levonorgestrel for medical treatment after sexual assault can be morally justified by a proper fulfillment of the traditional three fonts of morality. If the moral object of the act is self-defense against the unjust sexual aggression of the attacker, and the intention is to suppress ovulation in order to prevent an unjust pregnancy (and not to cause the death of a child which may have been conceived), and if the disposition of the morally relevant circumstances (such as what drug is given and its likely effects) is consistent with the object and intention, then the administration of the drug may proceed. If all these conditions are fulfilled, the morally certain judgment can be made that the hormonal intervention is not preventing implantation and is morally justified. Because of this morally certain judgment, there is no moral obligation to administer drugs such as levonorgestrel only if negative results have been obtained from both a pregnancy test and an LH or serum progesterone test. However, this fact does not preclude a hospital from offering ovulation testing as an option.

This conclusion represents the author's considered theological and ethical opinion. If this opinion is found in error by the magisterium or is found to be in any way inconsistent with the teaching of the magisterium, then it will gladly be retracted in order to uphold the teaching of the magisterium.

Notes

[1] See William E. May, *Catholic Bioethics and the Gift of Human Life* (Huntington, IN: Our Sunday Visitor Publishing Division, Our Sunday Visitor, Inc., 2000); Thomas J. O'Donnell, S.J., *Medicine and Christian Morality*, 3rd ed. (New York: Alba House, 1996), 195–196; Germain Grisez, *The Way of the Lord Jesus*, vol. 2, *Living a Christian Life* (Quincy, IL: Franciscan Press, 1993), 512; Edward J. Bayer, *Rape Within Marriage: A Moral Analysis Delayed* (Lanham, MD: University Press of America, 1985); John T. Noonan Jr., *Contraception: A History of Its Treatment by the Catholic Theologians and Canonists* (New York: New American Library, 1965), 440–442.

[2] See Grisez, *Living a Christian Life*, 512; Bayer, *Rape Within Marriage*, 9.

[3] See Benedict M. Ashley, O.P., and Kevin D. O'Rourke, O.P., *Health Care Ethics: A Theological Analysis*, 4th ed. (Washington, D.C.: Georgetown University Press, 1997), 303; Grisez, *Living a Christian Life*, 512; Francis J. Connell, C.Ss.R., "Is Contraception Intrinsically Wrong?" *American Ecclesiastical Review* 150.6 (June 1964): 434–439; Connell, "The Sterilization of a Retarded Girl," *American Ecclesiasti-*

cal Review 152 (January–June 1966): 280–281; L. L. McReavy, "The Dutch Hierarchy on Marriage Problems," *Clergy Review* 49 (February 1964): 113–115.

[4] Pope Pius XII, "Christian Principles and the Medical Profession," Allocution to the Italian Medical-Biological Union of St. Luke, November 12, 1944, in *The Human Body*, ed. Monks of Solesmes (Boston: Saint Paul Editions, 1960), 62.

[5] Congregation for the Doctrine of the Faith, *Quaecumque sterilizatio* (On Sterilization in Catholic Hospitals), March 13, 1975, *Origins* 10 (1976): n. 1, emphasis added, quoting Pope Paul VI, *Humanae vitae*, n. 10.

[6] Congregation for the Doctrine of the Faith, *Declaration on Certain Questions concerning Sexual Ethics* (December 29, 1975), n. 9, emphasis added, quoting Vatican II, *Gaudium et spes*, n. 51.

[7] U.S. Conference of Catholic Bishops, *Ethical and Religious Directives for Catholic Health Care Services*, 4th ed. (Washington, D.C.: USCCB, 2001), dir. 36.

[8] See O'Donnell, *Medicine and Christian Morality*, 196–197; Eugene F. Diamond, "Rape Protocol," *Linacre Quarterly* 60.3 (August 1993): 13–14; Diamond, "Ovral in Rape Protocols," *Ethics & Medics* 21.10 (October 1996): 2; and Steven P. Rohlfs, "Pregnancy Prevention and Rape: Another View," *Ethics & Medics* 18.5 (May 1993): 1–2. Arguments that the principle of double effect does not validly apply for cases in which drugs like levonorgestrel are used have been based largely on the assumption that there is no reliable method of determining the ovulatory phase of the sexual assault survivor. See also May, *Catholic Bioethics*, 149 note 44.

[9] For a summary and evaluation of the recent scientific literature on the question, see Nicanor Pier Giorgio Austriaco, O.P., "Is Plan B an Abortifacient? A Critical Look at the Scientific Evidence," *National Catholic Bioethics Quarterly* 7.4 (Winter 2007): 703–707. For critiques of Austriaco and his replies, see Marie T. Hilliard, "Plan B's Abortifacient Effect," *National Catholic Bioethics Quarterly* 8.1 (Spring 2008): 9–13; and Patrick Yeung Jr., Erica Laethem, and Joseph Tham, L.C., "Is Plan B Abortifacient? Further Responses," *National Catholic Bioethics Quarterly* 8.2 (Summer 2008): 217–221. On the moral status of foreseeing consequences of acts, see St. Thomas Aquinas, *Summa theologiae* I-II, q. 20, a. 5.

[10] This weak causal relation between act and effect is essentially why a double-effect analysis is not required for common, ordinary actions like the proper operation of a motor vehicle, as a result of which operation deaths nonetheless occur at a definite rate.

[11] A similar analysis can be made for the parallel acts of the health care professional.

[12] For a good description of the various mechanisms of oral contraceptives, see Walter L. Larimore and Joseph B. Stanford, "Postfertilization Effects of Oral Contraceptives and Their Relationship to Informed Consent," *Archives of Family Medicine* 9.2 (February 2000): 126–133.

[13] For other moral arguments in favor of anovulatory hormonal treatment, see Orville N. Griese, *Catholic Identity in Health Care: Principles and Practice* (Braintree, MA: Pope John Center, 1987), 336–337; Ashley and O'Rourke, *Health Care Ethics*, 303–307; Joseph J. Piccione, "A New Approach to Sexual Assault Treatment: Moral Considerations," in *Walk as Children of Light: The Challenge of Cooperation in a Pluralistic Society*, ed. Edward J. Furton (Boston: National Catholic Bioethics Center, 2003), 187–203.

[14] Aristotle, *Nicomachean Ethics*, trans. W. D. Ross, in *The Basic Works of Aristotle*, ed. Richard McKeon (New York: Random House, 1941), book I, ch. 3. See also Thomas Aquinas, *Commentary on Aristotle's* Nicomachean Ethics, trans. C. I. Litzinger, O.P. (Notre Dame, IN: Dumb Ox Books, 1993), book I, lecture 3, nn. 32–36.

[15] Utilizing some of the categories and criteria for moral certitude from the Catholic moral tradition of casuistry does not thereby endorse casuistry per se, or suggest that the categories of casuistry ought to dominate Catholic bioethics. Romanus Cessario, O.P., has demonstrated the deficiencies of casuistic theology as it relates to Catholic bioethics. See his "Towards an Adequate Method for Catholic Bioethics," *National Catholic Bioethics Quarterly* 1.1 (Spring 2001): 51–62. What is needed is a Catholic bioethics that properly integrates the complementarity between divine law and human liberty found in Pope John Paul II's *Veritatis splendor* (Boston: St. Paul Books & Media, 1993) with some of the practical guides from the casuistic tradition. The highly complex and often uncertain subject matter of some questions in bioethics can be aided by an application of notions such as the nature of moral certitude, the principle of double effect, or the principle of cooperation (see chapter 25), in an effort to secure the good of the human person in Catholic health care.

[16] John A. McHugh, O.P., and Charles J. Callan, O.P., *Moral Theology: A Complete Course*, vol. 1., rev. ed. (New York: Joseph F. Wagner, 1958), 259–260.

[17] Ashley and O'Rourke, *Health Care Ethics*; Griese, *Catholic Identity in Health Care*.

[18] See Larimore and Stanford, "Postfertilization Effects of Oral Contraceptives"; Walter L. Larimore and Randy Alcorn, "Using the Birth Control Pill Is Ethically Unacceptable," in *The Reproduction Revolution: A Christian Appraisal of Sexuality, Reproductive Technologies, and the Family*, eds. John F. Kilner, Paige C. Cunningham, and W. David Hager (Grand Rapids, MI: Wm. B. Eerdmans, 2000), 179–191; R. T. Mikolajczyk and J. B. Stanford, "Levonorgestrel Emergency Contraception: A Joint Analysis of Effectiveness and Mechanisms of Action," *Fertility and Sterility* 88.3 (September 2007): 565–571; and Susan A. Crockett et al., "Using Hormone Contraceptives Is a Decision Involving Science, Scripture, and Conscience," in *Reproduction Revolution*, ed. Kilner, Cunningham, and Hager, 192–201, for opposing positions from pro-life physicians on the question of the abortifacient effect of oral contraceptives. It might

be said that the "Statement on the So-Called Morning-After Pill" by the Pontifical Academy for Life (http://www.vatican.va/roman_curia/pontifical_academies/acdlife/documents/rc_pa_acdlife_doc_20001031_pillola-giorno-dopo_en.html) qualifies as authoritative. There are two points that can be made in response. First, the claims by the Pontifical Academy for Life that the abortifacient effect of emergency contraception is "supported by precise scientific data," or that emergency contraception "has a predominantly 'anti-implantation' function," or that "the final result" of the use of emergency contraception "will thus be the expulsion and loss of this embryo," or that the "'anti-implantation' action of the *morning-after pill*' is "proven" have not been demonstrated. None of these claims has been proved true; rather, the preponderance of evidence shows that levonorgestrel, specifically, is likely not to have an abortifacient effect. To the extent that the statement refers to mifepristone (RU-486), its claims are true. The second point is that while the Pontifical Academy for Life is an important advisory body, it does not carry any magisterial authority. Therefore, its con-

clusions as an advisory body should not be considered official Catholic teaching.

[19] See B. M. Landgren et al., "The Effect of Levonorgestrel in Large Doses at Different Stages of the Cycle on Ovarian Function and Endometrial Morphology," *Contraception* 39.3 (March 1989): 275–289; M. Durand et al., "On the Mechanisms of Action of Short-Term Levonorgestrel Administration in Emergency Contraception," *Contraception* 64.4 (October 2001): 227–234; L. Marions et al., "Emergency Contraception with Levonorgestrel and Mifepristone: Mechanism of Action," *Obstetrics and Gynecology* 100.1 (July 2002): 65–71; and K. Gemzell-Danielsson and L. Marions, "Mechanisms of Action of Mifepristone and Levonorgestrel When Used for Emergency Contraception," *Human Reproduction Update* 10.4 (July–August 2004): 341–348.

[20] See Tirelli et al., "Levonorgestrel Administration in Emergency Contraception: Bleeding Pattern and Pituitary-Ovarian Function," *Contraception* 77.5 (May 2008): 328–332.

✠

Editorial Summation: A woman who is sexually assaulted has the right to defend herself against this unjust aggression. She is free to act against any semen deposited in the reproductive tract as a result of the assault. Scientific evidence indicates that it is unlikely that levonorgestrel (Plan B) acts as an abortifacient. The remote possibility of a secondary mechanism occurring which might prevent implantation is morally justifiable under the proper circumstances and conditions of moral certitude using a three-moral-fonts approach. The moral object of the act is self-defense against the consequences of the unjust sexual aggression. The intention of the survivor is to suppress ovulation in order to prevent the unjust circumstance of the gametes meeting. The circumstances of the act produce a moral certitude that the hormonal intervention will not prevent the implantation of a fertilized ovum. As such, there is no moral obligation to first test for the ovulation phase of the survivor before administering levonorgestrel. The objection that one must always follow the safer course does not apply in this case, for what is at stake here is not whether what exists is a human being, but rather whether a human being exists at all.

Rebuttal

Patrick Yeung Jr., M.D., Erica Laethem, and Rev. Joseph Tham, L.C., M.D.

We thank Dr. Cataldo for his moral analysis of the issues surrounding the use of emergency contraceptives.

Dr. Cataldo's article is primarily a *moral analysis* based on the premise that "there is significant evidence both about the anovulatory effectiveness of the drug and its lack of an abortifacient effect" (132). Our article (chapter 11C) is an *original scientific analysis* of the available evidence on which the premise rests. Our analysis leads us to conclude that, when levonorgestrel is administered during the preovulatory phase of a woman's cycle (that is, in the five days leading up to ovulation), an abortifacient effect occurring at a significant rate cannot be ruled out.

When an action is evaluated by use of the three moral fonts approach, it is necessary to take into consideration the risks that accompany the means chosen as part of the moral object. In this case, the moral object includes choosing to take or to administer a pill which acts as an anovulant most of the time, but which also brings with it a risk of causing an abortion.

In order for an object that endangers human life to be pursued in the absence of life-threatening circumstances, the risk of such an effect must be truly minimal. In the following analysis, we will show why the risk of an abortifacient effect from preovulatory levonorgestrel can be neither ruled out nor considered rare.

To bring greater clarity to the scientific debate, we make two original contributions. First, we present a *physiological* model explaining how levonorgestrel emergency contraceptives, when given in the *preovulatory* period, can have post-fertilization effects that prevent implantation (an abortifacient effect). Second, we use updated clinical models to provide a *statistical estimate* of how often these post-fertilization effects occur. The remainder of our scientific analysis reviews systematically the most up-to-date evidence available from human studies on levonorgestrel emergency contraceptives. We conclude that the strength of evidence favors support for an abortifacient effect by the physiological model described, and that no evidence exists to contradict it.

In his article on the previous pages, Cataldo relies exclusively on an article published by Rev. Nicanor Austriaco, O.P., in the *National Catholic Bioethics Quarterly* for his premise that levonorgestrel does not have post-fertilization effects. In the Summer and Autumn 2008 issues of the *National Catholic Bioethics Quarterly*, we laid out the reasons why the studies that Austriaco cited do not refute the evidence that levonorgestrel has post-fertilization effects—specifically when it is administered during the preovulatory period. It is interesting to note that the authors of the main study cited by Austriaco to prove his case (N. Novikova et al.) recently acknowledged that they "cannot exclude a small post-fertilization effect of ECP."[1] Because our dialogue with Austriaco has already been published, we do not wish to present our discussion again here.[2] We would, however, like to highlight a few of the points from our present analysis that we consider to be most important:

1. We agree that when levonorgestrel emergency contraceptives are given in the early follicular phase (cycle day 10 or earlier), it is not expected to be abortifacient. Since the chance of conception resulting from intercourse during this time is near zero, this is not the period in which the moral issue arises.

2. The time in question is the preovulatory period (within five days of ovulation), when levonorgestrel emergency contraceptives can *either* prevent ovulation *or* not; it cannot do both. We agree that if preovulatory levonorgestrel prevents ovulation, it will not be abortifacient, and that there is good evidence that this mechanism occurs the majority of the time. If it does not prevent ovulation, however, then it appears to prevent implantation approximately 3 to 13 percent of the time; there is evidence to support this post-fertilization effect of preovulatory levonorgestrel, and no evidence to rule it out.

3. We agree that if levonorgestrel emergency contraceptives are given in the luteal phase (the time after ovulation), it will likely not disrupt a pregnancy. However, *please note* that studies that do not show a negative effect on implantation or pregnancy rates when levonorgestrel emergency contraceptives are given in the luteal phase *do not contradict* the evidence for a post-fertilization effect when levonorgestrel is given in the preovulatory phase.

4. The term "unlikely" confuses two distinct issues: likelihood and frequency. There is a difference between likelihood (which refers to the strength of evidence in favor of or refuting a particular effect), and frequency (which refers to the percentage of time an effect occurs). Our analysis shows that the available literature does not rule out post-fertilization effects that prevent implantation from preovulatory levonorgestrel emergency contraceptives (but rather, it supports such effects), and that the frequency by which this effect occurs is significant.

5. When considering the strength of evidence, the quality of the studies is more important than the number of studies. The strength of a study comes from the strength of its design. A single well-designed study can contradict several poorly designed studies. Although there are several studies, such as those cited by Austriaco, that seem not to be consistent with abortifacient effects, *none of them* have the methodological design to contradict those well-designed studies that support abortifacient effects.

6. The article by Tirelli et al.[3] also does not have the methodological design to contradict a post-fertilization effect. In fact, the results are consistent with a post-fertilization effect. Levonorgestrel given in the follicular phase of the study (defined as up to two days before ovulation) shortened the luteal phase, whereas levonorgestrel given in the periovulatory phase (on the day of the LH surge or after) did not. In other words, preovulatory levonorgestrel led to the equivalent of a luteal phase insufficiency.

Based on our scientific analysis of the mechanism of action of levonorgestrel emergency contraceptives, the following moral conclusions could be drawn:

1. For the use of levonorgestrel during the preovulatory phase to be considered ethically licit, the frequency of an abortifacient effect of levonorgestrel emergency contraceptives would have to be extremely rare. It is not enough that it merely prevents ovulation the *majority* of the time or that

it is more likely to prevent ovulation than to cause an abortion.

2. To administer levonorgestrel in the preovulatory phase knowing that the best available evidence suggests that it acts as an abortifacient in a significant proportion of cases is to *accept this effect as an aspect of the means chosen.* One must remember that the intention of the moral agent does not pertain only to the end or reason for which one acts, but also to the moral object, including the means one chooses. If someone freely administers or takes levonorgestrel knowing that the risk of an abortifacient effect is neither unlikely nor rare, he or she is morally responsible for this choice, regardless of whether or not the abortive consequence follows. Even if levonorgestrel is administered or taken with the end or purpose of preventing fertilization, the means chosen has an abortifacient effect as a direct effect in a significant proportion of cases. Therefore, levonorgestrel emergency contraception should not be used.

In summary, we think that it is most important to make clear that post-fertilization effects of levonorgestrel emergency contraceptives are not simply an intellectual possibility or logical speculation, but that the best-designed studies on human subjects suggest that the only way that the effectiveness of preovulatory levonorgestrel emergency contraceptives can be explained is by abortifacient effects in addition to anovulatory effects. To date, there are no well-designed studies on this phase of the ovarian cycle that provide any evidence to the contrary. Using the most accurate databases available, we estimate that the risk of abortion resulting from the administration of preovulatory levonorgestrel is approximately 3 to 13 percent. As a result, we cannot support the thesis that an abortifacient effect resulting from preovulatory levonorgestrel is practically nonexistent or rare, nor can we agree that its use is permissible.

Notes

[1] Ian S. Fraser, Response to letter to the editor, *Contraception* 77.6 (June 2007): 464, citing N. Novikova et al., "Effectiveness of Levonorgestrel Emergency Contraception Given Before or After Ovulation: A Pilot Study," *Contraception* 75.2 (February 2007): 112–118.

[2] Nicanor P. G. Austriaco, O.P., "Is Plan B an Abortifacient? A Critical Look at the Scientific Evidence," *National Catholic Bioethics Quarterly* 7.4 (Winter 2007): 703–707; our responses and Austriaco's replies are found in Patrick Yeung Jr., Erica Laethem, and Joseph Tham, L.C., "Is Plan B Abortifacient? Further Responses," *National Catholic Bioethics Quarterly* 8.2 (Summer 2008): 217–221; Yeung, Laethem, and Tham, "More on Plan B," *National Catholic Bioethics Quarterly* 8.3 (Autumn 2008): 418–424.

[3] Tirelli et al., "Levonorgestrel Administration in Emergency Contraception: Bleeding Pattern and Pituitary-Ovarian Function," *Contraception* 77.5 (May 2008): 328–332.

C. Argument Against the Use of Levonorgestrel in Cases of Sexual Assault

Patrick Yeung Jr., M.D., Erica Laethem, and Rev. Joseph Tham, L.C., M.D.

Women who are survivors of sexual assault suffer unspeakable pain and deserve compassionate and understanding care. Catholic moral tradition has held that a woman victim of rape may protect herself by using an agent or device that would prevent fertilization resulting from sexual assault. However, an agent that acts by an *abortifacient* mechanism may not be used. The *Ethical and Religious Directives for Catholic Health Care Services*, issued by the U.S. Conference of Catholic Bishops, articulates this tradition in the following way:

a female who has been raped should be able to defend herself against a potential conception from the sexual assault. ... It is not permissible, however, to initiate or to recommend treatments that have as *their purpose or direct effect the removal, destruction, or interference with the implantation of a fertilized ovum.*[1]

Levonorgestrel, a progestin-only regimen marketed as Plan B, has replaced the Yuzpe regimen, a combination estrogen and progestin hormonal regimen, to become the standard treatment for emergency contraception.[2]

The hormonal composition of the Yuzpe regimen and levonorgestrel differ, so it is necessary to consider the two mechanisms of action independently. The present analysis will pertain only to levonorgestrel emergency contraception, and is not necessarily applicable to other emergency-contraception regimens.[3] Levonorgestrel is now available to any adult over the counter,[4] and has recently been granted approval by some Catholic bishops and some Catholic hospitals to dispense.[5] The basis of such approval is the understanding that there is little to no evidence that levonorgestrel emergency contraception is abortifacient (as defined above). Even if the intent is to prevent fertilization, moral approval *cannot* be given to levonorgestrel emergency contraception if one of its effects is the "interference with implantation of a fertilized ovum."[6] Therefore, *the key question at hand is essentially a scientific one*: can an abortifacient effect of levonorgestrel be ruled out (or is it at least rare)? The answer is no.

The present scientific analysis will show that when levonorgestrel is given *before ovulation*, an effect that interferes with implantation *after fertilization* cannot be ruled out. Our approach will be to show that when levonorgestrel is administered in the *preovulatory* period (two to five days *before* ovulation), post-fertilization effects that interfere with implantation (1) make sense (by a *physiological* model), (2) are supported by several well-designed mechanistic studies in the literature, (3) are not considered rare (by an estimate using updated, well-designed statistical models), and (4) are not refuted by other studies (since no study has the methodological design to do so).

Physiological Model of Post-fertilization Effects from Preovulatory Levonorgestrel

Let us begin with a *physiological model* of how levonorgestrel might have post-fertilization effects that interfere with implantation when given in the *preovulatory* period. The fertile window, or the time in a woman's cycle when there is a significant chance of pregnancy, comprises of six days, which include the five days before ovulation and the day of ovulation itself.[7] Human spermatozoa can survive in the female cervical crypts for up to five days leading to ovulation, and the egg is fertilizable for approximately twenty-four hours after ovulation. Ovulation (denoted day 0 in the scientific literature) is triggered by the luteinizing hormone (LH) surge which occurs twenty-four hours prior on day -1. For our purposes, both ovulation and the LH surge will be

considered part of the ovulatory process. Thus, the time *before* ovulation that is within the fertile window comprises days -5 to -2 before ovulation and will be referred to as the "preovulatory" period. The administration of levonorgestrel during the preovulatory period will be called "preovulatory levonorgestrel."

Levonorgestrel given before the fertile window raises no moral issue, since the chance of pregnancy is near zero. Levonorgestrel given after ovulation (including the LH trigger) may not interfere with implantation, since levonorgestrel is a progestin,[8] a synthetic derivative of progesterone. Progesterone is the dominant hormone produced in a woman's cycle *after* ovulation (during the luteal phase[9]). This is why progestins are often used in artificial reproductive technology protocols to support a pregnancy,[10] and why from a physiological standpoint, levonorgestrel is not expected to interfere with implantation when given after ovulation. By contrast, the dominant hormone produced *before* ovulation (during the follicular phase[11]) is estrogen, not progesterone. Therefore, from a physiological standpoint, the *preovulatory* period is *precisely* the time in question when levonorgestrel administration might cause post-fertilization effects *after* ovulation that interfere with implantation.

The ability of the endometrium (lining of the uterus) to receive an embryo at implantation depends on the function of the corpus luteum, which in turn depends on the function of the follicle. *Post-fertilization effects of levonorgestrel that interfere with implantation could occur in the following way*: administration of levonorgestrel *before* ovulation does not prevent ovulation (that is, a "breakthrough" ovulation occurs) but interferes with the normal development and function of the corpus luteum; a dysfunctional corpus luteum then leads to an impaired endometrium that interferes with embryonic implantation. *Physiologically, post-fertilization effects that interfere with implantation when levonorgestrel is given in the preovulatory period make sense.*

Studies That Support Post-fertilization Effects from Preovulatory Levonorgestrel

Let us now see what scientific evidence exists to support this proposed physiological model of *post-fertilization* effects from *preovulatory* levonorgestrel emergency contraception. The most direct evidence in support of the model would be a study that demonstrated a decrease in implantation rates after levonorgestrel emergency contraception was given in the preovulatory period. The difficulty is that there is no direct test for fertilization prior to implantation. Standard pregnancy tests, which measure human chorionic gonadotropin (ß-hCG), detect pregnancy only after implantation (seven to ten days after ovulation). There is no test to determine if an embryo that has not yet implanted is present. Indirect evidence that supports post-fertilization effects of preovulatory levonorgestrel emergency contraception would include some *combination of* (1) studies that demonstrate the release of fertilizable eggs or "breakthrough ovulations," (2) studies that demonstrate a dysfunctional corpus luteum or decreased endometrial receptivity, and (3) studies that show a decreased pregnancy rate.[12]

Any mechanistic study addressing post-fertilization effects must have a reliable method of measuring ovulation. The most accurate and reliable method of determining whether ovulation has occurred is daily ultrasound tracking that shows actual rupture of the follicle. The next most reliable method of measuring ovulation (that results in a fertilizable egg) is an LH surge (the trigger for ovulation) with a peak concentration above 30 international units per liter (IU/L). A lower LH peak concentration has been associated with non-fertilizable eggs by the data of W. M. Verpoest.[13]

A well-designed study demonstrates that the larger the size of the follicle (or the closer the time to ovulation), the less chance preovulatory levonorgestrel will prevent ovulation. H. B. Croxatto et al. evaluated the effect of levonorgestrel at three different follicular sizes (12–14 mm, 14–17 mm, > 18 mm) measured by ultrasound.[14] Overall, ovulation was prevented or ineffective (determined by failure of follicular rupture or "ovulatory dysfunction"[15]) in 79 percent of cycles. When the follicle diameter was 12 to 17 mm, ovulation was prevented or ineffective in 91 to 94 percent of cycles. However, when the follicle was greater than 18 mm, ovulation was prevented or ineffective in only 47 percent of cycles. These data indicate that the larger the follicular size, the greater the chance of breakthrough ovulation. Furthermore, when ovulation did occur (determined by ultrasound follicular rupture), a fertilizable egg was released (indicated by a normal LH peak concentration above 30 IU/L preceding rupture) 29 to 38 percent of the time despite the administration of levonorgestrel. These data are consistent with post-fertilization effects since levonorgestrel given in the preovulatory period results in breakthrough ovulations.[16]

Three well-designed studies (using accurate methods of assessing ovulation) demonstrate post-fertilization effects that could interfere with implantation after the administration of preovulatory levonorgestrel. M. Durand

et al. evaluated the effect of levonorgestrel on ovulation and luteal phase function in ovulatory women with tubal ligation.[17] In this study, ovulation was determined by ultrasound follicular rupture. Participants were given levonorgestrel at different times in the menstrual cycle. When levonorgestrel was given on the day of LH peak concentration or later (groups B and C), there was no effect on luteal-phase hormone concentrations. However, when levonorgestrel was given in the preovulatory period (group D, late follicular phase, eight subjects), 100 percent of the women ovulated *and* had significantly reduced luteal phase length and luteal-phase progesterone serum concentrations (both daily and area under the curve). Luteal-phase length is a function of progesterone production which, in turn, is necessary to sustain a pregnancy at the time of implantation. This study by Durand et al. supports post-fertilization effects that interfere with implantation, since levonorgestrel given in the preovulatory period results in breakthrough ovulations *and* impaired luteal function.

In a later study, Durand et al. used a similarly strong study design where the timing of ovulation was determined by ultrasound.[18] When levonorgestrel was given in the preovulatory period (group 1, three to four days before LH surge, eight subjects), luteal phase length, serum progesterone levels, and endometrial glycodelin-A expression were all significantly reduced. The endometrial expression of glycodelin-A is mediated by luteal phase progesterone and is considered one of the most potent markers of endometrial receptivity.[19] Reduced levels of glycodelin-A in the endometrium indicate that it is less "receptive" to implantation.[20] This study by Durand again gives strong mechanistic support for post-fertilization effects that interfere with implantation, since levonorgestrel given in the preovulatory period results in breakthrough ovulations *and* impaired endometrial receptivity.

D. Hapangama et al. evaluated the effect of levonorgestrel administered before the LH peak.[21] In their study, ovulation was confirmed by a serum LH peak concentration greater than 30 IU/L. In seven of twelve women (58 percent) in whom levonorgestrel was given in the preovulatory period (on or before the first significant rise in urinary LH), luteal phase length and total luteal phase LH concentrations were significantly reduced. LH, produced in the luteal phase, is required for the proper function of the corpus luteum.[22] The data support post-fertilization effects that interfere with implantation, since levonorgestrel given in the preovulatory period results in breakthrough ovulations *and* impaired luteal function.

Estimation of the Frequency of Post-fertilization Effects from Preovulatory Levonorgestrel

Now let us turn to the question of how often the preovulatory administration of levonorgestrel causes post-fertilization effects that interfere with implantation. A statistical model to gain insight into the mechanism of action of emergency contraception based on its effectiveness was originally proposed by J. Trussell in 1999.[23] He compared estimates of the *observed* effectiveness of the Yuzpe regimen in published studies ("clinical effectiveness") to the *calculated* maximum theoretical effectiveness that could be obtained if the regimen worked only by preventing or delaying ovulation ("theoretical effectiveness"). Any significant difference in effectiveness (clinical effectiveness minus theoretical effectiveness) would lead to the conclusion that emergency contraception operates by mechanisms other than preventing or delaying ovulation and could be used to estimate the frequency with which post-fertilization effects occur.

To estimate post-fertilization effects of levonorgestrel, accurate estimates for both clinical and theoretical effectiveness are needed. *Clinical effectiveness* of levonorgestrel has been estimated to be between 58 and 95 percent, based on five large-scale levonorgestrel-effectiveness studies;[24] the effectiveness quoted in the Plan B labeling is 89 percent. Recently, however, E. Raymond and J. Trussell have argued that these studies have overestimated the clinical effectiveness of emergency contraception, mainly due to the way that expected pregnancies were calculated.[25] The overestimate of clinical effectiveness from these studies has been addressed in a recent methodological review by J. B. Stanford and R. T. Mikolajczyk.[26] In this review, the authors propose a method of calculating expected pregnancies per cycle day (the Mikolajczyk method) which incorporates the correction recommended by Trussell (the Trussell method) and estimates the clinical effectiveness of levonorgestrel emergency contraception to be 72 percent based on the pooled data.[27]

The first and only systematic statistical calculation of *theoretical effectiveness* of levonorgestrel emergency contraception was performed by Mikolajczyk and Stanford.[28] This represents a much more precise adaptation of the original model by Trussell, since it incorporates data from ultrasound on follicular diameter[29] and the Croxatto clinical data of the effect on levonorgestrel.[30] If levonorgestrel worked *only by* preventing ovulation or rendering ovulation ineffective, the maximum theoretical effectiveness would be 49 percent. To be more conservative, the effectiveness of levonorgestrel was also calculated assuming *complete* prevention of fertilization whenever levonorgestrel is taken before ovulation (this would include other mechanisms to prevent fertilization beyond preventing ovulation or rendering it ineffective). Even in this conservative estimate, the maximum effectiveness is still only 59 percent when levonorgestrel is taken within twenty-four hours of intercourse.

An estimation of the percentage of time that levonorgestrel effectiveness can be explained by post-fertilization effects when levonorgestrel is taken in the *preovulatory* period, can now be made on the basis of these updated estimates—based on well-designed models—of clinical and theoretical effectiveness. Even if the estimate for clinical effectiveness is adjusted downward by another 10 percent,[31] an estimate of post-fertilization effects of preovulatory levonorgestrel is clinical effectiveness minus overestimation minus maximum theoretical effectiveness, that is, 72 percent minus 10 percent minus 49 to 59 percent, equaling 3 to 13 percent post-fertilization effects that interfere with implantation. In other words, levonorgestrel is estimated to act as an abortifacient 3 to 13 percent of the time when it is administered in the preovulatory period. Notice that this is a *conservative* estimate of post-fertilization effects based on: (1) a recent recalculation of the clinical effectiveness that accounts for overestimation, and (2) published clinical data based on the effect of preovulatory levonorgestrel on ovulation.[32]

Studies That Seem Inconsistent with Post-fertilization Effects of Preovulatory Levonorgestrel

Studies that seem to be inconsistent with post-fertilization effects will now be addressed. While no study has the methodological design to rule out post-fertilization effects for preovulatory levonorgestrel, several studies have been cited. These studies will be categorized as follows: (1) studies that address preovulatory levonorgestrel and luteal phase function, (2) studies that address preovulatory levonorgestrel and pregnancy rates, and (3) studies that address the direct effect of levonorgestrel on embryo implantation or endometrial receptivity.

Three studies address preovulatory levonorgestrel and luteal phase function that are not consistent with post-fertilization effects that interfere with implantation. In L. Marions et al., levonorgestrel was given on day LH surge -2 (based on the control cycle), and ovulation was determined by ultrasound.[33] Preovulatory levonorgestrel delayed the LH surge in 33.3 percent of subjects (two of six) by two and five days, indicating that breakthrough ovulation occurred in 66.7 percent of subjects (four of six). However, in these cycles where breakthrough ovulations occurred, negative effects on luteal phase levels of urinary pregnanediol P4 (a metabolite of serum progesterone), luteal phase length, or markers of endometrial receptivity[34] were not observed. In another study, Marions et al. used a similar study design.[35] When levonorgestrel was given before ovulation, ovulation was either prevented (determined by a lack of ultrasound follicular rupture) or ineffective (indicated by a delay or inhibition of the LH surge) in all subjects. This time, however, a significant delay in the normal rise of urinary P4 levels was observed, indicating luteal phase dysfunction. Together, these studies are not consistent with post-fertilization effects that interfere with implantation, since they indicate that preovulatory levonorgestrel either does not result in breakthrough ovulations or results in breakthrough ovulations without impaired luteal function.

The problem with the two studies by Marions is that the sample sizes were extremely small (six subjects in the first study and seven in the second), so they cannot be used to disprove the studies by Durand.[36] In statistical analyses, sample size is important to demonstrate a lack of difference; the same is not true to demonstrate that a difference is due to an experimental intervention (preovulatory levonorgestrel for our purposes). If a statistical test shows that an observed difference is "significant," it means that the difference cannot be explained by random chance alone, but must be due to the experimental intervention. However, if a statistical test shows that an observed difference is "not significant," the difference may be due to random chance (and thus not ruled out) *unless* the sample size is large enough to have the statistical "power" to detect a real difference. The studies by Marions are too small to have the statistical power to rule out breakthrough ovulations and impaired luteal function after preovulatory levonorgestrel.

In a third study by J. A. do Nascimento et al., the effect of preovulatory levonorgestrel on luteal phase endometrial glycodelin-A levels was studied. Levonorgestrel was given twelve to thirty-six hours after intercourse in the presence of fertile cervical mucus and before ovulation as determined by ultrasound.[37] No significant difference in endometrial glycodelin-A levels between the control and treatment groups was observed. However, endometrial sampling was performed at twenty-four or forty-eight hours after levonorgestrel administration and thus at most two to three days after ovulation. Glycodelin-A is not expressed in the endometrium until six days after

ovulation,[38] so it is not surprising that no difference was measured in glycodelin-A levels. The results of this study do not disprove the results of Durand et al.[39]

One study uniquely addresses the effect of preovulatory levonorgestrel on pregnancy rates. In N. Novikova et al., levonorgestrel was given before and after ovulation, and expected pregnancy rates were compared to observed pregnancy rates.[40] A great weakness of this study is that ovulation was estimated using serum hormone levels to an accuracy of only about 80 percent. When intercourse occurred on or after the LH peak day (days -1 to 0, where day 0 is the day of ovulation), 3.5 pregnancies were expected, and three pregnancies were observed. Since this is not a significant difference, the authors conclude that levonorgestrel does not have post-fertilization effects. It is important to underscore, however, that in this study-group levonorgestrel was taken on day +2 in the luteal phase (after ovulation), so it could not have post-fertilization effects by the model described above.

When intercourse occurred and levonorgestrel was given in the preovulatory period (days -5 to -2), four pregnancies were expected, but no pregnancies were observed.[41] The reported differences between expected and observed pregnancies indicate that levonorgestrel is effective when given in the preovulatory period. However, since there was no ultrasound determination of ovulation and no LH peak concentration levels were reported, it is not possible to know whether the effectiveness of preovulatory levonorgestrel was due to pre-fertilization events (such as failed or ineffective ovulation) or to breakthrough ovulations and post-fertilization effects.

Now let us look at studies that address the direct effect of levonorgestrel on embryo implantation or endometrial receptivity. In vitro models were used both in P. G. Lalitkumar et al. to study the direct effect of levonorgestrel on the implantation of embryos (which would correspond to levonorgestrel given in the luteal phase in humans),[42] and in C. X. Meng et al. to study the effect of levonorgestrel on endometrial markers for receptivity (from samples taken on LH surge +4 or LH surge +5).[43] Remember that in the physiological model proposed above, levonorgestrel given in the luteal phase is not expected to interfere with implantation, since it is a progestin. For this reason, these studies that show a lack of difference in implantation rates, or endometrial receptivity, when levonorgestrel is given *after* ovulation do not disprove post-fertilization effects of levonorgestrel given *before* ovulation.

It is clear from our analysis of the studies which seem inconsistent with post-fertilization effects from preovulatory levonorgestrel that *none of the studies cited have the methodological design to rule out post-fertilization effects from preovulatory levonorgestrel.*

Ovulation Testing Is Not Useful in the Administration of Levonorgestrel

Finally, let us briefly address the proposed use of the ovulation test as a guide to determine whether or not to use levonorgestrel emergency contraception. The ovulation test is a test for urinary LH and, as such, can be used to determine when the LH surge is happening. Some have proposed to use the ovulation test in the following manner: if the test is positive, then ovulation is about to happen and levonorgestrel emergency contraception should be avoided since (if it works at all) it can do so only by post-fertilization effects; if the test is negative and the woman (by her own report) is thought to be in the follicular phase of her cycle (before ovulation), then levonorgestrel emergency contraception could be used to prevent fertilization *if* it did not have an abortifacient effect. Throughout our analysis of the current scientific studies available, we have found support for post-fertilization effects of preovulatory levonorgestrel. Therefore, it is not helpful to use an ovulation test at all. If the ovulation test is positive, then according to data from the two Durand studies, levonorgestrel will neither prevent ovulation nor have a negative effect on luteal phase function; that is, it will not work to prevent pregnancy at all.[44] If the test is negative, it cannot be accurately known whether the woman is in the luteal phase or the follicular phase of the cycle, since women's self-reports of ovulation are generally very inaccurate.[45] If a woman is in the luteal phase, levonorgestrel emergency contraception is not expected to prevent pregnancy according to the data of Novikova et al.[46] If the woman is in the follicular phase of the cycle, then she may be in the preovulatory period which, as we have seen, is *precisely* when levonorgestrel emergency contraception may act as an abortifacient. *The ovulation test is not a helpful guide* since, whatever the result, levonorgestrel emergency contraception will either not prevent pregnancy or will be potentially abortifacient.

Conclusions

In summary, post-fertilization effects that interfere with implantation when levonorgestrel is given two to five days *before* ovulation have been (1) shown to make sense by physiological principles, (2) shown to be supported by several well-designed studies, and (3) estimated to occur 3 to 13 percent of the time by updated models. Abortifacient effects can be neither ruled out nor considered rare.

No studies have the methodological design to disprove this abortifacient mechanism. Finally, the ovulation test is not a helpful guide for the use of levonorgestrel emergency contraception. For those who affirm that human life begins at fertilization, levonorgestrel emergency contraception should not be used.

Notes

The authors thank Joe Stanford, M.D., at the University of Utah, for his help and comments.

[1] U.S. Conference of Catholic Bishops, *Ethical and Religious Directives for Catholic Health Care Services*, 4th ed. (Washington, D.C.: USCCB, 2001), dir. 36, emphasis added.

[2] Task Force on Postovulatory Methods of Fertility Regulation, "Randomised Controlled Trial of Levonorgestrel Versus the Yuzpe Regimen of Combined Oral Contraceptives for Emergency Contraception," *Lancet* 352.9126 (August 8, 1998): 428–433; P. C. Ho and M. S. Kwan, "A Prospective Randomized Comparison of Levonorgestrel with the Yuzpe Regimen in Post-Coital Contraception," *Human Reproduction* 8.3 (March 1993): 389–392.

[3] Note that the previous edition of this publication focused on the Yuzpe regimen. See ch. 11, "Pregnancy Prevention After Sexual Assault," in *Catholic Health Care Ethics: A Manual for Ethics Committees*, ed. Peter J. Cataldo and Albert S. Moraczewski, O.P. (Boston: National Catholic Bioethics Center, 2001), 11/1–11/22.

[4] U.S. Food and Drug Administration, "FDA Approves Over-the-Counter Access for Plan B for Women 18 and Older, Prescription Remains Required for Women 17 and Under," *FDA News*, August 24, 2006, http://www.fda.gov/bbs/topics/news/2006/new01436.html.

[5] Connecticut Bishops, "Statement on Plan B and Catholic Hospitals," September 27, 2007, http://www.ctcatholic.org/Bishops-Statement-Plan-B.php.

[6] U.S. Conference of Catholic Bishops, *Ethical and Religious Directives*, dir. 36.

[7] A. J. Wilcox, D. Dunson, and D. D. Baird, "The Timing of the 'Fertile Window' in the Menstrual Cycle: Day Specific Estimates from a Prospective Study," *British Medical Journal* 321.7271 (November 18, 2000): 1259–1262.

[8] A progestin was originally defined as any hormone that supports a pregnancy in an oophorectimized animal.

[9] The luteal phase is named after the corpus luteum, which is what is left behind in the ovary after the follicle releases the egg at ovulation. The corpus luteum produces progesterone.

[10] E. A. Pritts and A. K. Atwood, "Luteal Phase Support in Infertility Treatment: A Meta-Analysis of the Randomized Trials," *Human Reproduction* 17.9 (September 2002): 2287–2299.

[11] The follicular phase is named after the follicle, or cyst, that nourishes and eventually releases the egg at ovulation. The follicle produces estrogen.

[12] Pregnancy rate, as emergency contraception researchers use the term, refers to the rate of implantation, not the rate of fertilization.

[13] W. M. Verpoest et al., "Relationship Between Midcycle Luteinizing Hormone Surge Quality and Oocyte Fertilization," *Fertility and Sterility* 73.1 (January 2000): 75–77.

[14] H. B. Croxatto et al., "Pituitary-Ovarian Function Following the Standard Levonorgestrel Emergency Contraceptive Dose or a Single 0.75-mg Dose Given on the Days Preceding Ovulation," *Contraception* 70.6 (December 2004): 442–450.

[15] In this study, "ovulatory dysfunction" was defined as follicular rupture not preceded by an LH peak or preceded by a blunted peak LH (LH < 21 IU/L), or not followed by elevation of serum progesterone over 12 nmol/L. It was assumed that ovulatory dysfunction represented ovulations of unfertilizable eggs given the data of Verpoest et al. on midcycle LH levels and fecundity in in vitro protocols.

[16] Although breakthrough ovulations are demonstrated in this study, no data were given on luteal function in these cycles.

[17] M. Durand et al., "On the Mechanisms of Action of Short-Term Levonorgestrel Administration in Emergency Contraception," *Contraception* 64.4 (October 2001): 227–234.

[18] M. Durand et al., "Late Follicular Phase Administration of Levonorgestrel as an Emergency Contraceptive Changes the Secretory Pattern of Glycodelin in Serum and Endometrium During the Luteal Phase of the Menstrual Cycle," *Contraception* 71.6 (June 2005): 451–457.

[19] M. Seppala et al., "Glycodelin: A Major Lipocalin Protein of the Reproductive Axis with Diverse Actions in Cell Recognition and Differentiation," *Endocrine Reviews* 23.4 (August 2002): 401–430.

[20] Since glycodelin-A acts as an inhibitor of "natural killer cells" present where implantation occurs, reduced levels "may indicate a weakened immunosuppressive microenvironment at the feto-maternal interface at the time of implantation."

[21] D. Hapangama, A. F. Glasier, and D. T. Baird, "The Effects of Peri-Ovulatory Administration of Levonorgestrel on the Menstrual Cycle," *Contraception* 63.3 (March 2001): 123–129.

[22] J. E. Hall et al., "Variable Tolerance of the Developing Follicle and Corpus Luteum to Gonadotropin-Releasing Hormone Antagonist-Induced Gonadotropin Withdrawal in the Human," *Journal of Clinical Endocrinology and Metabolism* 72.5 (1991): 993–1000.

[23] J. Trussell and E. G. Raymond, "Statistical Evidence about the Mechanism of Action of the Yuzpe Regimen of Emergency Contraception," *Obstetrics & Gynecology* 93.5 pt 2 (May 1999): 872–876.

[24] Task Force on Postovulatory Methods of Fertility Regulation, "Randomised Controlled Trial of Levonorgestrel"; Ho and Kwan, "Prospective Randomized Comparison"; H. Hamoda et al., "A Randomized Trial of Mifepristone (10 mg)

and Levonorgestrel for Emergency Contraception," *Obstetrics & Gynecology* 104.6 (December 2004): 1307–1313; H. von Hertzen et al., "Low Dose Mifepristone and Two Regimens of Levonorgestrel for Emergency Contraception: A WHO Multicentre Randomised Trial," *Lancet* 360.9348 (December 7, 2002): 1803–1810; A. O. Arowojolu, I. A. Okewole, and A. O. Adekunle, "Comparative Evaluation of the Effectiveness and Safety of Two Regimens of Levonorgestrel for Emergency Contraception in Nigerians," *Contraception* 66.4 (October 2002): 269–273.

[25] E. Raymond et al., "Minimum Effectiveness of the Levonorgestrel Regimen of Emergency Contraception," *Contraception* 69.1 (January 2004): 79–81; J. Trussell et al., "Estimating the Effectiveness of Emergency Contraceptive Pills," *Contraception* 67.4 (April 2003): 259–265.

[26] J. B. Stanford and R. T. Mikolajczyk, "Methodological Review of the Effectiveness of Emergency Contraception," *Current Women's Health Reviews* 1.2 (2005): 1–11.

[27] Notice that, based on the Trussell method for correcting overestimation, the clinical effectiveness of levonorgestrel emergency contraception is higher at 79 percent for the pooled data (see table 5 of Stanford and Mikolajczyk, "Methodological Review"). Thus, the Stanford estimation of clinical effectiveness is more conservative than Trussell would be.

[28] R. T. Mikolajczyk and J. B. Stanford, "Levonorgestrel Emergency Contraception: A Joint Analysis of Effectiveness and Mechanism of Action," *Fertility and Sterility* 88.3 (2007): 565–571.

[29] R. Ecochard et al., "Chronological Aspects of Ultrasonic, Hormonal, and Other Indirect Indices of Ovulation," *BJOG* 108.8 (August 2001): 822–829.

[30] Croxatto et al., "Pituitary-Ovarian Function."

[31] Raymond et al., "Minimum Effectiveness"; Trussell et al., "Estimating the Effectiveness."

[32] Croxatto et al., "Pituitary-Ovarian Function."

[33] L. Marions et al., "Emergency Contraception with Mifepristone and Levonorgestrel: Mechanism of Action," *Obstetrics and Gynecology* 100.1 (July 2002): 65–71.

[34] Durand et al., "Late Follicular Phase Administration," did show a difference in luteal phase glycodelin-A after preovulatory levonorgestrel. Notice that in Marions et al., "Emergency Contraception," glycodelin-A, a particularly strong marker of endometrial receptivity, was not measured.

[35] L. Marions et al., "Effect of Emergency Contraception with Levonorgestrel or Mifepristone on Ovarian Function," *Contraception* 69.5 (May 2004): 373–377.

[36] Marions et al., "Emergency Contraception"; Marions et al., "Effect of Emergency Contraception"; Durand et al., "On the Mechanisms of Action"; Durand et al., "Late Follicular Phase Administration."

[37] J. A. do Nascimento et al., "In Vivo Assessment of the Human Sperm Acrosome Reaction and the Expression of Glycodelin-A in Human Endometrium after Levonorgestrel-

Emergency Contraceptive Pill Administration," *Human Reproduction* 22.8 (August 2007): 2190–2195.

[38] Seppala et al., "Glycodelin."

[39] Durand et al., "Late Follicular Phase Administration."

[40] N. Novikova et al., "Effectiveness of Levonorgestrel Emergency Contraception Given Before or After Ovulation: A Pilot Study," *Contraception* 75.2 (February 2007): 112–118. Expected pregnancy rates were based on Wilcox calculations. See Wilcox, Dunson, and Baird, "Timing of the 'Fertile Window.'"

[41] Complete data on expected and observed pregnancies appear in Table 1 of Novikova et al., "Effectiveness of Levonorgestrel," 114.

[42] P. G. Lalitkumar et al., "Mifepristone, but Not Levonorgestrel, Inhibits Human Blastocyst Attachment to an In Vitro Endometrial Three-Dimensional Cell Culture Model," *Human Reproduction* 22.11 (November 2007): 3031–3037.

[43] C. X. Meng et al., "Effect of Levonorgestrel and Mifepristone on Endometrial Receptivity Markers in a Three-Dimensional Human Endometrial Cell Culture Model," *Fertility and Sterility* 91.1 (January 2009): 256–264.

[44] Durand et al., "On the Mechanisms of Action"; Durand et al., "Late Follicular Phase Administration."

[45] Novikova et al., "Effectiveness of Levonorgestrel."

[46] Ibid.

Editorial Summation: Catholic moral tradition holds that a victim of rape may protect herself by using an agent or device that would prevent fertilization resulting from sexual assault. However, an agent that acts by an abortifacient mechanism may not be used. Levonorgestrel is the standard treatment for emergency contraception, but moral approval cannot be given to levonorgestrel emergency contraception if one of its effects is the interference with implantation of a fertilized ovum. Scientific analysis shows that when levonorgestrel is given before ovulation, an effect that interferes with implantation after fertilization cannot be ruled out. The drug may interfere with the normal development and function of the corpus luteum. A dysfunctional corpus luteum leads to an impaired endometrium that interferes with embryonic implantation. According to three well-designed studies, levonorgestrel is estimated to act as an abortifacient 3 to 13 percent of the time when it is administered in the preovulatory period. This is a conservative estimate. Studies showing no post-fertilization effect have either extremely small sample sizes or suffer design flaws. The ovulation test is not a helpful guide since, whatever the result, levonorgestrel emergency contraception either will not prevent pregnancy or is potentially abortifacient.

Rebuttal

Peter J. Cataldo

I would like to thank Dr. Patrick Yeung, Erica Laethem, and Rev. Joseph Tham for their article. In the previous pages, they assert that the following text from directive 36 of the *Ethical and Religious Directives for Catholic Health Care Services* (*ERDs*) excludes use of a pharmacological agent "that acts by an abortifacient mechanism":

> A female who has been raped should be able to defend herself against a potential conception from the sexual assault. ... It is not permissible, however, to initiate or to recommend treatments that have as their purpose or direct effect the removal, destruction, or interference with the implantation of a fertilized ovum.

Yeung, Laethem, and Tham also claim that the "basis" for the approval of Plan B (a drug regimen using levonorgestrel) by some Catholic bishops and Catholic hospitals is "the understanding that there is little to no evidence that levonorgestrel emergency contraception is abortifacient."

What these claims by Yeung, Laethem, and Tham have in common is reflected in the central premise of their argument, which is that the issue of whether or not to allow the use of levonorgestrel in Catholic hospitals is a scientific one. They state, "*The key question at hand is essentially a scientific one*: can an abortifacient effect of levonorgestrel be ruled out (or at least be rare)? The answer is no" (original emphasis). For Yeung, Laethem, and Tham, levonorgestrel may not be morally approved for use in the treatment of rape survivors because the possibility of post-fertilization effects of the drug that interfere with implantation cannot be absolutely excluded.

The foundational premise of the argument by Yeung, Laethem, and Tham is a question-begging one. They assume the very thing in need of proof, and what they assume is false. Yeung, Laethem, and Tham assume that the type of certitude required to answer the question of the moral permissibility of levonorgestrel must be of the sort that excludes every possibility of error—that is, they assume a mathematical certitude—and this is why they believe the question is a scientific one. I have shown in the moral analysis of this chapter that in the practical realm of human action mathematical certitude is inappropriate because the nature of the subject matter is unclear, changeable, and variable. The subject matter of practical judgments cannot bear the precision expected from scientific or mathematical judgments. Given the imprecise nature of human action, the type of certitude in practical judgment is called moral or prudential certitude. Moral certitude precludes any prudent fear of erring. Such a judgment has the possibility of error, but the reasons against the judgment are inconclusive and are outweighed by the reasons in support of the judgment (see the aforementioned moral analysis). Yeung, Laethem, and Tham incorrectly assume that so long as there is any possibility of an abortifacient effect from levonorgestrel, what they consider the morally requisite certitude for approval of the drug does not obtain.

However, the nature of moral certitude is such that one cannot be morally responsible for the consequences of actions that cannot be reasonably foreseen. This has been a tenet of the Catholic moral tradition. St. Thomas Aquinas argued in the *Summa theologiae*, for example, that there is moral responsibility for some unforeseen consequences but not for others. If an effect does not follow from the nature of a cause and in the majority of cases, but instead follows accidentally and seldom, then it may be considered an unforeseen consequence that does not add any good or evil to the act that is attributable to the agent.[1] If, however, an unforeseen consequence follows from the nature of a cause and occurs in the majority of cases, then it should have been foreseen and the agent is responsible for the good or evil that it adds to the act. Aquinas makes the same point in the *Summa contra gentiles* where he discusses responsibility for morally defective effects of actions which are in themselves good.[2] He explains that such consequences, though apart from the intention of the agent (*praeter intentionem*), are morally evil if they always or frequently occur. The examples Aquinas cites are the man who drinks wine for the pleasure of its sweetness but becomes intoxicated, and the married man who engages in sex with a woman other than his wife for the pleasure of it but "to which pleasure is attached the disorder of adultery."[3] Such cases are distinct from the man who kills another man while shooting at a bird. In this case, the death of the man is both apart from intention and cannot be morally attributed to the shooter because it is not something that invariably or frequently occurs. Yeung, Laethem, and Tham do not account for the moral tradition on foreseen and unforeseen effects of actions, and they assume what needs proof. They incorrectly as-

sume that any possibility of death, as an evil effect in the circumstances in question, makes the use of levonorgestrel morally prohibitive. However, the theoretical possibility of an abortifacient effect from the use of levonorgestrel in rape treatment qualifies neither as a foreseen effect nor as an unforeseen effect for which the moral agents are responsible, should it actually occur.[4] This point is supported by the status of the evidence.

Nicanor Pier Giorgio Austriaco, O.P., has convincingly countered the claims by Yeung, Laethem, and Tham that levonorgestrel causes post-fertilization effects that interfere with implantation.[5] Austriaco has pointed to studies that counter the claims of their proposed physiological model. These studies indicate that levonorgestrel does not "dramatically alter the structure" of endometrial tissue, that there is a "vanishingly small" risk of impairment to the luteal function if levonorgestrel is taken during the periovulatory phase in any given case, and that levonorgestrel does not affect the ability of embryos to implant on endometrial tissue.[6] Moreover, the criticisms by Yeung, Laethem, and Tham of the studies by Marions et al., and their use of do Nascimento et al. to argue for adverse effects on endometrial function, are countered by the results of A. Tirelli, A. Cagnacci, and A. Volpe.[7] Austriaco points out that the Tirelli, Cagnacci, and Volpe study "suggests that Plan B taken prior to ovulation does not detrimentally impact endometrial function even when ovulation does occur."[8] Austriaco also shows that recent studies, which reveal a "substantially lower effectiveness rate" to levonorgestrel than in previous studies, "undermine the statistical argument that Plan B is an abortifacient."[9] These studies represent independent evidence countering the claims of R. T. Mikolajczyk and J. B. Stanford on which Yeung, Laethem, and Tham in part rely.[10] In addition, Austriaco points out how studies show that "it is unlikely that Plan B increases the risk of ectopic pregnancy … or kills an already implanted embryo."[11]

Yeung, Laethem, and Tham have begged the question on a second important aspect of the issue. They present studies in an attempt to show support for what they declaratively characterize as "post-fertilization effects that interfere with implantation." Prescinding from the question of the scientific merit of these studies, Yeung, Laethem, and Tham have begged the question about what constitutes interference with implantation, which is one of the central points at issue. First, they incorrectly assume that implantation is the same thing as endometrial receptivity. However, implantation is the embryo's penetration of and adherence to the uterine wall. Endometrial receptivity is the physiological receptivity of the endometrium to the invasive activity of the embryo. The fact that implantation and endometrial receptivity are coordinated does not entail that they are one and the same act. Yeung, Laethem, and Tham make another incorrect assumption based on their assumption about implantation and endometrial receptivity, namely, any alteration of endometrial receptivity is abortifacient, that is, prevents implantation. But this is true only if implantation is the same thing as endometrial receptivity. This conceptual error enables Yeung, Laethem, and Tham to view any study that indicates post-fertilization effects as being equivalent to showing a likelihood of abortifacient effects. However, as Austriaco's review of the literature shows, the scientific arguments by Yeung, Laethem, and Tham may be reliably countered, and the preponderance of evidence suggests that whatever alteration to endometrial function may happen as a result of levonorgestrel, this change is unlikely to be abortifacient. If Yeung, Laethem, and Tham were to argue that they are concerned only with alterations of endometrial receptivity that directly prevent implantation, they nevertheless erroneously equate endometrial receptivity with implantation for the purposes of their moral conclusion. In other words, for Yeung, Laethem, and Tham, any possibility of an endometrial effect is also the possibility of an abortifacient effect. If some endometrial alterations might possibly cause an abortifacient effect, then any possibility of such alterations must be ruled out in order to justify the use of a pharmacological agent. Thus, at a minimum, Yeung, Laethem, and Tham rely on an identification of endometrial alteration with prevention of implantation as the premise for their moral conclusion, which is another reason why they unqualifiedly cite any and all studies that indicate endometrial alteration as being supportive of an abortifacient effect.

Given the distinction between endometrial receptivity and implantation, the prohibition against the direct interference with implantation in directive 36 of the *ERDs* cannot legitimately refer simply and only to the alteration of the endometrium. This interpretation is supported by the wording of the proscription, which is against treatments whose "purpose or direct effect" is the interference with implantation. If a treatment solely and directly interferes with the implanting activity of the embryo, then it is designed to prevent implantation and is prohibited. But if a treatment indirectly alters the endometrium while directly doing something else, it does not for that sole reason fall under the *ERD* proscription.[12]

A moral agent is not responsible for consequences that are not reasonably foreseen. There are several compelling reasons why a possible abortifacient effect from levonorgestrel would be both unforeseen and of the sort that does not make the act evil. Some of these reasons are treated here in response to Yeung, Laethem, and Tham, and all are discussed in my moral analysis on pp. 128 to 133. Not only do these reasons show that a possible abortifacient effect from Plan B cannot be reasonably foreseen, they are also grounds for the conclusion that levonorgestrel may be administered for the prevention of pregnancy after rape with a moral certitude that it will not cause an abortifacient effect. Catholic hospitals should develop protocols for the dispensing of Plan B that incorporate proper informed consent and where possible specify the conditions under which its use is most effective.

Notes

[1] See *Summa theologiae* I-II, q. 20, a. 5.

[2] See *Summa contra gentiles*, trans. V. J. Bourke (Notre Dame, IN: University of Notre Dame Press, 1975), III, ch. 6, nn. 4 and 7

[3] Ibid., III, ch. 6, n. 7.

[4] If the mere possibility of death were sufficient to make an act morally unacceptable, then numerous actions of ordinary life would not be justified. Consider the many routine surgeries and medical and dental treatments in which the life of the patient is not in jeopardy but which entail the unforeseen possibility of death, or ordinary travel for which there is an unforeseen possibility of death. Examples include tonsillectomy, plastic surgery, flu vaccinations, routine dental work on someone with mitral valve prolapse, and the proper operation of a motor vehicle. The morally prohibitive value of possible death would certainly preclude any surgical operation in which death is foreseen but legitimately justified by the principle of the double effect, such as the hysterectomy of a cancerous uterus holding a living child. See Kevin L. Flannery, S.J., "The Field of Moral Action according to Thomas Aquinas," *Thomist* 69.1 (January 2005): 29–30, for Aquinas's distinction between the intentional and the voluntary as it applies to foreseen evil effects from actions by professionals such as physicians.

[5] For Austriaco's initial review of the scientific literature, his critics' views, and his replies to critics, see Nicanor Pier Giorgio Austriaco, O.P., "Is Plan B an Abortifacient? A Critical Look at the Scientific Evidence," *National Catholic Bioethics Quarterly* 7.4 (Winter 2007): 703–707; Marie T. Hilliard, "Plan B's Abortifacient Effect," *National Catholic Bioethics Quarterly* 8.1 (Spring 2008): 9–13; Patrick Yeung Jr., Erica Laethem, and Joseph Tham, L.C., "Is Plan B Abortifacient? Further Responses," *National Catholic Bioethics Quarterly* 8.2 (Summer 2008): 217–221; and Yeung, Laethem, and Tham, "More on Plan B," *National Catholic Bioethics Quarterly* 8.3 (Autumn 2008): 418–425. I am grateful to Father Austriaco and to Dan O'Brien, Ph.D., for their comments on Yeung, Laethem,

and Tham's "A Scientific Analysis of the Effects of Levonorg-estrel" (137–143 in this volume) and on an earlier draft of this rebuttal, the responsibility for which is solely my own.

[6] Austriaco, "More on Plan B," 422–423. Austriaco acknowledges the immorality of some of the experiments that have produced these data.

[7] A. Tirelli, A. Cagnacci, and A. Volpe, "Levonorgestrel Administration in Emergency Contraception: Bleeding Pattern and Pituitary-Ovarian Function," *Contraception* 77.5 (May 2008): 328–332.

[8] Austriaco, "More on Plan B," 424. Austriaco recognizes that additional studies are needed to confirm the results of Tirelli, Cagnacci, and Volpe.

[9] Ibid., 423; see also 421–422.

[10] Ibid., 424. R. T. Mikolajczyk and J. B. Stanford, "Levonorgestrel Emergency Contraception: A Joint Analysis of Effectiveness and Mechanism of Action," *Fertility and Sterility* 88.3 (2007): 565–571.

[11] Austriaco, "More on Plan B," 423; see also 422.

[12] The studies highlighted by Austriaco, which indicate an unlikely abortifacient effect from Plan B, show that whatever else may be known about the drug, its "purpose or direct effect" is other than prevention of implantation. In light of Aquinas's analysis of unforeseen effects, an abortifacient effect is unlikely to occur at all much less in the majority of cases. For this reason, this unlikely possible effect cannot be said to follow from its nature in the sense of being a direct effect or being ordered necessarily to this effect.

D. Moral Certitude and Emergency Contraception

Marie T. Hilliard, R.N.

A number of bioethicists have argued that a pregnancy-test-only protocol is morally sufficient before administering the emergency contraceptive levonorgestrel (sometimes referred to as the "morning-after pill," and the active substance in Plan B) in sexual assault protocols at Catholic hospitals.[1] In defense of this view, some offer various statistical assumptions and mathematical conjectures using the Bayesian method, which is controversial when applied to particular cases.[2] Others have cited animal and in vitro studies and have made unfounded inferences pertaining to the in vivo effects of emergency contraception.[3] Many agree that there is the possibility of a post-fertilization effect, but question whether an effect on the human endometrium from emergency contraception is sufficient to prevent implantation.[4] Most significantly, the Congregation for the Doctrine of the Faith has stated that "scientific studies indicate that *the effect of inhibiting implantation is certainly present*, even if this does not mean that such interceptives [intrauterine devices and the so-called morning-after pills] cause an abortion every time they are used, also because conception does not occur after every act of sexual intercourse."[5]

The question is whether the pregnancy-test-only protocol is sufficient to achieve moral certitude that emergency contraception will not have an abortifacient effect in *each specific victim* of sexual assault. Most would agree that, on the basis of findings from a thorough medical history and physical examination, not every victim of sexual assault would need to be given a predictive test of ovulation, that is, a test for luteinizing hormone (LH), before the administration of emergency contraception.[6] However, consistency with directive 36 of the *Ethical and Religious Directives for Catholic Health Care Services* (*ERDs*),[7] as promulgated by every diocesan bishop in the United States, requires moral certitude as to the effects of emergency contraception in *each particular victim* before it is administered. This moral certitude pertains to the well-formed prudential medical judgment that the administration of emergency contraception will have a properly contraceptive effect, which is the prevention of fertilization engendering a new human being, in *each specific victim* to whom it is administered.

Emergency contraception may have the potential to function as an abortifacient if fertilization has already taken place. It may do so by altering the uterine lining and thus preventing implantation. Since there currently is no readily available and accurate test for conception before implantation, the key is to know *with as much medical certainty as possible* whether conception is occurring or may take place shortly in a particular patient. Proponents of the pregnancy-test-only protocol claim that the negative pregnancy test affords one a sufficient level of moral certitude that an abortifacient effect will not occur. Under the pregnancy-test-only protocol, if the test result is negative (i.e., the test indicates that the victim was not likely to have been pregnant at the time of the sexual assault), then emergency contraception is administered. Proponents of the pregnancy-test-*plus*-ovulation-test protocol claim the two together are often necessary.[8] Since pregnancy test results become accurate only about ten to fourteen days after ovulation, and since victims of sexual assault usually are seen in an emergency department within seventy-two hours after the assault, a positive result in a pregnancy-test-only protocol indicates only that the victim was pregnant at least ten days before the sexual assault took place.[9] A pregnancy test performed within seventy-two hours after the assault cannot indicate whether conception has resulted or will result from the assault.

The purpose of an ovulation test is to indicate whether ovulation is imminent. Ovulation is stimulated by a sharp surge of LH one or two days prior to rupture of the ovarian follicle; an ovulation test detects the LH surge in the urine or blood. If the test result is positive, then ovulation is occurring or soon will occur, and conception is likely to take place.[10]

Once ovulation has been stimulated by the LH surge, emergency contraception alone normally cannot prevent ovulation from occurring.[11] Given that emergency contraception may function as an abortifacient if fertilization has occurred, Catholic hospitals have an obligation to ensure with moral certitude that the possibility of an abortion is excluded. The argument for the ovulation test is that it provides this certainty.

Furthermore, even if some researchers remain skeptical about whether the effect of emergency contraception on the endometrium is sufficient to prevent implantation, the administration of emergency contraception during or after ovulation serves no other medically validated purpose. The purpose of administering emergency contraception must be consistent with directive 36 of the *ERDs*, which stipulates that emergency contraception be given only to "prevent ovulation, sperm capacitation, or fertilization." Since evidence shows that emergency contraception alone is unable to prevent ovulation once there is evidence of the LH surge, and since current research indicates that the effect of emergency contraception on sperm capacitation is not rapid enough to prevent fertilization, the only reason for which emergency contraception can be given licitly is to prevent ovulation.[12] Thus, moral certitude pertaining to the administration of emergency contraception can be achieved only through the administration of the LH test.

Ovulation testing is not cumbersome, or burdensome, or even invasive, for it can be done by a simple and inexpensive urine test from a sample that already has been taken from the victim to test for pregnancy. When the test for pregnancy is done using a blood sample, that same sample likewise can be used to test for ovulation.[13] Furthermore, blood testing usually is done to provide a baseline for sexually transmitted diseases, and to assess major organ functioning before the administration of prophylaxis against sexually transmitted diseases.

What follows are arguments for moral certitude, not statistical probability, concerning the medical rationale for the administration of emergency contraception in human beings, not in vitro or in animals, specific to *each particular victim* of sexual assault. To administer emergency contraception when there is insufficient information as to its effect is not only morally illicit but medically unsound. In other words, if there is no known medically documented reason for administering the medication, so doing constitutes medical negligence. Finally, this argumentation will conclude with some observations on the present political circumstances that have brought the discussion over ovulation and pregnancy testing to the fore.

Scientific Certitude versus Moral Certitude

Some claim that those who advocate for a pregnancy test *plus* an ovulation test do so "because it has not been scientifically proven that [emergency contraception] never prevents early embryos (1–7 days old) from implanting in the wall of the uterus."[14] On the contrary, we make no claim that there must be scientific certitude that emergency contraception will not have an abortifacient effect before it is administered. Rather, there must be moral certitude that administration of the emergency contraceptive is consistent with directive 36 of the *ERDs*, that is to say, that there is "solid probability" that the emergency contraceptive will "prevent ovulation, sperm capacitation, or fertilization" in the specific victim of sexual assault. The ovulation test gives that level of moral certitude. "Solid probability" is based on the available scientific information about which significant favorable arguments are held by authorities, against which there are no decisive authoritative judgments or satisfactory authoritative refutations. There is no scientific research to support the claim that the administration of emergency contraception alone will prevent ovulation after the LH surge has stimulated ovulation. In fact, such an assertion has been scientifically refuted.[15]

Arguments supporting other mechanisms of preventing fertilization pertain to the effect of emergency contraception on cervical mucus and sperm capacitation.[16] There have been satisfactory authoritative refutations of this point. The effects of emergency contraception on cervical mucus and sperm capacitation can take up to nine hours. E. Kesserü et al. found that after the administration of 0.4 mg levonorgestrel, there is a decrease in sperm mobility beginning in five hours, and an increase in cervical mucus viscosity beginning in nine hours.[17] Sperm can reach the fallopian tubes within minutes of ejaculation, and are capacitated as early as five hours after entering the female reproductive track.[18] Furthermore, K. Gemzell-Danielsson and L. Marions conclude that data indicate that "levonorgestrel or mifepristone in doses relevant for emergency contraception have no direct effect on sperm function."[19] They observe that the effects reported by Kesserü et al. are probably seen when levonorgestrel is used as a regular contraceptive, but are unlikely to be its main action. Thus, any such effects of levonorgestrel on sperm function are from daily ingested oral contraceptives, not from two doses of emergency contraception administered within a sexual assault protocol.

The process used to assure moral certitude concerning the effects of the emergency contraceptive on each patient is to identify the three moral fonts: the intent of the act (to prevent the engendering of a new human being from an assault by an unjust aggressor); the object of the act (to prevent fertilization of an ovum by sperm), and the circumstances consistent with the intent and object. Circumstances consistent with the intent and object require that a health care provider know why the medication is being administered to each specific patient. This is not just a requirement of moral certitude; it is a requirement of non-negligent medical practice. The only scientifically agreed-on effect of emergency contraception in preventing fertilization is its anovulant effect. There is no evidence to show that emergency contraception alone can have such an effect after ovulation has been initiated through an LH surge. Thus, to achieve moral certitude as to the reason for administering emergency contraception, a test for the LH surge is required. Furthermore, while it is acknowledged that a number of researchers in the scientific community are skeptical concerning whether the effect of emergency contraception on the endometrium is sufficient to prevent implantation, there is sufficient debate concerning this matter, as addressed below, to require the non-administration of emergency contraception after ovulation has been initiated.

Some would argue, why then not also require a serum progesterone test, which would determine the pre- or post-ovulation day exactly?[20] Such testing is not readily available in all emergency departments. Furthermore, the life span of an ovum is twenty-four hours, thus reducing the probability that a viable ovum is present in the fallopian tube if emergency contraception is administered after the LH surge has occurred.[21] If undetected "breakthrough" ovulation does occur despite the administration of emergency contraception following a negative LH test result, the conditions for morally licit administration of emergency contraception under the principle of double effect would have been met. This is to say that the action itself would be good or morally neutral (to prevent the engendering of a new human being from an assault by an unjust aggressor); that the good effect (preventing fertilization of an ovum by sperm) would be intended, but not the possible bad effect (impending break-through ovulation leading to the engendering of an embryo whose implantation in the uterus is impeded); and that the circumstances were consistent with the intent and object. Circumstances consistent with the intent and object require that the health care provider have moral certitude concerning why the medication is being administered to each specific patient in question. The negative LH test result demonstrates with solid probability that emergency contraception can have its intended anovulatory effect. However, if this determination is not made through LH testing, the criteria for invoking the principle of double effect are not met, since the circumstance of administering emergency contraception (only after testing for the absence of a prior pregnancy) is inconsistent with determining that emergency contraception will function by preventing fertilization.

Furthermore, the typical life span of a sperm is seventy-two hours.[22] Thus, if a victim presents in the emergency department more than seventy-two hours after a sexual assault, there is a solid probability that emergency contraception cannot prevent fertilization, and in fact an undetected pregnancy (prior to implantation) from the sexual assault could already exist. Thus, administration of emergency contraception at that time, even with a negative LH test result, would not be able to "prevent ovulation, sperm capacitation, or fertilization" in a timely enough manner, consistent with the requirements of directive 36 of the *ERDs*. However, for the psychological well-being of a victim who wishes to receive emergency contraception even after it could have the aforementioned effects, and to assure that the timing of the victim's cycle indicates that ovulation has not already occurred, a serum progesterone test could be administered for such a determination.

Why Raise the Possibility of an Abortifacient Effect?

While this paper focuses on the necessity of achieving moral certitude that emergency contraception will have an anti-fertilization effect, and recognizes that there is a question concerning whether the effect on the endometrium is sufficient to prevent implantation with each administration, there are significant arguments to indicate a solid probability that emergency contraception can have an abortifacient effect. There are those who claim that "there is no credible evidence to date that [these drugs] ever prevent implantation."[23] However, two prominent scientific studies make this claim questionable.[24] The research of Hapangama, Glasier, and Baird suggests that possible mechanisms of levonorgestrel, in addition to its anovulatory effects, include a retardation of the endometrium. Mikolajczyk and Stanford conclude from an extensive analysis of numerous studies that the effectiveness of levonorgestrel also may be attributed to post-fertilization effects. More specifically, a comparative study of the effectiveness of emergency contraception with the abortifacient mifepristone (RU-486, acknowledged to prevent implantation as well as to abort an implanted embryo[25]) and with levonorgestrel found that "there was no significant trend in the pregnancy rates in the 5 successive days from the time of unprotected intercourse for the 2 groups ... although the number of women receiving emergency contraception beyond 72 and up to 120 hours after unprotected intercourse was small."[26] Ignoring such a scientific possibility within a sexual assault protocol indicates a willingness to accept all the possible effects of emergency contraception.

In addition, the U.S. Food and Drug Administration states publicly that "it is possible that Plan B [levonorgestrel] may also work by preventing fertilization of an egg (the uniting of sperm with the egg) or by preventing attachment (implantation) to the uterus (womb), which usually occurs beginning 7 days after release of an egg from the ovary."[27] The FDA did not arrive at this conclusion because there is no credible evidence to date that this drug ever prevents implantation; it arrived at this conclusion from an analysis of the relevant scientific data.[28] Likewise, the manufacturer of Plan B, Barr Pharmaceuticals, states in the full prescribing information that Plan B "may inhibit implantation (by altering the endometrium)."[29] Finally, and most importantly, the Congregation for the Doctrine of the Faith has concluded that

> it is true that there is not always complete knowledge of the way that different pharmaceuticals operate, but

scientific studies indicate that *the effect of inhibiting implantation is certainly present,* even if this does not mean that such interceptives [intrauterine devices and the so-called morning-after pills] cause an abortion every time they are used, also because conception does not occur after every act of sexual intercourse. It must be noted, however, that anyone who seeks to prevent the implantation of an embryo which may possibly have been conceived and who therefore either requests or prescribes such a pharmaceutical, generally intends abortion.[30]

There is currently no readily available and accurate test for conception before implantation. Hence, there cannot be certainty before implantation occurs that an abortion will result. However, to administer emergency contraception at the request of a victim or in response to a mandate from the government, either of whose intent is to prevent implantation,[31] may cause health care providers to cooperate in evil by way of immediate material cooperation. Thus, health care providers must have sufficient information when treating each victim of sexual assault to ensure that they do not engage in such cooperation with evil acts.

Arguments Based on Bayesian Statistical Probability

Some ethicists argue that the probability that emergency contraception has an unintended abortifacient effect when given in the pregnancy-test-only protocol is equivalent to the probability that it has an abortifacient effect when both the results of both the ovulation and pregnancy tests are negative. They claim that the probability of an unintended abortifacient effect from emergency contraception when administered in the pregnancy-test-only protocol is very low, that the inaccuracy of ovulation testing means that an unintended abortifacient effect could still occur after the testing, and that it is questionable whether emergency contraception functions as an abortifacient at all.[32]

Statistical probability arguments must start with accurate definitions and recent data on the frequency of pregnancy occurring after sexual assault, not data from 1979 (as were used by one advocate for a pregnancy-test-only protocol, who claimed the frequency was 1 percent[33]). For pregnancy to occur after a sexual assault, the assault must include genital-to-genital sexual contact. Thus, an accurate definition of terms is critical, i.e., "unwanted sexual intercourse."[34] More recent information on pregnancy resulting from sexual assault of women over eighteen years of age indicates a rate of 5 percent.[35]

Insofar as these studies were confined to women eighteen years old and older, the actual pregnancy rate may be higher. Data indicate that about 44 percent of sexual assault victims are under age eighteen, and 80 percent are under age thirty.[36] The peak of female fertility occurs before age thirty.[37] Therefore, the statistical probability that emergency contraception may be abortive must begin with *this latter statistic of 5 percent*, not the unfounded 1 percent, which is not simply exaggerated but false.

Furthermore, false assumptions can be made concerning the number of women who at the time of a sexual assault are already pregnant, assumptions resulting in inaccurate determinations of statistical probability of an abortifacient effect from administering emergency contraception. One proponent of a statistical probability approach states, "I assume, based on background prevalence rates for U.S. women of child-bearing age, that 1 percent already will have a positive pregnancy test from intercourse prior to the sexual assault," and then inaccurately deducts this rate from a 1979 resulting pregnancy rate of 1 percent, yielding a 0.99 percent pregnancy rate.[38] However, the rate of 1 percent for women who become pregnant because of sexual assault does not include women who are pregnant because of prior consensual sex. The pregnancy test in the emergency department already excludes them from these statistics.

Furthermore, women who arrive at an emergency department are less likely, statistically, to be a cross-section of those of child-bearing age. As referenced earlier, 80 percent of victims are under the age of thirty. The result is that the pre-existing pregnancy rate among these women is likely to be smaller than 1 percent. The sad fact is that in the United States, sexual activity and contraceptive use begin in the teenage years, with 35.6 percent of all ninth- to twelfth-grade girls reporting being currently sexually active, 54.9 percent indicating use of a condom during their last sexual intercourse, and 18.7 percent reporting use of oral contraceptives.[39] Ninety-eight percent of teens fifteen to nineteen years old who have had sex report using at least one method of birth control.[40]

In addition, more than 98 percent of sexually active women in the United States have used at least one contraceptive method.[41] This would render them less likely to be pregnant from a prior act of intercourse. However, the condom was found to be the third-leading method of contraception in the United States, used by about nine million women and their partners.[42] Such victim-protective methods are unlikely to be used by a rapist; thus, while the incidence of a prior pregnancy is greatly overestimated using the statistical probability method mentioned above, the probability that a woman will become pregnant from a sexual assault is greater than estimated by that same method. Specifically, among women nineteen to twenty-six years of age (the age group at which fertility is greatest and the incidence of being sexually assaulted is high), the probability of pregnancy resulting from unprotected intercourse, if occurring on a day relative to ovulation, may be as high as 50 percent.[43] Hence, the chance increases that a greater number of women who will become pregnant from sexual assault will present at the hospital.

Proponents of statistical probability arguments also attempt to be predictive of fertility periods without engaging in medical testing to determine such periods. Such inaccurate methodology assumes that 11 percent of the women who seek emergency contraception at a Catholic hospital will be in their fertile period.[44] Sperm, while having a standard viability of seventy-two hours, may remain potent for five days.[45] Thus, it is possible that a woman who is sexually assaulted five days prior to the three-day window in the middle of her cycle will become pregnant. Furthermore, the ovum can live for twenty-four hours, presenting a window of possibly nine days (32 percent) for conception to occur, instead of the figure of 11 percent.

Statistical probability using Bayesian methodology must rely on published research, such as that above, not on defective data and unfounded assumptions like those referenced earlier. This perpetuates a chain of erroneous reasoning, and each of the errors in this chain is built upon the previous errors, so that a miscalculation at the beginning is compounded as the error progresses and is joined to those made in later assumptions.

Even if all the data and assumptions are factually supported, the key question is whether mere statistical probability provides sufficient evidence to support the proposition that emergency contraception will not have an abortive effect in *this* victim. Bayesian method is applied validly when used to find correlations among events in general, as in the study by Mikolajczyk and Stanford which indicates that emergency contraception has a post-fertilization effect.[46] The difficulty is that mere statistical frequency, as delineated by the Bayesian method, will not justify this conclusion for a specific victim being treated.

To explicate this, consider the following example from L. Jonathan Cohen, who objects to using frequencies to justify beliefs:

> The criminal courts ... would do very well if 95 percent of their verdicts were correct: there is always the

risk of missing or perjured witnesses, incompetent advocates, perverse or corrupt juries, etc. So suppose the only evidence presented to the court in the trial of a man accused of possessing illegal drugs is that he possesses a rainbow-painted car and that 95 percent of those who possess rainbow-painted cars also possess illegal drugs. Would it be justice to condemn him? Should he be deprived of his liberty? No. But why not?[47]

Any prosecution would be ill-advised because there is not *enough* evidence, and because the evidence we do have is *irrelevant* to whether the person is guilty or not. Furthermore, using such a methodology is ineffective in determining appropriate treatment for a victim of sexual assault. Two facts prevent such an inference, the first being the problem of induction, i.e., there is no guarantee that the medical facts pertaining to each victim conform to the statistical frequencies; and second, statistical frequency alone does not indicate anything about the causal relationships between events.

Advocates of the statistical probability method of developing a sexual assault protocol would have the health care provider justified in believing that emergency contraception will not have an abortive effect in *this* victim on the basis of the statistical frequency of sexually assaulted women who need treatment, are fertile, and yet have a negative pregnancy test result (which, as noted earlier, indicates nothing about a pregnancy from the sexual assault). However, such a generalization does not indicate any linkage of cause and effect concerning a possible pregnancy in the present case. In order to move from premise to conclusion, one needs justification for the intervening premise: on the basis of relevant medical data, not statistical generalizations, emergency contraception will not act as an abortifacient in *this* victim.

False Claims about the Ovulation Test

Proponents of the pregnancy-test-only protocol make various claims about the inaccuracy of the ovulation test and the difficulty of its use. Concerning the supposed inaccuracy of the test, E. Guermandi et al. have demonstrated that urine LH testing is 100 percent sensitive and 96 percent accurate: "Urinary LH surge preceded follicular rupture assessed by ultrasonography in all cycles and showed concordance with ultrasound-evidenced ovulation in 98 of 101 cases."[48] Concerning the errors, the report continues, "in three cases, no evidence of follicular rupture at ultrasonography was found, despite positive LH readings." Furthermore, the report states, "the LH urinary surge showed ovulatory events in 99 cycles (four

false-positive findings)." The same article sets the positive predictive value of the LH urine test at 0.97.

However, in the event of a positive LH urine test result, a serum LH test could be administered. M. Durand et al., while demonstrating a higher level of false-positive results with a urine LH test than did Guermandi et al., indicate the value of LH serum testing:

> A highlight in this study was the possibility to identify the exact cycle day of [levonorgestrel] administration, particularly relative to the midcycle serum gonadotropin surge. Serum LH measurements helped us to assess the day of ovulation, adding a new dimension to data interpretation of our study. Urinary LH proved to be a poor guide to determine the day of ovulation, yielding 13.3 percent false positives (true LH surge in serum occurred later in the cycle).[49]

An important note is required on the last sentence of this quotation. Durand et. al. indicate that LH urine testing is not reliable, but this is a somewhat inaccurate reading of the evidence they site for this claim. The study Durand et. al. site actually says that their "analysis showed that, 95 percent of the time, ovulation can be expected to occur 14–26 hours after detection of LH surge in the urine."[50] These authors noted that of twenty-six subjects, only one showed a urine LH surge that was not followed by ovulation. Furthermore, if there remains a concern based on medical history and physical examination (e.g., the absence of ferning of cervical mucus[51]), serum progesterone testing to determine the day in the victim's cycle or ultrasound visualization of ovarian follicular rupture could be conducted.

The Present Political Circumstances

There is much more at stake here than winning an argument on which protocol achieves the moral certitude that directive 36 of the *ERD* expects. The debate has developed in response to legislative mandates on Catholic health care that attempt to dictate hospital policies in violation of the tenets of the Catholic Church. It would be fair to conjecture that a mind-set of accommodation to secular mandates has generated a willingness to settle for statistical probability over moral certitude in developing sexual assault protocols. But in making these accommodations, Catholic ministries are allowing ongoing erosion of their religious liberty. (For a comprehensive discussion of this phenomenon, see chapter 27, on state mandates.) By capitulating to such mandates, Catholic health care is paying tribute to secular law over the particular law of the Church contained in the *ERDs*.

In the debate over whether Catholic health care facilities should be obliged under the law to provide emergency contraception to victims of sexual assault, it should be noted that Catholic health care is fully prepared to do just that. Catholic hospitals have had compassionate and medically sound sexual assault protocols in place before many of their secular counterparts, in awareness of the potential of there being two victims from the sexual assault: the woman and her child who may be conceived by the act of unjust aggression. The sperm of the rapist is an unjust aggressor and the victim is fully entitled to defend herself from this prolongation of the original assault. Every woman who has not conceived as the result of sexual assault should receive drugs that will suppress ovulation and thus prevent fertilization. But when a pregnancy already exists, or when it is likely to soon occur and cannot be prevented, the use of these drugs cannot be called contraceptive.

Directive 36 of the *ERDs* is very specific as to the conditions which must be met for the administration of emergency contraception after a sexual assault: the administration may "prevent ovulation, sperm capacitation, or fertilization. It is not permissible, however, to initiate or to recommend treatments that have as their purpose or direct effect the removal, destruction, or interference with the implantation of a fertilized ovum." There are no data to confirm that emergency contraception can act quickly enough to prevent sperm capacitation or fertilization separate from an anovulatory action. There is evidence of post-fertilization effects of emergency contraception. Thus, it is necessary to know that the emergency contraceptive will have its proper anovulatory effect if the health care worker is to have the requisite moral certitude that its administration is consistent with the *ERDs*. This is the basis on which arguments for a pregnancy-test-*plus*-ovulation-test protocol are presented here, rather than unresolved arguments pertaining to potentially abortifacient effects of emergency contraception on the endometrium. However, if further research shows clearly that emergency contraception does have an abortifacient effect, Catholic health care already may have capitulated to a secular legal mandate, thus showing a willingness to compromise religious liberty in the delivery of health care. Such a capitulation bodes ill for the future of Catholic health care.

The path of least resistance always poses a temptation, especially when the media takes an active interest in such controversial issues as sexual assault protocols in Catholic hospitals. There are ongoing efforts in the political arena, at the federal level and in various states in this country, to use the force of law to compel Catholic health care facilities to violate the *Ethical and Religious Directives for Catholic Health Care Services*. The list of legal mandates affecting Catholic ministries continues to grow, from the proposed federal Freedom of Choice Act, which will require Catholic health care facilities to provide abortions, to the requirement that Catholic Charities be an agent for the adoption of children by same-sex couples.[52] These efforts are a pernicious trespass on the religious liberty of Catholics and on the right of every individual to follow the moral teachings of his or her own religious tradition.

Catholic health care, having attempted to accommodate secular legal mandates, and despite what may be temporary protections by the recent "conscience rule" of the U.S. Department of Health and Human Services (in December 2008),[53] now finds itself at a crossroad. There is no more room for legal accommodation as threats to religious freedom and Catholic identity reach a crisis. We cannot allow legislative and judicial efforts to override sound medical and moral decisions in Catholic health care.

If the participants in these debates are to use terms in the proper meanings, and not hide their true agendas behind euphemisms, then issues must be described as they truly are. Catholic institutions are not being asked to provide emergency contraception; they are being forced to accept all the potential effects of "emergency contraception," including its potential to act as an emergency abortifacient. It is to this that Catholic health care must say no.

Notes

The author thanks Stephen Napier and Edward Furton for their advice and assistance on this manuscript.

[1] "Emergency contraception" as used here refers to two administrations of high-dose (0.75 mg) levonorgestrel, the active ingredient in Plan B, twelve hours apart. See, for example, R. E. Wertheimer, "Emergency Postcoital Contraception," *American Family Physician* 62.10 (November 15, 2000): 2287–2292. It should be noted that Plan B is a different regimen than the so-called Yuzpe regimen, which uses a combination of ethinyl estradiol and norgestrel (Ovral).

[2] Daniel P. Sulmasy, "Emergency Contraception for Women Who Have Been Raped: Must Catholics Test for Ovulation, or Is Testing for Pregnancy Morally Sufficient?" *Kennedy Institute of Ethics Journal* 16.4 (December 2006): 305–331. Bayesian probability theory is a branch of mathematics that allows one to model uncertainty about the world and outcomes of interest to various agents by combining commonsense knowledge and observational evidence.

[3] M. E. Ortiz et al., "Postcoital Administration of Levonorgestrel Does Not Interfere with Post-Fertilization Events in the New-World Monkey *Cebus paella*," *Human Reproduction* 19

(April 22, 2004):1352–1356; and P. G. Lalitkumar et al., "Mifepristone, but Not Levonorgestrel, Inhibits Human Blastocyst Attachment to an In Vitro Endometrial Three-Dimensional Cell Culture Model," *Human Reproduction* 22.11 (November 2007): 3031–3137.

⁴ J. Trussell and E. G. Raymond, "Emergency Contraception: A Last Chance to Prevent Unintended Pregnancy," Princeton University Office of Population Research (October 2008), 5, http://ec.princeton.edu/questions/ec-review.pdf.

⁵ Congregation for the Doctrine of the Faith (CDF), *Instruction* Dignitas Personae *on Certain Bioethical Questions* (December 8, 2008), n. 23, original emphasis.

⁶ Dan O'Brien and John Paul Slosar, "A Sexual Assault Protocol for Catholic Hospitals," *Ethics and Medics* 27:6 (June 2002).

⁷ U.S. Conference of Catholic Bishops, *Ethical and Religious Directives for Catholic Health Care Services*, 4th ed. (Washington, D.C.: USCCB, 2001).

⁸ The blood serum test is an even more accurate means of determining whether a woman is about to ovulate, but in view of the difficulty of performing such a test in a timely fashion in some hospital settings, the urine ovulation test may be the best that can be done.

⁹ *Merck Manual of Diagnosis and Therapy*, 18th ed. (Whitehouse Station, NJ: Merck, 2006), s.v. "Introduction: Normal Pregnancy," rev. online June 2007, http://www.merck.com/mmpe/sec18/ch260/ch260a.html?qt=pregnancy&alt=sh.

¹⁰ Ovulation occurs twelve to twenty-four hours after urinary evidence of the luteinizing hormone surge. See Elaena Quattrocchi and Irene Hove, "Ovulation and Pregnancy: Home Testing Products," *U.S. Pharmacist* 23.9 (September 1998).

¹¹ At least one study, however, has indicated that levonorgestrel administered with an enzyme called cyclooxygenase-2 (Cox-2) can stop ovulation in the setting of an LH surge. M. R. Massai et al., "Does Meloxicam Increase the Incidence of Anovulation Induced by Single Administration of Levonorgestrel in Emergency Contraception? A Pilot Study," *Human Reproduction* 22.2 (February 2007): 434–439.

¹² N. Novikova et al., "Effectiveness of Levonorgestrel Emergency Contraception Given Before or After Ovulation: A Pilot Study," *Contraception* 75.2 (February 2007): 112–118; K. Gemzell-Danielsson and L. Marions, "Mechanisms of Action of Mifepristone and Levonorgestrel When Used for Emergency Contraception" *Human Reproduction Update* 10.4 (July–August 2004): 342.

¹³ The serum test is more difficult to perform than a urine test, and not all health care facilities are equipped to provide the results in a timely manner.

¹⁴ Sulmasy, "Emergency Contraception for Women," 307.

¹⁵ N. Novikova, "Effectiveness of Levonorgestrel Emergency Contraception."

¹⁶ M. Durand et al., "On the Mechanisms of Action of Short-Term Levonorgestrel Administration in Emergency Contraception," *Contraception* 64.4 (October 2001): 227–234.

¹⁷ E. Kesserü et al., "The Hormonal and Peripheral Effects of D-Norgestrel in Postcoital Contraception," *Contraception* 10.4 (October 1974): 411–424.

¹⁸ D. R. Coustan et al., *Human Reproduction: Growth and Development* (Lebanon, IN: Little, Brown, 1995), 22.

¹⁹ Gemzell-Danielsson, "Mechanisms of Action of Mifepristone and Levonorgestrel," 342.

²⁰ R. P. Miech, "Rape Protocol," letter, *Ethics and Medics* 27:12 (December 2002). The emergency contraceptive available at the time this article was written was a combination of both progestin and estradiol, and its abortifacient properties were more widely accepted.

²¹ K. M. Thies and J. F. Travers, *Human Growth and Development through the Life Span* (Thorofare, NJ: Slack, 2001), 32.

²² *Merck Manual*, s.v. "Introduction: Normal Pregnancy."

²³ Sulmasy, "Emergency Contraception for Women," 319.

²⁴ D. Hapangama, A. F. Glasier, and D. T. Baird, "The Effect of Peri-Ovulatory Administration of Levonorgestrel on the Menstrual Cycle," *Contraception* 63.3 (March 2001): 123–129; and R. T. Mikolajczyk and J. B. Stanford, "Levonorgestrel Emergency Contraception: A Joint Analysis of Effectiveness and Mechanism of Action," *Fertility and Sterility* 88.3 (September 2007): 565–571.

²⁵ Kristina Gemzell-Danielsson et al., "Implantation: Effects of a Single Post-Ovulatory Dose of RU486 on Endometrial Maturation in the Implantation Phase," *Human Reproduction* 9:12 (1994): 2398–2404.

²⁶ H. Hamoda et al., "A Randomized Trial of Mifepristone (10 mg) and Levonorgestrel for Emergency Contraception," *American College of Obstetrics and Gynecology* 104.6 (December 2004), 1307–1313.

²⁷ U.S. Food and Drug Administration, Center for Drug Evaluation and Research, "Plan B: Questions and Answers" (August 24, 2006, updated December 14, 2006), http://www.fda.gov/cder/drug/infopage/planB/planBQandA20060824.htm.

²⁸ Sulmasy, "Emergency Contraception for Women," 319.

²⁹ Barr Pharmaceuticals, full U.S. prescribing information for Plan B (levonorgestrel) tablets, 0.75 mg, rev. February 2004, http://www.barrlabs.com/proprietary/keyproducts/BRL_PIB-planb.pdf. See also the American College of Obstetrics and Gynecology (ACOG), "Emergency Contraception," pamphlet AP114, May 2007, http://www.acog.org/publications/patient_education/bp114.cfm.

³⁰ CDF, *Dignitas personae*, n. 23, original emphasis.

³¹ "Conception" historically and more accurately referred to fertilization, but the medical meaning was changed to refer to implantation. See ACOG Committee on Terminology, *Obstetric-Gynecologic Terminology, with Section on Neonatology and Glossary of Congenital Anomalies*, ed. Edward Hughes (Philadelphia: F. A. Davis, 1972).

[32] Sulmasy, "Emergency Contraception for Women."

[33] Ibid., 310–311, citing John R. Evrard and E. M. Gold, "Epidemiology and Management of Sexual Assault Victims," *Obstetrics and Gynecology* 53.3 (March 1979): 381–387.

[34] F. H. Stewart and J. Trussell, "Prevention of Pregnancy Resulting from Rape: A Neglected Preventive Health Measure," *American Journal of Preventive Medicine* 19.4 (November 2000): 228–229.

[35] M. M. Holmes et al., "Rape-Related Pregnancy: Estimates and Descriptive Characteristics from a National Sample of Women," *American Journal of Obstetrics and Gynecology* 175.2 (August 1996): 320–324; and Rape, Abuse, and Incest National Network (RAINN), "Statistics," http://www.rainn.org/statistics/.

[36] RAINN, "Statistics."

[37] *ADAM Medical Encyclopedia* (Atlanta, GA: ADAM, 2005), s.v. "Infertility," updated February 5, 2008, http://www.nlm.nih.gov/medlineplus/ency/article/001191.htm.

[38] Sulmasy, "Emergency Contraception for Women," 301.

[39] Danice K. Eaton et al., "Youth Risk Behavior Surveillance—United States, 2007," *Morbidity and Mortality Weekly Report* 57.SS-4 (June 6, 2008): 99, 101.

[40] J. C. Abma et al., "Teenagers in the United States: Sexual Activity, Contraceptive Use, and Childbearing, 2002," National Center for Health Statistics, *Vital and Health Statistics* 23.24 (December 2004): 1–48.

[41] William D. Mosher et al., "Use of Contraception and Use of Family Planning Services in the United States: 1982–2002," National Center for Health Statistics, *Advanced Data from Vital and Health Statistics* 350 (December 10, 2004), http://www.cdc.gov/nchs/data/ad/ad350.pdf.

[42] Ibid.

[43] D. B. Dunson, B. Colombo, and D. D. Baird, "Changes with Age in the Level and Duration of Fertility in the Menstrual Cycle," *Human Reproduction* 17.5 (May 2002): 1399–1403.

[44] Sulmasy, "Emergency Contraception for Women," 311.

[45] Mikolajczyk and Stanford, "Levonorgestrel Emergency Contraception."

[46] Ibid.

[47] L. Jonathan Cohen, "Bayesianism versus Baconianism in the Evaluation of Medical Diagnoses," *British Journal for the Philosophy of Science* 31.1 (March 1980): 54.

[48] E. Guermandi et al., "Reliability of Ovulation Tests in Infertile Women," *Obstetrics & Gynecology* 97.1 (January 2001): 92–95.

[49] Durand, "Mechanisms of Action," 232.

[50] P. B. Miller and M. R. Soules, "The Usefulness of a Urinary LH Kit for Ovulation Prediction during Menstrual Cycles of Normal Women," *Obstetrics and Gynecology* 87.1 (1996): 15.

[51] Ferning of cervical mucus, a distinct pattern of microscopic crystallization, occurs immediately before ovulation. See Adele Pillitteri, *Maternal and Child Health Nursing: Care of the Childbearing and Childrearing Family*, 5th ed. (Philadelphia: Lippincott, Williams & Wilkins, 2006), 86.

[52] The 110th U.S. Congress is considering a Freedom of Choice Act, which in fact will take freedoms away from states and all Americans, prevent citizens from enacting even the most modest limitations on abortion, and force taxpayers to pay for abortions. See *Freedom of Choice Act*, S. 1173 and H. R. 1964, 110th Cong., 1st sess. (April 19, 2007), and "Overview of State Adoption Laws," Lamda Legal, www.lambdalegal.org/our-work/issues/marriage-relationships-family/parenting/overview-of-state-adoption.html.

[53] On December 19, 2008, the U.S. Department of Health and Human Services published a final rule to ensure that HHS funds do not support practices or policies in violation of existing federal conscience protection laws. See "Ensuring That Department of Health and Human Services Funds Do Not Support Coercive or Discriminatory Policies or Practices in Violation of Federal Law; Final Rule," *Federal Register* 73.245 (December 19, 2008): 78071–78101. However, plans to rescind the rule are already in progress. "Rescission of the Regulation Entitled 'Ensuring That Department of Health and Human Services Funds Do Not Support Coercive or Discriminatory Policies or Practices in Violation of Federal Law'; Proposal," *Federal Register* 74.45 (March 10, 2009).

✠

Editorial Summation: Moral certitude, not statistical probability, is the proper rationale for the administration of emergency contraception in humans, consistent with directive 36 of the *Ethical and Religious Directives for Catholic Health Care Services*—a rationale that is specific to each particular victim of sexual assault. The data, as they currently exist, do not allow us to generalize about the endometrial effects of emergency contraception; however, before administering emergency contraception to a victim of sexual assault, Catholic providers must have moral certitude that there will not be two victims affected by emergency contraception, the sexual assault victim of the unjust aggressor and an unborn child who has already been engendered. There is no conclusive scientific data to support an anti-fertilization ability of emergency contraception if it is administered after ovulation has been initiated. To administer emergency contraception when there is insufficient information as to its effect is not only morally illicit but medically unsound. If there is no known medically documented reason for administering the medication during or after ovulation, doing so constitutes medical negligence.Those who argue that statistical probability equates to moral certitude gravely misunderstand the concept of moral certitude, as well as the concept of medical certainty. Before administering any medication to any patient, health care providers must know what action that medication will have on *that particular patient*. The Congregation for the Doctrine of the Faith has added that even though we do not possess complete knowledge of how "morning-after pills" operate, scientific studies show that they do have the effect of inhibiting implantation. Anyone who seeks to prevent the implantation of an embryo, and who therefore either requests or prescribes such a pharmaceutical, generally intends abortion. Thus, to administer emergency contraception at the request of the victim or in response to a mandate from government may cause the health care provider to cooperate in an evil by way of immediate material cooperation.

PART IV

END-OF-LIFE ISSUES

CHAPTER 12

Determining Death

James M. DuBois

Modern medicine has produced an ironic situation regarding the determination of death. Through the use of angiographies, electrocardiograms, and blood gas monitoring, we can now reliably determine when a brain lacks blood flow, when a heart ceases beating, and when respiration has discontinued. Yet in this age of advanced medicine, once again we find ourselves wrestling with the fear that we may be mistaken for dead while still alive. It is precisely modern medical technology that has given rise to such fears, specifically the ability to transplant organs and the ability to make early determinations of death. The connection between these two things is not coincidental: organs that have begun to decompose or grow necrotic cannot be transplanted; thus, death must be determined quickly when organ donation is desired.

Two common sets of criteria exist for determining death in the context of organ donation: circulatory–respiratory criteria, which are used in donation after cardiac death, or so-called non-heart-beating organ donation; and neurological criteria, also known as "brain death" criteria. All fifty U.S. states have adopted a variation of the Uniform Determination of Death Act (UDDA), formulated in 1981 by the President's Commission, which allows the use of either set of criteria: "An individual who has sustained either (1) irreversible cessation of circulatory and respiratory functions, or (2) irreversible cessation of all functions of the entire brain, including the brain stem, is dead. A determination of death must be made in accordance with accepted medical standards."[1] A 2002 survey of death criteria in eighty nations found that 86 percent had brain death practice guidelines in addition to traditional criteria for determining death.[2] Nevertheless, despite broad legal acceptance, criteria for determining

death are frequently controversial. This essay explores how the two most common sets of criteria can be used to generate specific tests for determining death that are consistent with a Catholic understanding of death.

Increasingly, we witness proposals to bypass the debates surrounding the determination of death by separating eligibility for organ donation from the determination of death. For example, some propose that patients who are permanently unconscious (e.g., patients in a persistent vegetative state or with anencephaly) should be allowed, with the consent of a surrogate, to donate vital organs prior to death even though doing so would cause death.[3] It should be clear that this approach would not be acceptable in Catholic health care. The *Ethical and Religious Directives for Catholic Health Care Services* (ERDs) express both a commitment to organ donation and a commitment to ensuring that individuals who donate vital organs are dead before procurement begins:

> Catholic health care institutions should encourage and provide the means whereby those who wish to do so may arrange for the donation of their organs and bodily tissues for ethically legitimate purposes, so that they may be used for donation and research after death. ... Such organs should not be removed until it has been medically determined that the patient has died.[4]

Determining that an individual has died in a manner that enables organ donation is challenging. But as the ERDs express, it is challenging work that we ought to pursue, at least as resources permit. Organ donation should be encouraged because, as Pope John Paul II has written, it is a "genuine act of love";[5] it can also significantly prolong and improve lives,[6] and it can bring meaning to grieving families.[7]

The Need for an Operational Definition of Death

In the Catholic tradition, death is conceptualized as "the separation of the soul from the body."[8] Philosophically, if one understands the soul as the life principle (in humans, the principle of life, motion, and rationality) then this definition amounts to little more than saying that a person ceases to be alive when the principle of life is lost. If one means that an immortal mind has separated from the body, then one clearly enters into theological concepts based on forms of "evidence" that medicine does not recognize. But in either case, the biggest problem for medicine is that we do not know when a soul leaves the body, that is, we cannot observe a precise moment of death. Thus, physicians need an operational definition based on what we can observe. As John Paul II taught,

> The death of the person, understood in this primary sense (i.e., the separation of the soul from the body), is an event which *no scientific technique or empirical method can identify directly*. Yet human experience shows that once death occurs *certain biological signs inevitably follow*, which medicine has learnt to recognize with increasing precision. In this sense, the "criteria" for ascertaining death used by medicine today should not be understood as the technical-scientific determination of the *exact moment* of a person's death, but as a scientifically secure means of identifying the *biological signs that a person has indeed died*.[9]

Viewed through this lens, death is an event, but the result of the event is a dead body (i.e., a body in the *state of death*), and physicians are better off determining the biological traits of dead bodies than trying to determine the actual moment that a soul leaves a body.

A Focal Description of Dead Bodies

In casuistry, or a case-based approach to ethics, it is quite common to begin with focal cases—those that are clear and convincing—before moving to more difficult cases through analogy. In a similar spirit, it may be wise to begin with noncontroversial descriptions of death that most people will recognize as accurate. Prescinding from specific etiologies, consider three possible ways of dying: cardiac arrest, asphyxia, and head trauma. In the case of cardiac arrest, circulation ceases. This means

that oxygenated blood is no longer flowing to the brain. Within about fifteen seconds, the brain loses functions. Because breathing is a brain-stem-mediated function, breathing discontinues. In the case of asphyxia, breathing ceases suddenly. Eventually, oxygen levels in the blood drop while carbon dioxide levels increase. This causes both the heart and the brain to lose their functions. In the case of head trauma, death may not immediately ensue. However, because the skull is a solid casing, if swelling of the injured brain cannot be successfully controlled, it will cut off circulation within the brain. As the brain stem dies from a lack of blood flow, it ceases to provide an impulse to breathe, and circulation is lost soon afterward as the heart becomes oxygen starved.[10]

In all three cases, merely restoring the initial lost function will be insufficient to restore the life of the human being, because the lack of oxygenated blood, at least at room temperature, causes cells to die quickly; as damage grows more extensive, the loss becomes permanent. Drawing from these few focal cases, one can offer the following: To call a body dead is to say that it is in *a state of widespread nonfunction—including a loss of neurological functions (particularly consciousness and brain-stem reflexes), circulation, and respiration—and this state naturally becomes permanent within minutes.* Because the key functions—neurological, circulatory, and respiratory—are interdependent, the state of death may be determined by focusing on any one of them, most commonly circulatory or neurological functions. If natural processes are allowed to run their course at normal temperatures, then the body quickly becomes flaccid, pale and cool, then stiff (rigor mortis), and then flaccid again prior to decomposing.

With interventions, which may include maintaining a body on a ventilator or cooling the body using cold solutions, it is possible to preserve some biological functions in a corpse. Nevertheless, common sense tells us that it is possible, even if sometimes difficult, to distinguish between the life of an organism and the life of isolated organs or cells. As D. Alan Shewmon and Elisabeth Seitz Shewmon have put it, "The understanding of certain comparisons as dichotomous, when viewed on a large scale, such as between a healthy organism and a putrefying corpse, is not invalidated by the fuzziness of the transition viewed on a small scale, any more than the representational meaning of an impressionist painting is vitiated by the fact that close-up one sees only brush strokes."[11]

Once an organism has died, all other "life activities" can be considered residual—the life activities of parts of a whole that no longer exist. Some of these residual functions are trivial, and explaining their insignificance is not particularly difficult. Other residual functions are more significant and have led some people to wonder whether they indicate the life of a human being. As we look at neurological and circulatory-respiratory criteria for death, we will examine the respective residual biological activities and consider whether they should prevent a determination of death.

Neurological Criteria

The term "brain death" typically refers to the irreversible loss of all functions of the entire brain, including the brain stem. However, despite the fact that neurological criteria focus only on the functions of the brain, they are used to determine the death of the human being, not merely an organ. Thus, the UDDA refers to neurological criteria for determining death, and the recent Institute of Medicine (IOM) committee advocated dropping the term "brain death" altogether, referring instead simply to death or neurological determinations of death. This is consistent with Pope John Paul II's statement made to the Transplantion Society. Referring to neurological criteria for determining death, he wrote that such criteria

> [do] not seem to conflict with the essential elements of a sound anthropology. Therefore a health worker professionally responsible for ascertaining death can use these criteria in each individual case as the basis for arriving at that degree of assurance in ethical judgment which moral teaching describes as "moral certainty." This moral certainty is considered the necessary and sufficient basis for an ethically correct course of action.[12]

This statement was consistent with the recommendations of the Pontifical Academy of Sciences, which in 1989 approved the use of neurological criteria for determining death of the human being.[13]

Key Features of Protocols

John Paul II, echoing a statement by Pope Pius XII, stated that, "with regard to the parameters used today for ascertaining death—whether the 'encephalic' signs or the more traditional cardiorespiratory signs—the Church does not make technical decisions."[14] The specific tests for determining death using neurological criteria will continue to change as technology develops and as the quality of our data improves. What follows is a very brief description of the typical findings when death is determined neurologically, and some of the variations of practice that currently exist.[15]

The "three essential findings in brain death are coma, absence of brain-stem reflexes, and apnea."[16] In the United States, a neurological determination of death may be entirely clinical because a bedside examination may confirm all three of these essential findings. Establishing the presence of deep coma requires "eyes-closed coma" and unresponsiveness to painful stimuli (e.g., nail-bed pressure). Establishing that it is irreversible ordinarily requires knowledge of the cause and exclusion of states that can mimic brain death, such as locked-in syndrome, hypothermia, and drug intoxication.[17] Among other things, clinical examination of brain-stem reflexes should indicate no pupil response to bright light, no ocular movement, no corneal reflexes, and no gag or cough reflex. Finally, an apnea test is conducted to demonstrate that there is no respiratory effort even when the patient is taken off the ventilator and carbon dioxide levels are allowed to drop into a range that should stimulate respiratory movement. Specific methods of testing for brain-stem reflexes and apnea vary across institutions, and practice guidelines typically allow for such variations. Ordinarily, when the diagnosis is clinical, then the examination is repeated after an interval. "Most experts agree that a 6-hour observation period is sufficient in adults and children over the age of 1 year. Longer intervals are advisable in young children."[18]

In some nations, a neurological determination of death requires a confirmatory test; in the United States, a confirmatory test is typically optional unless a complete clinical examination is not feasible (e.g., if the apnea test is contraindicated because of high levels of therapeutic barbiturates or etiology is unknown). A variety of confirmatory tests exist, including angiography (e.g., computed tomography, magnetic resonance, and radionuclide imaging), electroencephalography, nuclear brain scanning, and transcranial Doppler ultrasonography. Which test is used is often determined according to hospital policy, physician preference, medical contraindications, or simple availability. According to the guidelines provided by the New York State Department of Health (2005), "a cerebral blood flow study that demonstrates absent intracranial blood flow is consistent with the diagnosis of brain death even in the presence of [central nervous system] depressants."[19] Because many physicians use barbiturates to reduce cerebral swelling, and barbiturates can depress the CNS and take days to clear the blood system, blood flow studies can be useful in making a timely determination of death.

No one has ever recovered from brain death when it has been correctly determined.[20] Particularly in dealing with families at the time of death, it is important to be able to distinguish between death (brain death) and the persistent vegetative state (PVS). While some authors have advocated for the use of so-called higher-brain death criteria,[21] which focus only on the functions of the cerebrum, or higher brain (which are lost, for example, in the PVS), both the President's Commission and Pope John Paul II only sanctioned the use of "whole-brain death" criteria, which involve the irreversible loss of all brain functions including those of the brain stem. Patients with higher-brain death only may not have any of the essential findings of brain death (i.e., deep coma, apnea, and absent brain-stem reflexes). It is important for families to know that a determination of death using neurological criteria is not a quality-of-life judgment or a judgment about futility, but a determination of death.

The Problem of Residual Biological Functions

When mechanical ventilation and support are continued for a body declared dead using neurological criteria, "what usually follows is an invariant heart rate from a differentiated sinoatrial node, structural myocardial lesions leading to a marked reduction in the ejection fraction, decreased coronary perfusion, the need for increasing use of inotropic drugs to maintain blood pressure, and a fragile state that leads to cardiac arrest within days or weeks."[22]

Nevertheless, even if it is typically only for a period of days, bodies that are maintained on a ventilator do demonstrate numerous "signs of life": the heart is beating, the body is pink and warm, waste may be processed, and wounds may be healed. In some rare cases, with support to maintain blood pressure and to prevent or manage diabetes insipidus, female bodies have sustained a pregnancy until viability and a few bodies have been maintained for years.[23] This means that such bodies do not fully satisfy our "focal description" of death. To be perfectly clear, but for mechanical ventilation, all bodies pronounced dead using neurological criteria would immediately satisfy our focal description—there is no respiratory effort, hence all respiration and circulation would discontinue. However, mechanical ventilation is often used to support respiration and circulation in bodies pronounced brain dead, most frequently in order to enable organ donation.

Above I noted that deceased bodies may demonstrate some residual biological activities but that such activities are functionally meaningless. Is this really the case with brain death? In the case of a body sustaining pregnancy, one might say no, they are not meaningless, because the functions sustain the life of a human being, the gestating fetus. But apart from such rare cases, do the various

biological functions in brain-dead bodies have a similar meaning, that is, do they serve the purpose of sustaining the body of a living human being?

Ultimately, in answering this question—the key question—there is no avoiding an appeal to intuition. Kenneth Iserson offers the following analogy to support the intuition that an individual who has lost all brain functions is dead:

> In death by brain criteria, the body is physiologically decapitated. In an anatomic decapitation, the head is actually lopped off but the heart continues to beat for some time, spraying blood from the severed neck arteries. Yet, despite the continued pumping of the heart, there is no question that the person is irreversibly dead. Even in ancient times, the Talmud said, "the death throes of a decapitated man are not signs of life any more than is the twitching of a lizard's amputated tail."[24]

Moreover, if one rejects this notion that a physiologically decapitated body is a dead body, then one is left with a conclusion repugnant to common sense and good metaphysics, namely, that both a severed head and a decapitated body are living substances if separately maintained alive.[25] To be completely consistent, one would actually need to hold that they are *both* the *same* living human being that existed prior to the decapitation—a view that flatly contradicts the unity required to be a human being (or any substance, for that matter). If one claims that they are living substances, but that neither is the same living human being, then one has conceded that the living human being has ceased to exist or has died.

It is important to note that the acceptance of brain death criteria does not presuppose a dualistic, "Cartesian" notion of the human being, in which the loss of "mind" alone indicates the death of the human being. After all, the brain is not equal to consciousness; it is biological, it is a major part of the body. Far from assuming that human beings are distinct from their bodies, defenders of neurological criteria for determining death assert that the connection between mind and body is so tight that a mind cannot animate a body with a dead brain.

Circulatory–Respiratory Criteria

Circulatory–respiratory criteria are those criteria most familiar to the average person. In popular television shows, we commonly see an inspector checking for a pulse in the carotid artery before making an amateur pronouncement of death. In ordinary language, to breathe one's last breath is to die. Yet despite their familiarity, circulatory and respiratory criteria have again become controversial as they are applied in the context of donation after cardiac death.

Two common forms of donation after cardiac death (DCD) exist: controlled and uncontrolled. These modifying adjectives describe the timing of the death rather than the donation procedure. While they are both referred to as forms of DCD, they raise very different ethical issues.

Death Criteria in Controlled DCD

In "controlled" DCD, the death of the patient is expected. Candidates for controlled DCD are patients who are ventilator-dependent and were relatively healthy until their present illness. If a patient's surrogate decision makers determine that ongoing treatment is extraordinary, and accordingly decide to withdraw ventilation, then the patient becomes a candidate for DCD. If consent is given for donation, ventilation may be withdrawn in or near an operating room, and death is commonly declared between two and five minutes after circulation and respiration have discontinued. After death is declared, the transplant team is allowed to enter the operating room and begin organ recovery.[26]

Are DCD Donors Brain Dead?

Some have objected that controlled DCD criteria are problematic because a loss of circulation for a mere two to five minutes is insufficient to cause brain death, and without brain death an individual cannot be dead.[27] To be clear, in DCD one pronounces death using circulatory–respiratory criteria, not neurological criteria. This is important in understanding the legal basis of the pronouncement of death. However, even if the pronouncement is legal, one might still object that an individual cannot be dead if his or her brain is still alive. So have DCD donors lost all brain functions, and are they really dead when they are pronounced only two to five minutes after circulation is lost?

At the risk of oversimplifying, there are two fundamentally different kinds of biological signs one could look for in determining death: loss of functions and structural damage. As noted above, both the President's Commission and the Pontifical Academy of Science accepted death criteria that focus on a loss of functions, either all functions of the entire brain including the brain stem, or circulatory and respiratory functions. The critical functions that are referenced in contemporary death criteria are closely connected, which is why either neurological or circulatory–respiratory criteria may be used. Because the brain stem stimulates respiratory effort, breathing ceases

as soon as the brain stem loses functions; similarly, the brain cannot function without oxygen and accordingly stops functioning roughly fifteen seconds after circulation is lost.[28] Thus, if one focuses on a loss of brain functions rather than structural damage, then one finds that the brain has indeed lost all functions when loss of circulation has been verified for two to five minutes. It would be wrong to declare death in the presence of a functioning brain, but a patient simply cannot maintain neurological functions for more than fifteen seconds in the absence of circulation.

Focusing on biological functions has advantages. It avoids the need for invasive tests, thereby preserving the determination of death as a clinical diagnosis. It further avoids the arbitrariness of trying to establish how much biological damage is necessary to determine death. Finally, it allows death to be determined quickly and thereby enables organ transplantation, because a loss of functions in one vital organ system (e.g., the neurological or circulatory system) often precedes significant structural damage or necrosis in other organ systems (and typically precedes necrosis in the failing system itself).[29]

If one chooses to focus on structural damage—necrosis or death at a cellular level within organ systems—instead of functional losses, then one encounters all the corollary disadvantages: the determination of death becomes a highly technical, nonclinical diagnosis; no nonarbitrary amount of structural damage exists, because death blends seamlessly with decomposition when viewed through a purely biological-structural lens; and organ transplantation is made impossible.

So why would anyone insist on verifying structural damage? Typically, it is to ensure "irreversibility"—a concept that is embedded in contemporary death criteria, including those of the UDDA. Hence, the question arises, "What counts as an irreversible loss of key functions?"

Are Circulatory Functions Irreversibly Lost?

A number of commentators have questioned whether patients have irreversibly lost circulatory–respiratory functions when death is declared only two to five minutes following apnea and a loss of circulation. They note that patients in emergency settings are commonly resuscitated after circulation is lost for several minutes—sometimes with little or no neurological damage.[30] To paraphrase, there are possible worlds in which DCD donors have not irreversibly lost circulation when they are pronounced dead.

While all this is true, DCD donors do not live in such possible worlds. Rather, they live in the real world in which they or their families requested removal of life-sustaining treatments and they have elected to forgo resuscitation. Therefore, by today's legal and medical-ethical standards, it would be a violation of the doctrine of informed consent to attempt resuscitation on DCD donors following withdrawal of life-sustaining treatments. Accordingly, in establishing an *irreversible* loss of circulatory–respiratory functions, one does not need to consider the possibilities of modern resuscitative medicine, but rather the parameters for spontaneous recovery set by nature.

What are the parameters for recovery set by nature? The best available data indicate that patients do not spontaneously recover lost circulation after more than sixty-five seconds have elapsed.[31] Some have accused those who defend DCD criteria of ignoring "delayed spontaneous recovery in humans (called the Lazarus phenomenon)."[32] However, the standard cases cited on behalf of such claims involve resumption of functions following the discontinuation of attempted resuscitation (which is never attempted in controlled donation after cardiac death). In such cases, positive pressure with excessive ventilation can "cause pulselessness even with a beating heart ... cessation of ventilation in such cases allows the pressure to subside and palpable circulation to resume."[33] Further case reports exist of "pseudoelectromechanical dissociation," but these patients may "maintain circulation up to twelve minutes after loss of palpable femoral pulses."[34] Just as Lazarus did not come back to life without Jesus's help, there have been no instances of the so-called Lazarus phenomenon where a patient spontaneously resumed functions without the intervention of another. Thus, such cases do not challenge the current practice in DCD of waiting at least two but not more than five minutes after the loss of circulation before pronouncing death.

Ironically, transplantation itself suggests how arbitrary any other concept of irreversible loss is: the fact that we can transplant hearts and lungs indicates that they can retain the possibility of functioning even hours after being removed from the human body; yet surely the functioning of a transplanted heart is no evidence that its "original owner" continues to live. After reviewing the medical literature on controlled resuscitation studies, Michael DeVita concludes that, "if the diagnosis of death requires that the heart no longer has the potential to resume function (and that apnea and unresponsiveness are irreversible), then one might argue that death certification should never occur until hours have passed, as the heart retains the potential to resume function for up to hours after it has stopped."[35]

Nevertheless, as DeVita notes, requiring the heart to lose all potential for functioning—even in the face of resuscitative efforts—is "incompatible with the current practice of medicine [even outside the context of organ transplantation] and our social concept of death."[36] Moreover, in the document that explains the rationale behind the UDDA, the President's Commission repeatedly uses the term "permanent" loss as synonymous with "irreversible" loss. More significantly, the Commission explicitly states that

> several commentators have argued that organic *destruction* rather than cessation of functions should be the basis for declaring death. They assert that until an organ has been destroyed there is always the *possibility* that it might resume functioning. The Commission has rejected this position for several reasons ... [including that the] traditional cardiopulmonary standard relies on the vital signs as a measure of heart-lung function; the declaration of death does not await evidence of destruction.[37]

Thus, when a patient has a do-not-resuscitate order in place, verifying the irreversible loss of circulation and respiration requires only that one verify that the patient is not capable of "autoresuscitation," or the spontaneous recovery of function. Such a view is not an instance of ethical gerrymandering, for in general clinical practice there is no established waiting time following the loss of circulation, and such a notion of irreversible loss appears consistent with the intentions of those who framed the UDDA.

Some may find this concept of irreversibility problematic, because it implies that death is sometimes reversible. Yet the idea of a reversible state of death is not only consistent with certain theological concepts (such as the resurrection of the dead) and controversial reports of near-death experiences by those determined to be clinically dead, but it is simply logical. In order to determine that a body is permanently in a certain state (e.g., the state of being frozen, being comatose, or being dead), one must first be able to verify that the person is in the state. That is, the concept of being in a given state is necessarily prior to the concept of being irreversibly in that state.

Nevertheless, it is reasonable that the *determination of* death by a physician should involve some irreversibility or permanency criterion. But the primary reason for this is not metaphysical, but rather ethical: we do not want to treat a body as dead if we should attempt resuscitation (as in cases of unexpected cardiac arrest) or if there is a chance that nature has not yet run its course.

Uncontrolled DCD

A recent Institute of Medicine committee noted that of the more than two million people who die in the United States each year, only 10,500 to 16,800 are eligible donors if one restricts eligibility to a neurological determination of death.[38] At present, patients who are pronounced dead using neurological criteria (standard donors) make up about 93 percent of all deceased donors in the United States; controlled DCD accounts for most of the remaining 7 percent.

However, another large population of patients are eligible for organ donation using so-called uncontrolled DCD, or rapid-organ-recovery, protocols. (The 2006 IOM committee estimated this number to be in excess of 22,000.) Such protocols are rarely used in the United States, though they are commonly used in Spain and the Netherlands, and the Institute of Medicine urged local organ procurement organizations to pilot such programs. Rapid organ recovery involves a circulatory–respiratory determination of death following aggressive attempts at resuscitation. If resuscitation is unsuccessful at restoring circulation and respiration, then the patient may be pronounced dead in the usual manner. Because circulation is lost, and procurement cannot begin immediately (given the fact that death is unanticipated and typically occurs "in the field" or in the emergency room), organ preservation is necessary. This typically involves the use of a cooling blanket and the insertion of a catheter in the femoral artery to fill the abdominal cavity with cold solution.[39]

Ethical issues surrounding uncontrolled DCD include ensuring that resuscitation efforts are continued sufficiently long enough to establish futility, and determining whether explicit consent is needed to preserve organs.[40] However, the determination of death itself is not particularly controversial, since it proceeds exactly as it would in any other case with failed resuscitative efforts. The only exceptions to this rule typically involve a prolongation of resuscitative efforts—that is, a delayed pronouncement—so that death may be pronounced in an emergency room by a physician and with the opportunity for organ preservation. No one in the ethics literature appears to question whether such donors are deceased at the time of donation.

Moral Certainty

Much like the earliest hours and days of human life, when the transfer of DNA is still in progress and twinning is still possible, the end of life is shrouded in mystery, and it is almost impossible to determine, on the basis of medical evidence alone, when we are (still) in the presence of a human being. Within a theology that embraces the concept of an immortal rational soul, it is reasonable to assume that the indeterminacy is epistemological, not ontological. As Leon Kass has observed, if "the indeterminacy lies in nature ... then all criteria for determining death are arbitrary and all moments of death a fiction. If, however, the indeterminacy lies in *our* confusion and ignorance [not in nature], then we must simply do the best we can in approximating the time of transition."[41]

Out of deep respect for human dignity, it is not uncommon for Catholic moral theologians to default to the "precautionary principle" when a risk exists of terminating a human life. That is to say, when in doubt, err on the side of protecting human life. Thus, some might argue that in the context of organ donation, if we are not 100 percent certain that an individual is dead, then we should not procure vital organs. While this logic has some merit, two comments are in order.

First, the kind of certainty we can have regarding medical matters such as the diagnosis of death is merely moral certainty, not absolute certainty.[42] Second, there is always a cost to not acting. In the case of organ procurement, terminally ill patients will die who might otherwise enjoy years of life with a transplant. Moreover, individuals who would otherwise become organ donors are denied the opportunity to perform the charitable act of consenting to donation, and bereaved families are denied the opportunity of seeing some tangible good come from their loss. Thus, the precautionary principle ought to be invoked only after we have valiantly tried to establish certain relevant facts and failed. This article has attempted to indicate that we can indeed establish that an individual has died in a timely manner that enables organ donation—not perhaps with absolute certainty, but with that moral certainty necessary to act responsibly.

Notes

[1] President's Commission for the Study of Ethical Problems in Medicine and Biomedical and Behavioral Research, *Defining Death: Medical, Legal, and Ethical Issues in the Determination of Death* (Washington, D.C.: U.S. Government Printing Office, 1981), 73.

[2] E. F. M. Wijdicks, "Brain Death Worldwide: Accepted Fact but No Global Consensus Exists in Diagnostic Criteria," *Neurology* 58 (2002): 20–25.

[3] L. L. Emanuel, "Reexamining Death: The Asymptotic Model and a Bounded Zone Definition," *Hastings Center Report* 25.4 (July–August 1995): 27–35; R. D. Truog, "Is It Time to Abandon Brain Death?" *Hastings Center Report* 27.1 (January–February 1997): 29–37; R. M. Arnold and S. J. Youngner, "The Dead Donor Rule: Should We Stretch It, Bend

It, or Abandon It?" *Kennedy Institute of Ethics Journal* 3.2 (June 1993): 263–278.

[4] U.S. Conference of Catholic Bishops, *Ethical and Religious Directives for Catholic Health Care Services*, 4th ed. (Washington, D.C.: USCCB, 2001), nn. 63 and 64.

[5] John Paul II, Address to the 18th International Congress of the Transplantation Society (August 29, 2000), n. 3.

[6] Institute of Medicine (IOM), *Organ Donation: Opportunities for Action* (Washington, D.C.: National Academies Press, 2006).

[7] T. E. Burroughs et al., "The Stability of Family Decisions to Consent or Refuse Organ Donation: Would You Do It Again?" *Psychosomatic Medicine* 60.2 (March–April 1998): 156–162.

[8] *Catechism of the Catholic Church*, n. 997.

[9] John Paul II, Address to Transplantation Society, n. 4.

[10] For highly readable medical accounts of how we die, see Kenneth V. Iserson, *Death to Dust: What Happens to Dead Bodies?* 2nd ed. (Tucson, AZ: Galen Press, 2001); and Sherwin B. Nuland, *How We Die: Reflections on Life's Final Chapter* (New York: Vintage, 1995).

[11] D. A. Shewmon, and E. Seitz Shewmon, "The Semiotics of Death and Its Medical Implications," in *Brain Death and Disorders of Consciousness*, eds. C. Machado and D. A. Shewmon (New York: Springer Science, 2004), 106–107.

[12] John Paul II, Address to Transplantation Society, n. 5.

[13] R. J. White, H. Angstwurm, and I. Carrasco De Paula, eds., *Working Group on the Determination of Brain Death and Its Relationship to Human Death* (Vatican City: Pontificia Academia Scientiarum, 1992).

[14] John Paul II, Address to Transplantation Society, n. 5.

[15] Perhaps the most widely cited practice guidelines are those offered by the American Academy of Neurology, *Practice Parameters: Determining Brain Death in Adults* (St. Paul: AAN, 1994). However, despite being reaffirmed in 2007, they have not been updated since 1994, and they address only the determination of death in adults. Therefore, I have cited the New York State Department of Health, *Guidelines for Determining Brain Death* (2005), and E. F. M. Wijdicks, "The Diagnosis of Brain Death," *New England Journal of Medicine* 344.16 (April 19, 2001): 1215–1221, which are more comprehensive and consistent with the AAN guidelines.

[16] NY State Department of Health, *Guidelines*, 1.

[17] Wijdicks, "Diagnosis of Brain Death."

[18] NY State Department of Health, *Guidelines*, 6.

[19] Ibid., 4.

[20] Iserson, *Death to Dust*.

[21] R. M. Veatch, "The Whole-Brain Death Oriented Concept of Death: An Outmoded Philosophical Formulation," *Journal of Thanatology* 3.1 (1975): 13–30; S. J. Youngner and E. T. Bartlett, "Human Death and High Technology: The Failure of the Whole-Brain Formulations," *Annals of Internal Medicine* 99.2 (1983): 252–258.

[22] T. P. Hung and S. T. Chen, "Prognosis of Deeply Comatose Patients on Ventilators," *Journal of Neurology, Neurosurgery, and Psychiatry* 58.1 (January 1995): 75–80, quoted in Wijdicks, "Diagnosis of Brain Death," 1220.

[23] D. A. Shewmon, "Chronic 'Brain Death': Meta-analysis and Conceptual Consequences," *Neurology* 51 (1998): 1538–1545.

[24] Iserson, *Death to Dust*, 19.

[25] Perhaps no one has so ably defended a variety of views on death as D. Alan Shewmon, who in one article recognized that a rejection of brain death criteria probably committed one to such views. See his article from 2001, in which he writes, "*Both* the isolated brain *and* the mechanically ventilated brainless body in the thought experiment are living organisms." "The Brain and Somatic Integration: Insights into the Standard Biological Rationale for Equating 'Brain Death' with Death," *Journal of Medicine and Philosophy* 26.5 (October 2001): note 6 (original emphasis).

[26] In many cases, heparin (an anticoagulant) is administered at the time ventilation is withdrawn in order to prevent blood clots that could prove fatal to organ recipients. This has raised concerns about the effects of heparin and potential conflicts between caring for an individual as a dying patient and as a potential organ donor. These issues are discussed by J. M. DuBois, F. L. Delmonico, and A. M. D'Alessandro, "When Organ Donors Are Still Patients: Is Premortem Use of Heparin Ethically Acceptable?" *American Journal of Critical Care* 16.4 (July 2007): 396–400.

[27] J. Menikoff, "Doubts about Death: The Silence of the Institute of Medicine," *Journal of Law, Medicine and Ethics* 26.2 (Summer 1998): 157–165; and Truog, "Time to Abandon?" 29–37. Elsewhere, I have argued that it is a mistake to privilege one set of death criteria over the other. For example, some argue that brain death alone indicates death of the human being, and circulatory criteria should be used only to infer to brain death. This poses problems insofar as it might imply that a human being cannot be alive without a brain—even in the earliest stages of development. However, espousing brain death criteria as one set of criteria that is useful for determining death in no way suggests that the human embryo is not a living human being; we are developmental beings, and brains simply are not necessary for life at the earliest stages of our development. See J. M. DuBois, "Organ Transplantation: An Ethical Road Map," *National Catholic Bioethics Quarterly* 2.3 (Autumn 2002): 413–453.

[28] M. A. DeVita, "The Death Watch: Certifying Death Using Cardiac Criteria," *Progress in Transplantation* 11.1 (March 2001): 58–66. In stating that all functions are lost, I assume the validity of the distinction the President's Commission made between functions and residual activities: "After an organ has lost the ability to *function* within the organism, electrical and metabolic *activity* at the level of individual cells or even groups of cells may continue for a period of time. Unless this cellular activity is organized and directed, however, it cannot contribute to the operation of the organism as a whole. Thus,

cellular activity alone is irrelevant in judging whether the organism, as opposed to its components, is 'dead.'" President's Commission, *Defining Death*, 75.

[29] President's Commission, *Defining Death*.

[30] Menikoff, "Doubts about Death"; and J. L. Verheijde, M. Y. Rady, and J. McGregor, "Recovery of Transplantable Organs after Cardiac or Circulatory Death: The End Justifying the Means," *Critical Care Medicine* 35.5 (May 2007): 1439–1440.

[31] DeVita, "Death Watch"; E. F. M. Wijdicks and M. N. Diringer, "Electrocardiographic Activity after Terminal Cardiac Arrest in Neurocatastrophes," *Neurology* 62.4 (February 24, 2004): 673–674.

[32] Verheijde, Rady, and McGregor, "Recovery of Transplantable Organs."

[33] J. M. DuBois, and M. DeVita. "The Authors Reply [to Verheijde, Rady, and McGregor]," *Critical Care Medicine* 35.5 (May 2007): 1440.

[34] DeVita, "Death Watch," 60.

[35] Ibid., 62.

[36] Ibid.

[37] President's Commission, *Defining Death*, 75–76.

[38] IOM, *Organ Donation*, 2006.

[39] Ibid.

[40] These ethical issues extend beyond the scope of this essay, but are discussed in the Institute of Medicine's (2006) report.

[41] L. R. Kass, "Death as an Event: Commentary on Robert Morison," *Science* 173.3998 (August 20, 1971): 700.

[42] John Paul II, Address to Transplantation Society.

⚜

Editorial Summation: The actual event of death may be hidden from view, but we can identify the signs that death has occurred. The key functions of the body—neurological, circulatory, and respiratory—are interdependent; therefore, death may be determined by the loss of any one. Death occurs when the function of the organism as a whole has been lost. The term "brain death" typically refers to the irreversible loss of all functions of the entire brain, including the brain stem. These are the criteria accepted by Pope John Paul II in his August 2000 address to the Transplantation Society. No one has ever recovered from brain death when it has been correctly determined. The existence of residual biological functions (e.g., heart beat) in the brain-dead body conflicts with our general concept of death, but it makes no sense to say that a severed head and a decapitated body, if both kept alive, are living substances. Far from assuming that human beings are distinct from their bodies, defenders of neurological criteria for determining death assert that the connection between mind and body is so tight that a mind cannot animate a body with a dead brain. The two common forms of donation after cardiac death (DCD) are controlled and uncontrolled. In controlled DCD, the death of the patient is expected. If one focuses on a loss of brain function rather than structural damage, then the brain has indeed lost all functions when loss of circulation has been verified for two to five minutes. In establishing an irreversible loss of circulatory–respiratory functions, one does not need to consider the possibilities of modern resuscitative medicine but the parameters for spontaneous recovery set by nature. In the determination of death, it is important to recall that we can obtain only moral certainty, not absolute certainty.

CHAPTER 13

Physician-Assisted Suicide and Euthanasia

Edward J. Furton

Physician-assisted suicide and euthanasia are two forms of unjust killing. In the first, the physician assists in the patient's own act of self-destruction; in the second, someone directly kills the patient either with or without consent. Both actions are characterized by their proponents as moral means of ending the misery and suffering of others, although it is euthanasia that usually receives the designation "mercy-killing."

Like physician-assisted suicide, euthanasia may be carried out at the patient's request, but it may also be proposed for those who lack decision-making capacity. Advocates of euthanasia ("euthanasiasts") hold that certain lives are not worth living—or, less delicately put, that some people are better off dead. These people typically include not only those in the end stages of terminal illness, but also those in a persistent vegetative state, the aged, the mentally incompetent, and children who suffer serious fetal anomalies.

The leading edge of this movement is in the Netherlands, where the practice of euthanasia is legal for patients over the age of twelve years. Under the 2005 Groningen Protocol, the country decriminalized the euthanizing of children of even lesser ages. The principal criteria for the direct killing of a child is the determination that he or she is enduring "hopeless and unbearable suffering." This is obviously a vague standard. Two defenders of the protocol, Hilde Lindemann and Marian Verkerk, observe that its aim is to bring "within its compass babies who are in no danger of dying—and indeed, with proper care could live into adulthood."[1] They explain that "it is precisely those babies who could continue to live but whose lives would be wretched in the extreme who stand in most need of the interventions for which the protocol offers

guidance." The protocol may even permit the killing of infants who are not necessarily suffering at present, but may suffer in the future, either through physical or mental disabilities. "This forward-looking feature of the protocol is justified on the grounds that it is inhumane to keep a baby alive until it begins to experience intolerable suffering."

General Overview

The Catholic Church condemns both suicide and murder. The *Catechism of the Catholic Church* describes suicide as a contradiction of the natural human inclination to self-preservation and declares it an act "gravely contrary to the just love of self" (n. 2281). Similarly, voluntary cooperation in the suicide of another is "contrary to the moral law" (n. 2282). As for euthanasia, the *Catechism* reminds us, with the lines of Genesis 4:10, that "those who cooperate voluntarily in murder commit a sin that cries out to heaven for vengeance" (n. 2268). Both suicide and murder are violations of the Fifth Commandment, "Thou shalt not kill."

Efforts to advance physician-assisted suicide and euthanasia in the United States through state legislatures and ballot initiatives have generally not been successful, although the proponents continue to actively promote these practices and may eventually find success. What acceptance has materialized often rests on a failure to understand the difference between the legitimate refusal of unnecessary means of prolonging life and direct killing. Many mistakenly hold that when a patient or health care proxy ends extraordinary or useless means of treatment, this qualifies as euthanasia. A misunderstanding of terms—as well as a misunderstanding of the moral reasoning behind their use—has thus increased the impression that physician-assisted suicide and euthanasia are more widespread than they actually are.

There can be little question that advanced technologies have enabled physicians to preserve human life beyond what is morally obligatory, and their use has led some to embrace physician-assisted suicide and euthanasia. Only a few decades ago, physicians were likely to overtreat patients and perhaps ignore the desire to end burdensome courses of therapy. Today, the pendulum has swung to the opposite extreme, with patients now exerting a degree of autonomy over their own treatment that sometimes makes it difficult for conscientious physicians to give them the best possible care. Increasingly, some patients are demanding that physicians assist in their deaths.

The prospect of a prolonged and painful illness, under the dominance of technological devices that only extend the dying process, rightly alarms all who wish to die a peaceful and natural death. Catholic moral teaching recognizes that there is a definite limit to the medical treatment that a patient is morally bound to accept. The governing principle is "that no moral obligation to have recourse to extraordinary measures exists; and that, incidentally, a doctor must follow the wishes of a sick person who refuses such measures."[2] As a rule, extraordinary means of preserving life may be abandoned at any time (whether or not one is dying), and the use of comfort measures that unintentionally hasten death may sometimes be permissible.

Medical Tradition Past and Present

The medical community has traditionally refused to participate in any act of physician-assisted suicide or euthanasia. The Oath of Hippocrates, dating from the fourth century BC, states, "I will neither give a deadly drug to anybody who asked for it, nor will I make a suggestion to this effect." The American Medical Association's policy H-140.952 reflects this same standard. Physician-assisted suicide is "fundamentally incompatible with the physician's professional role."[3] The AMA emphasizes the need for physicians to recognize and understand the true meaning of a request for any assistance in suicide:

> It is critical that the medical profession redouble its efforts to ensure that dying patients are provided optimal treatment for their pain and other discomfort. The use of more aggressive comfort care measures, including greater reliance on hospice care, can alleviate the physical and emotional suffering that dying patients experience. Evaluation and treatment by a health professional with expertise in the psychiatric

aspects of terminal illness can often alleviate the suffering that leads a patient to desire assisted suicide. Physicians should not withdraw "physically or emotionally" from their patients when treatment goals inevitably shift from cure to comfort care.

The AMA offers a similar condemnation of euthanasia in policy E-2.21, which observes that euthanasia is "fundamentally incompatible with the physician's role as healer, would be difficult or impossible to control, and would pose serious societal risks."[4] The policy notes that "the physician who performs euthanasia assumes unique responsibility for the act of ending the patient's life," and states that "patients near the end of life must continue to receive emotional support, comfort care, adequate pain control, respect for patient autonomy, and good communication."

Currently, a physician who administers a lethal dose with the intention of ending a patient's life is subject to prosecution under laws prohibiting homicide. Oregon and Washington, the only two U.S. states to permit physician-assisted suicide, are no exception to this rule. There the physician may only prescribe, but not administer, the lethal dose. This may yet change, for the proponents of a "right to death" argue that if the law permits individuals to request and receive drugs that will enable them to kill themselves, then it ought to allow physicians to actively put to death those who are too weak or otherwise unable to complete the suicide without help. The slippery slope thus leads from an initial permission to allow the individual to kill himself to a later demand that the medical profession take up the task.

Teachings of the Church

The most important statement of Church teaching on euthanasia remains the 1980 *Declaration on Euthanasia* issued by the Congregation for the Doctrine of the Faith. Here the Church reminds the world community of "the lofty dignity of the human person" and the Second Vatican Council's condemnation of all acts of unjust killing.[5] The declaration makes its appeal across denominational lines to those "who, philosophical or ideological difference notwithstanding, have nevertheless a lively awareness" of the centrality of human dignity to all moral reasoning.

Of special note is the document's rejection, as illegitimate and ill-founded, of any argument that seeks to justify euthanasia and physician-assisted suicide on the grounds of "political pluralism or religious freedom." The universal standards of the natural law, the declaration avers, transcend particular political and religious affiliations; thus, the claim that respect for the diversity of opinion or religious belief requires that we tolerate the direct killing of the innocent is unacceptable. Those who ask to be put to death do not truly seek death, but are making appeals for appropriate medical treatment to alleviate their pain and depression. These appeals also express the universal need of the human heart for warmth and love from those who care for them.

Of greatest value in the Congregation's statement is its description of four general principles governing "due proportion in the use of remedies," summarized here:

- If other alternatives are not available, one may make use of the most advanced, even if still experimental, medical procedures.

- One may also refuse or cease to use extraordinary means if the benefits they provide fall short of expectations.

- One may make do with the ordinary means available and refuse all extraordinary means. "Such a refusal is not the equivalent of suicide; on the contrary, it should be considered as an acceptance of the human condition, or a wish to avoid the application of a medical procedure disproportionate to the results that can be expected, or a desire not to impose excessive expense on the family or the community."

- When death is imminent one may "refuse forms of treatment that would only secure a precarious and burdensome prolongation of life."[6]

These four points provide an excellent thumbnail sketch of the proper grounds for refusal of burdensome treatment. The *Ethical and Religious Directives for Catholic Health Care Services* (*ERDs*), issued by the U.S. Catholic bishops, reiterate these four principles.[7] Directive 60 states, among other things, that "Catholic health care institutions may never condone or participate in euthanasia or assisted suicide in any way."

Pope John Paul II placed the stamp of magisterial authority on the condemnation of euthanasia in his 1995 encyclical *Evangelium vitae* (The Gospel of Life).[8] There he states that "euthanasia in the strict sense is understood to be an action or omission which of itself and by intention causes death, with the purpose of eliminating all suffering" (n. 65). Such an act is distinguished from the refusal of "aggressive medical treatment" in which medical procedures are employed that no longer correspond to reasonable prospects for continued life in the patient. Refusal of medical procedures is permissible either when the benefits are disproportionate to the difficulties incurred or when they would pose an excessive burden on the patient or his family: "To forgo extraordinary or disproportionate means is not the equivalent of suicide or euthanasia; it rather expresses acceptance of the human condition in the face of death" (n. 65).

Pope John Paul concludes this important article 65 with the following pronouncement:

> Taking into account these distinctions, in harmony with the magisterium of my predecessors and in communion with the bishops of the Catholic Church, *I confirm that euthanasia is a grave violation of the law of God*, since it is the deliberate and morally unacceptable killing of a human person. This doctrine is based upon the natural law and upon the written word of God, is transmitted by the Church's Tradition and taught by the ordinary and universal magisterium. (original emphasis)

The wrongfulness of all participation in euthanasia could not be stated in a more forceful or definitive way.

Terms of the Debate

Advocates of euthanasia claim that Catholics already permit the direct killing of patients through their recognition of the right to refuse burdensome treatment ("passive euthanasia"), which leads them to further observe that Catholics should also permit the direct killing of patients through the administration of a "lethal medication" ("active euthanasia"). This blurring of the fundamental distinction between forgoing extraordinary treatment and killing a human being was a central theme in the so-called Philosophers' Brief, submitted in favor of a constitutional right to commit suicide.[9] In *Washington v. Glucksberg*, the U.S. Supreme Court rejected these and similar arguments, emphasizing instead the countervailing interests of the states to enact laws protecting the lives of their residents, as well as the states' long-standing practice of prohibiting suicide.[10]

Physicians like Dr. Timothy Quill, who shocked the medical community with his report on how he assisted in a patient's death and then lied to the medical examiner,[11] have also tried to portray permitting a terminal patient to die as a form of direct killing. The principle of double effect is central to the Catholic understanding of the difference between foreseeing that removal of extraordinary means will lead to death, and intentional killing. Advocates of physician-assisted suicide and euthanasia have therefore sought to undermine this distinction.[12] Removal of extraordinary means, we are told, should not be described as allowing the patient to die from an underlying disease, but as "passively" putting someone to death. These authors, in short, hold that it is false to say that a death can be foreseen as an unintended side effect of removing treatment. Similarly, the unwillingness to provide an extraordinary level of treatment is described as yet another type of intentional killing.

If Catholic physicians, nurses, and other health care workers are to oppose this encroachment on good medicine, they must be able to distinguish clearly between the refusal of extraordinary means and direct killing. Certainly the news media regularly show themselves unable to maintain even the more obvious distinctions—for example, that brain dead patients are in fact dead, and therefore cannot die when removed from "life support." Of course, there are some very difficult cases in which the standard distinctions may appear vague or confusing at best, and it is these cases which are often exploited by advocates of physician-assisted suicide and euthanasia. This challenges us to be very careful in our use of terms, especially when we consider that the debate is over more than linguistics, and concerns whether the actions of a physician and staff actively contribute to the death of a patient. Catholic health care workers, above all, need to be fully informed on the key distinctions.

To die a good death is a well-founded hope in Christian moral theology. The original meaning of the word *euthanasia* was simply "good death," from the Greek *eu* ("well") and *thanatos* ("death"). Use of the term to mean forgoing extraordinary treatment and allowing an individual to die of natural causes is still legitimate; traditionally, to allow death was understood as "passive euthanasia."[13] However, those who favor "mercy-killing" have corrupted the meaning of this phrase for political advantage. In today's political parlance, the term "passive euthanasia" is often used to signify killing by omitting a morally obligatory means. It has thus become necessary to abandon this phrase to avoid confusion in the public debates.

Standard Cases

To provide clarity on the distinction between the refusal of extraordinary means and direct killing, the remainder of this article focuses on some standard cases that concern applying treatment, removing treatment, and allowing a patient to die. Examples of a moral and an immoral decision are given for each category. No one, general distinction covers all cases. For example, there is a difference between removing extraordinary means of treatment and allowing someone to die, but some removals, while not expressly immoral, will nonetheless not be prudent, and some instances of allowing to die will clearly not be moral. Thus, one cannot say that the

removal of extraordinary means is always advisable or that allowing the patient to die is always permissible. As with most matters of ethics, it is the particulars of the cases that determine the correct course of action.

Applying a Treatment

The standard case of applying treatment is the administration of strong painkillers that unintentionally hasten death through the suppression of respiration. Their administration for the relief of pain in a patient who is dying is permissible under the principle of double effect, for even though the hastening of death is foreseen, death is not intended by the physician who provides proper palliative care. Obviously, in such cases it is crucial to be able to distinguish between the primary aim of the action (relief of pain) and the secondary effect (suppression of breathing).

It is simply inaccurate to say that one who seeks to relieve pain is also intending to hasten the death of the patient. Of course, a physician or nurse could use strong painkillers with the intention of shortening the life of the patient, only indirectly intending to alleviate the pain, but then the principle of double effect would no longer apply and the action would be immoral. This is why it is so important to strictly maintain the correct dosages in palliative care. Incorrect dosages indicate an immoral intention.

Removing a Treatment

In removing a treatment it is important to understand that a patient may refuse extraordinary (or disproportionate) means of treatment at any time, whether or not one is actively dying.[14] Thus, an elderly woman who suffers lung cancer may refuse a difficult program of chemotherapy in view of her age or concurrent complications in her condition. She may not be dying, and may indeed have many years of life remaining, and yet this does not prevent her from making the decision to refuse further treatment in good conscience. Consider a similar case. Suppose an unconscious patient on a ventilator suffers serious complications and has no hope of recovery. If the patient's health care proxy decides that further use of the ventilator is useless, and if the patient has previously expressed a desire to become an organ donor, then the ventilator may be removed and organs may be donated under the protocol for non-heart-beating donors. Here the cause of death is clearly the condition of the patient, not the removal of the ventilator or the desire to donate organs. The proxy is simply refusing extraordinary measures on the patient's behalf.

Sometimes, however, prudence demands that we pursue what would otherwise seem to be extraordinary treatment. For example, if a particularly difficult course of surgery would enable a patient to return to full health, especially if the patient has many long-term moral obligations, like a wife and children with no other means of support, then it would be the more prudent course to undergo the procedure despite the very considerable challenges. Or perhaps a patient, by enduring a difficult course of therapy for a considerable but limited period of time, could achieve some great good, such as reconciliation with an estranged relative or the fulfillment of an important social obligation. Although no one could say that the person who refused the surgery or therapy was committing an intrinsically immoral act, the refusal would still be a wrong decision in the circumstances. Although actions that are intrinsically immoral are always forbidden, there are a range of other actions that may or may not be moral, depending on the character, time of life, and particular circumstances of the patient.

Allowing to Die

Of particular complexity are cases involving a decision not to act. How can one discriminate between legitimate decisions to allow nature to take its course and very similar cases of not taking action when there is a moral obligation to do so? Are there any clear markers that can distinguish these cases into the good and the bad? Most of the proponents of physician-assisted suicide and euthanasia argue that if one is willing to let a patient die on the grounds of mercy, then one ought to be willing to actively kill the patient for the same reason. These arguments are not easily met, and require careful thinking.

Consider the case of a patient who has suffered head trauma and has descended into a persistent vegetative state. Should food and water be provided? By rule, we may say that it ought to be provided, for there should always be a presumption in favor of providing nutrition and hydration unless its administration presents some particular difficulty.[15] Conscious patients who repeatedly pull out the tubes, or who are otherwise violently uncooperative, pose another difficult case. Although drugs may calm these patients, and the use of physical restraints is a possibility, it would not seem appropriate to insist on these measures in all cases; they infringe too much on human freedom and do not change the fact that the patients are refusing the care. In still other cases, when repeated infections occur at the site of tube entry, the food and water are not being assimilated, the tube exacerbates aspiration pneumonia, or other complicating factors are present, then allowing the patient to die may indeed be the correct course of action.

When none of these problematic factors prevails, an examination of the likely cause of death can be very instructive. A patient in a persistent vegetative state, for example, typically is not dying and is in a stable medical condition, albeit with severely diminished cognitive capacity. When such a patient dies from a lack of food and water that could easily have been provided, the death cannot be attributed to an underlying disease, but results instead from the failure of the medical staff to perform a fairly simple surgical procedure. No one has ever died of a persistent vegetative state. The true cause of death is the dehydration or starvation that results from the inaction of the proxy and the caregivers.

Quality-of-Life Considerations

Another difficult area of consideration is indicated by the much-abused phrase "quality of life." If we could rid ourselves of this term, it would be much to the better; however, it is obvious that quality-of-life considerations are a relevant aspect of moral reflection when considering whether a patient may abandon a particular treatment. For example, a patient who is already suffering multiple complications, such as congestive heart failure, stroke, and persistent bed sores, will not be a good candidate for a risky course of surgery. Even if the patient survived the surgery, the prospects for a reasonable quality of life are so greatly diminished by the complicating factors that the surgery would be inadvisable. The potential benefits simply do not outweigh the burdens.

This is very different from saying that those who are seriously disabled do not have lives worth living. Talk about quality of life should never suggest that the life of any patient has no value. Life itself is an intrinsic good and so always possesses value. What is at issue is the condition of the patient, the state of disease, and the resources that are available to combat it, or if necessary, continue to live with it. If we distinguish between the good of life that always belongs to the patient, and the condition of life that the patient currently experiences, it is possible to make a quality-of-life assessment without denigrating the person.

The problem arises when the value of the person is called into question by those who would say that life becomes "worthless" when it is not of a sufficient quality, usually meaning that the patient has lost some or all higher cognitive abilities. We cannot associate loss of consciousness with the loss of value.

Another difficult area for judgment concerns patients whose lives can be saved after a traumatic event but who are not likely to return to a meaningful level of recovery.

Here again it would seem unnecessarily rigorous to hold that measures must always be taken so long as there is any possibility of continued life. If the means to preserve the life of the patient require minimal effort, then these means must be employed. But it is also reasonable to hold that if the patient cannot hope for a meaningful level of recovery, then the measure of an ordinary course of treatment diminishes considerably. Although a permanent loss of consciousness is not a reason to diminish the value of a person, the decision to restrict care to comfort measures can be an appropriate and justifiable response to this diminished quality of life. Cognitive powers are vital to our personal identity; their loss cannot help but affect an assessment of what treatment options should be pursued.

Terminal Sedation

Of recent concern has been the promotion of terminal sedation as a means of assisted suicide. Under terminal sedation, a patient is given strong doses of narcotic painkillers to eliminate all experience of suffering at the end of life. The procedure has a legitimate use in medicine, but is also easily open to abuse by those who favor the active killing of patients.

California recently enacted a bill requiring physicians to provide patients with "comprehensive information and counseling regarding legal end-of-life care options."[16] These options include the use of terminal sedation as a method of suicide or euthanasia, causing the patient's death by the removal of food and water. The bill provides no legal safeguards against such use of terminal sedation and no conscience protections for physicians and other health care providers who object to such use. Obviously, when the cause of death in such a case is dehydration or starvation, those who did not provide the patient with food and water are responsible for the resulting death. There is no question that the use of terminal sedation to hasten the death of a patient is medically inappropriate and immoral; those who propose that a right to terminal sedation be guaranteed in law also want to ensure that physicians and other health care providers can be coerced to violate their conscience.

Terminal sedation does have a proper role in medical practice when a patient near the end of life is enduring extreme pain, as in the terminal stages of cancer. Then the use of strong painkillers is perfectly appropriate and advisable, and food and water may be removed if death is sufficiently near to ensure that their removal will not be its cause. Although the Catholic Church calls on us to experience our deaths consciously, if that is at all possible, it also allows for the proper amelioration of pain in every

case where physical or emotional distress goes beyond what can ordinarily be expected of a patient. In cases where the patient is unable to respond to requests for direction on palliative care, the medical personnel and health care proxy should assume that remedy for pain is desired.

Notes

[1] Hilde Lindemann and Marian Verkerk, "Ending the Life of a Newborn: The Groningen Protocol," *Hastings Center Report* 38.1 (January–February 2008): 46.

[2] Pontifical Council *Cor Unum*, "Questions of Ethics regarding the Fatally Ill and the Dying" (June 27, 1981), n. 2.4.3, reprinted in *Conserving Human Life*, ed. Russell E. Smith (Braintree, MA: Pope John Center, 1989), 286–304.

[3] American Medical Association, *Policies of the AMA House of Delegates*, policy H-140.952, "Physician Assisted Suicide" (reaffirmed 1999), in *Health and Ethics Policies of the AMA*, 213–214, http://www.ama-assn.org/ad-com/polfind/Hlth-Ethics.pdf.

[4] American Medical Association, *Code of Medical Ethics*, policy E-2.21, "Euthanasia" (updated June 1996), in *Health and Ethics Policies of the AMA*, 887.

[5] Congregation for the Doctrine of the Faith (CDF), *Declaration on Euthanasia* (May 5, 1980), introduction, citing Vatican Council II, *Gaudium et spes*, n. 27.

[6] CDF, *Declaration on Euthanasia*, part IV.

[7] U.S. Conference of Catholic Bishops, *Ethical and Religious Directives for Catholic Health Care Services*, 4th ed. (Washington, D.C.: USCCB, 2001). See, in particular, Part 5, "Issues in Care for the Dying."

[8] John Paul II, *Evangelium vitae* (March 25, 1995) (Boston: Pauline Books, 1995).

[9] See "Brief of Ronald Dworkin, Thomas Nagel, Robert Nozick, John Rawls, Thomas Scanlon, and Judith Jarvis Thomson as *Amici curiae* in Support of Respondents," *Issues in Law & Medicine* 15.2 (Fall 1999): 183–198.

[10] *Washington v. Glucksberg*, 521 U.S. 702 (1997).

[11] Timothy E. Quill, "Death and Dignity: A Case of Individualized Decision Making," *New England Journal of Medicine* 324.10 (March 7, 1991): 691–694.

[12] See Timothy E. Quill, Rebecca Dresser, and Dan W. Brock, "The Rule of Double Effect: A Critique of Its Role in End-of-Life Decision Making," *New England Journal of Medicine* 337.24 (December 11, 1997): 1768–1771.

[13] See Stanley Joel Reiser, "The Dilemma of Euthanasia in Modern Medical History: The English and American Experience," in *Ethics in Medicine: Historical Perspectives and Contemporary Concerns*, ed. Stanley J. Reiser, Arthur J. Dyck, and William J. Curran (Cambridge, MA: MIT Press, 1977), 488–494; and, in the same volume, Carl F. Marx, "Medical Euthanasia," 495–497.

[14] The terms "ordinary" and "extraordinary" have the same meaning in this essay as "proportionate" and "disproportionate,"

although some now use the first pair of terms to refer to medical facts and the second to refer to the personal circumstances of the patient. Although this change in terminology is not reflected in this essay, what are ordinary and extraordinary in the medical sense are certainly not the same as what are ordinary and extraordinary in the moral sense. The first concerns any procedure that is scientifically established, statistically successful, and reasonably available; the second refers to what does not impose excessive burdens on the patient, holds out a sufficient prospect of appropriate benefits, and incurs costs that are within the financial means of the individual, the family, or society. See chapter 3B, "Ordinary and Extraordinary Means."

[15] John Paul II, Address to the Participants in the International Congress on Life-Sustaining Treatments and the Vegetative State (March 20, 2004), n. 4, reprinted in *National Catholic Bioethics Quarterly* 4.3 (Autumn 2004): 574–575; and CDF, "Responses to Certain Questions of the United States Conference of Catholic Bishops concerning Artificial Nutrition and Hydration" (August 1, 2007), reprinted in *Ethics & Medics* 32.11 (November 2007): 1–3.

[16] *Terminal Patients' Right to Know End-of-Life Options Act*, AB 2747 (Berg-Levine), 2008 Cal. Stat. 683. Notably, this bill provides no conscience protection for physicians who refuse to engage in this practice.

Editor's Summation: Physician-assisted suicide and euthanasia are two forms of unjust killing. Success in enacting laws that favor these wrongs has been limited, but efforts to legalize them continue. Much of the support for these practices flows from misunderstanding the difference between refusing extraordinary means of treatment and direct killing. The Catholic Church teaches that the patient has the freedom to refuse burdensome forms of treatment, and rejects the view that such decisions are suicidal. Such decisions are, rather, a recognition of the fundamental limitations of the present life. The medical tradition has long rejected physician-assisted suicide and euthanasia and continues to do so today. Proponents of these wrongful actions seek to confuse the debate by denying the difference between intending and foreseeing, by arguing that allowing to die means the same as putting to death, and by claiming that there is no proper remedy for pain and suffering short of killing the patient. Catholic health care workers should educate themselves in the nuances of this debate if they are to respond to it effectively. Among the distinctions that are necessary to a proper understanding of end-of-life decisions are those of applying and removing treatments, allowing to die, and assessing quality of life. Terminal sedation, when properly applied, has a legitimate use in palliative care, but it is sometimes advocated as a means of advancing physician-assisted suicide and euthanasia.

CHAPTER 14

Hospice Care

Helen Stanton Chapple, R.N.

Central to the United States and its health care system is the idea that death is an invader from whom all patients should have an equal opportunity to be rescued. Rescuing and stabilizing patients "buys time" to resolve uncertainty, even if it may not succeed in reversing the effects of injury or advanced illness. The cultural dominance of rescue and its high elaboration in the United States relates to hospice and ethics in two ways: it both encourages the existence of hospice as a countercultural foil, and it encroaches upon hospice's formulations of the good. These influences suggest that the discussion of hospice and ethics should be framed by culture and health care economics rather than by bedside dilemmas only.

This wider context is relevant to hospice ethics committees for at least two reasons, outlined by Spencer et al.[1] Many ethics dilemmas regarding individual patient management require some level of attention from the institution in the form of policies regarding informed consent, for instance. Even more fundamental is the challenge of reconciling the institution's mission with its conflicting interests and commitments. By sketching the U.S. cultural landscape, this discussion enables hospice ethics committees to become familiar with the external ethical climate in which the institution must operate.[2] With a foothold in this territory, hospice ethics committees can facilitate moral reflection within the organization as it formulates ethical responses to multiple pressures and stakeholders.

This chapter concerns both hospice and palliative care. By hospice I mean the hospice interdisciplinary model of care which assumes an open awareness of death's imminence and often takes place at home or in skilled nursing settings.[3] By palliative care I mean interdisciplinary symptom control according to a hospice model,

administered to patients for whom a dying process may or may not be acknowledged, usually in the hospital.

The moral goods of hospice care for individuals are not absolute (see below), but the significance of the unique position that hospice and palliative care together occupy in the American health care landscape is clear: they assert that value can and must be found in vulnerability itself. This stance questions the premise that cultural respect emanates only from attempts to overcome adversity. It rejects rescue's required focus on body compartments and asserts the importance of wholes. Ironically, this countercultural position has assisted the expansion of what might be called the medical-industrial complex by providing a place of refuge for those who have had enough of it. But this position as counterpoint to the behemoth of rescue medicine is not one of comfort.

As the quintessential example in U.S. health care of not rescuing from death, hospice encounters obstacles to delivering its good care to the dying that are not unlike the problems faced by other sidelined groups in the U.S. health care system. Payers exert economic pressure on health care services which stand outside the paradigm, services whose mandate is something other than rescue. As this pressure shrinks delivery options and access to rehabilitation, mental health services, and long-term care generally, it also threatens hospice's moral premises and its existence. Unlike hospice, however, these services cannot be construed so directly as a safety valve for the medical project's top priority of producing "more time alive." Nonetheless, the pressures are very real.

Individual hospices may wish to avoid patients whose illnesses are resource-heavy, such as those with HIV/AIDS, while seeking patients who are a better fit with their capitated payment system, such as those with chronic obstructive pulmonary disease (COPD).[4] By expanding their awareness of these issues, hospice ethics committees may find themselves examining the stance of their organization among others in the community, especially others delivering hospice and palliative care, and wondering whether all classes of eligible hospice patients are able to access the care they need.

This chapter will also consider the problem of autonomy as a good offered by hospice to the individual and the good that hospice provides to the society at large. The dominant position of the rescue paradigm in American health care has resulted in peculiar foregrounding of parts versus wholes. The good of the organic parts of the patient are given preference over the good of the patient as a whole. This causes tensions that constrain the function of hospice and palliative care and that relate to the problems of non-crisis health care delivery in the United States generally. The chapter concludes by considering the delicate cultural balance hospice and palliative care strike with the rescue paradigm.

Hospice and the Good

Autonomy in Dying

If being ethical means promoting what is humanly good, it is helpful to consider the characteristic good hospice advocates represent. Bruce Jennings defines the human good in hospice as having three moral "faces": palliation, autonomy, and healing.[5] He asserts that the third face, healing (in the sense of making whole) carries more significance than the first two, maintaining control of physical discomfort and honoring patient preferences. Healing includes sustaining relationships, the integrity of the self, and appropriate life closure.[6] Jennings correctly identifies a tension between this beneficent view of healing and the moral face of autonomy, even when he constrains the latter in terms of relationship and dependency. In a culture where individualism trumps other ideals most of the time, to impose a "hospice-preferred" view of proper healing on particular patients can interfere with their personal autonomy.[7]

Autonomy occupies an important strategic position in hospice. Prioritizing the idea of personal autonomy in the face of death allows hospice to ally itself with the values of individualism and control, so important to the American outlook. In the United States, this is a critical issue, because respect for autonomy signals the central ideological concept in the culture, that of self-reliance, and its twin, abhorrence of dependency.[8] Self-reliance, as Francis Hsu describes it, is a militant individualism characterized by

equality, self-determination, fear of dependence, and a pervasive insecurity about one's position in the world, reflecting the true inability to achieve self-reliance. Hsu points out that in America, old-age dependence on the largesse of one's offspring could never be a reason to take pride in the child's wherewithal, as it might be in China. Instead, it would be a source of personal shame. Hsu's idea of self-reliance does not match up exactly with the more nuanced descriptions of autonomy which acknowledge its contextualization and the possibility of its absence.[9] But the centrality of *respect* for autonomy in ethics discussions (rather than autonomy itself) reflects its strong cultural grounding in the United States and the stigmatization of dependency that Hsu identifies as central. Hospice's emphasis on maintaining patient autonomy minimizes the horror of dying's dependency, and maintains an illusion of order and control attractive to America's worried well. By foregrounding the concept of autonomy, hospice positions itself as a clear extension of the American health care system.

But there are problems with the assertion of autonomy within hospice. In analyzing the revival of the death movement, Tony Walter explores the unease between honoring individual choice and hospice's prescriptions of how dying can indeed be "good."[10] He points out that many hospice advocates (Bruce Jennings included) fail to notice an underlying assumption: that the dying process is "better" when it conforms to an ideal of social ordering. Hospice advocates believe that dying can deliver a greater good when it can be made orderly, often defined in terms of the hospice experts' concept of order. But in fact the territory of dying is aleatory, very often fraught with unpredictability and unknowns, even in hospice.

Both orderliness and autonomy rely on a further assumption common to conceptualizing the good of hospice: that its patients enjoy a reasonably intact sense of self, at least on admission. Much of the good that hospice promises relies on this premise. A predictable trajectory of physical decline, such as what may occur with many cancers, fits with the assumptions of order and persistence of the self. Julia Lawton's hospice research has shown, however, that the deterioration of the physical body brings a disintegration of one's sense of self that can accelerate as death approaches.[11] Negotiating autonomy through the lens of dependency and relationship becomes more complex as a disease claims more physiological territory.[12]

Hospice may enact its good most effectively for the largely white, middle-class, elderly patients who have traditionally dominated its demographic: persons who can remain at home with their advanced cancer, a set of able caregivers, and an agreement to forgo further aggressive treatments. These patients and families may have had routine access to a level of health care that enabled diagnosis to occur before the final stages of the disease.[13] Further, in their lifetimes they may have had the luxury to reflect and question the wisdom of unlimited aggressive care, rather than having to focus their attention on day-to-day survival.[14] The good of hospice and palliative care may be far more difficult to realize for the many dying patients who do not fit the traditional hospice model, such as those propped up by life support in the hospital, exhausted by both their illnesses and by the efforts to save them, who may not be recognized as dying at all. They are undergoing a "ritual of intensification" in an effort to resolve this prognostic uncertainty.[15]

Hospice in a Rescue Culture

While hospice's assertion of the good it represents for the dying patient may not be unassailable, its role in the rescue-dominated culture deserves closer examination. Its holistic values present an alternative model with implications for vulnerable populations of all types. Despite its emphasis on patient autonomy, hospice is a more communitarian model of care than it is individualistic, seeking to serve not only the patient but also those in the patient's coterie. Because hospice prioritizes a fidelity of accompaniment, Daniel Sulmasy points out that it attempts to bridge the power gap between the sick and the well.[16] He argues that hospice contributes to the common good through relationship. The important hospice message is that neither dependency nor vulnerability need be alienating experiences, but rather that they become so as society marginalizes them. Dorothee Soelle points out that to join in such marginalization is to become alienated from one's own humanity.[17] Hospice offers this ethical connection with vulnerability to society as a cultural good. The radical nature of this orientation becomes clear when we juxtapose it with the dominance of the rescue paradigm.

The Rescue Paradigm

Recalling Hsu's identification of the American pursuit of self-reliance and the insecurity that results, the onset of dependency may be the most abhorrent feature of death and dying. This would align with the rescue orientation of the U.S. health care system, which operates as if death is an attacker from the outside to be resisted, rather than originating from within as a part of the human condition.[18] If the battle against death is the ultimate morality play in American ideology, then

hospice proposes a different denouement, one that looks for meaning not in seeking to vanquish the attacker, but in offering a way to come to terms with inborn finitude. Zygmunt Bauman describes the logic of the prevailing view of death from the outside: even though one cannot overcome death in the abstract, one can certainly fight the particular causes of death that present themselves.[19] This dramatic and heroic project demands and obtains more health care resources than more mundane work around chronic illness, such as preserving function, minimizing pain, tapping reserves of resilience, and learning to hope for things other than recovery or even a return to baseline. How has this dominance become so pervasive?

Development and Dominance of Rescue

Since World War II, the dream that the medical project should save Americans from death would seem to have come true, in at least some isolated cases. The first successful cardiopulmonary resuscitation in the 1960s built directly on the invention of the mechanical ventilator the decade before. The capability to both stabilize the airway and control the breathing of the individual in extremis added recovery possibilities to the restoration of a heart rhythm and blood pressure. Rescue technology in the United States exploded thereafter. Rescue and stabilization have been universalized in U.S. hospitals as the default mode for most patients. Together they have come to epitomize the gold standard of acute care, a benchmark against which other forms of care are measured. Before treatment can be given, the patient must be stable. Rescue and stabilization as a form of triage ally seamlessly with the hospital imperative of "moving things along,"[20] the medical-industrial complex and its dazzling technological interventions, and the twin values of individualism and equal opportunity for all.[21] They gain untold reinforcement from these enmeshments as they address American insecurity about dependency as a state of being.

Economic and Moral Influence of Rescue

In a health care system skewed toward acute care, parts of persons, such as their organ systems, have acquired more legitimacy in the biomedical purview than the persons themselves. Indeed, disorders of heart, lungs, and brain command hegemonic prestige. As the primary targets of rescue and stabilization,[22] they are hardwired to the major thresholds of death avoidance. More diffuse diseases which affect the whole body command less interest, and their specialists receive less professional respect.[23] To declare that a patient is terminally ill and eligible for hospice care not only places body parts beyond the reach of medicine, both now and after death (since whole organ donation is unlikely), but it also shifts the focus of attention away from puzzle-solving to the surprisingly less compelling person-as-a-whole.

The rescue orientation exerts moral as well as professional dominance. The duty to care becomes the duty to stabilize first, a prerequisite to the system's implicit promise to confer "more time alive." Such a promise does not seem open to question or hesitation in the first moments when it is most efficacious. It acquires further legitimacy by appearing as an "equal opportunity" application. Cardiopulmonary resuscitation and advanced life support are default treatments to which every collapsed patient is immediately entitled.

The power to apply the accoutrements of rescue augments the distance and the potential for alienation between the able-bodied and the deathly sick. Further, patients with a "rescuable" malady enjoy a greater moral legitimacy in such a system, in congruence with both the direct lines to reimbursement they represent and the drama of immediate positive reinforcement if and when the harm is reversed. By the same token, economic outlay is more easily justified for such crisis intervention than for less heroic purposes. Hope, technology, and rescue intensify one another, evading moral criticism in an American ideology that prizes heroism, drama, and overcoming adversity.

Further evidence for unequal cultural legitimacy can be seen in payment patterns in the U.S. health care system. Reimbursement for rescue activities and discrete procedures is straightforward and reliable, even if it is often inadequate.[24] Payment for interventions aimed at the whole person, such as prevention, chronicity, disability, and mental illness—none qualifying as a "fix" for a discrete ailment or particular risk of death—is much more complicated to obtain.

Hospice's arrival in the United States in the 1960s coincided interestingly with the invention of successful CPR, so that rescue elaboration and the hospice movement have grown up side by side. It is possible that the presence of its antithesis enabled each to galvanize support for its cause. Taking as its model advanced cancer with its predictable trajectory of deterioration, the hospice movement found grassroots acceptance in a middle-class, white demographic. The passage of the Medicare hospice benefit in the mid-1980s marked an important cultural acknowledgment that rescue efforts could have limits, that dying could and should occupy its own space, and that the hospice vision for the "good death" carried significant social weight. The motivation for its passage was the rising

expense of end-of-life rescue.[25] It established a "separate but unequal" dichotomy requiring that patients give up curative treatment in order to obtain this once-in-a-lifetime benefit. This dualism reflected not only a prevailing belief that a clear line could be drawn between rescuable conditions and dying patients, but also that a reimbursement setup based on the discrete treatments and procedures was less appropriate in hospice than a daily rate (capitation).[26] This economic arrangement closed hospice out of the legitimacy conferred by higher-level patterns of reimbursement in health care, which privileged attention to parts of patients rather than whole persons.[27] Further, it said that on the one hand, dying should be supported with excellent care and accorded interdisciplinary attention; on the other hand, it should enjoy that support and accompaniment in spaces that would not interfere with the important work of rescue and stabilization.

This arrangement provided a necessary cultural and economic escape valve for the rescue endeavor, enabling it to burgeon without questioning its own fundamental assumptions, because hospice and rescue could each occupy its own domain. The ethical and practical boundaries between the two are under increasing stress, however, and the outcomes are uncertain.

Marginalized by Rescue

Chronic vulnerability and dependence are anathema to a health care system built around the priority of reversibility and an economy increasingly fueled by the technology that drives rescue. The reach of rescue and stabilization's dominance includes discrete procedures and technological interventions such as radiation, surgery, and pharmaceuticals. When these are covered by insurance or private pay, they are the chief contributors to hospitals' and the health care industry's bottom line. As reimbursable care in these narrow fields becomes more elaborated, the list of health needs pushed to the sidelines expands. Non-rescuable conditions include chronic illnesses (from which most Americans die[28]), many mental illnesses, disability, and the state of dying itself. Persons with such maladies who lack full access to the health care system through insurance or private means are doubly afflicted. If the system caters to the eradication of reversible and life-threatening conditions, people lacking these problems also lack care.

Hospice's Cultural Voice for the Good

The dichotomous arrangements set forth in the 1983 Medicare endorsement of hospice are under strain both culturally and financially. As the medical project of rescue consumes more of the U. S. gross domestic product (GDP), reimbursement for non-rescue medical activities seems to require more justification, if the alarms sounded by regulatory agencies over long-lived hospice patients are any indication. Hospice programs are denied payment when patients live "too long," a common consequence of the good care they receive.[29] Meanwhile, the culture's predominant interest in rescue continues unabated, placing hospices in a difficult position. The designation of "terminal" has fallen out of fashion, since it too is a determination about whole bodies rather than their parts. The illnesses that now precede death (including cancer and HIV/AIDS) are chronic and complex, often lacking a clear trajectory of deterioration that would give the appearance of order and provide a reference point for categorizing the patient as dying. Without a "dying process," no motivation exists to deny a given patient the gold standard of rescue interventions. Indeed, to do so may be seen as inequitable (as discussed below). Extending the linear metaphor for the patient's clinical experience, proponents of palliative care talk of moving it "upstream," that is, implementing it prior to any decision to designate a patient as officially dying, so that it becomes a feature of the patient's total care.[30]

As these developments push the needs of the (possibly) dying into mainstream medicine's sphere of attention, equal pressures from the curative side encroach into hospice territory. With ever-wider options for seeking "more time alive," even patients with advanced cancer who are interested in hospice care are less willing to give up all aspects of curative treatment in order to gain its benefits. Such care options are not only culturally appealing to patients, but they also carry a level of reimbursement that discourages referral to hospice and palliative care. Patients and physicians are reluctant to close down the clinical narrative, even when the ultimate outcome of terminality becomes clear. This blurring of the boundaries in both directions means that dying will not keep to its "place," becoming a source of cultural and economic discomfort. How might the impending failure of its confinement threaten the good of hospice and palliative care? What are its impacts on the operational ethics of hospice providers?

These specific tensions are visible in several overlapping domains discussed below: attempts to mix therapies, differential access to hospice care, the pressure for data, and the unrelenting regulatory pressure from Medicare in administering the Medicare hospice benefit. Facing these challenges may compel hospice and palliative care providers to engage not only in institutional reflection,

but also regional networking and even political action regarding balancing their responsibilities to various stakeholders within their missions.[31]

Mixing Dichotomous Therapies

The life circumstances of patients with advanced illness are ambiguous and chaotic. Options for different kinds of intervention expand continuously. Examples of attempts to combine rescue and comfort domains can be seen in calls for CPR in hospice[32] and in "concurrent care," which would combine hospice with the option of participation in phase I clinical trials.[33] A very bold example of mixing therapies occurred when palliative care was implemented while a patient with end-stage liver disease waited for the transplant that could save the person's life.[34] Maintaining clear bright lines between paths that seek to reverse the course of disease and those that seek only to mitigate its effects has become less realistic and more arbitrary. The forced "choice" between the good of hospice, which offers a blanket of services at a daily rate, and the heroic possibilities of separable interventions would appear to serve patients, their illusion of ultimate autonomy, and hospice poorly. The existence of the choice illustrates a cultural phenomenon at work. To frame advanced illness in the language of choice, autonomy, and advance care planning dignifies it with a particularly American illusion of orderliness, indicating that some things must happen before other things can be allowed to happen. The push to mix therapies reflects the true untidiness of this territory.

A few patients work this untidiness to their advantage. They exert their autonomy by rejecting the defined sequence, choosing instead to customize their clinical journey according to available options. Evidence of such empowerment among dying patients is the exception rather than the rule, however. "Dying Americans remain neglected, and as a group, their pain is undertreated, their access to services is limited, and their preferences for care are often ignored."[35] The traditional white, middle-class woman with cancer continues to dominate the hospice demographic.[36] This reflects compartmentalization by social class and by class of disease, and both are barriers to obtaining hospice or palliative care. Groups of people who have less opportunity to experience hospice care in the United States are often the same as those who have trouble gaining access to health care in general: people of color, those who speak English poorly or not at all, the urban or rural poor. Further, terminally ill patients without solid tumors, such as those suffering from HIV/AIDS, congestive heart failure, mental illness, or dementia, are less likely to seek or obtain access to hospice or palliative care services. As its advocates seek to move hospice and palliative care "upstream," they encounter resistance from rescuing clinicians who accuse them of "being on the side of the disease," that is, lacking fidelity to the "right" cause. It is not only dying itself but chronic illness and vulnerability in populations of all stripes which rescue can neither cure nor contain.

Pressure for Measurement and Data

As hospice and palliative care negotiate their positions in the field of U.S. health care, they must cope with the tyranny of the measurable. Research and development fuels mainstream medicine and vice versa. The currency for both real legitimacy and funding in mainstream medicine relies on research and the production of data. Investigating vulnerable subjects such as people who are terminally ill is difficult ethically and methodologically,[37] and the NIH State-of-the-Science Conference reported the difficulty of obtaining hard data in this area.[38] Further, much of the good of hospice and palliative care resists measurement by conventional investigational models.[39] The gold standard of validity in investigational research (large double-blind randomized clinical trials) is a rigid model that reinforces the gold standard of acute care, rescue, and stabilization. Such a perception of hierarchy based on discrete pieces of data puts hospice and palliative care (which have traditionally emphasized such intangibles as process, relationship, and meaning) at a disadvantage in the competition for funding and the legitimacy and status that such funding confers.

Tension of Reimbursement Patterns

If these pressures were not enough, hospice and palliative care must also contend with a hierarchy in reimbursement structures. In the history of U.S. health care, the passage of the Medicare hospice benefit represented an unprecedented financial endorsement of end-of-life care. It also affirmed the legitimacy of hospice's grassroots origins. At the same time it reinforced the divide between dying patients, whose finitude was openly declared and who would spend down their single hospice benefit by paying a daily charge to hospice; and "viable" patients, whose more legitimate futures qualified them for the higher rates of "piecework" reimbursement for discrete interventions delivered by mainstream medicine.[40]

Hospices can be crushed by complex palliative care needs or by too many patients who die shortly after admission, before the program has had a chance to recoup the high costs of the patient's first days. Even as the difficulty of prognostic line-drawing has increased over time, Medicare has ramped up its oversight mechanisms and infrastructure, a direct indication of the pressure that the dominant medical model of rescue places on the nonconforming system when faced with the need for belt-tightening. Frequently, hospices must deny admission to or even discharge home patients whose needs for supportive care exceed the hospice's budget. If hospice ethics committees confine themselves to dilemmas regarding admitted patients, they may miss the ethical implications of organizational policies that refuse admission to categories of patients, such as those on tube feedings.[41] Medicare's fiscal intermediaries deny payments, the local medical review policies have been instituted to oversee implementation of the Medicare hospice benefit, and the Office of the Inspector General's efforts to root out Medicare fraud have caused disruption in care for hospices and patients.[42] If receiving felicitous care through hospice interrupts the patient's deterioration, the person may face discharge, even though the terminality of the clinical condition is unchanged. Joanne Lynn describes the attitudinal shift regarding the six-month requirement of the Medicare hospice benefit from a "more likely than not" prediction to a "damn sure you're going to die by then" prognosis.[43]

The Center to Advance Palliative Care recommends that programs incorporate tracking and financial mechanisms to show their institutions the economic viability of palliative care. If hospitals believe that palliative care is a cost-saving measure, then they are more likely to embrace it.[44] This is a pragmatic move, but it implies that if care for dying patients is less costly, then they themselves carry little value. Further, it ignores the fact that the more comprehensive care that hospice patients receive can paradoxically lengthen life.

Attempts at Cultural Balance

Even as it faces enormous challenges, the hospice movement continues to gain supporters and patients, showing consistent and steady growth. With all the difficulties and pressures exerted on hospice and palliative care by the dominance of the rescue paradigm, it is instructive that in March 2008, the Joint Commission (formerly the Joint Commission on Accreditation of Healthcare Organizations, or JCAHO) called for comment on a proposed set of standards for palliative care.[45] This national accrediting organization's decision to require ethics consultation placed a needed stamp of validity on ethics processes in hospitals in 1991. In 1995, it produced standards for organization ethics. The current initiative will put palliative care squarely "on the map" of acute care territory.[46] Such a development illustrates that while many forces in the culture put up barriers to hospice and palliative care, other movements can apply pressure to open doors. Such conflicting signals provide further evidence of the cultural push to find equipoise between "more time alive" and its antithesis.

Why is this balance so difficult to achieve, and why is it important? One answer relates to the different perspectives on social justice positions that hospice and rescue present in the configuration of U.S. health care. Hospice attends to a particular subaltern population: persons who are close to their own deaths, persons who not only epitomize powerlessness and isolation, but also betray to the American culture the inescapability of dying. Their fates can be seen as the most universal of human conditions, and because of this, among the most marginalized. The delivery of hospice and palliative care is an example of the Church's preferential option for the poor,[47] that is, it models a way for Americans to face up to ultimate vulnerability by providing excellent, multidimensional care and by actively exploring the possibilities of vulnerability as a state of being. This model instantiates the belief in a countercultural ethical good: that value must be sought and found in vulnerability itself.

Daniel Sulmasy uses universality as a way to connect the values of hospice and social justice.[48] He cites three aspects of the human condition that overlap with norms of social justice: socialness (recalling Paul Ramsey's expression, "solidarity in mortality"),[49] acknowledgement of inborn finitude, and a "radically equal intrinsic social worth or dignity that commands the respect of others."[50] In his view, this prestige has nothing to do with respect for autonomous preferences. For Americans otherwise compelled by self-reliance to fight illness to the death while vigorously suppressing insinuations of their own weaknesses, hospice offers a place of safety through what Ira Byock calls "the covenantal framework of community."[51] Only in the context of acknowledged interdependency can one gingerly put self-reliance aside. Hospice and palliative care suggest that to find oneself on the receiving end of others' ministrations can be nontoxic.

In one sense it is exactly the universal aspect of vulnerability that rescue denies. For Americans to valorize rescue in the health care system is to assert that because it is *sometimes* possible to hold off death, it is permissible to pretend that not all human beings are its carriers. If death were always an outside invader, society could be justified in uniting to protect itself. But this would be solidarity around a fiction, reflecting a need to affirm that death comes only to the other guy, the one whose poor body failed to respond to the applied technology. Rescue is not only a way to deny mortality but also to deny that it is shared.

What, then, is the social justice position of rescue? The style of rescue's deployment in the United States demonstrates the core value that must complement self-reliance: that of equal opportunity. Having designed a national emergency response system to emphasize speed and universality rather than medical acumen,[52] Americans use the various components of rescue (the 911 emergency response system, universal CPR as default, and guaranteed treatment in the emergency department) to assert how equitable they are in making the most important and dramatic medical treatments available to all. Rescue is therefore not only individualized but also all-inclusive, giving it enough of a social justice claim to stay culturally afloat. This "safety net" is, in fact, inadequate, deeply discriminatory, and inordinately expensive.[53] It perpetuates a myth that if one is sick enough in the United States, one can get access to the most advanced health care in the world. As such, universal rescue is a primary symbol of equal access to the salvatory aspects of American technology. Any alternative would require meaningful universal access to a U.S. health care system that accounts for the chronicity of human frailty across the life span. Until this becomes a reality, it is ethically questionable to deny access to the possibility of rescue, even in the face of death.

Hospice's grounding in social justice, then, is an equality in finitude common to the human condition, unappealing to Americans at first blush. Rescue's cultural pretense of social justice works to make the pursuit of individuality palatable. It promises equal opportunity for the chance at "more time alive," a powerful and alluring concept. From a cultural standpoint, the existence of hospice itself becomes the emergency backup, the safety net for times when the more attractive belief in rescue fails to deliver. Both, therefore, have an important role to play in the present U.S. health care system.

Hospice and palliative care offer another cultural value regarding the human condition that is unavailable to the rescue orientation, with its strong motivation to overcome mortal limitations: being open to the unknowable. Within rescue it is often necessary to stabilize patients long enough to resolve uncertainty about their prognoses. This is a benefit derived from skillful, highly elaborated medical care applied to patients who would expire without it. But rescue's tolerance of ambiguity regarding the cause of a collapse or the patient's ultimate outcome can be short-lived. Triage is based on stabilization rather than cure, and stable patients must be "stepped down" to places removed from intensive or urgent care. Aggressive care then makes room for uncertainty, but it cannot afford to open itself to the truly unknowable, such as why this occurred, what it could mean to those affected, or how the community will cope. The pressure to "move things along," to free up the bed in order to apply rescue to the next patient in extremis is too great.

But the unknowable will not go away. It cannot be banished through medical advances. It is true that neither hospice nor the rescue project can answer the important questions of individual patient frailty and survival. But within hospice and palliative care, the fact of human limitation and the need for community is unquestioned. The presence of hospice in the United States invites Americans to go deeper, to explore the possibilities for finding value in vulnerability. To be open to the unknowable as a matter of course makes it possible to visualize a different cultural strength that comes not from overcoming individual limitations, but from seeking out the possibilities for human resiliency in community. Hospice and palliative care hold out this cultural good, underutilized in American health care, as a method of delivering services to living persons, since all their patients are fully engaged in living until the moment of their deaths.

Notes

[1] E. M. Spencer et al., *Organization Ethics in Health Care* (New York: Oxford University Press, 2000).

[2] Ibid., 93.

[3] B. G. Glaser and A. L. Strauss, *Awareness of Dying* (Chicago: Aldine Publishing, 1965).

[4] "HIV/AIDS and Hospice," Hospice Blog, December 13, 2004, http://www.hospiceblog.org/2004/12/hivaids-and-hospice.html.

[5] Bruce Jennings, "Individual Rights and the Human Good in Hospice," in *Ethics in Hospice Care: Challenges to Hospice Values in a Changing Healthcare Environment*, ed. Bruce Jennings (Philadelphia: Haworth Press, 1997), 1–8.

[6] Ibid., 4.

[7] R. S. Loewy, "Honouring the Age-Old Commitment to 'The Patient's Good': The Promise—and Peril—of Hospice," *Wiener Medizinische Wochenschrift* 153.17–18 (September 2003): 392–397.

[8] Francis L. K. Hsu, "American Core Value and National Character," in *Psychological Anthropology: Approaches to Culture and Personality*, ed. F. L. K. Hsu (Homewood, IL: Dorsey Press, 1961), 209–229.

[9] T. L. Beauchamp and J. F. Childress, *Principles of Biomedical Ethics*, 4th ed. (New York: Oxford University Press, 1994); D. Callahan, "Autonomy: A Moral Good, Not a Moral Obses-

sion," *Hastings Center Report* 14.5 (October 1984): 40–42.

[10] T. Walter, *The Revival of Death* (New York: Routledge, 1994).

[11] J. Lawton, *The Dying Process: Patients' Experiences of Palliative Care* (New York: Routledge, 2000).

[12] Jennings, "Individual Rights," 5.

[13] M. T. Halpern et al., "Insurance Status and Stage of Cancer at Diagnosis among Women with Breast Cancer," *Cancer* 110.2 (July 15, 2007): 403–411; C. H. Shiboski, B. L. Schmidt, and R. C. Jordan, "Racial Disparity in Stage at Diagnosis and Survival among Adults with Oral Cancer in the United States," *Community Dentistry and Oral Epidemiology* 35.3 (June 2007): 233–240.

[14] I am grateful to Richard O'Brien for this insight.

[15] H. S. Chapple, "Dying to be Rescued: American Hospitals, Clinicians, and Death" (Ph.D. diss., University of Virginia, 2007).

[16] D. P. Sulmasy, "Health Care Justice and Hospice Care," *Hastings Center Report* 33.2 (March–April 2003) suppl: S14–S15.

[17] D. Soelle, *Suffering*, trans. E. R. Kalin (Philadelphia: Fortress Press, 1975), 178.

[18] Sulmasy, "Health Care Justice."

[19] Z. Bauman, *Mortality, Immortality, and Other Life Strategies* (Cambridge, UK: Polity Press, 1992), 137.

[20] S. R. Kaufman, *And A Time to Die: How American Hospitals Shape the End of Life* (New York: Scribner, 2005).

[21] Bauman, *Mortality, Immortality*, 112.

[22] D. Album and S. Westin, "Do Diseases Have a Prestige Hierarchy? A Survey among Physicians and Medical Students," *Social Science and Medicine* 66.1 (January 2008), 182–188.

[23] Ibid.

[24] P. A. Taheri et al., "The Cost of Trauma Center Readiness," *American Journal of Surgery* 187.1 (January 2004): 7–13.

[25] C. A. Robinson, T. Hoyer, and C. Blackford, "The Continuing Evolution of Medicare Hospice Policy," *Public Administration Review* 67.1 (January/February 2007): 127–134.

[26] A. Gawande, "Piecework: Medicine's Money Problem," *New Yorker*, April 4, 2005.

[27] Other residential health services reimbursed by capitation share this lower status, such as nursing home and home health services.

[28] J. Lynn, "Living Long in Fragile Health: The New Demographics Shape End of Life Care," *Hastings Center Report* 35.6 (November–December 2005) Special Report: S14–S18.

[29] S. R. Connor et al., "Comparing Hospice and Nonhospice Patient Survival among Patients Who Die within a Three-Year Window," *Journal of Pain and Symptom Management* 33.3 (March 2007): 238–246; B. Jennings et al., "Access to Hospice Care: Expanding Boundaries, Overcoming Barriers," *Hastings Center Report* 33.2 (March–April 2003) Supplement: S3–S7, S9–S13, S15–S21.

[30] E. F. Pitorak, M. B. Armour, and H. D. Sivec, "Project

Safe Conduct Integrates Palliative Goals into Comprehensive Cancer Care," *Journal of Palliative Care* 6.4 (August 6, 2003): 645–655.

[31] J. A. Gallagher, and J. Goodstein, "Fulfilling Institutional Responsibilities in Health Care: Organizational Ethics and the Role of Mission Discernment," *Business Ethics Quarterly* 12.4 (October 2002): 433–450.

[32] P. G. Fine and B. Jennings, "CPR in Hospice," *Hastings Center Report* 33.3 (May–June 2003): 9–10; S. Henderson, J. J. Fins, and E. H. Moskowitz, "Resuscitation in Hospice," *Hastings Center Report* 28.6 (November–December 1998): 20–22.

[33] D. J. Casarett et al., "Must Patients with Advanced Cancer Choose between a Phase I Trial and Hospice?" *Cancer* 95.7 (October 1, 2002): 1061–1604.

[34] L. Rossaro et al., "A Strategy for the Simultaneous Provision of Pre-Operative Palliative Care for Patients Awaiting Liver Transplantation," *Transplant International* 17.8 (September 2004): 473–475

[35] I. R. Byock, "End-of-Life Care: A Public Health Crisis and an Opportunity for Managed Care," *American Journal of Managed Care* 7.12 (December 2001): 1130.

[36] T. Walter, *Revival of Death*; S. R. Connor et al., "Measuring Hospice Care: The National Hospice and Palliative Care Organization National Hospice Data Set," *Journal of Pain and Symptom Management* 28.4 (October 2004): 316–328; R. L. Rhodes, "Racial Disparities in Hospice: Moving from Analysis to Intervention," *Virtual Mentor, American Medical Association* 8.9 (September 2006), http://virtualmentor.ama-assn.org/2006/09/oped1-0609.html.

[37] M. C. Dobratz, "Issues and Dilemmas in Conducting Research with Vulnerable Home Hospice Participants," *Journal of Nursing Scholarship* 35.4 (2003): 371–376; D. J. Casarett and J. H. Karlawish, "Are Special Ethical Guidelines Needed for Palliative Care Research?" *Journal of Pain and Symptom Management* 20.2 (August 2000): 130–139.

[38] "Improving End-of-Life Care," *NIH Consensus and State-of-the-Science Statements* 21.3 (December 6–8, 2004): 7, http://consensus.nih.gov/2004/2004EndOfLifeCareSOS024PDF.pdf.

[39] Casarett et al., "Must Patients with Advanced Cancer Choose?" and C. Zimmermann et al., "Effectiveness of Specialized Palliative Care: A Systematic Review," *Journal of the American Medical Association* 299.14 (April 9, 2008): 1698–1709.

[40] Gawande, "Piecework."

[41] For a discussion of the advantages and challenges facing institutional ethics committees that wish to expand their vision to include organization ethics, see Spencer et al., *Organization Ethics*, 166.

[42] Jennings et al., "Access to Hospice Care," S29–33.

[43] Joanne Lynn, speaking at the National Hospice and Palliative Care Organization Research Conclave, April 13, 2003, NHPCO edited transcript, 38.

[44] S. K. Payne, P. Coyne, T. J. Smith, "The Health Economics of Palliative Care," *Oncology* 16.6 (June 2002): 801–802; National Hospice and Palliative Care Organization, "Hospice care saves money for medicare, new study shows," November 8, 2007, http://www.nhpco.org/i4a/pages/Index.cfm?pageID=5386.

[45] Joint Commission, "The Joint Commission introduces draft palliative care standards available for comment," press release, March 11, 2008.

[46] Ethics processes are often provided on a volunteer basis, so that a regulatory mandate for hospitals to provide them would have required a relatively small investment. Palliative care services require payment, however, and even in facilities with established palliative care units, the mechanisms for reimbursement are far from straightforward. The effect of the Joint Commission's prioritizing here remains to be seen. This movement to set forth standards is a lesser threshold of legitimacy than was the establishment of the Medicare hospice benefit, but it is still significant.

[47] P. Farmer, *Pathologies of Power: Health, Human Rights and the New War on the Poor* (Berkeley: University of California Press, 2003), 138.

[48] Sulmasy, "Health Care Justice."

[49] P. Ramsey, *The Patient as Person: Explorations in Medical Ethics* (New Haven: Yale University Press, 1970), 129.

[50] Sulmasy, "Health Care Justice," S14.

[51] I. R. Byock, "Rediscovering Community at the Core of the Human Condition and Social Covenant," *Hastings Center Report* 33.2 (March–April 2003) Supplement: S40–S41.

[52] S. Timmermans, *Sudden Death and Myth of CPR* (Philadelphia: Temple University Press, 2004).

[53] G. Becker, "Deadly Inequality in the Health Care 'Safety Net': Uninsured Ethnic Minorities Struggle to Live with Life-Threatening Illnesses," *Medical Anthropology Quarterly* 18.2 (June 2004): 258–275.

╬

Editorial Summation: The cultural dominance of the rescue ideal in American medical practice both encourages the existence of hospice as a countercultural foil and encroaches upon hospice's formulations of the good, which assert that value can and must be found in vulnerability itself. The U.S. health care system operates as if death is an attacker from the outside to be resisted, rather than originating from within as a part of the human condition. Its heroic project demands and obtains more health care resources than more mundane work around chronic illness, such as preservation of function, minimizing pain, tapping reserves of resilience, and learning to hope for things other than recovery. In a health care system skewed toward acute care, parts of persons, such as their organ systems, have acquired more legitimacy in the biomedical purview than the persons themselves. Further evidence for unequal cultural legitimacy can be seen in payment patterns. Reimbursement for rescue activities and discrete procedures is straightforward and reliable, even if often inadequate. Payment for interventions aimed at the whole person, such as prevention, chronicity, disability, and mental illness—none qualifying as a "fix" for a discrete ailment or particular risk of death—is much more complicated to obtain. Even as it faces enormous challenges, the hospice movement continues to gain supporters and patients, showing consistent and steady growth. The delivery of hospice and palliative care is an example of the Church's preferential option for the poor. Hospice and palliative care offer a cultural value regarding the human condition that is unavailable to the rescue orientation: being open to the unknowable. The unknowable will not go away. It cannot be banished through medical advances.

CHAPTER 15

Palliative Care, Pain Management, and Human Suffering

Suzanne Gross, F.S.E., and Marie T. Hilliard, R.N.

The *Catechism of the Catholic Church* identifies "Christ's compassion toward the sick and his many healings of every kind of infirmity. ... His compassion toward all who suffer goes so far that he identifies himself with them: 'I was sick and you visited me'" (n. 1503). Those who follow in Christ's footsteps are called to be compassionate and to be aware of the healing processes that are available for persons.

Palliative care (from Latin *palliare*, meaning "to cloak") is any form of care or medical treatment that concentrates on reducing the severity of disease symptoms rather than providing a cure. Palliative care involves a comprehensive plan for serving the needs of persons who are ill, who usually are living with a terminal or chronic diagnosis for which care can be provided but for which a cure is not anticipated. The World Health Organization calls palliative care "an approach that improves the quality of life of patients and their families facing the problems associated with life-threatening illness, through the prevention and relief of suffering by means of early identification and impeccable assessment and treatment of pain and other problems, physical, psychosocial and spiritual."[1] The phrase "quality of life" needs to be used with caution, because it can denote an individual interpretation of what constitutes "quality" in the meaning and living of one's life. It is important that proper ethical principles be applied to the use of the word "quality." The Church has always advocated for the life of the person no matter how small or how fragile.

Rev. Romanus Cessario, O.P., discusses the understanding of "quality of life" in his article "Catholic Considerations of Palliative Care."[2] In interpreting the National Hospice and Palliative Care Organization's description of palliative care, Cessario states that the "test of palliative care lies ... in the agreement between the individual, physician(s), primary caregiver, and hospice team that the expected outcome is relief from distressing symptoms, the easing of pain, and the enhancement of quality of life." He adds, "The moral theologian will observe with caution, if not alarm, the amenability of this description to be put at the service of moral expediency." Non-hospice palliative care is not dependent on prognosis, and is offered in conjunction with curative and all other appropriate forms of medical treatment. It should not be confused with hospice care, which delivers palliative care to those at the end of life.

In 2005, data showed that one in four U.S. hospitals had a palliative care program.[3] The National Palliative Care Research Center reports that the number of hospital-based palliative care programs in the United States continues to grow. All medical schools in the United States are required to provide training in palliative medicine.[4] A relatively recent development is the concept of a dedicated health care team that is entirely geared toward palliative treatment, called a palliative care team.

There is often confusion between the terms hospice care and palliative care. In the United States, hospice services and palliative care programs share similar goals of providing symptom relief and pain management. However, one of the most important distinctions between hospice and palliative care programs is that hospice is a Medicare Part A benefit, which requires enrollment in a hospice regulated by the U.S. federal government.[5] Non-hospice palliative care does not require such enrollment. Furthermore, palliative care is appropriate for anyone with a serious or complex illness, whether or not the patient is expected to recover fully, to experience disease progression, or to live with a chronic illness for an extended time.[6]

History of Palliative Care

Palliative care began in the hospice movement and today is no longer limited to hospice care. Hospices were originally places of rest for travelers in the fourth century. In the late nineteenth and early twentieth century, the Irish Sisters of Charity established hospices for the dying in Ireland and London. The modern hospice originated and gained momentum in the United Kingdom after the founding of St. Christopher's Hospice in 1967 by Dame Cicely Saunders. She is widely regarded as the founder of the modern hospice movement.

Hospice care in the United States has grown from a volunteer-led movement to improve care for people dying alone, isolated, or in hospitals, to a significant part of the health care system. In 2005, more than 1.2 million individuals and their families received hospice care.[7] Hospice is the only Medicare benefit that includes pharmaceuticals, medical equipment, continuous access to care, and support for loved ones following a death. The majority of hospice care is delivered at home. It is also available to people in home-like hospice residences, nursing homes, assisted-living facilities, veterans' facilities, hospitals, and prisons.

Hospice is a philosophy of care in situations when no cure is possible but care is needed for the patient and the family. The hospice care interdisciplinary team (care team) develops the plan of care. The team consists of the hospice nurse, the hospice director, the medical director, the pastoral care person, the social worker, and the pharmacist. For those individuals who are eligible for Medicare, funding for hospice care within a nursing home setting is also available if the nursing home has a written agreement with a certified Medicare hospice provider. For a patient to be eligible for hospice services, the patient's attending physician must determine that the patient has six months or less to live. In general practice, however, the patient chooses hospice services when it becomes apparent that death will ensue in only a few months or even a few weeks. Thus, the care team often has a short period of time to assess the needs of the patient and family.

Spiritual Care

There are many examples of how hospice care as a ministry participates in the salvific meaning of human suffering. Hospice caregivers meet the patient with terminal illness when the patient is most vulnerable and when the family often appears helpless. Western culture attempts to avoid suffering, while fostering ideologies that not only aim to eliminate suffering, but sometimes the sufferer. Through hospice, those with a Christian belief in the meaning of suffering are offered a horizon of opportunity to support the sufferer.

Rev. Bede Jarrett, O.P., offers this thought: "And Life is eternal and Love is immortal, and death is only an horizon, and an horizon is nothing save the limit of our sight."[8] The patient who has been told they have less than six months to live needs assistance in facing death and in examining the limitations of personal perceptions of death. When death is imminent, patients can benefit from an assisted exploration of their perceptions of eternal life. People of faith "live to die." For the believer, the moment of death is the most important moment of "earthly" life. However, many people fear and wish to avoid death. So, too, there are families who do not want their loved one to be told that death is near. It should be understood that the one who is dying has a right and a need to know that death is imminent. The *Ethical and Religious Directives for Catholic Health Care Services* requires that persons in danger of death be provided with opportunities to prepare for death. This entails being provided with information to help them understand their condition, as well as the opportunity to receive the sacraments to prepare well for death.[9]

Pain Management

Many patients will have pain and will need the physician and the attending nurse to provide effective pain management. With advances in medicine, pain management is readily achieved. The physician needs to have the professional knowledge and communication skills to assure effective pain management.

Pope Pius XII affirmed that it is licit to relieve pain by narcotics, even when the result is decreased consciousness and a shortening of life, "if no other means exist, and if, in the given circumstances, this does not prevent the carrying out of other religious and moral duties."[10] In *Evangelium vitae* (The Gospel of Life), Pope John Paul II encourages caregivers to develop programs of palliative care and to provide proper pain management to patients:

> In modern medicine, increased attention is being given to what are called "methods of palliative care," which seek to make suffering more bearable in the final stages of illness and to ensure that the patient is supported and accompanied in his or her ordeal. Among the questions which arise in this context is that of the licitness of using various types of painkillers and sedatives for relieving the patient's pain

when this involves the risk of shortening life. ... In such a case, death is not willed or sought, even though for reasonable motives one runs the risk of it: there is simply a desire to ease pain effectively by using the analgesics which medicine provides. All the same, "it is not right to deprive the dying person of consciousness without a serious reason" as they approach death people ought to be able to satisfy their moral and family duties, and above all they ought to be able to prepare in a fully conscious way for their definitive meeting with God.[11]

The U.S. Conference of Catholic Bishops states clearly in the *Ethical and Religious Directives* that no patient should experience intense pain and that medications should be provided as comfort measures:

> Patients should be kept as free of pain as possible so that they may die comfortably and with dignity, and in the place where they wish to die. Since a person has the right to prepare for his or her death while fully conscious, he or she should not be deprived of consciousness without a compelling reason. Medicines capable of alleviating or suppressing pain may be given to a dying person, even if this therapy may indirectly shorten the person's life so long as the intent is not to hasten death.[12]

Achieving these ends of alleviating pain while allowing patients to satisfy their moral and family duties requires intense listening skills. A hospice patient diagnosed with esophageal cancer was asked by the hospice nurse to describe her pain level on a scale of one to ten. The patient responded, "Dare I say fifteen?" The hospice nurse, recognizing the intensity of her pain, assured the patient that she would manage her pain to a comfortable level. The patient requested that her pain management be determined by a level of consciousness and be measured this way: she wanted to be conscious enough to be able to recognize her husband of forty years. The patient's pain was managed without undue diminishment of consciousness, and her wish to maintain the bond with her husband was respected.

Meaning of Suffering

In addition to physical suffering, the patient in hospice care often experiences spiritual suffering, emotional suffering, psychological suffering, and moral suffering. When faced with a terminal illness, questions arise concerning the meaning of suffering. The *Ethical and Religious Directives* states, "Patients experiencing suffering that cannot be alleviated should be helped to appreciate the Christian understanding of redemptive suffering."[13] Suffering is a deep mystery. There is meaning in suffering because through it we share in Christ's suffering. Pope John Paul II, in his powerful apostolic letter *Salvifici doloris*, helps to clarify the meaning of suffering: "Love is also the richest source of the meaning of suffering, which always remains a mystery: we are conscious of the insufficiency and inadequacy of our explanations."[14] Patients facing death often seek answers concerning their sufferings in the following domains:

- *Spiritual suffering*: What do I really believe? Am I ready to meet my God? What is my unfinished business? What can I do to make peace with my God? Will God be merciful?[15]

- *Emotional suffering*: What bothers me the most? What relationships are unreconciled? Whom do I need to see and talk to before I die? How have I loved? How could I have been a better mother or father?

- *Psychological suffering*: Who am I? Who have I become? Have I used the talents God gave me? Did I share them with others?

John Paul II states further in *Salvifici doloris* that Sacred Scripture "is a great book about suffering."[16] Christ is the center of Sacred Scripture—this tells us that suffering is a key theme in his life. In the New Testament, Christ shows his concern consistently to those who suffered. He "heals the sick, consoles the afflicted, feeds the hungry, frees people from deafness, from blindness, from leprosy, from the devil."[17] He is very sensitive to human suffering. Jesus washes the feet of his disciples. It is precisely through suffering, through his own suffering, that Christ saves us and opens the way to eternal life. This is the catechesis to offer to patients with terminal illness—to assure them that their suffering has meaning.

In hospice, there are young mothers with breast cancer and brain tumors; there are fathers with lung cancer and liver disease; there are senior adults with end-stage heart disease and bone cancer. As the pain is managed, the questions about human suffering are raised: Why is it my time to die? What meaning is there in this process? Why do I have to leave my spouse and my children? All are examples of human suffering. One can only find the answer to these questions in the suffering of Christ. Christ suffers voluntarily and suffers innocently. Suffering is the way to "mount the Cross," the way to unite with the love of Christ. This is the message to give to those receiving hospice care or palliative care. The powerful mandate to co-suffer, to be a companion to another, is the opportunity that hospice care in the home offers. Pope Benedict XVI in his encyclical letter on hope, *Spe salvi*, offers a deep understanding of co-suffering and compassion:

> The true measure of humanity is essentially determined in relationship to suffering and to the sufferer. This holds true both for the individual and for society. A society unable to accept its suffering members and incapable of helping to share their suffering and to bear it inwardly through "com-passion" is a cruel and inhuman society.[18]

Hospice care and palliative care offer persons the possibility to co-suffer with another.

What about the caregiver, whether a member of the hospice team, palliative care team, or family? The spouse, the family, and the caregiver are given the opportunity to suffer with another. Being at the bedside of a patient or loved one who is dying is an invitation to co-suffer with that person.

Nathaniel Hawthorne wrote a short story titled "The Birthmark" (1843), in which a scientist named Alymer grows troubled by a birthmark on his wife Georgiana's face. He wants his wife, in his mind, to be perfect and beautiful. Georgiana tells him, "You cannot love what shocks you." He goes to the extreme to rid her face of this birthmark, at the expense of her life. The caregiver needs to be an apostle of love, one who can care for and be a companion to the one who is dying. Sometimes there are physical changes in the body; sometimes the patient's disposition changes; sometimes breathing becomes labored; or sometimes there is weight loss. At all times it is important to remember those words, "You cannot love what shocks you." All of these are examples of the invitation to co-suffer. The caregiver too is invited to carry the Cross, like Simon of Cyrene on the way to Calvary, to support the Other.

A young mother in her forties was diagnosed with terminal cancer. She was cared for at home by her very devoted husband, with the professional support of a home hospice agency around the clock. With time, this wife and mother died. When her husband was in the receiving line at the funeral home, a very concerned friend commented to the husband, "I am so sorry; I do not know why your wife had to get sick and die." The husband offered a remarkable answer: "If my wife had not gotten sick, I would never have really gotten to know her; I would never have learned how to care for her. I discovered my wife in ways that I never knew. Because of her illness, I learned what it meant to be a husband." In the spirit of Simon of Cyrene, this husband co-suffered with his beloved wife, and with her he carried her cross.

There are those who wish never to suffer, and reject co-suffering with others. To eliminate any obligation to co-suffer, or their own experience of suffering, they advocate the right to eliminate the person who suffers through euthanasia or assisted suicide. The *Ethical and Religious Directives* provide the real answer to such suffering: "Dying patients who request euthanasia should receive loving care, psychological and spiritual support, and appropriate remedies for pain and other symptoms so that they can live with dignity until the time of natural death."[19] In St. Peter's Basilica in Rome, there is a powerful sculpture, the *Pieta*, in which Michelangelo captures the meaning of co-suffering. This sculpture is so counter-cultural that its meaning can be missed. Mary holds her Son after he has suffered and given humankind every ounce of energy and love. Mary co-suffered. It is unthinkable that she would have done anything to eliminate Christ's suffering by hastening his death, taking his life, which is so much the theme of this culture. Jesus was totally given, no matter how intense the suffering. Mary was totally given, no matter how great the cost.

Notes

[1] World Health Organization, "WHO Definition of Palliative Care," www.who.int/cancer/palliative/definition/en/.

[2] Romanus Cessario, "Catholic Considerations of Palliative Care," *National Catholic Bioethics Quarterly* 6.4 (Winter 2006): 642.

[3] R. S. Morrison et al., "The Growth of Palliative Care Programs in United States Hospitals," *Journal of Palliative Medicine* 8.6 (December 2005): 1127–1134.

[4] "Why Is Palliative Care Research Needed?" National Palliative Care Research Center Web site, http://www.npcrc.org/about/about_show.htm?doc_id=374985.

[5] U.S. Department of Health and Human Services, Centers for Medicare and Medicaid Services, *Medicare Hospice Benefits,* CMS publ. no. 02154 (Baltimore: CMS, 2008), 3.

[6] "Palliative Care vs. Related Services," Center to Advance Palliative Care Web site, http://www.capc.org/building-a-hospital-based-palliative-care-program/case/definingpc/designing/presenting-plan/pc_vs_other/.

[7] "NHPCO's Facts and Figures—2005 Findings," National Hospice and Palliative Care Organization, http://www.alfa.org/files/public/NHPCO2005-facts-and-figures.pdf.

[8] Prayer attributed to William Penn and used by Rev. Jarrett, http://www.poeticexpressions.co.uk/POEMS/Prayer of father Bede Jarrett.htm.

[9] U.S. Conference of Catholic Bishops, *Ethical and Religious Directives for Catholic Health Care Services*, 4th ed. (Washington, D.C.: USCCB, 2001), n. 55.

[10] Pius XII, "To an International Assembly of Doctors and

Surgeons" (February 24, 1957), in *AAS* 49 (1957), 147.

[11] John Paul II, *Evangelium vitae* (March 25, 1995), n. 65.

[12] *Ethical and Religious Directives*, n. 61.

[13] Ibid.

[14] John Paul II, *Salvifici doloris* (February 11, 1984), n. 13.

[15] Many Catholics receive the sacraments of Reconciliation and Anointing of the Sick, which provide powerful support for the one suffering. Directives 15 and 16 of the *Ethical and Religious Directives* speak to the role of pastoral care in making available the Anointing of the Sick and Viaticum.

[16] *Salvifici doloris,* n. 6.

[17] Ibid., n. 16.

[18] Benedict XVI, *Spe salvi* (November 30, 2007), 38.

[19] *Ethical and Religious Directives,* n. 60.

Editorial Summation: Palliative care (from Latin *palliare*, meaning "to cloak") is any form of care or medical treatment that concentrates on reducing the severity of disease symptoms rather than providing a cure. Hospice care differs from palliative care. Hospice is a Medicare Part A benefit, which requires enrollment in a hospice regulated by the U.S. federal government. Non-hospice palliative care does not require such enrollment. Furthermore, it is appropriate for anyone with a serious or complex illness, whether or not the patient is expected to recover fully, to experience disease progression, or to live with a chronic illness for an extended time. Hospice is the setting in which much palliative care is administered. Hospice care in the United States has grown from a volunteer-led movement to improve care for people dying alone, isolated, or in hospitals, to a significant part of the health care system. The majority of hospice care is delivered at home. It is also available to people in home-like hospice residences, nursing homes, assisted-living facilities, veterans' facilities, hospitals, and prisons. Hospice is a philosophy of care in situations when no cure is possible but care is needed for the patient and the family. As a ministry, hospice care participates in the salvific meaning of human suffering. People of faith "live to die." For the believer, the moment of death is the most important moment of "earthly" life. However, many people fear death and wish to avoid it. In addition to physical suffering, the patient in hospice care often experiences spiritual suffering, emotional suffering, psychological suffering, and moral suffering. As the pain is managed, questions about human suffering arise: Why is it my time to die? What meaning is there in this process? Why do I have to leave my spouse and my children? One can only find the answer to these questions in the suffering of Christ, who suffers voluntarily and innocently.

CHAPTER 16

Medical Facts and Ethical Decision Making

A. Assessing Benefits and Burdens

Rev. Albert S. Moraczewski, O.P., and Greg F. Burke, M.D.

To treat or not to treat, that is the question! In a hospital or outpatient setting it is not only a frequent question, but also a lament. Is one, in a particular circumstance, morally obligated to initiate treatment or withhold it? A more difficult issue, at least emotionally, is whether or not an ongoing treatment may be terminated or withdrawn. Are the decision maker and the person "who pulls the plug" in such a situation responsible for the death of the patient?

At the core of all these decisions is the rational assessment of the benefits and burdens of a specific treatment for a specific patient. Such an assessment is based on the best medical evidence and the unique circumstances of a particular case. Those circumstances may include medical comorbidities, psychological reserve, and family and financial resources. There are, of course, many others. The clinician and patient are both responsible for bringing clarity to the final course of action, from each of their own perspectives. In the event of incompetence on the part of the patient, a surrogate will be asked to make similar determinations in consultation with the physician. It cannot be overstated that the Catholic physician must be continually aware of his absolute obligations to sustain his patient's life and oppose any act of euthanasia or assisted suicide.

Identifying Benefits and Burdens

Because it is difficult for most persons to terminate a treatment, especially if death results promptly, it may be easier to begin here by discussing the ethical issues surrounding the withholding of treatment. As a matter of fact, ethicists recognize that ethically there is no difference between the withholding and the withdrawal of treatment. The conditions required for an ethically acceptable withholding apply equally to withdrawal of treatment.

Although ethical questions surround any sort of treatment termination, the focus here is on terminations resulting in the death of the patient. Whether one may stop using a cough medicine, for example, or discontinue medication given to control moderate hypertension, or use a medication to get a better night's sleep are questions that have an ethical dimension involving the general responsibility to maintain one's personal health ... but they are not life-and-death decisions.

Before entering the ethical arena per se, an essential issue is to correctly identify the patient's medical condition. What is the diagnosis, and how secure is it? For example, does the patient have cancer and, if so, what type? Has it been properly identified and perhaps confirmed by a second opinion? With regard to prognosis, one can ask, What is the natural course of the disease if treatment were not to be instituted? What is the likelihood that the current treatment will be effective? What are the short-term and long-term effects of the treatment? What are the survival rates for this particular treatment modality? Are there other treatment modalities available, and what is involved in their use? How effective are they? What would the course of the disease be if the treatment were to be terminated? The answer to these and related questions depends on the personal experience of the physician as well as the cumulated experience of other physicians.

It is incumbent on the clinician, therefore, to maintain certification in his specialty, review the relevant literature, and consult colleagues when appropriate. Modern medicine is blessed with what is perhaps the most extensive and accessible record of specialized experiences that has ever been available. Hence, it is possible for a physician to find instant peer-reviewed information that can help in the diagnosis and treatment of diseases. With the help of online computer searches, the physician can obtain the required information without leaving his office or hospital. Armed with evidence-based medical information, the physician is able to offer sound information to the patient or family. The physician must be prudent, however, given the staggering amount of readily available data. He must choose his sources wisely and not be too prone to accept what often amounts to "medical hearsay." This attribute is what distinguishes a truly excellent physician from a mediocre physician. Moreover, the description and analysis of burdens must be tempered by the clinician's avoidance of personal bias. The information may be technical, statistical, or experiential. The clinician will need to master his communication skills to deliver such information in an intelligible way. Recent studies suggest that discussions based on the "number needed to treat" or the "number needed to harm" may be helpful in such dialogue.

Finally, the clinician needs to approach such discussions with humility and be willing to change his mind on the basis of new data, and never be "married" to a diagnosis. An incorrect or incomplete diagnosis is an acceptable reason for divorce!

Jerome Groopman, M.D., in his bestseller *How Doctors Think*, seeks to offer insight into the reasoning processes of physicians.[1] Such reasoning is often used in the clinician's assessment of benefits and burdens in patient care. It may be surprising to know that such judgments are often arrived at in a matter of seconds, perhaps a minute at most! Practitioners arrive at a "gestalt" diagnosis and prognosis based on a number of factors. The essential ones include

1. A review of the medical facts of the case
2. Pattern recognition based on prior experience and statistical odds
3. The presence or absence of key historical features, physical examination findings, and laboratory data
4. In more complex cases, discussions with colleagues and a quick review of the medical literature
5. In the assessment of the benefit–burden ratio, a full appreciation of the patient's values and goals balanced against the clinician's own ethical and moral beliefs

It should be obvious that it is paramount, if possible, for a patient to choose his physician with due diligence. He should find a doctor who values the sanctity of life while simultaneously avoiding "vitalism," an extreme approach that may subject the patient to harmful or disproportion-

ate treatments. In the art of medical practice, the physician must be proficient in advising those seeking his counsel and be vigilant in making the correct diagnosis, knowing the best treatment options, and finally standing with the patient in solidarity as a companion throughout the duration of illness. Diagnostic and therapeutic perfection are beyond human hope, but the patient still expects the doctor to remain faithful to his calling of service.

Medical-Moral Decision Making

The patient or surrogate is now in a position to make an ethical analysis of the situation. With the general ethical obligation to maintain life and health as background, one has to inquire whether or not there is a moral obligation to initiate or continue the current treatment. Recall that the presumption here is that the patient has a lethal disease and that the treatment is to be (or has been) instituted to treat the condition in order that the patient may improve, even to the point of full recovery.

In "The Prolongation of Life," Pope Pius XII stated a basic principle from Catholic teaching:

> Natural reason and Christian morals say that man (and whoever is entrusted with the task of taking care of his fellow man) has the right and duty in case of serious illness to take the necessary treatment for the preservation of life and health. ... But normally one is held to use only the ordinary means—according to circumstances of persons, places, times, and culture—that is to say, means that do not involve any grave burden for oneself or another."[2]

This teaching means that there are limits to the obligation to use a life-sustaining treatment. If the foreseen burdens of the treatment exceed the benefits that can be reasonably expected from it, then one has no obligation to proceed with it; the treatment is optional. Alternatively, of course, one may also decide to initiate the treatment unless there is a clear obligation not to.

The Congregation for the Doctrine of the Faith's *Declaration on Euthanasia* (1980) repeated the earlier teaching and suggested the terms "proportional" and "disproportional" to replace "ordinary" and "extraordinary," respectively (n. 4), which some considered ambiguous terms. Some clarifications were also made in this document. Financial considerations could enter into the ethical analysis, that is, if the cost of treatment (and its consequences) were prohibitive for the family, patient, or community. However, the statement does not define who is included in the term "community"; presumably, "community" could include the hospital as well as the various civil communities, like city, county, state, and nation. In light of both documents, the notion of burden is to be understood as applying not only to the patient but to others, such as family, hospital, and civic community, and could include those such as third-party payers. It is important that such assessments of burdens themselves be proportional and always balanced against the intrinsic value of human life. One must not overstate the burdens of treatment, just as much as one must avoid an irrational belief in the benefit of a medical intervention.

A Case Analysis

Having identified both the expected benefits and the foreseen (or experienced) burdens to the patient and others, the next task in the ethical analysis is to determine whether the burdens of the treatment exceed the benefits or, in other words, whether the burdens are disproportionately large in comparison with the expected benefits. The difficulty is, how does one weigh or compare benefits and burdens belonging to different categories of reality? For example, the treatment for cancer of the mandible (jaw bone) involves removal of half the mandible, removal of the tongue, and loss of at least one eye, with the hope of a one-year survival of only 25 percent. Is the burden of this treatment less or greater than the hoped-for benefit of survival for one year? Notice that not only are the surgical or medical procedures considered in the determination of burdens, but also the consequences of the procedure, namely, in what condition has the intervention left the patient?

One way to approach the question of how to weigh benefits and burdens is to compare the hoped-for good with the good that would be lost by the surgery and its consequences. The goods lost by this surgery are (at least) binocular vision, speech, auditory acuity, facial or cosmetic integrity, and identity. The goods gained include life for one year (at least)—albeit seriously impaired—and whatever other benefits may accrue from a that one-year extension of life.

Clearly, given the goods saved and the goods lost, one could expect a difference as to how different persons will evaluate and compare them. A person might want to live long enough to witness the marriage of a daughter, the birth of a first grandchild, or the graduation from medical school of one of his children. With an important goal in view, one person might opt for the "heroic" surgery. But another person might be horrified by the prospect of such disfigurement and linguistic limitation for what he judges to be relatively little gain. Or the expense could exceed what an underinsured (or uninsured) patient is capable of handling. Hence, using the same ethical principles and reasoning, different persons of equal knowledge and vir-

tue could decide on opposite courses of action. The ethical principle is the same for both, but the application of values in a prudent decision may well differ markedly.

Suppose, however, that in a similar example, the patient opts initially for treatment but matters take a turn for the worse, so that the reasonable expectations of benefit held before treatment began are now clearly unrealistic. Now the question arises, should treatment be continued or may it be terminated?

As mentioned earlier, it is easier emotionally to withhold life-supporting treatment than to withdraw it. When it is withdrawn and the patient dies, the decision maker may feel that he contributed to the patient's death. The old Latin axiom *post hoc, ergo propter hoc* applies here. Just because B follows A, it does not mean that A caused B. Because life support was stopped and the patient died soon after does not mean that the cause of death was the removal of life support. Nor does it mean that the person who made the decision to remove life support and the person who physically "pulled the plug" are guilty of killing the patient. The cause of death is the condition that originally required the patient to be placed on a mechical ventilator or other form of life support. The human intervention with the initiation of life-support technology is to provide time for a better assessment of the patient's condition. When it becomes clear that life support is not providing any benefit to the patient, or that the burdens (to all concerned) exceed the few benefits to the patient, the decision can be made to withdraw life support.

It is critical to remember that the moral analysis of benefits and burdens is uniquely related to a patient's personal circumstances, but in Catholic understanding all decisions must be viewed against such absolute norms as the protection of the sanctity of human life and the rejection of euthanasia. For instance, it is almost impossible to justify not doing an appendectomy on a healthy seventy-year-old because of the burden of transient pain related to the procedure, and equally hard to explain putting an eighty-nine-year-old with terminal cancer on dialysis to extend life for several days in a comatose state. These, of course, are the "easy" cases in terms of ethics, and should remind us of the basic principles used in the assessment of proportionality. The difficult cases require more thoughtful analysis, but the vast majority can come to a satisfactory resolution.

A final word is necessary to address one of the most controversial areas in judging medical benefits and burdens. Nothing in clinical practice seems to cause as much confusion, and in some situations emotional turmoil, as the use of assisted nutrition and hydration (ANH) via feeding tubes. Our late Holy Father's allocution in March 2004 concerning the provision of ANH to patients in a persistent vegetative state (PVS) adds much clarity and guidance. The Pope endorsed the routine utilization of ANH to patients in a PVS and spoke of it in terms of ordinary care. However, there are cases of patients in a PVS in which the use of ANH can be disproportionate—for instance, when there is a concomitant terminal illness (such as cancer), when the patient is unable to assimilate the nutrition and hydration (because of a bowel obstruction, for example), or when the provision of ANH is implausible (as in a developing country where ANH is not available).

Thorough and prayerful deliberation on the benefits and burdens of ANH in a patient in a PVS can be soundly accomplished as well. Furthermore, it must be empha-

sized that the Pope's statement did not refer to patients with malignancy, stroke, or end-stage dementia. His focus was only on patients in a PVS. Such cases must be evaluated on a case-by-case basis, with the guidance of Catholic principles rooted in the protection of human dignity and life and tempered by a legitimate consideration of proportionality.

Notes

[1] Houghton Mifflin, 2007.

[2] Pius XII, "The Prolongation of Life," address to an International Congress of Anesthesiologists (November 24, 1957), in *The Pope Speaks* 4.4 (Spring 1958): 393–398, reprinted in *National Catholic Bioethics Quarterly* 9.2 (Summer 2009): 327–332.

Editorial Summation: A clear distinction must be made between the medical facts of a case and the ethical analysis. All the relevant facts (medical and otherwise) of the case must be known and understood. The ethical issue or question need to be clearly stated so that a correct answer can be formulated and recognized as such. ("A clear statement of the question is half the answer.") To determine whether it is ethically right to withhold or withdraw a life-sustaining treatment, one has to determine whether, given all the relevant items to be considered in a particular case, the expected benefits are greater than the anticipated burdens. This is done by comparing the goods obtained (or retained) and the goods lost. Because of differences among human beings, these goods may be weighed differently by different persons. This may lead to different ethically correct conclusions, even among those who agree on the ethical principles and even though a decision may be followed by a patient's death (without the patient's or decision maker's direct involvement). As discussed in chapter 3, every person has the ultimate responsibility for his life and health to the extent that he has the requisite knowledge, power, and freedom to act. Granting this general principle, it remains that individual circumstances introduce important considerations. A treatment may not be available to an individual at a particular place and time. An available treatment may not be sufficiently effective, that is, the burdens of the treatment may exceed its anticipated benefits. There may be conflicting obligations, so that an otherwise nonobligatory procedure (i.e., one that is morally optional) may become obligatory. Hence, in making a decision about continuing, withholding, or terminating treatment, a number of factors need to be considered: the patient's diagnosis and the prognosis, the availability of treatment, the expected effectiveness of a treatment, and the burdens of the treatment to the patient and others.

B. *Providing Assisted Nutrition and Hydration*

Rev. Germain Kopaczynski, O.F.M. Conv.

In his article "Caring for Persons in the 'Persistent Vegetative State' and Pope John Paul II's March 20, 2004, Address on Life-Sustaining Treatments and the Vegetative State,"[1] Professor William E. May has

chronicled the fact that some Catholic moralists have presented the views of Pope Pius XII on ordinary and extraordinary means of prolonging life and Pope John Paul II's views on providing nutrition and hydration to persons in a vegetative state as contrasting rather than complementary. Indeed, some might go so far as to claim that John Paul II betrays the legacy of his predecessor.

On November 24, 1957, Pius XII delivered his allocution "The Prolongation of Life" to a group of anesthesiologists assembled in Rome to discuss developments in medicine. The address is rightly regarded as a watershed moment in Catholic medical-ethical reflection for spelling out in some detail what is meant by ordinary and extraordinary means of prolonging life. It contains the *locus classicus* for Catholic teaching on the matter:

> Normally one is held to use only ordinary means—according to circumstances of persons, places, times, and culture—that is to say, means that do not involve any grave burden for oneself or another. A more strict obligation would be too burdensome for most men and would render the attainment of the higher, more important good too difficult. Life, health, all temporal activities are in fact subordinated to spiritual ends. On the other hand, one is not forbidden to take more than the strictly necessary steps to preserve life and health, as long as he does not fail in some more serious duty.[2]

Pius XII died a year after giving this speech, on October 9, 1958.

Almost half a century later, John Paul II spoke to a group of physicians and other experts gathered in Rome to discuss life-sustaining treatments and the vegetative state.[3] The Pope's allocution was delivered on March 20, 2004; in it the Holy Father confronts head on what was becoming a divisive issue in Catholic health care, namely, the provision of nutrition and hydration to patients in the so-called vegetative state. The Pope came down solidly on the side of providing nutrition and hydration to these profoundly disabled human beings:

> The obligation to provide the "normal care due to the sick in such cases" includes, in fact, the use of nutrition and hydration. The evaluation of probabilities, founded on waning hopes for recovery when the vegetative state is prolonged beyond a year, cannot ethically justify the cessation or interruption of minimal care for the patient, including nutrition and hydration. Death by starvation or dehydration is, in fact, the only possible outcome as a result of their withdrawal. In this sense it ends up becoming, if done knowingly and willingly, true and proper euthanasia by omission. (n. 4)

A year after the papal address was delivered, John Paul II died, on April 2, 2005.

General Observations

It is a truism, of course, but one worth repeating, that each of us is a child of our own age. Each Pope speaks to the health care practitioners of his own era, with its attendant problems and issues. When Pius XII addressed the anesthesiologists in 1957, it was simply unthinkable for physicians to withhold food and water from any of their patients, comatose or otherwise. It was not an issue, and it was not done. Indeed, as Pius answers the three questions posed to him by the doctors, he makes no mention of food and water, nutrition and hydration. He is interested in the ordinary and extraordinary means of prolonging life, and his focus is on medical treatments that may or may not prolong life and how they do so. Pius assumes that medical care will be given while the course of treatment is being discussed and evaluated. In a word, Pius takes care for granted. John Paul II did not have that luxury.

The medical world that John Paul II faced was much changed from that of Pius XII. What was unthinkable in 1957, the withholding of food and water from severely compromised patients, was no longer unthinkable. How did this sea change in attitudes come about in such a relatively short time? I think that Rev. Richard John Neuhaus is on mark when he tries to answer this question: "Thousands of ethicists and bioethicists, as they are called, professionally guide the unthinkable on its passage through the debatable on its way to becoming the justifiable, until it is finally established as the unexceptional."[4] Aware that the ethical landscape had been altered dramatically by such changes in thinking, John Paul II exhorts physicians to remember their moral roots when he observes, "Medical doctors and health care personnel, society and the Church have moral duties toward these persons from which they cannot exempt themselves without lessening the demands of both professional ethics and human and Christian solidarity" (n. 4). He is compelled to address the issue clearly and *sine glossa*:

> The sick person in a vegetative state, awaiting recovery or a natural end, still has the right to basic health care (nutrition, hydration, cleanliness, warmth, etc.), and to the prevention of complications related to his confinement to bed. He also has the right to appropriate rehabilitative care and to be monitored for clinical signs of eventual recovery. (ibid.)

William May mentions in his article that when some Catholics juxtapose the allocutions of Pius XII and John Paul II, Pius comes off in a favorable light because he warns of obligations being too onerous; John Paul has to remind physicians in particular and society in general that they must not shirk their obligations to their severely compromised brothers and sisters. In a word, Pius is seen as lightening our load, while John Paul, on the other hand, is seen as adding to our burdens. Guess who wins that battle in the poll of public opinion?

The Nub of the Issue

When the Second Vatican Council tells us to feed the hungry in *Gaudium et spes*, n. 69, we nod our heads in agreement and say, "But of course. It's the very least we can do." And the same holds true in the health care setting as well. There would seem to be no major problems so far.

What happens, however, when the hungry person happens to be unconscious, or comatose, or in a vegetative state that is long lasting and perhaps even permanent, and cannot feed himself or herself? Since the condition is so dire and the prognosis seemingly so bleak, are food and water still to be given? In the words of John Paul II, "The person in a vegetative state, in fact, shows no evident sign of self-awareness or of awareness of the environment, and seems unable to interact with others or to react to specific stimuli" (n. 2). Do not these conditions change our obligation to feed the hungry? Is not such feeding futile? Is it not overly burdensome?

Some will try to argue that providing assisted nutrition and hydration in such cases is indeed to be eschewed. How valid is their case? Richard Doerflinger, deputy director of the Secretariat for Pro-Life Activities of the U.S. Conference of Catholic Bishops, makes an important point when he observes,

> Bioethicist Daniel Callahan warned in the *Hastings Center Report* in October 1983 that many of his colleagues favored broad policies for withdrawing feeding tubes not because of special burdens involved in such feeding, but because "a denial of nutrition may in the long run become the only effective way to make certain that a large number of biologically tenacious patients actually die."[5]

The Pope is aware that some have tried to impugn the full humanity of vegetative and other "biologically tenacious" individuals. He comes to their defense in these memorable words:

> In opposition to such trends of thought, I feel the duty to reaffirm strongly that the intrinsic value and personal dignity of every human being do not change, no matter what the concrete circumstances of his or her life. *A man, even if seriously ill or disabled in the exercise of his highest functions, is and always will be a man*, and he will never become a "vegetable" or an "animal." (n. 3)

The Most Scrutinized Paragraph

While many no doubt applauded the Pope for his ringing defense of the full humanity of persons in the vegetative state, some were nevertheless convinced that providing food and water to such patients simply had to be a medical treatment rather than ordinary care, and as such was not morally obligatory. A recent court decision from Australia, adjudicated by a Justice of the Supreme Court of Victoria, represents this line of thinking:

> Justice Morris determined that the use of a [percutaneous endoscopic gastrostomy tube] for artificial nutrition and hydration is a "medical procedure," because it involves "protocols, skills and care which draw from, and depend upon, medical knowledge. ... Viewed in this way, PEG feeding and hydration fall within the scope of 'medical treatment.'"[6]

Pope John Paul II in his March 2004 address does not go along with this line of thinking, a point the authors themselves note at the end of their article.

In a world so bedazzled by technology, it is not perhaps surprising that some are led to believe that the act of providing food and water to patients (ordinary care) is somehow transformed into a medical treatment when that food and water has to be delivered by means of tubes which must be inserted and perhaps even monitored by trained medical personnel. I, for one, totally lack the skills necessary to attach the tubes and make the incisions, and must rely on medical personnel to see that they are effectuated. But is this dependence of the layman on the health care technician to attach the tubes morally relevant enough to change care into treatment?

Though some may indeed think so, John Paul II does not agree and, in the most scrutinized paragraph of his address, insists,

> I should like particularly to underline how the administration of water and food, even when provided by artificial means, always represents a *natural means* of preserving life, not a medical act. Its use, furthermore, should be considered, in principle, *ordinary* and *proportionate*, and as such morally obligatory, insofar as and until it is seen to have attained its proper finality, which in the present case consists in providing nourishment to the patient and alleviation of his suffering. (n. 4)

While John Paul II is grateful to the medical profession for its labors on behalf of the sick, he nevertheless insists that the provision of food and water—no matter the manner of their delivery—to all patients, including those in vegetative conditions, remains a human act of caring, not a feat of technological prowess, and certainly not a medical treatment to be provided or not provided as the condition of the patient requires. As the Holy Father notes toward the end of his address, "The true task of medicine is 'to cure if possible, always to care'" (n. 7).

The Pope is saying that the tubes by which the food and water are delivered, and the medical skills needed to insert them, do not change the nature of what is taking place, namely, an act of providing ordinary care, which is mandatory unless the pathological situation dictates otherwise. In this regard, we should note his use of the expression "in principle." I believe he means that providing food and water to all who require them is—if I may use a computer analogy—the default position of Catholic health care, the starting point, if you will.

In a sense, the Pope may be seen as delivering a helpful commentary on the precise meaning of directive 58 of the USCCB's *Ethical and Religious Directives for Catholic Health Care Services* (2001): "There should be a presumption in favor of providing nutrition and hydration to all patients, including patients who require medically assisted nutrition and hydration, as long as this is of sufficient benefit to outweigh the burdens involved to the patient."

Considering the latest medical findings at the time, the Holy Father cautions against a lax reading of what is truly "burdensome" to the patient when he notes, "Moreover, it is not possible to rule out *a priori* that the withdrawal of nutrition and hydration, as reported by authoritative studies, is the source of considerable suffering for the sick person" (n. 5).

In "A Catholic Guide to End-of-Life Decisions," The National Catholic Bioethics Center assesses the burdens associated with tube feeding in the following way:

> There should be a presumption in favor of providing food and water to all patients, even to those in a comatose state, but there are exceptions. Obviously, when the body can no longer assimilate food and water, they provide no benefit and may be withdrawn. Sometimes placement of a tube may cause repeated infections. Some patients may display agitation at the sight of a tube and may pull it out repeatedly. Certain patients experience burdensome complications, such as repeated aspiration and the constant need for suctioning of the throat. All of these are factors that may cause one to reevaluate the placement of a feeding tube.

The Pope did not say that food and water must be provided in each and every case, but that it must always be provided unless it fails to achieve its principal aims of hydrating and nourishing the body and alleviating suffering.

No More Doubt

In 1992, speaking of the Catholic debates regarding patients in a PVS, the Committee for Pro-Life Activities of the National Conference of Catholic Bishops observed that "further complicating this debate is a disagreement over what responsible Catholics should do in the absence of a final resolution of this question."[7] Likewise, the American Catholic bishops wrote in the introduction to Part 5 of the most recent edition of the *Ethical and Religious Directives for Catholic Health Care Services*,

> Some state Catholic conferences, individual bishops, and the USCCB Committee on Pro-Life Activities … have addressed the moral issues concerning medically assisted hydration and nutrition. The bishops are guided by the Church's teaching forbidding euthanasia, which is "an action or an omission which of itself or by intention causes death, in order that all suffering may in this way be eliminated." These statements agree that hydration and nutrition are not morally obligatory either when they bring no comfort to a person who is imminently dying or when they cannot be assimilated by a person's body. The USCCB Committee on Pro-Life Activities' report, in addition, points out the necessary distinctions between questions already resolved by the magisterium and those requiring further reflection, as, for example, the morality of withdrawing medically assisted hydration and nutrition from a person who is in the condition that is recognized by physicians as the "persistent vegetative state."

The "final resolution" and that "further reflection" took place on March 20, 2004.

Let us return to the question of whether Pius XII and John Paul II stand in opposition to each other. The Congregation for the Doctrine of the Faith addresses this matter directly in a recent statement, "Responses to Certain Questions of the USCCB concerning Artificial Nutrition and Hydration." The CDF first notes that Pius XII was responding to questions about resuscitation, not about providing nutrition to those in a vegetative state.

The case in question has nothing to do with such techniques [of resuscitation]. Patients in a vegetative state breathe spontaneously, digest food naturally, carry on other metabolic functions, and are in a stable condition. But they are not able to feed themselves. If they are not provided artificially with food and liquids, they will die, and the cause of their death will be neither an illness nor the vegetative state.[8]

Thus Pius XII and John Paul II are not at odds over what constitutes the proper care of patients, but are discussing very different cases.

Notes

¹ Available on the Christendom Awake Web site, at http://www.christendom-awake.org/pages/may/caringforpersons.htm. A shorter version was published in *Medicina e Morale: Rivista internazionale di Bioetica* 55 (May–June 2005): 533–555.

² Pius XII, "The Prolongation of Life," address to an International Congress of Anesthesiologists (November 24, 1957), in *The Pope Speaks* 4.4 (Spring 1958): 393–398, reprinted in *National Catholic Bioethics Quarterly* 9.2 (Summer 2009): 327–332.

³ Reprinted in *National Catholic Bioethics Quarterly* 4.2 (Summer 2004): 367–370.

⁴ Richard John Neuhaus, "The Return of Eugenics," Commentary 85.4 (April 1988): 19. See also his "The Politics of Bioethics," *First Things* 177 (November 2007): 23–28.

⁵ Richard Doerflinger, "Pope John Paul II Affirms Obligation to Feed Patients in the 'Vegetative' State," *National Right to Life News*, http://www.nrlc.org/euthanasia/Pope032004.html.

⁶ Michael A. Ashby and Danuta Mendelson, "Gardner; re BWV: Victorian Supreme Court Makes Landmark Australian Ruling on Tube Feeding," *Medical Journal of Australia* 181.8 (October 18, 2004): 442–445, http://www.mja.com.au/public/issues/181_08_181004/ash10074_fm.html.

⁷ NCCB Committee for Pro-Life Activities, "Questions about Medically Assisted Nutrition and Hydration," in *Nutrition and Hydration: Moral and Pastoral Reflections* (Washington, D.C.: USCCB, 1992), n. 6.

⁸ Reprinted in *Ethics & Medics* 32.11 (November 2007): 2.

Editorial Summation: Pope Pius XII and Pope John Paul II do not stand in contradiction to each other on the question of whether food and water constitute ordinary or extraordinary means of treatment, as some scholars have suggested. Pope Pius was not addressing artificial nutrition and hydration in his 1957 address, "The Prolongation of Life," for it was not a relevant issue at the time; he was instead examining the question of resuscitation. Pope John Paul was obliged to address the question of whether food and water, even when administered by artificial means, is an ordinary or extraordinary treatment, in his March 20, 2004, statement, "On Life-Sustaining Treatments and the Vegetative State." His conclusion was that this provision was not a treatment at all, but rather a form of care due to all patients regardless of their physiological condition. The fact that the provision of food and water sometimes requires medical skills does not change what is basically a form of ordinary human care into a medical act. So long as the provision of food and water, even if by artificial means, achieves its primary aims of providing sustenance and alleviating pain, it is obligatory.

C. The Persistent Vegetative State

Greg F. Burke, M.D., and Rev. Germain Kopaczynski, O.F.M. Conv.

The tragic death by dehydration of Terri Schiavo in March 2005 brought end-of-life ethics into the public discourse in a most profound way. Ethicists, clergy, politicians, and pundits alike all contributed to this critical debate. The right-to-life and the death-with-dignity movements were in an exhaustive media campaign to sway public opinion. As Catholics, we are graced with the Church's teaching authority to guide us in these highly emotional and tremendously difficult situations.

While addressing the Eighth Bishops' Workshop in Dallas, Texas, organized by The National Catholic Bioethics Center in 1989, Fred Plum, M.D., observed that the question of the persistent vegetative state (PVS) is part of a larger and even more fundamental question:

what is human consciousness? Plum described various altered states of human consciousness, such as coma and the vegetative state, which he divided into two sorts: temporary and persistent (chronic), distinguishing them from other altered states such as delirium, dementia, psychiatric pseudo-coma, and the locked-in state.

Recently, the International Congress on Life-Sustaining Treatments and Vegetative State: Scientific Advances and Ethical Dilemmas further clarified the issue. In their final statement, the Congress participants reminded us that in general, patients in a vegetative state "do not require any technological support to maintain vital functions" and "cannot in any way be considered terminal patients, since their condition can be stable and enduring."[1] The Congress, which met in Rome in March 2004 under the guidance of the Pontifical Academy for Life, also reminded us that "no single investigation method available today allows us to predict, in individual cases, who will recover and who will not" among patients in a vegetative state.[2]

Clinical Aspects

What is the condition known as PVS? True, as Plum intimated, the PVS is not an easy condition to diagnose even for trained medical personnel; yet since there may well be nonmedical persons serving on the ethics committees of Catholic health care facilities, it may be helpful to give a definition of this condition that is understandable in layman's terms. The PVS is a "condition in which the patient is awake without being aware. In this state the *brainstem* is functioning but the cerebral cortex is not, and the patient lies with his eyes open, looks around, but has no meaningful interaction with the environment."[3]

Plum described the condition in medical terms:

The vegetative state describes a condition in which cyclic arousal, i.e., waking and sleeping, remains (or returns after injury or acute disease), but no evidence of self-awareness or purposeful behavior can be elicited. … Many patients transiently go through a temporary vegetative state lasting a few hours or days on their way to recovery following an event causing acute coma. A few, however, for weeks or months, fail to regain any evidence that they are aware of themselves or their specific surroundings or that they can learn even the most simple acts. This we call a *persistent* or *chronic vegetative state*. … It can last unchanged for many months or years until the rest of the body finally dies of some independent cause.[4]

The Multi-Society Task Force on PVS has undertaken important medical work on this condition and published "Medical Aspects of the Persistent Vegetative State."[5] More needs to be done, but on two points, at least, there seems to be consensus among medical personnel:

- Assuming the condition is correctly diagnosed, few patients emerge from a PVS state after six months, and,

- Those in PVS cannot suffer.

Nonetheless, a determination of suffering is much less a medical determination and more a philosophical and spiritual question. Recent studies suggest the possibility of some degree of rudimentary awareness in patients in a PVS. Such studies have used neuroimaging techniques, including those which demonstrate metabolic activity, to establish degrees of consciousness in these patients with severebrain injuries.[6] These ongoing inquiries may prove pivotal in the debate over the management of patients in a PVS. In a clear contradiction of reason, those who supported the removal of assisted nutrition and hydration (ANH) for Terri Schiavo said it would bring an end to Terri's suffering, while at the same time they assured us that Terri was incapable of physical perceptions and ultimately incapable of suffering!

These observations on patients diagnosed with a PVS should be read in close conjunction with the other sections of this manual that are meant to guide those who serve on ethics committees in Catholic health care facilities, especially the previous section (chapter 16B) treating the artificial delivery of nutrition and hydration. Many of the Church's statements in that chapter will also be relevant to the present discussion of PVS.

Moreover, John Paul II's March 2004 allocution concerning the provision of nutrition and hydration to patients in a PVS adds much to the Church's proclaimed teaching. Despite ongoing divisions among Catholic moralists, one can state with clarity that the Church favors the provision of ANH to patients in a PVS. In his statement to the International Congress, John Paul II unambiguously declared,

the administration of water and food, even when provided by artificial means, always represents a *natural means* of preserving life, not a *medical act*. Its use, furthermore, should be considered, in principle, *ordinary and proportionate*, and as such morally obligatory, insofar as and until it is seen to have attained its proper finality, which in the present case consists in providing nourishment to the patient and the alleviation of suffering.[7]

In the very phrase PVS, the word "vegetative" speaks much about the condition. While "vegetative" is not meant to be pejorative, it can be and often is used that way. Terms like "vegetables" and "brain-dead" are frequently used to describe—incorrectly—those in this condition. John Paul II clearly did not endorse the term "vegetable." He reminds us of this in his statement to the International Congress, "*A man, even if seriously ill or disabled in the exercise of his highest functions, is and always will be a man*, and he will never become a 'vegetable' or an 'animal.'"[8] These are strong words from a man who suffered from a severe neurologic disorder.

The *Ethical and Religious Directives for Catholic Health Care Services* explicitly mentions this condition:

The NCCB Committee on Pro-Life Activities report, in addition, points out the necessary distinctions between questions already resolved by the magisterium and those requiring further reflection, as, for example, the morality of withdrawing medically assisted hydration and nutrition from a person who is in the condition which is recognized by physicians as the "persistent vegetative state."[9]

The bishops acknowledge that the problem surrounding patients in a PVS is one "requiring further [moral] reflection." If this is true for the bishops, it is also true for those who serve on ethics committees in Catholic facilities. One approach to the problem has been to present the pros and the cons, and let the stronger side prevail as far as argumentation is concerned. Ethics committee members in Catholic health care facilities should consider themselves under a serious obligation to become informed about these arguments and to reflect on them. One reason for this is that the PVS raises a host of other difficult, complex issues: the definition of death for one, euthanasia and physician-assisted suicide for others.

In September 2007, the Congregation for the Doctrine of the Faith (CDF) responded to questions put forth by the USCCB in July 2005, shortly after the death of Terri Schiavo. When asked if there is a moral obligation to provide food and water to a patient in a PVS, except in cases where assimilation could not occur or would result in significant physical discomfort, the CDF responded with an unequivocal yes. Furthermore, when asked whether it is permissible to discontinue ANH to a patient in a PVS if there is moral certainty the patient will not recover consciousness, the CDF replied no. It would appear that the Church's magisterial teaching on this clinical condition is becoming more solidified, with a greater sense of clarity.

As a careful reading of the medical literature will attest, the medical diagnosis of PVS is difficult to make, since the condition itself can at times appear to be like several others, most notably coma. The National Catholic Bioethics Center has, in several of its publications, attempted to deal with the complexities of this medical condition. So, too, did the President's Commission for the Study of Ethical Problems in Medicine and Biomedical and Behavioral Research (1981) and, more recently, the President's Council on Bioethics. While the Catholic and the President's groups are united in their presumption for life, they do not agree on everything.

There are differences of opinion even among Catholic moralists on the issue. Some favor discontinuing the provision of food and water to patients in a PVS. Others,

however, are troubled by such a procedure, seeing it as an abdication of one of our most solemn duties. At the risk of oversimplifying their very nuanced positions, perhaps we can say that the former position is largely pragmatic, and the latter view is predominantly metaphysical. This having been said, the first ought not to be seen as unreflective, and the second must not be regarded as unemotional. However, the most recent Church declarations on this issue place the former opinion on much weaker magisterial ground than previously, and have given renewed support to the latter opinion. It is important to understand the historical development of the opposing arguments.

Arguments Against Providing Assisted Nutrition and Hydration

Pope Pius XII's 1957 address to a congress of anesthesiologists is often cited by proponents of the termination of food and water to those in conditions such as the PVS. Here is the text in question:

> Normally one is held to use only ordinary means—according to circumstances of persons, places, times, and culture—that is to say, means that do not involve any grave burden for oneself or another. A stricter obligation would be too burdensome for most men and would render the attainment of the higher, more important good too difficult. Life, health, and all temporal activities are, in fact, subordinated to spiritual ends. On the other hand, one is not forbidden to take more than the strictly necessary steps to preserve life and health, as long as he does not fail in some more serious duty.[10]

Since those correctly diagnosed with this condition will not be able to fulfill the higher, spiritual aims of life, it is acceptable, on this reading of Pius's view, to discontinue food and water.

To pursue the spiritual aims of life, one must have a minimum of cognitive and affective functions. If such abilities are lacking in the correctly diagnosed PVS, some moralists would allow the ANH to be discontinued for the the PVS patient. Granted, feeding the sick does possess a great symbolic meaning, yet this ought not to be seen as so great as to categorically keep caregivers from withholding food and water in cases such as the PVS. If it is acceptable for the mother of a family to forgo chemotherapy in order to provide for her family, cannot the same reasoning hold true for those diagnosed in a PVS?

Catholic teaching on ethically ordinary and extraordinary means of preserving life is also brought to bear: it is regarded as acceptable for competent adults to refuse care which they find burdensome or futile, and this can be done by those who inform their loved ones in advance, as in the case of firefighter Paul Brophy.[11] Is this not the precise situation of a PVS? On this account, the Catholic view is one of authentic realism: pro-life, yes, but death is always regarded as a reality, an ineluctable part of the human condition.

These arguments were articulated prior to the papal statement of 2004, however, and need to be addressed in that light. Perhaps in rare cases of a PVS, ANH could be seen as burdensome or futile if some other terminal pathology or extreme financial or family burdens were involved. Can we expect the same standard of care for a patient in in PVS the United States as in a developing country? Perhaps in the ideal, but clearly practical and technical issues may intervene to limit this ideal. Of course, it is best not to start an ethical debate from difficult cases, but from the norm. The vast majority of patients in a PVS do not have co-terminal conditions and the administration of hydration and nutrition via a gastric tube is not painful or financially prohibitive. Unfortunately, the patient in a PVS is often thought to have lost dignity, leading to the judgment that it would be best if he were relieved of his suffering condition. It is frequently the family who, with a true sense of compassion, asks to remove basic support. Yet this is based on a dualistic vision of man, ignoring the inherent worth of the human person as an embodied spirit, not spirit alone. Our bodies matter, even when injured or irreversibly disabled.

Arguments in Favor of Providing Assisted Nutrition and Hydration

Some moralists, Catholic as well as Protestant, profess a certain uneasiness with granting that food and water can ever be regarded as medical treatment. The distinction between the spiritual and the corporeal ends of life, adumbrated in the position of those who use Pius XII's comments to support the removal of ANH from patients in a PVS, raises in the minds of these ethicists the specter of dualism. Our worth cannot be defined by our capacity for spiritual actions alone. Then again, if we define medical treatment as "an action or group of actions performed to alleviate or neutralize some sort of pathological condition or disease,"[12] the logical question arises, if food and water are medical treatment, what precisely do they treat? Patients can be weaned from respirators, to be sure, but they cannot be taken off nutrition and hydration. With all due respect to the contention of the President's Commission that there is no distinction between tube feeding and other forms of life-sustaining treatment, such as ventilation or dialysis, these moralists ask, Can we withdraw food

and water from a patient and say at the same time that this action is not a direct killing?

If there is one argument frequently cited by those who are against the removal of ANH from patients in a PVS, it is their contention that such a move places society on a slippery slope in matters of life and death. The fact that slope argumentation is not easy to prove (or disprove, for that matter) does not thereby mean that it is false. Indeed, many of the moralists who have qualms about keeping food and water from patients in a PVS find it a most weighty consideration. With the strength of the recent papal teaching on this subject, the clear presumption of duty is that nutrition and hydration should be provided in all cases of PVS. This should be the normative approach in any Catholic health care facility.

It would be a mistake to lump together those who are against removing food and water from patients in a PVS and dismiss them as "vitalists" (i.e., committed to keeping a person alive at all costs.) Those who are against removing food and water from PVS patients know that there may be objective conditions that would allow the withdrawal of food and water without thereby intending a direct killing, but they advise extreme caution:

> In judging whether treatment of an incompetent person is excessively burdensome, one must be fair. Great care should be taken not to employ a double standard, by which consciously or unconsciously one attributes greater weight to burdens imposed by the treatment and less to benefits provided by it, because the patient is cognitively impaired or physically debilitated.[13]

Catholic teaching proclaims the inherent dignity of the human person, even one in a PVS, and with clarity affirms a presumption to assist those with the condition in the reception of nutrition and hydration through assisted means. Only the development of a coterminal condition, such as an incurable malignancy, or, less likely, the technical inability to deliver ANH could alter the moral imperative to sustain life in these vulnerable human persons. They are, after all, our brothers and sisters in the Lord.

Notes

[1] Pontifical Academy for Life and the World Federation of Catholic Medical Associations, "Joint Statement on the Vegetative State," from the International Congress on Life-Sustaining Treatments and Vegetative State: Scientific Advances and Ethical Dilemmas, Rome, March 10–17, 2004, n. 3 and 4.

[2] "Joint Statement on the Vegetative State," n. 7.

[3] Mikel A. Rothenberg and Charles F. Chapman, *Dictionary of Medical Terms for the Nonmedical Person*, 4th ed.

(Hauppauge, NY: Barron's Educational, 2000), s.v. "PVS."

⁴ Fred Plum, "Artificial Provision of Nutrition and Hydration: Medical Description of Levels of Consciousness," in *Critical Issues in Contemporary Health Care*, ed. Russell E. Smith (Braintree, MA: Pope John Center, 1989), 48.

⁵ Multi-Society Task Force on PVS, "Medical Aspects of the Persistent Vegetative State," part 1, *New England Journal of Medicine* 330.21 (May 26, 1994): 1499–1508; part 2, 330.22 (June 2, 1994): 1572–1579.

⁶ See, for example, S. Laureys, A. M. Owen, and N. D. Schiff, "Brain Function in Coma, Vegetative State, and Related Disorders," *Lancet Neurology* 3.9 (September 2004): 537–546.

⁷ John Paul II, Address to the Participants in the International Congress on Life-Sustaining Treatments and Vegetative State: Scientific Advances and Ethical Dilemmas (March 20, 2004), n. 4 (original emphasis).

⁸ John Paul II, Address on Life-Sustaining Treatments, n. 3 (original emphasis).

⁹ U.S. Conference of Catholic Bishops, *Ethical and Religious Directives for Catholic Health Care Services*, 4ᵗʰ ed. (Washington, D.C.: USCCB, 2001), pt. 5, intro.

¹⁰ Pius II, "The Prolongation of Life," address to an International Congress of Anesthesiologists (November 24, 1957), in *The Pope Speaks* 4.4 (Spring 1958): 395–396.

¹¹ Paul Brophy was a Massachusetts firefighter who entered the persistent vegetative state after suffering from an aneurism in 1983. His food and water were stopped after a court ruled that Brophy, before he became ill, expressed a wish that he not be kept alive by artificial means. See Matthew L. Wald, "Court Says Feeding May Stop for a Man in a Vegetative State," *New York Times*, September 12, 1986, A10.

¹² Stephen J. Heaney, "'You Can't Be Any Poorer Than Dead': Difficulties in Recognizing Artificial Nutrition and Hydration as Medical Treatments," *Linacre Quarterly* 61.2 (September 1994): 79.

¹³ William E. May et al., "Feeding and Hydrating the Permanently Unconscious and Other Vulnerable Persons," *Issues in Law & Medicine* 3.3 (Winter 1987): 203–217.

Editorial Summation: There have been two approaches advocated by Catholic moralists concerning assisted nutrition and hydration for patients in a persistent vegetative state (PVS). Following Pope Pius XII's famous statement on ordinary and extraordinary means, some have said that, since those correctly diagnosed with this condition will not be able to fulfill the higher, spiritual aims of life, it is acceptable to withdraw nutrition and hydration. A recent Church declaration places this opinion on much weaker magisterial ground. In September 2007, the Congregation for the Doctrine of the Faith (CDF) responded to questions put forth by the USCCB in July 2005, shortly after the death of Terri Schiavo. The document stated with clarity that the Church favors assisted nutrition and hydration for patients in a PVS, thus supporting the arguments of those moralists who had said that there should be a clear presumption in favor of providing these basic needs. If a medical treatment is an action or group of actions performed to alleviate or neutralize some sort of pathological condition or disease, food and water are not treatments. Patients can be weaned from respirators, but they cannot be taken off nutrition and hydration. This presumption in favor of food and water for patients in a PVS should be the normative approach at any Catholic health care facility.

D. Do-Not-Resuscitate Orders

Rev. Albert S. Moraczewski, O.P.

In a scene commonly viewed on television and movie screens, a person has a heart attack and a rush of medical personnel attempt to resuscitate him. Electrode paddles are placed on his chest and a jolt of electricity is used to jump-start the heart, and mouth-to-mouth efforts are performed or an oxygen mask is placed over his face in an attempt to restore respiration once the heart is functioning. No question that the scene is dramatic and to a great extent realistic, and lives are saved. But is this process, cardiopulmonary resuscitation (CPR), always in the best interests of the patient? As a protection against unwanted CPR, the practice has risen of writing do-not-resuscitate orders (DNR) when requested by the patient or appropriate proxy. Experience has shown that CPR is not always in the patient's best interest, in part because of the ambiguity of what DNR orders really mean in any particular case.¹

Catholic Teaching and Do-Not-Resuscitate Orders

One can raise a series of questions regarding DNR orders. How to decide on medical grounds whether it is of benefit to the patient to initiate CPR? Who decides when to initiate it and when to terminate it? By what criteria and by what principles are such decisions to be made? What is to be done when there is a conflict between physician and family regarding whether to initiate or to withdraw? And then there is a basic question as to whether DNR is compatible with the teaching of the Church.

We can begin with the last question first, because if the answer is no, then the other questions are rendered moot. DNR orders are part of a larger issue about withholding and terminating treatment. Under what conditions may lifesaving procedures be withheld (e.g., in the case of DNR orders).

While Church teaching has not directly addressed the issue of DNR, there are teachings in place that address the issue. In chapter 3 it was established as part of Catholic teaching that under the appropriate conditions, summarized in the principle of ethically ordinary and extraordinary means of sustaining life, life-supporting interventions are or can become optional. It is understood that supporting life is always obligatory unless certain conditions are met, namely, that the intervention (or its consequence) has become excessively burdensome to the patient or others, or that there is a disproportion between the burden of the intervention and the hoped-for benefit.[2]

Since every person has the basic right and obligation to maintain and preserve his or her life and has the right to those means necessary to carry out responsibly that obligation, the person can decide whether or not to have CPR performed on them, even antecedently to the actual time of need. Some form of advance directive is often used to document in writing the desire of the patient. These directives usually state the conditions under which CPR or other life-supporting procedures are to be used or withheld.

Since the Church's teaching does not prohibit the use of DNR orders, under what conditions may it be invoked? A good general rule in a Catholic hospital is that any intervention into a person's life should be an expression of Christian love, it should really be of eternal benefit to that individual, and generally that same love would also consider the temporal well-being of the individual so long as it does not interfere with the person's eternal welfare. For example, it is important that a patient is at peace with God and has fulfilled his temporal obligations to the extent that his condition permits this. In particular, when a Catholic patient is sufficiently conscious, opportunity should be given for him to receive the sacraments and to meet with family and friends (and others as desired) so that he can bring proper closure to his life.

All of the above are necessary so that if and when DNR is invoked, the patient is prepared for death. But just when is DNR invoked? It is invoked when the patient has a cardiac arrest or sudden respiratory failure so that immediate lifesaving action is imperative. But that is not sufficient. If a DNR is placed, the condition of the patient must be such that the intervention would be of no significant benefit. If the patient is already dying from an untreatable cancer, for example, the CPR will not remedy that condition and will give the patient no improvement of his condition. In most cases that would represent an unacceptable return to an excessively burdensome condition. There is no moral obligation incumbent on the patient or proxy to insist that all be done to restore him to the dying condition in which he had been. However, to help clarify and exemplify the principle, the following case will be used.

A Case Application: Resolving Possible Conflicts

The patient is a thirty-five-year-old white man with advanced multiple sclerosis, whose condition is progressively declining. He requires respiratory support in the form of a mechanical ventilator. Nutrition and hydration are provided by a nasogastric tube, and because of previous painful contractions of the lower extremities, he requires narcotics for pain relief. The patient is blind and unable to speak, but he is able apparently to communicate by means of eye blinks. He is essentially quadriplegic. The attending physician asserts that the patient previously expressed the wish to end his suffering and die in peace. On the basis of that communication, the physician has ordered a DNR after consultation and discussion with the family. (No written advance directives were found.) Was it a morally acceptable decision on the part of the physician to order a DNR status for the patient?

It must be assumed here, for lack of other evidence, that although the patient expressed a desire to die in order to escape the severe chronic suffering, he did not want or expect the physician to kill him with an overdose of the narcotic which he has already been receiving for managing his pain. But he was asking that nothing be done to unduly prolong his life and suffering. If he should happen to have a cardiac arrest, he did not want "heroic" efforts (i.e., CPR) to be made to restore him to his previous condition. He was saying, in effect, "Do not resuscitate me—I have had enough! Anymore will be futile!"

Would the CPR cure him and relieve him of his multiple disabilities? He has not directly willed to bring about his death; rather, he has declined any treatment that will not truly benefit him medically. Could one argue that his return to pain and suffering would have been to his spiritual benefit? More likely it could have been to his detriment. He could well have hated those who brought him back and similarly have cursed God. It is true that some heroic individual might want to offer his suffering in imitation of Christ on the Cross, but that would have to be a freely chosen option. Most human beings would choose the DNR.

Sometimes a conflict may arise between the physician and family because of their different understandings of a DNR. A situation can arise where the family wants "everything done for the patient." In lieu of a patient-signed document, they may deny that the patient would have, or could have, requested a DNR. In addition, they may interpret the DNR order as meaning that the medical staff will abandon the patient, that even comfort care will not be given.

Some sources of such conflicts between physician and family over DNR orders are differences in perspective, differences in values, and differences in expectations. The physician's perspective includes his understanding of his obligation to practice good medicine; to resuscitate the patient when there is no discernible medical benefit would be, for the physician, not practicing good medicine. He wants to restore the patient to good health, not return to life a patient who is medically deteriorating and has no reasonable hope for improvement.

The family, on the other hand, is more focused on its sick member and hopes or wishes for a miraculous recovery. They may have guilty feelings arising from previous poor relationships with the sick member. This would aggravate the misperception that if they permitted the DNR they would singly and collectively be responsible for his death. "We killed him because we did not take every medical means to keep him alive." In addition, their particular religious values may significantly influence the treatment. For example, they could believe that God would work a miraculous cure if only the sick member would be kept alive long enough for God to have time to work a miracle and for the family to manifest its collective faith in God's power. Another factor which could color their decision is the possible material benefit that would result from the patient's demise or survival.

Different values may be at stake. For the physician it is important that the medical problem not only be correctly diagnosed but also effectively treated. In the current atmosphere of managed care in which most physicians have to work, it is economically important for the physician that patients be discharged in a timely fashion. The physician is expected to deal effectively but tactfully with families who obstruct the "correct" management of a patient. If the situation calls objectively for a DNR, then a DNR is fully expected.

The family's values call for a full cure of the patient and a return home in "mint condition." If it takes a little longer, that's all right. "But don't let him die!" A DNR is not treatment but an escape, a giving up, the family may hold. Life is precious and should be retained as long as possible.

A third possible source of conflict between the physician and family in the matter of a DNR is their respective expectations. From personal experience and medical literature review, the physician not only is aware, much more than the family, of the limitations of the treatment the patient is currently receiving, but also has a realistic view of the downhill course of the patient (as described in the case cited above). Often the physician fully expects that his or her opinion and recommendation to the family will be fully respected and accepted ("Doctor knows best").

The family's expectations often may not be in tune with the reality, and they expect that the patient will somehow, perhaps by virtue of a medical miracle, fully recover and come home. "After all, we saw on television how a patient who was much sicker than Dad recovered and came home fully cured to a loving joy-filled family!" And "If it happened once, why could it not happen twice?" The family, too, expects the physician to be a paragon of medical professionalism: competent, compassionate, understanding, with plenty of time to listen to their fears, concerns, and hopes. The family usually expects that third-party payers will cover all or a major part of the medical expenses—so why worry about extra time in the hospital? It is likely that many families have not yet well understood the constraints that current medical fiscal policy places on hospitals and physicians.

When there is a conflict between the family and the physician (and hospital) regarding the implementation of DNR orders, some or all of the above factors may be operative. A knowledge of them will help medical personnel deal more effectively and smoothly with such conflicts when they arise. It should be noted that for some physicians, hospitals, and ethicists it is the physician who makes the decision about DNR orders, and the patient (or family) is subsequently notified. But this is not the understanding in the Catholic moral tradition. When the conditions are met for the ethically optional use of life-supporting procedures and when DNR orders are properly obtained and executed in keeping with the local hospital's policy, DNR orders pose no ethical problem relative to the Church's teaching.

Notes

[1] See Tom Tomlinson and Howard Brody, "Ethics and Communication in Do-Not-Resuscitate Orders," *New England Journal of Medicine* 318.1 (January 7, 1988): 43–46.

[2] See U.S. Conference of Catholic Bishops. *Ethical and Religious Directives for Catholic Health Care Services*, 4th ed. (Washington, D.C.: USCCB, 2001), nn. 56 and 57.

Editorial Summation: The DNR order is morally acceptable according to Catholic teaching if in the particular case it has been properly determined that resuscitation would be ethically extraordinary means of sustaining life. The DNR order is like an advance medical directive, in which the patient's wishes regarding future health care decisions are articulated before the need for these decisions, in case the patient lacks the capacity to make the decisions later. In the case of a DNR order, the advance directive is specifically about resuscitation measures. It is very important that the patient's family and surrogate decision maker are clear about what constitutes resuscitation and why it would not be ethically obligatory under the circumstances. There are other issues that relate to DNR orders in specific contexts, such as DNR orders in the operating room and in pediatric intensive care, and how physicians and nurses communicate information about DNR orders to patients and their families.

CHAPTER 17

Health Care Proxies and Advance Directives

Matthew P. Lomanno

A health care proxy is an individual ("the agent") designated to decide what medical procedures should be undertaken if a patient ("the principal") becomes incapacitated or incompetent. Typically, a proxy is chosen while the principal is healthy and under no duress of illness, but a proxy may need to be assigned after the patient becomes unable to make decisions if none was chosen previously. A hospital's ethicist or ethics committee may be charged with determining a patient's proxy (e.g., a spouse or relative) if one is not readily available or if there is a dispute among parties who claim to be the legitimate proxy.

An advance directive (or "living will") is a document signed by an individual, while fully aware and under no duress, that indicates wishes for medical treatment at the end of life, should the patient be unable to express desires at that time. Often created with the assistance of a lawyer, an advance directive provides general guidelines for treatment and describes what means the patient wishes to be used to preserve life.

Both of these methods of determining medical care—a health care proxy and an advance directive—can be legally binding. However, the two options are not equivalent in supporting effective decision making. An advance directive is limited to a statement of the most basic and general desires of the patient, whereas actual circumstances are typically far more complicated and nuanced than can be anticipated. This leaves the burden of interpretation on the patient's family and health care providers. The proxy decision maker, in contrast, usually knows the patient well and not only has a personal, intimate knowledge of the patient's desires, but he is also fully and unambiguously vested as a legal agent to determine what medical means should be provided or withheld. The proxy is effectively given full moral and legal rights by the principal to exercise judgment in any given situation.[1]

A Fuller Explanation

As a legal document expressing a patient's desires for medical treatment at the end of life, an advance directive attempts to give general guidance to the health care proxy, who may be chosen by the patient but, in an emergency or if no other proxy has been officially named, could be a health care provider or other agent. A patient, for example, might request that no life-saving treatment be given as death approaches. Unless this request is made specifically through a description of various particular scenarios, it provides almost no assistance to the proxy, as it is open to wide interpretation. If the patient is near death because of an infection, should antibiotics be provided? What if the patient could recover via an induced temporary coma and a few days on a ventilator to allow his body to heal? What about receiving one-time dialysis to restore kidney function? A strict interpretation of this patient's advance directive precludes the use of any of these means to restore health.

By necessity, an advance directive, as a set document written before health care decisions need to be made, must be general enough to be applicable in a number of circumstances. Not only is it impractical to make an advance directive more specific, but it is often impossible: one cannot even imagine the multitude of medical conditions and prognoses that are possible for any given patient. Furthermore, descriptions of the treatments the patient does or does not want may actually not be accurate at the time direction is needed—and precisely when the patient cannot express a desire otherwise. A preference expressed by the patient in the document may in fact be the exact opposite of what the patient would choose today if competent and able to make the decision.

The result is that, while advance directives offer some guidance to family members and health care professionals, they are often impractical because of their inherent generality and because they still need someone to interpret their proper application. The designation of a health care proxy can resolve both of these problems. Ideally, a proxy knows the patient's desires and is willing to choose on the patient's behalf. A health care proxy, if not an immediate associate of the patient (spouse, family member, or close friend), should discuss with the patient in some detail what he or she may want in the event of incapacity. If called on to exercise this function, the proxy should act as the patient would act if competent to choose, even if what the patient has requested is not what the proxy would choose for himself. This is the "substituted judgment" standard. When the proxy is genuinely not sure what the patient would want, he should follow the "best-interests" standard on the patient's behalf. The best-interests standard should take into account the entire physical, moral, spiritual, and emotional good of the patient.

Ordinary versus Extraordinary Means

What medical treatments ought to be allowed or rejected is the primary moral question for any patient, proxy, or health care professional. Health is a moral good and thus to be pursued (as its contrary, disease and illness, is to be avoided). Medicine is an activity that pursues health and seeks to eradicate disease. Thus, medicine itself is an activity that pursues a moral good. Any medical decision is a moral decision. This is presumed in every medical act, whether by a patient or medical professional. As most medical decisions have become routine, this moral underpinning often becomes explicit only in the difficult cases, especially when various and exclusive goods are presented or when there are particular evils that cannot all be avoided. Since health is not (and ought not to be) an absolute or highest good, some medical procedures can be deemed extraordinary for a number of reasons, whether due to the art of medicine itself (e.g., availability) or due to a patient's individual (e.g., spiritual, financial, or psychological) circumstances.

The language of "ordinary" and "extraordinary" often has different meanings for those involved in a medical decision than it does in its moral sense.[2] Physicians, for example, usually take these words to mean what is medically available or advisable, including the likelihood that a procedure will succeed, given a patient's medical condition, history, and prognosis. The long tradition of moral thinking about this topic, however, has given us a much broader understanding of "ordinary" as beneficial, useful, and not burdensome. "Extraordinary" has assumed the opposite meaning. For example, standard medical treatment for cancer might include a number of lengthy, painful, and financially costly options; only the patient and his family, however, under the guidance of experienced medical and moral advice, can determine whether this treatment is ordinary or extraordinary in the moral sense. To know this, the patient must judge prudently by incorporating into his decision the multitude of circumstances that affect them, some of which are external to the field of medicine.

Such decisions often fall to the health care proxy. We can say that in principle a treatment becomes morally extraordinary if it provides little or no physical benefit to the patient, if it is excessively stressful to the psyche, or if it is too expensive, painful, or otherwise burdensome. Medical expense can include costs to the patient, the family, and society at large. We must recall that death is not the end of life and that there is no obligation to preserve life at all costs. Some physical, mental, and financial burdens are beyond what any reasonable moral agent can be expected to endure. The patient is always free to pursue extraordinary means of treatment on his own volition, but the proxy has a duty to be wary of overtreatment at the expense of the patient's overall well-being. The proxy should favor extraordinary means of extending life only of the patient has clearly indicated that heroic measures should be taken.

The provision of food and water (nutrition and hydration) at the end of life, especially for those in reduced states of consciousness, has become a subject of increased attention in recent years. There are few cases in which nutrition and hydration (administered by whatever means, naturally or artificially) become extraordinary.[3] All living persons will die if sustenance is withheld from them, so its removal can almost never be for the benefit of a patient. The few cases in which nutrition and hydration may be licitly withheld arise when the harm caused by its administration is greater than the corresponding benefit. Reasonable factors in any consideration not to provide or to suspend the provision of nutrition and hydration are repeated local infections at the entry site, continued aspiration pneumonia, inability to assimilate fluids, and the desire to avoid using restraints in patients who pull out the tubes. The argument that patients with advanced dementia do not benefit from tube-feeding continues to be defended.[4]

In legitimate cases, the removal of nutrition and hydration is not intended to bring about the death of the patient but is a recognition that continued treatment causes more pain and illness than benefit. It should be kept in mind, however, that nutrition and hydration often bring comfort and relief from pain that a patient would otherwise experience at the end of life, and they generally should not be considered useless measures for the dying.

Problematic Directives

Many advance directives in common use today encourage or allow agents to reject ordinary means of preserving life. One popular version of such an advance directive is the *Five Wishes*.[5] It has been marketed nationally as a comprehensive, simply organized, legally binding means for a patient to name a health care proxy and lay out advance directives for future decision makers. Various options regarding medical treatment are listed, and the principal checks the appropriate boxes to indicate preferences and crosses out unwanted measures.

Five Wishes and documents like it typically fail to distinguish between morally licit and illicit medical treatments and decisions: every option is considered simply as the patient's choice, as if any decision is good so long as it has the autonomous agent as its source. Such a supposition conveys the moral relativism rejected in toto by the Church (and especially by Pope John Paul II). Examples abound in *Five Wishes*: a patient can choose to reject any life-saving treatment, including the most basic life-sustaining resources of food and water, if in a debilitated conscious state. Such a directive, then, can effectively instruct the patient's family and health care professionals to euthanize him—a gravely illicit act that any proxy would be morally obliged to reject.

A difficult question arises when an advance directive or a health care proxy requests a course of action that clearly conflicts with Catholic teaching. Patient directives that conflict with the values of the Catholic institution should not be followed, but the patient must be offered the opportunity for discharge in order to seek out another facility. The same difficulty may occur for individual Catholics who are asked to be health care proxies for those who do not follow the teachings of the Church. Those who are asked to serve as health care proxies must be morally certain that the directives they are asked to carry out are acceptable in conscience and Church teaching. Agreeing to carry out actions that are

contrary to sound ethics is typically a form of illicit cooperation with evil. A Catholic institution by its very nature commits itself to upholding these truths both in theory and (more importantly) in practice, and the charge of the ethics committee is often to decide the most difficult and challenging cases, in which the proper course of action is not entirely clear. If a patient or his proxy presents any request or advance directive that opposes these teachings, the hospital is under no obligation to fulfill it, given the hospital's prior commitment to moral medical practices and its proper vision of the human good.

Preserving Human Dignity

Many secular-minded individuals and institutions view the moral teachings of the Church as archaic, restrictive, and authoritarian. In an age when people are increasingly sympathetic to the siren call of the "death with dignity" movement, which promotes euthanasia, many hold a similar view of Church teachings on moral questions concerning the end of life. On the contrary, the Church seeks to understand, preserve, and protect the dignity of the human person at the end of life, knowing that the value of physical life is not the highest good. An act or omission that directly causes the death of a patient—even if requested by a proxy or in an advance directive—is morally illicit. Such an act violates the patient's personal dignity, the mission of the hospital, and goals and values of medicine itself.

Notes

[1] William E. May, *Catholic Bioethics and the Gift of Human Life*, 2nd ed. (Huntington, IN: Our Sunday Visitor, 2008), 303.

[2] Ibid., 277.

[3] For a brief list, see Congregation for the Doctrine of the Faith, "Responses to Certain Questions of the USCCB concerning Artificial Nutrition and Hydration" (August 1, 2007), reprinted in *Ethics & Medics* 32.11 (November 2007): 3.

[4] Peter J. Gummere, "Assisted Nutrition and Hydration in Advanced Dementia of the Alzheimer's Type: An Ethical Analysis," *NationalCatholic Bioethics Quarterly* 8.2 (Summer 2008): 291–305; Greg F. Burke, "Advanced Dementia," *Ethics & Medics* 26.3 (March 2001): 1–2.

[5] *Five Wishes* (Tallahassee, FL: Aging with Dignity, 2007). See Edward J. Furton, "A Critique of the *Five Wishes*: Comments in the Light of a Papal Statement," *Ethics & Medics* 30.3 (March 2005): 3–4.

✠

Editorial Summation: A health care proxy is an individual ("the agent") designated to decide what medical procedures should be undertaken if a patient ("the principal") becomes incapacitated or incompetent. An advance directive (or "living will") is a document signed by an individual that indicates wishes for medical treatment at the end of life should the patient be unable to express desires at that time. What medical treatments ought to be allowed or rejected is the primary moral question for any patient, proxy, or health care professional. We can say that in principle a treatment becomes morally extraordinary if it provides little or no physical benefit to the patient, if it is excessively stressful to the psyche, or if it is too expensive, painful, or otherwise burdensome. Nutrition and hydration often bring comfort from pain otherwise experienced at the end of life and generally should not be considered useless measures for the dying. Many advance directives in common use today encourage or allow agents to reject ordinary means of preserving life. Such directives can instruct the patient's family and health care professionals to euthanize—a gravely illicit act that any proxy would be morally obliged to reject. Patient directives that conflict with the values of the Catholic institution should not be followed, but the patient must be offered the opportunity for discharge in order to seek out another facility.

PART V

SELECTED CLINICAL ISSUES

Ethical Issues in Organ Donation and Transplantation

Marie T. Nolan, R.N.

The teachings of the Catholic Church have supported organ and tissue transplantation that is carried out in accordance with the moral law. Respect for life, human dignity, bodily integrity, and the desire to relieve suffering should guide transplantation care.

As early as 1956, Pope Pius XII addressed the ethics of transplantation. Speaking to a group of eye specialists, the Pope discussed the potential use of animal tissues, such as corneal tissue, as a source for human transplantation. Pius XII asserts that not every transplantation of tissues that is biologically possible between individuals of different species is morally wrong. But he also says that it is still less true that any heterogeneous transplantation which is "biologically possible is not forbidden or is not objectionable." He continues, "The transplantation of the sexual glands of an animal to man is to be rejected as immoral. On the contrary, the transplantation of a cornea from a nonhuman being to a human being would not raise any moral difficulty if it were biologically possible and were warranted."[1]

On November 24, 1957, addressing the International Congress of Anesthesiologists, Pius XII charged the group to clearly define death: "It remains for the doctor, and especially the anesthesiologist, to give a clear and precise definition of 'death' and the moment of 'death' of a patient who passes away in a state of unconsciousness."[2]

At a 1990 meeting of the Pontifical Academy of Sciences, Pope John Paul II again asked for "the exact moment and indisputable sign of death" for the purpose of removing organs for transplantation.[3] Acknowledging the shortage of available donors for patients awaiting transplantation, John Paul II explained that "'no solution will be forthcoming without a renewed sense of human solidarity' based on

Christ's example, which can 'inspire men and women to make great sacrifices in the service of others.'"[4]

The *Ethical and Religious Directives for Catholic Health Care Services* places important restrictions on the transplantation of tissues from living donors:

> The transplantation of organs from living donors is morally permissible when such a donation will not sacrifice or seriously impair any essential bodily function and the anticipated benefit to the recipient is proportionate to the harm done to the donor. Furthermore, the freedom of the prospective donor must be respected, and economic advantages should not accrue to the donor.[5]

Similar concern for the living donor is expressed in the *Catechism of the Catholic Church*:

> *Organ transplants* are in conformity with the moral law if the physical and psychological dangers and risks to the donor are proportionate to the good that is sought for the recipient. Organ donation after death is a noble and meritorious act and is to be encouraged as an expression of generous solidarity. It is not morally acceptable if the donor or his proxy has not given explicit consent. Moreover, it is not morally admissible directly to bring about the disabling mutilation or death of a human being, even in order to delay the death of other persons.[6]

Organ Procurement

Brain Death

Brain death is defined as the irreversible loss of function of the brain, including the brain stem.[7] (See chapter 12 above.) In a statement to participants in the

221

Eighteenth International Congress of the Transplantation Society, Pope John Paul II stated that

> the criterion adopted in more recent times for ascertaining the fact of death, namely the *complete* and *irreversible* cessation of all brain activity, if rigorously applied, does not seem to conflict with the essential elements of a sound anthropology. Therefore a health-worker professionally responsible for ascertaining death can use these criteria in each individual case as the basis for arriving at that degree of assurance in ethical judgment which moral teaching describes as "moral certainty."[8]

The danger in using brain death as a definition of death is that confusion remains about the clinical application of this concept. In an examination of the brain death protocols at fifty highly rated neurological centers in the United States, David Greer and his colleagues found great variability in the extent to which the institutional brain death protocols adhered to those recommended by the American Academy of Neurology.[9] For example, although AAN guidelines stipulated the involvement of a neurologist or a neurosurgeon in determining brain death, this was required in only 42 percent of the institutional guidelines for determining brain death.

Another problem in the application of brain death criteria is the risk involved in confirming this diagnosis. Many problems can occur during the apnea test which is done to determine whether the patient has spontaneous respiration. Arrhythmia, hypotension, and cardiac arrest are all potential side effects of the apnea test. One study found that of 129 patients diagnosed as brain dead, clinical problems occurred during the apnea test in more than two thirds.[10] These problems included arterial hypotension (12 percent), acidosis (68 percent), and hypoxemia (23 percent). Four patients developed major complications, including pneumothorax, cardiac arrest, bradycardia, atrial fibrillation, and myocardial infarction. The authors noted that apnea testing was not innocuous and recommended following AAN guidelines for conducting these tests.

Non-Heart-Beating Organ Donors

In 1992, the University of Pittsburgh Medical Center, one of the leading transplant centers in the United States, announced that it had developed a new protocol for obtaining organs from patients whose end-of-life care included a planned removal of life support.[11] Because the protocol called for retrieving organs two minutes after cardiac functioning ceased, the donors became known as "non-heart-beating donors." Similar non-heart-beating donor protocols have been adopted by transplant centers in the United States and Europe, some requiring longer periods of cardiac cessation prior to organ retrieval. However, these protocols have not been universally accepted. Some people view non-heart-beating donors as similar to anencephalic donors—persons who are dying but not dead.[12] The distinction in this case hinges on the irreversibility of the cardiac arrest. A review of conflicting views on this protocol is provided by Thomas Huddle and his colleagues.[13] They report that in the most recent evolution of these protocols, some institutions permit the use of extracorporeal membrane oxygenation (ECMO) prior to the death of the donor for the purpose of maintaining the individual's organs in the best possible condition for transplantation. The authors conclude that while they can accept non-heart-beating donor protocols that involve obtaining organs after cardiac functioning has permanently ceased, they view the use of ECMO as extending life and creating a situation in which organs are taken from the dying rather than the dead.

Canadian critical care specialists Christopher James Doig and Graeme Rocker called for a national moratorium on non-heart-beating donor protocols until Canadian citizens could more carefully examine ethical issues such as the use of ECMO, intravenous heparin, and even the placement of catheters directly into kidneys prior to the death of the anticipated organ donor.[14] They also noted that the separation of family from the patient at the time of death seemed to be the antithesis of quality end-of-life care and contributed to a loss of the dignity in the dying process.

Persons in a Persistent Vegetative State as Donors

Some have proposed using patients who are in a persistent vegetative state as organ donors. (See chapter 16C.) Elysa Koppelman suggests that to follow an advance directive to remove organs from a person in PVS is respecting the autonomy of the individual.[15] Robert Veatch calls the whole-brain oriented definition of death "old-fashioned" and suggests that, for human life to be present, integrated functioning of mind and body must be present.[16] He proposes allowing individuals to decide, through their advance directives or surrogate decision makers, whether to accept "whole brain" criteria for death (brain death) or whether to accept "higher brain death" criteria (PVS).[17] Lainie Ross, however, argues that persons in a PVS are living and therefore cannot donate, because of the requirement that living donors should experience some benefit from a donation, such as the satisfaction of helping a loved one.[18] She also argues that surrogate decision makers cannot designate a person in PVS as an organ donor, as this would violate the person's right to bodily integrity and the right to be respected as an individual and not as a means to an end.

Ethicist Jocelyn Downie notes the utilitarian appeal of using patients in a PVS as organ donors: "Thousands of organs could become available for those requiring transplantation to stay alive ... and we would not incur the cost of maintaining [patients in a PVS] for a number of years."[19] Nevertheless, she provides three compelling reasons for rejecting patients in a PVS as organ donors. First, the diagnosis of PVS is not reliable enough to prevent the possibility of a patient who is not in a PVS being mistakenly killed to obtain organs for transplantation. Second, "if we start off by killing of PVS patients in order to use their organs for transplantation, we will (because of psychological slippage) end up killing demented, handicapped, or otherwise vulnerable human beings for their organs." Third, designating patients in a PVS as dead will further confuse the public, contributing to fear that patients will not be dead before their organs are removed. It has been shown that this fear already exists and serves as a barrier to organ donation.[20]

Another negative consequence of using patients in a PVS as organ donors is cited by M. Keatings. He cautions that if we redesign death to include those patients in PVS, "this definition must be absolute, since it is not our practice to care for and nurture the dead."[21] Therefore, care would have to be withdrawn from all patients who are in PVS, not just those who indicated a desire to serve as organ donors.

Anencephalic Infants as Donors

The use of anencephalic infants as organ donors has also been proposed as a means to decrease the shortage of transplantable organs.[22] The Council on Ethical and Judicial Affairs of the American Medical Association once supported using anencephalic infants in this manner by stating, "It is normally required that a person be legally dead before removal of their life-necessary organs (the 'dead donor rule'). The use of the anencephalic neonate as a live donor is a limited exception to the general standard because of the fact that the infant has never experienced, and will never experience, consciousness."[23] D. Shewmon and colleagues countered this when they explained, "Whether those [anencephalic infants] with relatively intact brain stems have any subjective awareness associated with their responsiveness to the environment is inherently unverifiable, but what is known about the functional capabilities of the brain stem, particularly in newborns, suggests at least keeping an open mind."[24] The public outcry against

using anencephalic infants as sources of organs for transplantation was so great that the American Medical Association reversed its previous statement emphasizing that anencephalic infants must meet brain death criteria before becoming organ donors.[25]

D. Medearis and L. Holmes note important clinical features of anencephaly: "Evidence indicates that anencephaly is a heterogeneous condition anatomically and functionally, that the diagnosis of anencephaly cannot be made with sufficient accuracy, and that the condition cannot be distinguished well enough from other severe intracranial disorders to justify changing the law. Anencephalic infants are alive and the length of their lives cannot be predicted accurately."[26] A. Capron adds, "Classifying anencephalic infants as dead before they meet generally applicable standards is wrong beccause it denies their humanity and treats them solely as a means (without their consent) to others' ends."[27]

Since the natural cause of death in anencephaly is ultimately hypoventilation, which renders vital organs unsuitable for transplantation, ventilatory support is required until the infant deteriorates to the point of brain death.[28] Physicians at Loma Linda Hospital in California developed a protocol to provide this type of ventilatory support for anencephalic infants who were designated as potential organ donors.[29] When, after six months of the protocol, only two of twelve infants met the criteria for brain death, the protocol was suspended. Physicians in the Loma Linda protocol noted with amazement the number of infants with less severe anomalies referred to them as potential organ donors. These included infants with hydrocephaly and infants born without kidneys but with a normal brain. Dr. Joyce Peabody, chief of neonatology at Loma Linda said, "I have become educated by the experience. ... The slippery slope is real."[30]

Fetuses as Donors

The transplantation of tissue from fetuses was first undertaken in the 1980s and 1990s as a treatment for patients with Parkinson's disease, while later experiments included patients with Alzheimer's disease and diabetes.[31] In more recent years, fetal cell transplantation in Parkinson's disease is rarely performed, as controlled trials have failed to demonstrate positive outcomes.[32] Kim Moore and colleagues have noted that adult stem cells have been used as an effective substitute for tissue derived from the fetus or embryo and recommend further study with these adult cells, as there is no moral objection to their use.[33]

The Church clearly defines the moral status of the fetus when it describes "every human being's right to life and physical integrity from the moment of conception until death."[34] As with anencephalic infant donation, fetal tissue donation does not serve the good of the fetus. Neurosurgeon Dr. Keith Crutcher points out that some fetuses may still be alive when fetal brain tissue is removed, suggesting the possibility of a painful death.[35] The *Ethical and Religious Directives for Catholic Health Care Services* state, "Catholic health care institutions should not make use of human tissue obtained by direct abortions even for research and therapeutic purposes."[36] A detailed discussion of complicity with evil is provided by Judith Lee Kissell and Edmund Pellegrino.[37]

Minority Donors

African Americans, who make up 12 percent of the population of the United States, account for over 30 percent of the patients with end-stage renal disease. However, only 27 percent of cadaveric organ recipients and only 15 percent of living organ recipients are African American.[38] One reason for this disparity is an insufficient number of African American donors. Due to differences in HLA antigens, 20 percent of African Americans would have greater transplant success by having an African American donor.[39] Waiting times are long for the affected 20 percent of African Americans, because African Americans make up fewer than 10 percent of organ donors nationally.[40] One response to the disparity in organs available for African American donors has been living donation. Living related donations have greatly increased during the last decade to meet the demand for transplantation, which far outstrips the availability of organs from deceased donors.

Living Related Donors

In considering living related donation, a transplant team may be guided by the principles of beneficence, nonmaleficence, and autonomy. Clearly, the team is obligated to act for the good of the recipient, but what are their obligations toward the donor? Nonmaleficence directs health professionals to do no harm. Harm is minimized by selection criteria which require donors to be in a good state of health prior to donation. For example, a parent without a smoking history was chosen over a parent with a smoking history for partial lung donation.[41] Despite these precautions, however, donors incur some risks. The mortality for renal donors was reported as 0.06 percent, while the mortality associated with liver donation was estimated as 0.8 percent.[42] Also, because of limited follow-up studies, much is not known about the risks to living organ donors. For example, regarding living kidney donation, follow-up studies had small sample sizes, did not adequately account for donors who were reported as lost to follow-up, and did not measure health status before the transplant surgery. Therefore, studies were not designed to measure the change in the health status of individual donors from before the transplant surgery to after.[43]

Benedict Ashley, O.P., and Kevin O'Rourke, O.P., propose four criteria which should be met prior to permitting living donation:

- There is a serious need on the part of the recipient that cannot be fulfilled in any other way.

- The functional integrity of the donor as a human person will not be impaired, even though anatomical integrity may suffer.

- The risk taken by the donor as an act of charity is proportionate to the good resulting for the recipient.

- The donor's consent is free and informed.[44]

Donors should be informed not only of the risks for physical harm but also the risks for psychological harm. S. Russell and R. Jacob described two suicides and one suicide attempt among renal donors who became despondent following the graft rejection and death of the organ recipients. They also describe several cases where the spouses of donors were upset by the donation, "as if giving an organ to someone outside of the nuclear family threatened its boundaries."[45] Health professionals who work closely with families, donors, and recipients during the recovery period should assess psychological distress relating to the transplant. Psychiatric intervention prior to and after transplantation should be provided if it appears that donors or their families are experiencing any psychological turmoil.

Ensuring that a potential donor is free from coercion may be difficult. N. Scheper-Hughes notes that family members may be made to feel guilty if they do not donate and that this pressure can come from other family members or from transplant professionals.[46] In fact, Scheper-Hughes reports that the desire to avoid coercing family members to donate has led some transplant recipients to travel to underdeveloped nations to illegally purchase kidneys for donation.

Concerning liver transplantation, R. Busuttil asked, "How can a parent be expected to make an informed, uncoerced, free choice when asked to consider donating an organ to his or her dying child?"[47] A. Dennison and colleagues stated that directly approaching a potential donor should not be permitted unless the recipient is critically ill and in urgent need of transplantation.[48] They propose that the family should be informed of the donor problem and the transplant team should then await a spontaneous volunteer.

Some have supported the concept of an advocate to protect the donor's interests.[49] Arthur Caplan resolves the tension between the autonomy of the person who chooses to donate an organ and the desire of the transplant team to avoid donor harm by advising "transplant centers [to] make sure that unreasonable risks are not presented to those who could not possibly refuse to accept them lest they see themselves as failing their moral duties to families or friends."[50]

The Impact of Scientific Developments on Organ Procurement

Since the number of organs available for transplantation is not sufficient to meet the growing demand, we are obligated to continue to seek out other ways to restore health to persons with organ failure. Each issue of *The International Journal of Artificial Organs* provides new research concerning the development of artificial means to replace organs. Also, refinement in surgical techniques may make some transplants unnecessary. For example, the number of heart transplantations needed could decrease if partial left ventricular resection, dynamic cardiomyoplasty, and left ventricular assist devices continue to be advanced as successful alternatives. Annette Vegas provides an overview of the most recent pharmacologic, surgical, and mechanical alternatives to heart transplantation.[51]

Innovations in preserving organs after death may increase the number of organs available for transplantation. T. Hauet and M. Eugene review the role of new molecules such as polyethylene glycol in preserving organs.[52] These innovations result in successful transplantation after longer ischemic times. One investigator has reported success in using hearts from non-heart-beating donors in an animal study.[53] Although it is difficult to estimate the potential impact, some families may consent to donation from a non-heart-beating family member more readily than they would from a brain-dead family member.

Finally, advancements in cellular therapy hold promise for curing illnesses previously treatable only with transplantation. In 1994, investigators first demonstrated that by transplanting adult mouse liver cells into mice with failing livers, up to 80 percent of the liver can be regenerated.[54] Scientists continue to explore cell therapy for liver disease with the hope of eliminating the need for liver transplants.[55]

Organ Allocation

Severity of Illness

In the United States the current method of determining the order of patients on waiting lists for a cadaveric donor takes into consideration the patient's severity of illness and predicted mortality.[56] Giving priority to more critically ill patients is viewed by some as an injudicious use of a scarce health care resource, because more critically ill patients have higher mortality rates after transplantation. For example, G. Mudge and colleagues reported that critically ill heart-transplant patients have an operative mortality rate of 14 percent compared with 6 percent for transplant patients in stable condition prior to surgery.[57]

Culpability of the Recipient

In the case of liver transplantation, some support transplanting the most critically ill patient but would give a lower priority to patients who acquired their end-stage liver disease through alcoholism. Initially, alcoholics may have been excluded from liver-transplant programs because of a belief that a high rate of relapse would be inevitable and survival limited. In contrast, T. Starzl and others reported that survival rates of liver transplant patients with alcohol-related end-stage liver disease were no different than those of patients with end-stage liver disease from other causes.[58] Nevertheless, A. Moss and M. Siegler argue that "it is only fair that patients who have not assumed equal responsibility for maintaining their health ... should be treated differently."[59] The authors also point out that since alcoholism is present in all socioeconomic levels, it is not discrimination against the poor when patients with alcohol-related liver disease are left off the list. T. Killeen counters this by asserting that patients from lower socioeconomic strata with alcohol-related liver disease are at a greater disadvantage because of an inability to afford treatment for their disorder.[60]

C. Cohen and M. Benjamin also argue against penalizing those with alcohol-related end-stage liver disease by stating, "We could rightly preclude alcoholics from transplantation only if we assume that qualification for a new organ requires some level of moral virtue."[61] The authors note that we do not attempt to determine whether transplant candidates are abusive parents, cheat on their income tax, or lie. Because it would be impossible to fairly judge the moral character of all in need of a transplant, Cohen and Benjamin suggest that it is fair to treat all in need of scarce resources by the same standard. "Public confidence in medical practice in general, and in organ transplantation in particular, depends on the scientific validity and moral integrity of the policies adopted."[62]

Efficacy

Retransplantation

Another challenge to the policy of giving the most severely ill patients priority in transplantation arises when a patient is in need of a second or third transplant. A study of cardiac transplant patients at Stanford University Hospital over a nearly thirty-year period revealed an 8 percent rate of re-transplantation.[63] The authors, who include cardiac transplant surgeons, noted that although the survival rate of patients undergoing re-transplantation was lower than that of patients undergoing their first transplantation, the surgeons felt conflicted between their desire to not abandon a patient who needed a second transplant and the desire to promote distributive justice so that others waiting for a heart transplant had a chance at this life-saving procedure.

P. Ubel and colleagues note that 10 to 20 percent of hearts and livers donated for transplantation are used for re-transplantation.[64] They cite three issues which affect the decision to have a patient undergo two or more transplantations: first, the obligation of the team not to abandon patients on whom they have already performed a transplant; second, the fairness of allowing patients to get multiple transplants while others die awaiting their first; and third, the difference in efficacy between primary transplantation and re-transplantation. They dismiss the transplant team's obligation not to abandon a transplant patient as feelings of attachment which should not alter allocation priorities.

While they make an important point, that allocation of scarce resources should not be based on emotion, they may not have given proper weight to the obligation of the transplant team to act for the good of the patient. Patients rightly expect that their physician or nurse will act for their good and not as a double agent acting on behalf of all of society. With their obligation to a particular patient in mind, it is understandable that a team may seek a second, third, or additional transplant if to do so would benefit their patient.

On the issue of fairness, Ubel and colleagues hold that allowing only one transplant per person requires a very narrow view of health care. They point out that other factors affect health, such as income, education, and access to primary care, and these are not fairly distributed among transplant patients. They conclude that only the difference in efficacy justifies giving preference to primary recipi-

ents. In the United States, primary liver transplantation recipients have a five-year survival rate of 67 percent, compared with 46 percent for those receiving a repeat liver transplant. Recipients receiving their first heart transplant have a five-year survival rate of 72 percent, compared with 58 percent for those receiving a repeat heart transplant.[65] Ubel and colleagues conclude that if we are to continue to limit access to transplants by referring to factors related to efficacy, such as blood type, we must also consider the decreased efficacy of retransplantation as justification for limiting access to transplantation.

Futility

One final concern regarding the efficacy of transplantation deals with the dilemma of when to stop treatment. It is generally assumed that patients who consent to transplantation are consenting to an aggressive venture. Although the science of transplantation has advanced rapidly in the past decade, some problems remain insurmountable. Informed consent is routinely obtained from patients at the outset of transplantation. It is less frequently confirmed throughout the transplant experience.

One mother recounted the experience of her thirteen-year-old daughter undergoing bone-marrow transplantation. While she and her daughter had hopes for a cure at the start of her treatment, in the end, their hopes were unrealized. The side effects, setbacks, and disappointments led this mother to write after her daughter's death, "Consumers of health services generally believe doctors honor their own code 'to do no harm.' It is my contention that the failure rate in bone-marrow transplants does not merit this assumption by consumers."[66]

Sensitivity and immediate attention to the amelioration of side effects can help make the transplant experience more tolerable. But respect and support should be given to the patient who chooses to stop treatment.

Health professionals who practice in the area of transplantation will continue to experience sorrow in the loss of patients awaiting transplantation who die for lack of donor organs, and joy in helping those who live. However, respect for the life and bodily integrity of all persons will help caregivers avoid treating persons as a means to an end and to act for the good of all who come under their care.

Transplantation Tourism

The practice of persons from wealthy countries traveling to poor countries to purchase organs is known as transplantation tourism. This practice is becoming more prevalent as organ donations in wealthy countries are not matching the demands. For example, in 2006, foreigners received two thirds of the two thousand kidneys transplanted in Pakistan.[67] In response to the growing practice of buying organs for transplant internationally, scientists, health professionals, and representatives of transplant societies from countries all over the world, including the Vatican, met in Istanbul, Turkey, in May 2008. The *Declaration of Istanbul on Organ Trafficking and Transplant Tourism*, which was issued by this group, calls on all nations to develop a legal and ethical framework to guide organ transplantation and prevent the exploitation of the vulnerable. In the United States, it is illegal to pay a donor for an organ or otherwise coerce an individual to donate an organ. The declaration also calls for transplantation practices that ensure informed consent of donors, adequate follow-up care for donors, and a fair and equitable distribution of organs for transplantation.

Notes

[1] Pius XII, "Tissue Transplantation," in *The Human Body*, ed. Monks of Solesmes (Boston: St. Paul Editions, 1960), 374.

[2] Pius XII, Address to International Congress of Anesthesiologists (November 24, 1957), in *The Pope Speaks* 4.4 (Spring 1958): 393–398.

[3] John Paul II, "Discourse to the Working Group," in *Working Group on the Determination of Brain Death and Its Relationship to Human Death*, eds. R.J. White, H. Angstwurm, and I. Carrasco de Paula (Vatican City: Pontifical Academy of Sciences, 1989), 10–14.

[4] John Dietzen, "The Church's Position on Organ Donations," *Catholic Review*, November 3, 2005, A11.

[5] U.S. Conference of Catholic Bishops, *Ethical and Religious Directives for Catholic Health Care Services*, 4th ed. (Washington, D.C.: USCCB, 2001), n. 30.

[6] *Catechism of the Catholic Church*, 2nd ed., trans. U.S. Conference of Catholic Bishops (Vatican City: Libreria Editrice Vaticana, 1997), n. 2296 (original emphasis).

[7] For a thorough description of its diagnosis, see Quality Standards Subcommittee of the American Academy of Neurology, "Practice Parameters for Determining Brain Death in Adults," *Neurology* 45.5 (May 1995): 10112–1014, and E.F. Wijdicks, "Determining Brain Death in Adults," *Neurology* 45.5 (May 1995): 1003–1011.

[8] John Paul II, Address to the 18th International Congress of the Transplantation Society (August 29, 2000), n. 5 (original emphasis).

[9] David M. Greer et al., "Variability of Brain Death Determination Guidelines in Leading U.S. Neurologic Institutions," *Neurology* 70.4 (2008): 284–289.

[10] Gustavo Saposnik et al., "Problems Associated with the Apnea Test in the Diagnosis of Brain Death," *Neurology India* 52.3 (2004): 342–345.

[11] M.A. Devita, "Development of the University of Pittsburgh Medical Center Policy for the Care of Terminally Ill Patients Who May Become Organ Donors after Death following the Removal of Life Support," *Kennedy Institute Ethics* 3.2 (June 1993): 131–143.

[12] See David Wainwright Evans, "Seeking an Ethical and Legal Way of Procuring Transplantable Organs from the Dying without Further Attempts to Redefine Human Death," *Philosophy, Ethics, and Humanities in Medicine* 2, article 11 (June 29, 2007), http://www.peh-med.com/content/2/1/11, and Michael Potts, "Truthfulness in Transplantation: Non-Heart-Beating Organ Donation," *Philosophy, Ethics, and Humanities in Medicine* 2, article 17 (August 24, 2007), http://www.peh-med.com/content/2/1/17.

[13] Thomas Huddle et al., "Death, Organ Transplantation and Medical Practice," *Philosophy, Ethics, and Humanities in Medicine* 3.5 (February 4, 2008).

[14] Christopher James Doig and Graeme Rocker, "Retrieving Organs from Non-Heart-Beating Organ Donors: A Review of Medical and Ethical Issues," *Canadian Journal of Anesthesia* 50 (2003): 1069–1076.

[15] Elysa Koppelman, "The Dead Donor Rule and the Concept of Death: Severing the Ties That Bind Them," *American Journal of Bioethics* 3.1 (Winter 2003): 1–9.

[16] Robert M. Veatch, "The Impending Collapse of the Whole-Brain Definitions of Death" *Hastings Center Report* 23.4 (July–August 1993): 18–24.

[17] Robert M. Veatch, "Abandon the Dead Donor Rule or Change the Definition of Death?" *Kennedy Institute of Ethics* 14.3 (September 2004): 261–276.

[18] Lainie Friedman Ross, "Should a PVS Patient be a Live Organ Donor?" *Medical Ethics* 13.1 (Winter 2006): 3.

[19] Jocelyn Downie, "The Biology of the Persistent Vegetative State: Legal, Ethical, and Philosophical Implications for Transplantation," *Transplantation Proceedings* 22.3 (June 1990): 995–996.

[20] José Maria Dominguez-Roldán et al., "Psychological Aspects Leading to Refusal of Organ Donation in Southwest Spain," *Transplantation Proceedings* 24.1 (February 1992): 25–26.

[21] M. Keatings, "The Biology of the Persistent Vegetative State, Legal and Ethical Implications for Transplantation: Viewpoints from Nursing," *Transplantation Proceedings* 22.3 (June 1990): 998.

[22] R.D. Troug and J.C. Fletcher, "Anencephalic Newborns: Can Organs Be Transplanted Before Brain Death?" *New England Journal of Medicine* 321.6 (August 10, 1989): 388–391.

[23] Council on Ethical and Judicial Affairs report for the American Medical Association, "The Use of Anencephalic Neonates as Organ Donors," CEJA report 5–I94 (December 1994), http://www.ama-assn.org/ama1/pub/upload/mm/369/ceja_5i94.pdf.

[24] D. A. Shewmon et al., "The Use of Anencephalic Infants as Organ Sources: A Critique," *Journal of the American Medical Association* 261.12 (March 24, 1989): 1776.

[25] Anna Schlotzhauer and Bryan A. Liang, "Definitions and Implications of Death," *Hematological Oncology Clinics of North America* 16.6 (December 2002): 1397–1413.

[26] D. N. Medearis Jr. and L. B. Holmes, "On the Use of Anencephalic Infants as Organ Donors," *New England Journal of Medicine* 321.6 (August 10, 1989): 393.

[27] Alexander Capron, "The Criteria for Determining Brain Death Should Not Be Revised to Place Anencephalic Infants into the Category of Dead Bodies," *Journal of Heart and Lung Transplantation* 12.6 (1993) S375.

[28] Shewmon et al., "Use of Anencephalic Infants."

[29] Joyce L. Peabody, J. R. Emery, and S. Ashwal, "Experience with Anencephalic Infants as Prospective Organ Donors," *New England Journal of Medicine* 321.6 (August 10, 1989): 344–350.

[30] Shewmon et al., "Use of Anencephalic Infants," 1775.

[31] L. M. Sanders, L. Giudice, and T. A. Raffin, "Ethics of Fetal Tissue Transplantation," *Western Journal of Medicine* 159.3 (September 1993): 400–407.

[32] G. Miller, "Parkinson's Disease: Signs of Disease in Fetal Transplants," *Science* 320.5873 (April 11, 2008): 167.

[33] Kim Moore, Jeanette F. Mills, and Melissa M. Thorton, "Alternative Sources of Adult Stem Cells: A Possible Solution to the Embryonic Stem Cell Debate," *Gender Medicine* 3.3 (September 2006): 161–168.

[34] *Catechism of the Catholic Church*, n. 2273.

[35] Keith Crutcher, "Fetal Tissue Research: The Cutting Edge?" *Linacre Quarterly* 60.2 (May 1993): 10–19.

[36] USCCB, *Ethical and Religious Directives*, n. 66.

[37] See Judith Lee Kissel, "Cooperation with Evil: Its Contemporary Relevance," *Linacre Quarterly* 62 (February 1995): 33–45, and Edmund Pellegrino, "Cooperation, Moral Complicity, and Moral Distance: The Ethics of Forensic, Penal, and Military Medicine," *International Journal of Law and Ethics* 2 (1993): 373–391.

[38] Laura Siminoff, R. H. Lawrence, and R. M. Arnold, "Comparison of Black and White Families' Experiences and Perceptions regarding Organ Donation Requests," *Critical Care Medicine* 31.1 (2003): 146–151.

[39] N. N. Reitz and C. O. Callender, "Organ Donation in the African-American Population: A Fresh Perspective with a Simple Solution," *Journal of the National Medical Association* 85.5 (May 1993): 353–358.

[40] M. K. Norris, "Disparities for Minorities in Transplantation: The Challenge to Critical Care Nurses," *Heart and Lung* 20.4 (July 1991): 419–420.

[41] S. A. Kirchner, "Living Related Lung Transplantation: A New Dimension in Single Lung Transplantation," *AORN Journal* 54.4 (October 1991): 703–714.

[42] R. M. Ghobrial, "Donor Morbidity after Living Donation for Liver Transplantation," *Gastroenterology* 135.2 (August 2008): 468–476.

[43] Marie T. Nolan et al., "Living Kidney Donor Decision Making: State of the Science and Directions for Future Research," *Progress in Transplantation* 14.3 (September 2004): 201–209.

[44] Benedict M. Ashley and Kevin D. O'Rourke, *Health Care Ethics: A Theological Analysis*, 4th ed. (Washington, D.C.: Georgetown University Press, 1997), 334 (original emphasis).

[45] S. Russell and R. G. Jacob, "Living Related Organ Donation: The Donor's Dilemma," *Patient Education and Counseling* 21.1–2 (June 1993): 92.

[46] Nancy Scheper-Hughes, "The Tyranny of the Gift: Sacrificial Violence in Living Donor Transplants," *American Journal of Transplantation* 7.3 (March 2007): 507–511.

[47] R. W. Busuttil, "Living-Related Liver Donation: Con," *Transplantation Proceedings* 23.1 (February 1991), pt.1: 44.

[48] A. R. Dennison, D. Azoulay, and G. J. Maddern, "Living Related Hepatic Donation: Prometheus or Pandora's Box?" *Australian New Zealand Journal of Surgery* 63.11 (November 1993): 835–839.

[49] Connie L. Davis and Francis L. Delmonico, "Living-Donor Kidney Transplantation: A Review of Current Practices for the Live Donor," *American Society of Nephrology* 16 (2005): 2098–2110.

[50] Arthur Caplan, "Must I Be My Brother's Keeper? Ethical Issues in the Use of Living Donors as Sources of Liver and Other Solid Organs," *Transplantation Proceedings* 25.2 (April 1993): 1999.

[51] Annette Vegas, "Assisting the Failing Heart," *Anesthesiology Clinics* 26.3 (September 2008): 539–564.

[52] T. Hauet and M. Eugene, "A New Approach in Organ Preservation: Potential Role of New Polymers," *Kidney International* 74.8 (October 2008): 998–1003.

[53] R. W. Illes et al., "Recovery of Nonbeating Donor Hearts," *Journal of Heart and Lung Transplantation* 14.3 (May–June 1995): 553–561.

[54] Johnathon A. Rhim et al., "Replacement of Diseased Mouse Liver by Hepatic Cell Transplantation," *Science* 263 (February 25, 1994): 1149.

[55] Philippe A. Lysy et al., "Stem Cells for Liver Tissue Repair: Current Knowledge and Perspectives," *World Journal of Gastroenterology* 14.6 (February 14, 2008): 864–875.

[56] G. Santori et al., "Potential Predictive Value of the Meld Score for Short-Term Mortality after Liver Transplantation," *Transplantation Proceedings* 36.3 (2004): 533–534.

[57] G. H. Mudge, "Twenty-fourth Bethesda Conference: Cardiac Transplantation. Task Force 3: Recipient Guidelines/ Prioritization," *Journal of the American College of Cardiology* 22.1 (July 1993): 21–31.

[58] T. E. Starzl et al., "Orthotopic Liver Transplantation for Alcoholic Cirrhosis," *Journal of the American Medical Association* 260.17 (November 4, 1998): 2542–2544.

[59] A. H. Moss and M. Siegler, "Should Alcoholics Compete Equally for Liver Transplantation?" *Journal of the American Medical Association* 265.10 (March 13, 1991): 1298.

[60] Theresa K. Killeen, "Alcoholism and Liver Transplantation: Ethical and Nursing Implications," *Perspectives in Psychiatric Care* 29.1 (January–March 1993): 7–12.

[61] C. Cohen and M. Benjamin, "Alcoholics and Liver Transplantations," *Journal of the American Medical Association* 265.10 (March 13, 1991): 1299.

[62] Ibid., 1301.

[63] S. A. Hunt et al., "A Single Center Experience with Heart Retransplantation: The 29 Year Experience at a Single Institution," in *Retransplantation: Proceedings of the 29th Conference on Transplantation and Clinical Immunology,* eds. J. L. Touraine et al. (Dordrecht, The Netherlands: Kluwer Academic, 1997), 229–228.

[64] Peter A. Ubel, Robert M. Arnold, and Arthur L. Caplan, "Rationalizing Failure: The Ethical Lessons of the Retransplantation of Scarce Vital Organs," in *The Ethics of Organ Transplantation*, eds. Arthur L. Caplan and Daniel H. Coelho (Amherst, NY: Prometheus Books, 1998), 260–274.

[65] Percentages based on the Organ Procurement Transplant Network (OPTN) data as of October 31, 2008.

[66] S. G. Connell, "An Experimental Bone Marrow Transplant Experience," *Transplantation Proceedings* 22.3 (June 1990): 956.

[67] International Summit on Transplant Tourism and Organ Trafficking, "The Declaration of Istanbul on Organ Trafficking and Transplant Tourism," *Clinical Journal of the American Society of Nephrology* 3.5 (September 2008): 1227–1231.

Editorial Summation: The teachings of the Catholic Church have supported organ and tissue transplantation carried out in accordance with the moral law. Respect for life, human dignity, and bodily integrity and the desire to relieve suffering should guide transplantation care. At a 1990 meeting of the Pontifical Academy of Sciences, Pope John Paul II again asked for "the exact moment and indisputable sign of death" for the purpose of removing organs for transplantation. Ashley and O'Rourke state, "When the whole brain is dead, the person is dead, since the organ that is the source of unified activity no longer functions, even though there may still be signs of residual cellular activity in the brain and other parts of the body." The *Ethical and Religious Directives for Catholic Health Care Services* place important restrictions on the transplantation of tissues from living donors. A living organ donation should not jeopardize the donor's essential bodily functions, and harm to the donor should be proportionate to the benefit to the recipient. Also, the donor's freedom must be respected, and there should be no economic benefit for the donor. A number of sources have been proposed for organ donation, but each has reasons for and against its use: patients in a persistent vegetative state, those with anencephaly, human fetuses, living related and unrelated persons, and deceased persons. Ashley and O'Rourke propose four criteria which should be met prior to permitting living donation: (1) serious need, (2) no loss of functional integrity of donor, (3) risk to donor proportionate to good to recipient, and (4) free and informed consent of donor. A major issue is that of allocation. There are more requests for organs than there are organs available. Several factors must be equitably balanced. Among these are urgency, efficacy, and the health status and prognosis of the recipient.

CHAPTER 19

Vaccination Refusals

Edward J. Furton

A common problem faced by the physician is immunization refusals, especially by parents on behalf of their children. The decision often places the health of the children at risk and weakens the general immunity of the public at large to commonly transmitted diseases. Typically, parents either have reservations about the risk of an adverse reaction in their child or they have moral concerns about vaccines that have an association with past abortions. At other times, vaccines associated with sexual promiscuity are refused because they are judged to be a poor substitute for chastity and sexual restraint. This article will examine the moral issues connected with these concerns, arguing that the risk of adverse reaction is the price that society must pay for the enormous benefits that derive from immunization; that immunization with vaccines derived from cell lines that originated in abortion is acceptable because of the distant character of that association; and that the use of vaccinations to prevent the spread of sexually transmitted diseases is morally acceptable but should not be mandated by law.

Justice and the Risks of Adverse Reaction

Immunization against disease has been one of the most effective medical advances of the twentieth century. Consider rubella (German measles). This disease is usually mild in children, causing a rash on the face and neck that lasts only two or three days. Teenagers and young adults may also experience swollen glands in the back of the neck and some swelling and stiffness in the joints. Most recover quickly from these symptoms without any aftereffects. The primary danger of harm from rubella is to the unborn. A woman who contracts rubella in the early stages of her pregnancy has a significant chance

of miscarrying or giving birth to a deformed baby. The Centers for Disease Control and Prevention estimate that mothers infected with rubella have a 20 percent chance of giving birth to a child with defects.[1] Birth defects range from deafness, blindness (atrophic eyes, cataracts, chorioretinitis), and damaged hearts to unusually small brains and mental retardation.

The purpose of vaccinating young children against rubella, therefore, is not simply to protect against the discomfort of a fairly mild childhood disease, but to prevent the unborn children of pregnant women from suffering serious birth defects or death through contact with those who are infected. Children who are immune to rubella generally cannot spread the disease to others, although it is important to realize that one who is vaccinated can still sometimes be infected.[2] A vaccinated girl who attains adulthood will also be protected against contracting this disease and transmitting it to her unborn child. The closer society comes to universal immunization against a particular disease, such as rubella, the smaller the danger of an outbreak in the future.

Thanks to the efforts of primary care physicians and public health officials, rubella has been virtually eliminated in the United States. The last large-scale outbreak occurred in 1964, when almost twenty thousand babies were born with birth defects.[3] Today the possibility of such devastation is much reduced, although given the global nature of the world economy, the reintroduction of a disease into a previously uninfected community always remains a possibility. When individuals refuse immunizations, they increase the chances for a return of the disease, and every new refusal increases the odds again. Various areas of the United States have suffered recent resurgences of epidemic disease because of parental refusals to vaccinate their children.[4]

Some parents believe that their children can avoid the minimal risks associated with immunization and still enjoy the benefits of "herd immunity," that is, the safety that comes from living in a community that is generally immunized. Such reasoning runs counter to the virtue of justice. Among the cardinal virtues, justice alone is directed toward the good of others.[5] The equality of our human nature obliges each of us to respect the right to life and health that belongs to each and every other human being. Therefore, the primary reason why we should use vaccines is for the general protection of society. Those who refuse immunizations without good reason harm the common good. For Catholics, this is especially problematic in the case of rubella, because rubella primarily afflicts the unborn. If the Church recognizes any distinction in justice among our fellow citizens at all, it is that preference ought to be given to the weakest and most vulnerable among us. Those who are unborn, and subject to the possibility of contracting a devastating disease while in the womb, are special members of this class.

Every immunization carries with it some measure of risk for an adverse reaction. These reactions can be severe in some cases, but the chances of a severe reaction occurring are small. Nonetheless, in those cases where there is good medical evidence of increased probability of an adverse reaction, caution—and sometimes outright refusal—may indeed be appropriate.[6] For the average person, however, the minimal risks do not justify refusal. The claim that some vaccines are responsible for autism and other serious childhood diseases have not been confirmed in the scientific literature. The signs of autism typically show themselves at about the same age when many childhood vaccines are given, leading some understandably anxious parents to accept the fallacy of *post hoc, ergo propter hoc* (literally, "after this, therefore because of this"). The incidence of autism has grown significantly in recent years and its cause is unknown, but the fact that one event follows another in the order of time is not evidence that the earlier event is the cause of the other. Until there is definitive evidence, these associations remain speculative.

Associations with Abortion

Another reason for refusal is the well-established fact that many vaccines in common use today are grown in cell lines that had their origin in aborted fetal tissue.[7] For example, the two cell lines commonly used to manufacture the vaccine for immunization against varicella, MRC-5 and WI-38, were both derived from procured abortions. In some cases, the virus itself that is grown in the cell culture has been derived from an aborted fetus. Such was the case with the rubella virus strain RA 27/3, which was taken from an aborted child infected with rubella.[8] These are tragic and regrettable facts, and even more distressing is that we can expect scientific researchers to continue to use the remains of deliberately destroyed human beings as biological material in future research.[9] Every effort should be made to ensure that all future products for general medical use are not compromised by immoral origins. Open and repeated pleas to the scientific community for a change in these practices have been ignored. The current vaccine against varicella was produced using not one but two compromised cell lines, long after complaints were expressed by those who oppose the intentional destruction of human life.

The problem of using material that has any connection with abortion is addressed in the *Ethical and Religious Directives for Catholic Health Care Services* in directive 66: "Catholic health care institutions should not make use of human tissue obtained by direct abortions even for research and therapeutic purposes."[10] Although the cell lines MRC-5 and WI-38 are not themselves aborted tissue, but are cells grown in culture that descend from a past abortion, this does not seem to be a relevant distinction for the *Directives*. Clearly, these lines are "human tissue" and "obtained by direct abortion." Thus they and other cell lines produced from deliberately destroyed human beings would be inappropriate for research use in Catholic health care facilities. The same is true of the use of embryonic stem cell lines derived from the destruction of human embryos.[11] Embryo destruction is not the same as abortion, but it is nonetheless the moral equivalent. Each involves the direct taking of human life. Thankfully, the rise of alternative and more promising sources of these pluripotent stem cells have made this question moot for all but the most dogmatic champions of embryo destruction.[12]

A Catholic parent who is asked to immunize a child with one of these products is in a very different situation from that of the researcher. The vaccine presented to the parent has been manufactured using the problematic cell line, removed from that medium, purified, and offered for routine use in health care. The parent is not responsible for the research that created the problematic cell line, nor is he or she responsible for the decision of the manufacturer to use that line in the production of the vaccine. In those cases where there is no alternative available on the market, it is generally acceptable for Catholic parents to use the vaccine to immunize their children against a serious disease.[13] Parents should ask for alternatives when these are available, and Catholic physicians and health care facilities should keep these alternatives in stock for patient use, but immunization with this product does not signal approval of how it was manufactured, nor does it promote the further spread of the insidious idea that aborted tissues are appropriate materials for use in scientific research. Indeed, parents have an ideal opportunity on these occasions to express their opposition to this idea when speaking with their family physician.

The Pontifical Academy for Life (PAV), an advisory body to the Holy See, has emphasized the importance of making one's objections known in connection with these products, but it has also stated that, even though the use of these vaccines does involve some measure of material cooperation in the evil of abortion, the degree of cooperation is sufficiently small—and the benefits from immunization sufficiently great—to justify their use until such time as an alternative is made available.[14] The PAV expresses its concern that "the use of such vaccines contributes in the creation of a generalized social consensus to the operation of pharmaceutical industries which produce them in an immoral way."[15] Nonetheless, it holds that when the risks to the health of children, and to the general population as a whole, are appreciable, it is appropriate to use them:

> The moral reason is that the moral duty to avoid passive material cooperation is not obligatory if there is grave inconvenience. Moreover, we find, in such a case, a proportionate reason, in order to accept the use of these vaccines in the presence of the danger of favoring the spread of the pathological agent, due to the lack of vaccination in children. This is particularly true in the case of German measles [rubella].[16]

In a strongly worded footnote, the PAV adds that parents who refuse vaccination in the case of rubella bear some moral responsibility for the fetal defects and abortions that follow from the contraction of this serious disease.[17] The clear implication of the PAV document is that use is permissible, but that our willingness must vary according to the seriousness of the disease. Thus, the recently produced vaccine against varicella—given its less serious implications and more odious production—would appear to offer more reasonable grounds for refusal than the vaccines offered against rubella.

In recent years, there have been efforts to claim a general "Catholic" exemption from all immunization with products that have a distant association with abortion, on the grounds that the teaching authority of the Catholic Church opposes this use. There is no specific doctrinal teaching of the Church on this matter. The *Catechism of the Catholic Church*, for example, does not speak to this or any other specific medical question. Parents, therefore, cannot claim a "religious" exemption on specifically Catholic grounds. They can, at best, claim a general right to follow the Church's teaching on the inviolability of conscience. The Church holds that we have a moral obligation to follow conscience even when it errs, but the exercise of conscience should not be confused with a claim to an exemption. For example, an exemption to a school policy that obliges parents to vaccinate their children prior to admission is not implied by the exercise of conscience.[18] Parents who refuse to vaccinate their children exercise their right of conscience, and do so freely, even if their children are subsequently denied an exemption. School administrators must also follow their consciences and look to the health and well-being of all their students. In such cases, they may legitimately decide to refuse an exemption to children who are not properly immunized.

Vaccination for Sexually Transmitted Diseases

A different conclusion must be reached concerning state mandates for vaccination for human papillomavirus and other sexually transmitted diseases. The use of the HPV vaccine can be an effective means of reducing the rate of cervical cancer among women. Its use does not signal that a young woman is destined to engage in sexually inappropriate conduct. One who is chaste and enters into marriage may still contract HPV as a result of a spouse's prior sexual activity. Also, and tragically, there are women and girls who are sexually assaulted. Nonetheless, despite these considerations, it would be wrong to use the power of the state to compel parents to have their children immunized against HPV contrary to their own best judgment.

Parents are being asked to draw a parallel between vaccinations against diseases such as rubella and a new line of vaccines that will protect their children against various sexually transmitted diseases. But are these two cases the same? To mandate immunization against rubella makes perfect sense. We have a duty to ensure that we are not the cause of harm to others. This is a duty under the principle of justice, as noted above. Coughing or sneezing is an involuntary activity that may happen on a public bus, in a school cafeteria, or at a movie theater. The same is not true of sexual activity—or at least we hope not. This is a voluntary activity. An element of consent plays a role in the spread of sexually transmitted diseases; hence, a logical response to the problem is to focus on the possibility of changing behavior.

Human nature is always hopeful that science or technology will relieve us of the difficult work of living moral lives. We see this in many areas. Every year there are new fads in dieting, with lots of money spent on books, prepared meals, exercise machines, and the like. We are told to eat nothing but meat, take herbal products, or swallow diet pills, when all that is really needed to reduce our weight is to eat a little less each day, and to engage in a minimal amount of exercise, such as a regular thirty-minute walk. But we like to deceive ourselves—to think that there is some magic formula, some pill, or some technological device that will resolve what may in fact be a moral problem, and do so without any need for self-discipline. What we need to do is change our behavior.

The HPV vaccine proposes a technological solution for a moral problem, but we solve moral problems through moral means, specifically, through an improvement in our individual choices and in our general social condition. Technology can be an aid in that effort, but it can also offer us the appearance of an easy solution, and thus thwart genuine progress. Even worse, it can undermine the legitimate efforts of parents, teachers, clergy, and other concerned citizens to encourage the young to lead healthy moral lives. If the problem of sexual promiscuity is approached by receiving a series of shots or taking various pills, then we are not asking ourselves to exercise self-control, but are using medicine to palliate our vices.

Parents who have chosen to refuse vaccination of their children for sexually transmitted diseases have taken on the challenging task of trying to raise children in a world that pretends that no one practices sexual restraint. They are simply asking others to leave them alone as they attempt to give their offspring the best possible upbringing they can. They do not understand why government finds it necessary to interfere with their own considered judgment in personal matters. Sexual education is a responsibility of the family. To a great many parents, working toward a reform of sexual mores seems a far more sensible approach—even if it is only one child at a time—than getting onto an endless treadmill of new vaccines, therapies, and other technological devices designed to contain an increasingly wide range of sexually transmitted diseases brought about through our own inappropriate choices.

Notes

[1] See Centers for Disease Control and Prevention of the U.S. Department of Health and Human Services (CDC), "Vaccines and Preventable Diseases: Rubella Disease In-Short (German Measles)," last modified September 28, 2008, http://www.cdc.gov/vaccines/vpd-vac/rubella/in-short-adult.htm.

[2] For an example of infection of those vaccinated against mumps, see CDC, "Multi-State Mumps Outbreak," CDC Health Update, last modified April 15, 2006, http://www2a.cdc.gov/HAN/ArchiveSys/ViewMsgV.asp?AlertNum=00244.

[3] CDC, "Basics and Common Questions: What Would Happen If We Stopped Vaccinations?" June 12, 2007, http://www.cdc.gov/vaccines/vac-gen/whatifstop.htm#rubella.

[4] For example, Indiana suffered the worst resurgence of measles in a decade, brought about by a group of home-schooling parents who refused immunization for their children. See Salynn Boyles, "Teens Carried Measles Back from Romania: Unvaccinated Kids at Teen's Church Caught Up in Indiana Outbreak," Web MD, August 2, 2006, http://www.webmd.com/parenting/news/20060802/teen-carried-measles-back-romania. For an in-depth medical study, see Daniel A. Salmon et al., "Health Consequences of Religious and Philosophical Exemptions from Immunization Laws: Individual and Societal Risk of Measles," *Journal of the American Medical Association* 282.1 (July 7, 1999): 47–53. This study indicates that as the number of exemptions to vaccination increases, the incidence of infection among those who have been properly vaccinated also increases.

[5] Thomas Aquinas, *Summa theologica* II-II, q. 58.

[6] CDC, "Vaccines and Preventable Diseases: Who Should NOT Get Vaccinated with These Vaccines?" last modified November 10, 2008, http://www.cdc.gov/vaccines/vpd-vac/should-not-vacc.htm.

[7] Rene Leiva, "A Brief History of Human Diploid Cell Strains," *National Catholic Bioethics Quarterly* 6.3 (Autumn 2006): 443–451.

[8] Ibid., 447.

[9] For a thorough study of this entire area, see the Autumn 2006 issue of *National Catholic Bioethics Quarterly* (6.3), devoted to "Ethics in Cell Research." The issue is examined in some detail by Timothy P. Collins, "Human Technology Manufacturing Platforms," 497–515.

[10] U.S. Conference of Catholic Bishops, *Ethical and Religious Directives for Catholic Health Care Services*, 4th ed. (Washington, D.C: USCCB, 2001).

[11] See, in particular, the response to the third ethical problem addressed in Pontifical Academy for Life, "Declaration on the Production and the Scientific and Therapeutic Use of Human Embryonic Stem Cells" (August 25, 2000).

[12] See Kazutoshi Takahashi and Shinya Yamanaka, "Induction of Pluripotent Stem Cells from Mouse Embryonic and Adult Fibroblast Cultures by Defined Factors," *Cell* 126.4 (August 25, 2006): 663–676. This paper was the first in a long

line of remarkable discoveries showing that adult stem cells can be reprogrammed to become the practical equivalent of embryonic stem cells. This progress in the field of regenerative medicine has completely eliminated the need for destructive embryonic stem cell research.

[13] Angel Rodríguez Luño, "Ethical Reflections on Vaccines Using Cells from Aborted Fetuses," *National Catholic Bioethics Quarterly* 6.3 (Autumn 2006): 453–459.

[14] Therefore, doctors and parents have a duty to take recourse to alternative vaccines (if they exist), putting pressure on political authorities and health systems so that other vaccines without moral problems become available. They should take recourse, if necessary, to the use of conscientious objection with regard to the use of vaccines produced by means of cell lines of aborted human fetal origin. Equally, they should oppose by all means (in writing, through the various associations, mass media, etc.) the vaccines which do not yet have morally acceptable alternatives, creating pressure so that alternative vaccines are prepared which are not connected with the abortion of human fetuses, and requesting rigorous legal control of the pharmaceutical industry producers. With regard to the diseases against which no alternative vaccines are available and ethically acceptable, it is right to abstain from using these vaccines if it can be done without causing children, and indirectly the population as a whole, to undergo significant risks to their health. However, if the latter are exposed to considerable dangers to their health, vaccines with moral problems pertaining to them may also be used on a temporary basis. See Pontifical Academy for Life, "Moral Reflections on Vaccines Prepared from Cells Derived from Aborted Human Fetuses" (June 5, 2005), reprinted in *National Catholic Bioethics Quarterly* 6.3 (Autumn 2006): 547–548.

[15] Ibid., 547.

[16] Ibid., 548.

[17] Ibid., footnote 16: "This is particularly true in the case of vaccination against German measles, because of the danger of congenital rubella syndrome. This could occur, causing grave congenital malformations in the fetus, when a pregnant woman enters into contact, even if it is brief, with children who have not been immunized and are carriers of the virus. In this case, the parents who did not accept the vaccination of their own children become responsible for the malformations in question, and for the subsequent abortion of fetuses, when they have been discovered to be malformed."

[18] Edward J. Furton, "Vaccines and the Right of Conscience," *National Catholic Bioethics Quarterly* 4.1 (Spring 2004): 53–62. See also Furton, "Vaccines Originating in Abortion," *Ethics & Medics* 24.3 (March 1999): 3–4.

✠

Editorial Summation: Immunizations are refused for various reasons. An adverse reaction to a vaccine may indeed be a serious concern, but for most of us the risk posed by vaccines is not appreciable. The enormous health benefits of immunization are well documented; therefore, justice demands that we immunize for the sake of others. We should refuse vaccines that have a distant connection with abortion when an alternative product is available. When there is no alternative, we may use these products until such time as a non-problematic product appears on the market, but we should also express our objections to their origins. Parents who claim an exemption to immunization cannot do so under any specific Catholic teaching but are free to appeal to the general right of conscience. Immunization against sexually transmitted diseases is certainly permissible but should not be mandated by the state. Sexual promiscuity is a moral problem, not a medical one.

CHAPTER 20

Genetic Medicine

Rev. Albert S. Moraczewski, O.P., and John B. Shea, M.D.

The genetic dimension of medicine has become increasingly important as our knowledge of basic genetic sciences has expanded. Before entering a discussion of that part of genetic medicine that would be most relevant to a hospital, this chapter will provide a brief overview of the field of genetics as applicable more directly to human beings.

Genes are the smallest units of an organism that are able to transmit information for the production of inheritable traits. A gene is a sequence of deoxyribonucleic acid (DNA) that occupies a specific location on a chromosome and controls transmission and expression of one or more traits by specifying the structure of a particular protein. It is possible now to diagnose a genetic disorder in an individual before birth (*prenatal diagnosis*). Closely related to prenatal diagnosis and often paired with it is *genetic counseling*. The former involves the acquisition of information necessary to determine the genetic condition of the infant before birth (or the possible genetic makeup of an infant even before conception), while the latter is concerned with communicating that information to the prospective parents together with the options available to them for managing the condition, while also providing them with psychological support in their decision. Complex ethical questions are associated with genetic diagnosis and genetic counseling. These will be identified and discussed later in this chapter.

Prenatal Diagnosis

Prenatal diagnosis is of two kinds: preimplantation genetic diagnosis, and diagnosis during pregnancy. In preimplantation diagnosis, embryos are conceived by in vitro fertilization. They are examined by the removal of a cell from the inner cell mass of the embryo. If the embryo is found to be normal, it is implanted in the woman's uterus. Abnormal embryos and extra normal embryos are discarded. This procedure is not morally acceptable for several reasons, most importantly because it substitutes a technological procedure for the marital act and because it destroys human life.

Methods of diagnosis during pregnancy include radiography, ultrasonography, amniocentesis, chorionic villus sampling, and measurement of maternal serum alpha-fetoprotein, beta hCG, and estriol. Morally legitimate uses of prenatal diagnosis include managing the remaining weeks of pregnancy and planning for possible complications of pregnancy, the birth process, and the newborn. It is morally illegitimate to use prenatal diagnosis for the purposes of procuring an abortion.

Radiography and sonography have many legitimate uses. Because of the relatively high rate of abortion induced by amniocentesis and chorionic villus sampling, their use is justified only in relatively rare circumstances, such as to diagnose intrauterine infection, to facilitate blood transfusion of a fetus with Rh blood disease [rhesus D hemolytic disease of the newborn], and in the diagnosis of some rare treatable metabolic fetal diseases. Amniocentesis is associated with 0.5 to 1.0 percent fetal death rate, and chronic villus sampling is even more dangerous, with a 1.0 to 1.5 percent fetal death rate. Chorionic villus sampling is also associated with abnormality of fetal limbs.

Advances in genetic knowledge and technology have made it possible to treat some genetic diseases radically. This means that the treatment is not merely management of the symptoms but is an actual correction of the genetic defect by replacement (physically or functionally) of the abnormal gene with a normal one (*genetic therapy*). This is still in the early experimental stage and has been performed successfully only on a small number of children.[1]

Somatic Cell Gene Therapy

Somatic cell gene therapy is the insertion of genes into an individual's cells and tissues to treat hereditary diseases, by replacement of a defective mutant allele with a functional one. A carrier called a vector, usually a virus, is used to deliver the therapeutic gene. This therapy has met with some success in the treatment of cystic fibrosis, muscular dystrophy, and SCIDS (severe combined immunodeficiency syndrome). The use of this treatment should be based on careful assessment of its safety and efficiency, alternative treatments, the patient's prognosis, and the balance of risk and benefit for the patient. It may be justified in cases of inevitably fatal or life-threatening disease for which no alternative treatment is available. Complications may include tumor formation, altered immune response, inflammation, and infection. Some authorities have noted that somatic cell gene therapy would need to be observed for decades to monitor long-term effects of therapy on future generations. It is simply assumed, but not proven, that this therapy will not affect the germ-line cells. A proposal to administer somatic cell gene therapy would have to be judged in the light of the above facts and Catholic Church teaching.

Closely related to gene therapy, and in a sense prior to it, is *genetic engineering*. This area of genetics involves the modification of the DNA molecule, a small segment of which is the chemical substance which constitutes the gene. DNA, or deoxyribonucleic acid, is a generic term for the very large and long molecules that are each made up of a long chain of smaller compounds. These chains include four subunits that are repeated in various combinations, which constitute the instructions by which the biochemical "machinery" of the cells synthesizes the various proteins that make up the enzymes, tissues, and organs of the body.

The role of genes in inheritance is not simple; it is not a direct one-to-one relationship, such that one gene corresponds to one physical or behavioral characteristic. Usually a characteristic appears with some modification because two parents are ordinarily involved in producing the one child. Physical characteristics such as color of the eyes, hair, and skin, shape of the face, and height, are the result of the interaction of genes from the two parents.

Relatives and friends gazing at a child will say, "He has his father's chin or his mother's eyes or his grandmother's smile." (Poor kid, nothing is his own!).

Genes also influence behavior patterns. But because these are much more complex (multifactorial, meaning that there may be several genes as well as environmental influences that account for the final "product"), the respective contributions of the genetic component and of subsequent environmental factors, as well as the transmission, are often less evident. The transmission of the predisposition to certain disorders such as diabetes, cystic fibrosis, and Huntington's disease also involves genes; in fact, there are over four thousand recognized disorders that have a genetic component. More controversial is the genetic role in sexual orientation. It is claimed, but has not been established, for example, that there is a genetically based predisposition for homosexuality, and that early environmental factors contribute to its expression.

The Principle of Totality

Among the more important recent statements of the Church on the prospects and limits of genetic medicine is that of the International Theological Commission, *Communion and Stewardship: Human Persons Created in the Image of God* (July 2004). In this document, the Commission first lays out some of the general principles governing this area, noting that the Catholic Church teaches that

> the exercise of a responsible stewardship in the area of bioethics requires profound moral reflection on a range of technologies that can affect the biological integrity of human beings. ... A right to dispose of something extends only to objects with a merely instrumental value, but not to objects which are good in themselves, i.e., ends in themselves. The human person, being created in the image of God, is himself such a good. The question, especially as it arises in bioethics, is whether this also applies to the various levels that can be distinguished in the human person: the biological-somatic, the emotional, and the spiritual levels.[2]

Although the image of God that exists within us cannot be changed, this prohibition does not necessarily apply to the whole of our nature. What role genetic medicine ought to play in that nature remains at issue.

The Church has always recognized that parts of the human body may be sacrificed for the sake of the whole when there is no other means of preserving life or health:

A limited form of disposing of the body and certain mental functions in order to preserve life … is permitted by the principle of totality and integrity. The lower functions are never sacrificed except for the better functioning of the total person, [and] the fundamental faculties which essentially belong to being human are never sacrificed, except when necessary to save life.[3]

For the application of the principle of totality and integrity, the following conditions must be met: (1) there must be a question of intervention in the part of the body that is either afflicted or is the direct cause of the life-threatening situation; (2) there can be no other alternatives for preserving a life; (3) there is a proportionate chance of success in comparison with drawbacks; and (4) the patient must give assent to the intervention.

Germ-Line Genetic Therapy and Enhancement

Germ-line genetic engineering is part of the eugenics project designed to "improve" the human race through enhancement of physical attributes such as hair, eye color, height, weight, body fat, muscle mass, strength, or mental attributes such as intelligence, memory, logic faculty, critical thinking, and temperament. The procedure involves recombinant gene transfer to a sperm or oocyte or foreign gene transfer to chromosomes, pronuclei, or to an early embryo. Many scientists admit that there is no convincing case to be made for human germ-line therapy and that such experimentation would involve significant risks and unproven benefits for subjects who cannot consent:

> Germ-line genetic engineering with a therapeutic goal in man would in itself be acceptable were it not for the fact that it is hard to imagine how this could be achieved without disproportionate risks, especially in the experimental stage, such as huge loss of embryos and the incidence of mishaps, and without the use of reproductive technologies.[4]

Germ-line genetic engineering for enhancement purposes is not morally acceptable and would unlawfully impinge on the evolutionary process.

> Enhancement genetic engineering aims at improving certain specific characteristics. The idea of man as "co-creator" with God could be used to try to justify the management of human evolution by means of such genetic engineering. But this would imply that man has a full right of disposal over his own biological nature. Changing the genetic identity of man as a human person through the production of an infrahuman being

is radically immoral. The use of genetic modification to yield a superhuman being with essentially new spiritual faculties is unthinkable, given that the spiritual life principle of man—forming the matter into the body of the human person—is not a product of human hands and is not subject to human engineering.[5]

Many of the plans of "transhumanists," who seek to wrest biological development from the control of nature and bring it under human control, overlook the fact that the uniqueness of each human being flows in part from the individual's distinctive biogenetic characteristics. These cannot be instrumentalized.

The Human Genome Project

The Human Genome Project is another aspect of genetics that needs to be mentioned, albeit briefly (because it is not immediately relevant to a hospital, even though the data banks which are being generated will have a great influence on hospital and medical practice). The objective of the project is to determine the location and the DNA sequence of all the genes, that is, the genome of the human cell. This has meant mapping the entire packet of the twenty to twenty-five thousand genes that are found in the nucleus of each human cell (except red blood cells, which have no nucleus when they are mature). The successful conclusion of this project means that the location of a particular gene on a specific chromosome can be known, as well as its locus on a specific DNA chain. This permits the identification of genetic disorders associated with specific genes, and may allow much more effective and radical treatment of such genetically related disorders.

A little reflection reveals the potential for abuse. In the near future one can see that the government or other agencies could obtain the genetic constitution of every individual, much like fingerprints, which could affect the jobs one could hold, the education one could receive, the person one could marry, and the children that a couple would be permitted to conceive. On the basis of personal genetic information, insurance companies could disqualify many claims for coverage on the ground that the diseases were pre-existing, because the disordered genes were already present, even if the disorders or diseases had not yet manifested themselves. The Genetic Information Non-Discrimination Act was signed into law in 2008 to forbid these types of abuse.[6]

When the Human Genome Project was started in 1990, it was expected to require fifteen years for completion at an estimated cost of three billion dollars; it was completed in 2003, two years ahead of schedule.

Specific Ethical Concerns

Preimplantation diagnosis, diagnosis during pregnancy, and genetic counseling all involve a number of ethical issues. At the outset let it be noted that one may not directly terminate an innocent human life under the excuse that the child is severely anatomically and physiologically challenged by virtue of a genetic defect or, for that matter, for any reason whatever. Pope John Paul II was most emphatic on the matter of abortion:

> Therefore, by the authority which Christ conferred upon Peter and his Successors, in communion with the bishops … , *I declare that direct abortion, that is, abortion willed as an end or as a means, always constitutes a grave moral disorder*, since it is the deliberate killing of an innocent human being.[7]

Prenatal diagnosis includes a number of specific procedures for obtaining information about the parents, which in turn will provide information about the genetic status of the unborn or to-be-conceived infant. In addition, a variety of tests can be done to obtain information about the fetus: fetoscopy, amniocentesis, sonography, and others. Some of these carry risks for the fetus, and the parents' decision to have the tests done should depend on the degree of risk of injury to the infant and on whether the risk is outweighed by the possible benefit to the fetus.

A genetic counselor seeks to aid the couple (or individual) to deal well with the genetic information obtained from the parents' history as well as, when so indicated, the result of prenatal diagnostic testing. Questions of truth-telling, confidentiality, directive versus nondirective counseling, the sacredness of life, individual worth, social responsibility, and the role of faith arise and need to be dealt with honestly by both the counselor and the parents who, after all, have the final decision.

A Case Study

Mr. and Mrs. D. consulted a geneticist because of the occurrence of Down syndrome in two siblings of Mrs. D. The siblings were of the type 14/21 translocation Down syndrome, and Mrs. D., who was nine weeks' pregnant at the time of the consultation, had heard that this condition could be hereditary. It was explained that chromosome analysis on blood would have to be done on Mrs. D. to see whether she was a carrier (a person who does not manifest the disease symptoms but has the abnormal chromosome and can transmit it to her offspring). Chromosome analysis revealed forty-five chromosomes with a 14/21 translocation. This means that she was a carrier for Down syndrome and has a 10 percent observed risk of producing Down syndrome in the fetus. Mrs. D. wanted to undergo amniocentesis, and later delivered a normal, healthy male child. The couple decided not to have more children because of the tremendous worry, frustration, and deliberation that surrounded the birth of the first child.

The consultation of the geneticist was morally appropriate. There is a small but real risk to the child in the performance of an amniocentesis. (Alpha-fetoprotein tests can also detect the disease.) The test was not performed with the intention of aborting the child if it revealed that the child had Down syndrome. The Congregation for the Doctrine of the Faith's *Instruction on Respect for Human Life in Its Origin and on the Dignity of Procreation* (*Donum vitae*) speaks clearly to the ethics of prenatal diagnosis:

> This diagnosis is gravely opposed to the moral law when it is done with the thought of possibly inducing an abortion, depending upon the results: a diagnosis which shows the existence of a malformation or a hereditary illness must not be the equivalent of a death sentence. Thus a woman would be committing a gravely illicit act if she were to request such a diagnosis with the deliberate intention of having an abortion should the results confirm the existence of a malformation or abnormality. The spouse or relatives or anyone else would similarly be acting in a manner contrary to the moral law if they were to counsel or impose such a diagnostic procedure on the expectant mother with the same intention of possibly proceeding to an abortion. So too the specialist would be guilty of illicit collaboration if, in conducting the diagnosis and in communicating its results, he were deliberately to contribute to establishing or favoring a link between prenatal diagnosis and abortion.[8]

But if the reason is to benefit the child in some significant way, then it can be done by experienced personnel, providing the couple is properly informed about the risks to the child and to the mother.

In this case, the couple decided not to have more children; natural family planning procedures should be carefully explained and suitable training provided.

Papal Reflections on Genetics

In the first creation account of the Book of Genesis, it is written: "God blessed them, saying: 'Be fertile and multiply; fill the earth and subdue it. Have dominion over the fish of the sea, the birds of the air, and all the living things that move on the earth'" (Gen. 1:28, NAB).

These words have been understood as a divine mandate to humans to till the soil; to use plants and animals for food, clothing, and other needs; to explore, migrate, and populate the world; to use the various mineral and water resources for human purposes; and to discover, invent, and probe the secrets of nature. All these activities are carried on to satisfy the multifarious needs and drives of human beings.

But contrary to some opinions, the divine command did not confer unlimited power to the human race. This given power is a *limited* dominion, and it necessarily includes accountability, primarily to God and secondarily to human society. In the second creation account, that limitation and the consequence for its violation are poetically stated: "The Lord God gave man this order: 'You are free to eat from any of the trees in the garden except the tree of knowledge of good and bad. From that tree you shall not eat; the moment you eat from it you are surely doomed to die'" (Gen. 2:16–17, NAB). The first sentence sets before us the limitation on our power over nature. The second recounts the punishment for transgressions, and, by implication, indicates our accountability for all actions that breach the natural moral order.

The possibility of genetic manipulation became a reality only in the last half of the previous century. Pope John Paul II addressed this issue briefly several times. His remarks were generally supportive; in an address to the Pontifical Academy of Sciences on October 23, 1982, for example, he stated, "It is also to be hoped, with reference to your activities, that the new techniques of modification of the genetic code, in particular cases of genetic or chromosomic diseases, will be a motive of hope for the great number of people affected by those maladies."[9] At the same time, while encouraging research and the clinical application of the results of genetic research, the Pope reminded his auditors and readers that there is a "priority of ethics over technology."[10]

He also expressed concern that genetic alteration should not result in a further marginalization of human beings. Respect for the individuality of our bodily nature is a critical element in the moral evaluation of genetics for John Paul II:

> The biological nature of every human is untouchable, in the sense that it is constituent of the personal identity of the individual throughout the course of his history. Each human person, in his or her absolutely unique singularity, is not constituted only by the spirit, but also by the body. Thus, in the body and through the body, one touches the person himself, in his concrete reality. Respecting the dignity of man consequently

comes down to safeguarding this identity of man *corpore et anima unus* (one in body and soul).[11]

It is one thing to seek a cure for a disease or to rectify a congenital abnormality, and it is quite another to seek an alteration of the normal human soma or psyche with the intent of "improving" human nature. What would constitute an improvement? Who would decide? On whom would the changes initially be made? These are complex problems, but their complexity does not necessarily mean that there is no way forward.

Pope John Paul II, in an address to the Pontifical Academy of Sciences (October 28, 1994), noted that

> genome research will enable man to understand himself to an unprecedented degree. In particular, it will be possible to perceive genetic influences more clearly and to distinguish them from those stemming from the natural and cultural surroundings and those associated with the individual's own experience … Scientific progress such as that involving the genome is a credit to human reason.[12]

The Pope also noted that,

> as regards interventions in the human genome sequencing, it would be appropriate to recall certain basic moral norms. All interferences in the genome should be done in a way that absolutely respects the specific nature of the human species, the transcendental vocation of every [human] being and his incomparable dignity. The genome represents the biological identity of each subject; furthermore, it expresses a part of the human condition of the being desired for its own sake through the mission entrusted to his parents.[13]

Finally, he added this caution:

> On this subject, we rejoice that numerous researchers have refused to allow discoveries made about the genome to be patented. Since the human body is not an object that can be disposed at will, the results of research should be made available to the whole scientific community and cannot be the property of a small group.[14]

The Church holds that any genetic changes brought about by human art should truly improve the human condition for some without worsening life for others. Knowledge about a person's genetic makeup should not be used in a kind of "search and destroy mission" that would be prejudicial in the person's seeking employment or health insurance coverage. Even worse is when it leads to the deliberate destruction of life.

May we all have the wisdom to discern what is right and good in the area of genetic research and medicine!

Notes

[1] See Albert S. Moraczewski, "Pastoral Hope and Genetic Medicine," in *The Bishop and the Future of Catholic Health Care: Challenges and Opportunities*, ed. Daniel P. Maher (Braintree, MA: Pope John Center, 1997).

[2] International Theological Commission, *Communion and Stewardship: Human Persons Created in the Image of God* (July 2004), nn. 81 and 82.

[3] Ibid., n. 83.

[4] Ibid., n. 90.

[5] Ibid., n. 91.

[6] *Genetic Information Non-Discrimination Act of 2008*, Public Law 110-233, 110th Cong., 2nd sess. (May 21, 2008).

[7] John Paul II, *Evangelium vitae* (March 25, 1995), n. 62 (emphasis added).

[8] Congregation for the Doctrine of the Faith, *Donum vitae* (February 22, 1987), I, 2; see also U.S. Conference of Catholic Bishops, *Ethical and Religious Directives for Catholic Health Care Services*, 4th ed. (Washington, D.C.: USCCB, 2001), n. 50.

[9] John Paul II, Address to Members of the Pontifical Academy of Sciences (October 23, 1982), n. 5.

[10] John Paul II, *Redemptor Hominis* (March 4, 1979), n. 16.

[11] John Paul II, "The Ethics of Genetic Manipulation," Address to the World Medical Association (October 29, 1983), n. 6, in *Origins* 13.23 (November 17, 1983), 385, 388–389.

[12] John Paul II, "The Human Person: Beginning and End of Scientific Research," Address to the Pontifical Academy of Science (October 28, 1994), n. 3, in *The Pope Speaks* (March–April 1995): 80–84.

[13] Ibid., n. 4.

[14] Ibid.

⟨✠⟩

Editorial Summation: Catholic teaching in the area of genetics affirms whatever respects human life and dignity from the moment of conception and is genuinely therapeutic for the individual. The teaching is not opposed to prenatal diagnosis or genetic counseling so long as these activities do not result in the direct destruction of human life and respect the unitive and procreative purposes of the conjugal act in marriage. Prenatal diagnosis is of two kinds: preimplantation genetic diagnosis, and diagnosis during pregnancy. In preimplantation diagnosis, embryos are conceived by in vitro fertilization. They are examined by means of the removal of a cell from the inner cell mass of the embryo. If the embryo is found to be normal, it is implanted in the woman's uterus. Abnormal embryos or extra normal embryos are discarded. Methods of diagnosis during pregnancy include radiography, ultrasonography, amniocentesis, chorionic villus sampling, and measurement of maternal serum alpha-fetoprotein, beta hCG, and estriol. The genetic counselor seeks to aid the couple (or individual) to deal well with the genetic information obtained from the parents' history as well as the result of prenatal diagnostic testing. Somatic cell gene therapy is the insertion of genes into an individual's cells and tissues to treat hereditary diseases in which a defective mutant allele is replaced with a functional one. Closely related to gene therapy is genetic engineering. Germ-line genetic engineering is part of a eugenics project designed to "improve" the human race through the enhancement of physical attributes such as hair, eye color, height, weight, body fat, muscle mass, strength, and mental attributes like intelligence, memory, logic faculty, critical thinking, and temperament. The divine command of dominion over the earth announced in *Genesis* did not, however, confer unlimited power to the human race. This power is a limited dominion, and it necessarily includes accountability, primarily to God and secondarily to human society.

CHAPTER 21

Human Experimentation and Research

Stephen R. Napier

Most health care institutions have institutional review boards (IRBs) that are in charge of reviewing research on human subjects. Some research projects, however, are either not federally funded or take place at a clinic that is nonetheless not "engaged" in research. In either case, ethics committees at these clinics, or those overseeing non–federally funded research, may bear the task of reviewing research.

This article is written to assist committees with that task, but the recommendations made here should not take the place of reviewing the regulations governing human subject protection. Even if research is not federally funded, the regulations offer a good guide by which to review it.

A review committee must look at several important items in order to determine the permissibility of a research project. The following items outline the core task of the review committee: (1) identify the benefits and risks, (2) determine that the research design minimizes the risks, (3) determine that the benefits outweigh the risks, and (4) assure that potential subjects will understand the research project including its purpose and the risks and benefits. This last requirement is typically referred to as the informed consent requirement. In addition, the review committee must ensure that (5) sufficient safeguards are in place to protect the privacy and confidentiality of the subjects, and (6) if the subject population is particularly vulnerable, other safeguards may need to be considered.[1] As one can see, this is quite a list, but thankfully it is nearly exhaustive. The items are easy to enumerate, but hard to put into practice.

Risks

The first task of reviewing research is to identify the risks and benefits. Risks are of different sorts. They include not just harms per se, but the *kind* of harm, the *probability* of the harm, and the *duration* of the harm. Suppose a study carries with it the risk of death, but the probability of this occurrence is very minute. Suppose another study carries with it a risk of vomiting, and the probability of this occurrence is very high. The second study may have a higher risk factor than the first, even though the first carries a risk of death and the second only a risk of vomiting.

Second, if there are risks to subjects, there *must be* benefits to those very same subjects as well. The only exception to this general rule is if the risks are minimal or the benefits to society *clearly* outweigh the risks to a few subjects. One should notice here that the risk–benefit assessment and the informed consent criterion are two different and independent areas of research protocol assessment. If a study presents high risk and low benefit to subjects, even obtaining their informed consent will not justify the study.

In identifying the risks, one needs to look at the risks of the research interventions alone. If a research project piggybacks on clinical interventions, one does not include the risks of those other interventions in reviewing the research risks. There is also research design. Risks can come from various sources, and the very design of a study may present risks. For example, many placebo-controlled trials carry with them risks for the placebo group, since there are risks to withholding treatment from subjects.

243

Also, a double-blind study may pose risks to subjects in that future therapy may require knowing whether the patient received the research drug. Notice that the source of risk is the design itself.

In addition, the research intervention is a source of risk, but more alarmingly, the knowledge gained from the research may be a source of risk as well. For instance, suppose a study aims to discover a possible link between a genetic disorder (for which there is no cure) and oppositional defiant disorder (ODD). The research interventions involve a simple blood test and taking confidential and well-validated psychological tests for ODD—both of which qualify as minimal risk. Since there is no cure for the genetic disorder, simply knowing that it also causes ODD poses only a risk of stigmatization to those with the genetic disorder, without any promised benefit. Notice that the source of the risk is the knowledge gained, not the research interventions themselves. To justify such studies, the researcher should ask what significance to human health is gained by carrying out the research. As the example indicates, knowledge alone is not a good enough answer.

Minimization of Risks

In addition to identifying the risks, the review committee should look at whether the risks identified could be minimized. This requirement looks primarily at the study design and other sources of risk, and at whether the scientific objectives could be met without the sources of risk. Here are several sample questions: Is the sample size large enough to obtain statistically significant results? If not, then the same research would have to be done again to get valid results, thus putting more human subjects at risk for no overriding reason. If the sample size exceeds what is required for statistical significance, then the "extra" subjects are put at unnecessary risk. Is the hypothesis testable? Without a testable hypothesis, subjects are exposed to the risks of research interventions for no reason. Is the researcher experienced in the research intervention? A research project which had an undergraduate psychology major conducting sensitive interviews on sexual abuse history would pose greater risk to subjects than the same project conducted by a well-seasoned interviewer. Does the recruitment of subjects protect their confidentiality?

Suppose the recruitment procedures were via referral from other subjects, and the subject population were HIV-infected professionals. Clearly, the recruitment procedures present ripe opportunity to violate the confidentiality of some subjects. Are there notable risks to the placebo group if the study is placebo-controlled? If so, could the study be made into a cross-over study to minimize such risks and still be scientifically valid?[2] Are there stopping rules in place if a series of unexpected events occur? Those conducting a study with no stopping rules may continue conducting research when the research intervention has clearly indicated statistically significant risks. Is there independent data monitoring if risks are high? If deception is involved in the study, is there a debriefing? If risks are realized during the research interventions (for example, psychological interventions may uncover suppressed memories which may need addressing) are referrals in place? Is unblinding a possibility in case adverse reactions occur, so that medical personnel will know whether the subject received the study intervention? These are just some questions the review committee must consider vis-à-vis the minimization of risks. In sum, risks can be minimized by looking at the researcher (e.g., experience, potential conflicts of interest), the research intervention (e.g., data monitoring, referrals, follow-up/debriefing), and design (e.g., sample size, exclusion criteria, testability of the hypothesis, placebo-controlled).

Benefits

There are three types of benefits: those accruing to the subjects directly, those accruing indirectly, and those accruing to society. Direct benefits to the subjects means that there is some probability that the research intervention itself will benefit the subjects in the way the intervention was intended. I say "in the way the intervention was intended" because other benefits accrue to subjects, through increased monitoring, for example, which may elevate the mood of the subjects. This may occur even though the research intervention aims to decrease tumor size or enhance coping skills vis-à-vis sexual abuse history. The elevation of a subject's mood due to increased monitoring is not due to the research *intervention*, but is a function of the subject's being in the research. The reduction in tumor size or enhanced coping skills are due to the research intervention. Indirect benefits are those accruing to the subject because he is in the research, direct benefits are those accruing to the subject because of the research intervention. Compensation, increased monitoring, and compassionate attention during a sexual abuse interview are all indirect benefits. Decrease in tumor size and enhanced coping skills qualify as direct benefits. Benefits to society are typically confined to increased medical knowledge.

When adjudicating whether the benefits justify the risks to the subjects, the review committee needs to look primarily at direct benefits. Indirect benefits are inconsequential, and benefits to society alone will not justify exposing even a few human beings to risks.

Informed Consent

Informed consent is a separate ethical requirement for permitting a research study. Even if the informed consent process is airtight and checks are in place to ensure that the participants understand the protocol, the project is still not permitted if it has a very high risk and minimal benefit. Likewise, if a research project has minimal risks associated with it, but there are no provisions for procuring the consent of the subjects, again, the study is impermissible. There are certainly exceptions to this latter rule; for instance, if the study has minimal risk, and the research could not be practicable if consent were obtained, then the research may go forward. An example of this type of research would be retrospective medical chart reviews. Such reviews count as research on human subjects, they have minimal risk, and because the reviews are retrospective, it is not practical to get consent from the subjects. Few people have an ethical problem with these studies.

The informed consent process comprises several elements. They are an explanation of the purposes and aims of the study; a description of any relevant foreseeable risks; a description of the *direct* benefits or, if no direct benefits are promised, an explicit statement to that effect; a statement describing alternative treatments; a statement indicating how confidentiality will be maintained; information concerning a contact person (e.g., the investigator); and a statement that participation is voluntary and will not affect the care of the subject or delimit his legal and moral rights.

In reviewing an informed consent document, the review committee should look not only at whether these eight elements are present but at their content. Of particular importance is the risk section of the document. The committee should think about what a potential subject might want to know concerning the risks of the intervention. A researcher may think that the risks associated with sex-abuse questionnaires are quite small, but to the subjects who live with such memories and may experience symptoms of post-traumatic stress syndrome, even a small risk is relevant. In addition to the content of the document, there is also the way in which the information is presented. The informed consent document should be written in a language suitable to the target subject population.

The informed consent process is just that, a process; it is not reducible to giving the subjects a written form to sign or not sign. No guarantee can be given that every subject will make a fully informed voluntary choice—we cannot peer into another's head, so to speak. We can, however, aim to remove barriers to voluntary informed consent. Ongoing communication should be standard, and should include the nature of the research interventions (if a longitudinal study), the risks associated with the interventions, and information about any new risks discovered at other sites. Furthermore, the review committee should consider potential points of coercion if, for example, the research involves subjects drawn from the researchers' own patients, the researcher is a professor approaching his or her own students as subjects, the research is to be done on military personnel, or the research will enroll subjects who are chronically ill and desperate for a cure. In such cases, the review committee may require additional procedures by which to assure that the informed consent process is noncoercive and removes as many impediments to informed voluntary decision making as possible. Examples of additional procedures may include impartial observers to the consent process, consent testing if the risks are high, audiovisual aids, and increased minimum time intervals to think about research involvement.

Notes

[1] These items are taken from Robin Levin Penslar, *Institutional Review Board Guidebook* (Washington, D.C.: Office of Human Research Protections, 1993), chapter 3, "Basic IRB Review," http://www.hhs.gov/ohrp/irb/irb_chapter3.htm.

[2] A cross-over study involves the initial placebo group and experimental group exchanging roles after some period of time. The result is that the placebo group begins to undergo the research intervention and the experimental group becomes the placebo group.

✠

Editorial Summation: Most health care institutions have institutional review boards that are in charge of reviewing research on human subjects. Ethics committees may also participate in research review. The following items outline the core task of the review committee: (1) identify the benefits and risks,

(2) determine that the research design minimizes the risks, (3) determine that the benefits outweigh the risks, and (4) assure that potential subjects will understand the research project including its purpose and the risks and benefits. This last requirement is typically referred to as the informed consent requirement. In addition, the review committee must ensure that (5) sufficient safeguards are in place to protect the privacy and confidentiality of the subjects, and (6) if the subject population is particularly vulnerable, other safeguards may need to be considered.

CHAPTER 22

Religious Freedom and Pastoral Care

Rev. Albert S. Moraczewski, O.P.

It should come as no surprise that at least ten of the *Ethical and Religious Directives for Catholic Health Care Services* (*ERDs*)—nn. 10, 11, and 22, for example—merit analysis and commentary under the discussion of the principle of religious freedom.[1] Catholic hospitals and other health facilities constitute an essential segment of the missionary role of the Church as emphasized in the concluding canon of the *Code of Canon Law*: "the salvation of souls ... always the supreme law of the Church" can. 1752). The hospital setting is ideal for turning the hearts and minds of patients to a consideration of the primacy of spiritual needs, and for promoting the importance of spiritual reconciliation if required (see *ERDs*, part 2). Depending on the urgency of the situation, all the sacraments except Holy Orders can be administered in a hospital setting. For the proper utilization of these spiritual treasures, however, a proper understanding of the phrase "religious freedom" is required.

Human Freedom

The danger of confusing that precious word "freedom" with the abuse of freedom known as licentiousness is manifested by the immoral lifestyles of many people (such as cohabitation in place of marriage, infidelity in marriage, and unjust business practices). These will say, "But I am free, and have no qualms of conscience." They choose to forget, or to deny, that freedom carries with it the obligation to seek the truth and to live accordingly. Human beings are free, after all, in order to reach the goal of life. It is significant that Vatican II's *Declaration on Religious Liberty* (Dignitatis humanae) avoids the use of the popular phrase "freedom of conscience." It establishes

the right to religious freedom on the basis of our common human dignity, defined as personal responsibility:

> It is in accordance with their dignity as persons ... that all men should be both impelled by nature and bound by a moral obligation to seek the truth, especially religious truth. They are also bound to adhere to the truth, once they come to know it, and to direct their whole lives in accordance with the demands of truth.[2]

Although the individual has the obligation to seek religious truth, all others, however, must refrain from interfering in any way with the individual's reaction or response to that obligation (to seek the truth). In other words, all human beings must be free to follow or not to follow the light of truth as they know themselves to be *obliged* to act. This sets the parameters for attention to the spiritual needs of all patients in a Catholic health facility. The human dignity of every patient must be reverenced even to the extent of seeing the Lord Jesus in those who wear the mantle of suffering and anxiety, regardless of their religious affiliation (or lack thereof), and yet without exerting any pressure or coercion which would violate the patient's right to religious freedom. The principle of religious freedom is adapted from Vatican II's *Declaration on Religious Liberty*:

> The Vatican Council declares that the human person has a right to religious freedom. Freedom of this kind means that all men should be immune from coercion on the part of individuals, social groups, and every human power so that, within due limits, nobody is forced to act against his convictions in religious mat-

ters in private or public, alone or in associations with others. The council further declares that the right to religious freedom is based on the very dignity of the human person.[3]

But what are the "due limits?" Such limits would include the protection of the rights of third parties. The more fundamental these are (like the right to life), the stronger the restraining limits. These limits will be discussed below.

A Loving and Caring Community of Spiritual Service

Proper appreciation and recognition of the role of the priest who is appointed by the bishop as chaplain of the hospital community is basic to the very concept of spiritual service. Even though he may not be assigned charge of the department of pastoral care by the hospital authorities, his spiritual authority and responsibilities by virtue of the appointment by the bishop cannot be curtailed or appropriated by any other member of the hospital staff. He is charged with the responsibility of attending to the spiritual needs of the hospital community, both patients and staff, "in a stable manner," with all due faculties from the bishop to meet that challenge (cann. 564–566). In a sense, he is the pastor or spiritual father of that select community, not only in his concern for the spiritual welfare of all members of that community, but also in celebrating or in overseeing liturgical functions (can. 567, §2).

The Church could hardly be more understanding and caring in facilitating reconciliation with God than she is with regard to all who are victims of sickness and anxiety. The chaplain or visiting priest is encouraged to motivate even a patient who is not in danger of death, so that the patient finds it hard to remain in a state of serious sin, as from abortion. Such a conversion justifies the priest in absolving that individual from the sin in the internal sacramental forum (can. 1357). Some formalities remain if the patient has incurred the censure of abortion, but interior peace and reconciliation may be achieved. If the patient can be said to be in danger of death (to be interpreted widely), reconciliation is possible for the patient regardless of the type of sin involved. This consoling gesture of forgiveness is conveyed in the noted "any priest—any sin" canon of the Church's *Code of Canon Law*: "Any priest, even though he lacks the faculty to hear confessions, can validly and licitly absolve penitents who are in danger of death from any censures and sins, even if an approved priest is present" (can. 976).

Many invalid marriages come to light in the hospital setting. The general rule is that invalid marriages should be "fixed up" or convalidated in a parish setting. In danger-of-death situations, providing that there is no impediment of the natural law (for example, impotence) or of the divine positive law (for example, the existing bond of a previous valid marriage), the place and time must be here and now (in the hospital). The procedure is simplified considerably (cann. 1068, 1079, 1081). If the marriage cannot be convalidated, peace of mind and of conscience may be restored by investigating the possibility of a brother-and-sister arrangement in marital life. If one of the parties cannot be persuaded to renew consent to a former civil marriage, a radical sanction (as long as mutual consent continues, the marriage bond is constituted in spite of some original defect) or "retroactive validation" is possible (cann. 1161–1165). The chaplain or attending priest must proceed with prayer and diplomacy, however, lest he exceed the bonds of prudent persuasion and become guilty of coercion or pressure in his efforts to bring the straying faithful back into the fold. The patient who refuses to reach out for the comfort and graces of any of the sacraments, including the reception of *viaticum* (can. 921), must be handled with prayer. Any undue pressure would be a violation of the right to religious freedom.

The Spiritual Needs of Non-Catholic Patients

There is no need to stress again that non-Catholic patients may receive the sacraments of penance, the Eucharist, and the anointing of the sick *only* in certain well-defined circumstances.[4] This would obtain in a situation when the non-Catholic patient is unable to get in touch with the minister of his own denomination. Designated staff members of a Catholic hospital are committed to Christian concern in informing non-Catholic ministers of the presence of members of their congregations in the hospital; all staff members are to consider themselves as members of the welcome committee in affording non-Catholic ministers every facility for visiting members of their congregation and in providing them with spiritual and sacramental ministrations. The Catholic Church would be in violation of the spirit of ecumenism if she looked upon her hospitals and health facilities as sources of "making converts" to the Catholic faith. If a non-Catholic patient voluntarily expresses an interest in learning more about the Catholic faith, and exhibits proper motivation for such a request (not based merely on criticism of his or her own denomination), the Catholic pastor of that individual's residential area should be informed and, if time allows, even invited to the hospital to become acquainted with the patient. In addition, there exist a veritable army of "fallen-away" Catholics and of patients with no religious affiliation whatsoever. There is no wisdom in risking offense to the sensitivities of our "separated brethren" by giving rise to possible suspicions that Catholic hospitals are used for proselytism.

Respect for Personal Beliefs and Preferences

The principle of religious freedom must be applied when, for example, a nurse in a Catholic hospital refuses to participate in a particular procedure on the basis of conscientious objection (convinced, for example, that the patient's insistence on a hysterectomy was for contraceptive purposes only), or when an elderly patient insists on cessation of substitute treatments such as artificial respiration or renal dialysis because of conscientious judgment of lack of balance between benefits and burdens. The situation becomes very difficult and delicate if a non-Catholic patient in a Catholic hospital refuses a lifesaving procedure which is standard in current medical practice, and refuses that procedure on religious grounds. In end-of-life cases where there is an irreconcilable conflict between the patient's decision and Catholic teaching, the only way to respect the wishes and religious freedom of the patient is to transfer the patient out of the Catholic facility.[5] The classic example is that of a member of the sect known as Jehovah's Witnesses who is convinced that allowing a blood transfusion would be contrary to religious beliefs.

Over five hundred thousand Jehovah's Witnesses in the United States do not accept blood transfusions. They believe that blood transfusions are prohibited by scriptural passages, such as "Only flesh with its lifeblood still in it you shall not eat" (Gen. 9:4) and the injunction of the Apostles, writing to the Gentile converts in Antioch, Syria, and Cilicia, "It is the decision of the Holy Spirit and of us not to place on you any burden beyond these necessities, namely, to abstain from meat sacrificed to idols, from blood" (Acts 15:28–29). Because Jehovah's Witnesses also believe that blood removed from the body must be properly disposed of (see Lev. 17:13), blood may not be taken from a person with the intention of later injecting it into the same individual.

These restrictions have inhibited many surgeons from operating on Jehovah's Witnesses and, in cases of minors, have sometimes led a physician or hospital to seek a court order that would permit the giving of blood transfusions over the objections of a child's parents. Some Jehovah's Witnesses have expressed the concern that such a legal procedure could result in lasting psychosocial harm to the persons involved.

Studies have shown that improvements in surgical procedures have permitted the successful performance of surgery—elective and emergency—on a large number of adult and minor Jehovah's Witnesses without the use of blood transfusions. Increasing numbers of surgeons see the restriction on the use of blood transfusions simply "as only one more complication challenging their skill."[6]

Many persons are uncomfortable with the idea of overriding parents' religious beliefs with a court order that removes the child from the custody of the parents so that a presumably lifesaving blood transfusion can be administered. It is good news that improved surgical techniques and non-blood substitutes now make it possible to perform safely a variety of surgical procedures without reliance on blood transfusions.[7]

The respect of an individual's conscience is a central aspect of a person's dignity, particularly when that conscience is concerned with a religious belief. The Church's official teaching is clear, as the quotations above from the *Declaration on Religious Liberty* illustrate. Accordingly, the beliefs of Jehovah's Witnesses must be respected. But are there any limits?

In practice, if a religious belief is harmful to other persons, then many feel that the application of that belief could be suspended by legal action if necessary. Particularly difficult is the case of the child who needs a blood transfusion to live. Do the parents have the moral right to withhold a potentially lifesaving procedure because of a religious prohibition? The child has a basic right to life and health; accordingly, the parents may not compromise that right but are obligated to promote it. Since the child is not yet capable of assenting freely to the religious belief regarding blood transfusions, the parents speak for the child. But their decision making should be for the *best interests of the child*. The *child's* conscience would *not* be violated if "forced" to accept a lifesaving transfusion.

With the willingness of more surgeons to operate without giving blood transfusions, however, it may be possible to avoid this particular conflict. What is important is that when a Jehovah's Witness, adult or child, is in need of surgery, an open discussion be held among the key figures: the patient (and parents when appropriate), surgeon, nurses, a mediating person (such as a pastoral care person or social worker), and others as appropriate.

The purpose of such a discussion would be to allow the participants to understand the medical and religious dimensions so that all can appreciate the reasons for the restriction as well as the risks (and benefits) associated with surgery performed without the support of blood transfusions. With such a careful preparation, the patient and family can approach the impending operation with less fear, and the surgeon and nurses with less tension, confident that the family would be able to deal constructively with a mishap should it occur.

The improvement in surgical procedures, partially under the stimulus of the bloodless surgery requirement, is an example of how medical advances may result from the need to respect a religious belief. Another example is found in the restriction against contraception. Improvements in natural family planning methods resulted, in part at least, from the need to control procreation without resorting to contraceptive sterilization or artificial means for preventing conception or birth.

Whether we agree or not with the interpretation of the biblical passages which undergird the Jehovah's Witnesses' religious belief that blood and blood components may not be transfused into a person, it is vital that respect for their conscience be strictly maintained by health care personnel so long as a basic right of a third party is not seriously violated. But what if a patient wants, or demands, a tubal ligation, claiming that her religious beliefs would permit such sterilizing procedure if her health or life were being threatened? A Catholic hospital would have to respond that to permit such a procedure would violate its own religious freedom. In such a conflict, the party for whom it would be morally wrong to do the procedure (the Catholic hospital) has precedence over the party for whom it would be permissible, because the hospital is not guilty of wrongdoing.

Notes

[1] U.S. Conference of Catholic Bishops, *Ethical and Religious Directives for Catholic Health Care Services*, 4th ed. (Washington, D.C.: USCCB, 2001).

[2] Vatican Council II, *Dignitatis humanae* (December 7, 1965), n. 2.

[3] Ibid.

[4] Orville N. Griese, "Reverend Humanity," *Ethics & Medics* 12.3 (March 1987): 2.

[5] See *Ethical and Religious Directives*, n. 28.

[6] J. L. Dixon and M. Gene Smalley, "Jehovah's Witnesses: The Surgical/Ethical Challenge," *Journal of the American Medical Association* 246.21 (November 27, 1981): 2471–2472.

[7] Ibid.

✠

Editorial Summation: The salvation of souls remains the principal goal of the Catholic Church; therefore, attending to the spiritual and pastoral needs of patients is a critical part of Catholic health care. The Church recognizes that the hospital setting is a special time to respond to the spiritual needs of the patient. In keeping with the *Declaration on Religious Liberty* of the Second Vatican Council, the Church respects the liberty of conscience that is founded on the innate dignity of every human being. The hospital, therefore, is not a time to engage in proselytizing. Nonetheless, the priest has a unique role in the hospital setting, regardless of whether or not he is a member of the pastoral team. He should be accorded the freedom necessary to fulfill his spiritual functions. End-of-life care provides unique opportunities for reconciliation to the faith, especially among fallen-away Catholics, but in the spirit of ecumenism, the priest should avoid any coercive use of his authority. Patients who refuse life-saving treatments for religious reasons, such as Jehovah's Witnesses, pose special challenge for Catholic health care. Oftentimes the medical challenges these patients present can be met, but in cases where there is a clear and irreconcilable conflict between a patient request and Catholic moral teaching, the Catholic health care facility must follow the teachings of its faith.

CHAPTER 23

The Professional–Patient Relationship

Marie T. Nolan, R.N.

> In some of us the ceaseless panorama of suffering tends to dull that fine edge
> of sympathy with which we started. A great corporation cannot have a
> very fervent charity; the very conditions of its existence limit its exercise.
> Against this benumbing influence, we physicians and nurses, the immediate
> agents of the Trust, have but one enduring corrective—the practice towards
> patients of the Golden Rule of Humanity as announced by Confucius:
> What you do not like when done to yourself, do not do to others—
> so familiar to us in its positive form as the great Christian counsel of
> perfection in which alone are embraced both the law and the prophets.
>
> — WILLIAM OSLER, *Aequanimitas*

William Osler, one of the founding physicians of the Johns Hopkins Hospital at the turn of the century, understood that it is not the role of the hospital but of health professionals to care for patients. He further proposed that this care must be grounded in Christianity. In our era of managed care, where multimillion-dollar contracts and even hospital survival are dependent upon corporate agreements to provide minimal care for multitudes of patients, health professionals must retain their identity as "agents of the Trust."

The Fiduciary Relationship

Trust is at the heart of the medical relationship with the patient. Edmund Pellegrino has asserted that the promise to provide competent help to the patient represents "beneficence-in-trust" from which all medical obligations are derived.[2] Pellegrino is careful to point out that beneficence, properly understood, is not synonymous with paternalism, in which the patient's nature as an autonomous being is disregarded. Although patient autonomy is commonly pitted against the beneficence of the health professional in the medical literature, Pellegrino demonstrates that this conflict is misplaced. He defines beneficence as that which seeks the good of the patient. This good is defined by Pellegrino as having four components in a descending order of importance starting with (1) the ultimate good of human life as perceived by the patient, (2) the good of a patient as a human person (3) the patient's subjective assessment of what is good; and (4) the biomedical or clinical good.

The ultimate good of human life is the patient's view of the meaning of human existence with reference to other human beings, the world, and God. The good of the patient as a human person represents his ability to reason and be self-determined. Interventions of health professionals which do not respect patients' autonomy therefore, are not consistent with beneficence. The patient's subjective assessment of a particular treatment will be based upon his own life goals and may be in conflict with the biomedical good. This final biomedical good represents the restoration of physiologic and psychological functioning.[3]

Informed Consent and Treatment Decisions

Although respecting the patient's autonomy is an important part of acting for the good of patients, E. Chevien warns that obtaining informed consent from patients is more complicated than simply providing them with treatment information and awaiting their decision to accept or decline the treatment.[4] Chevien recounts the story of a fifty-eight-year-old man dying of lymphoma who rejected all forms of chemotherapy, asking only for "natural" therapies. After spending time with the patient to understand his views, Chevien offered the patient "natural chemotherapy." By explaining to the patient the origins of the chemotherapeutic agents (i.e., adriamycin is from a fungus growing along the Adriatic Sea), he was able to persuade the patient to accept conventional and successful treatment. Was this paternalistic or manipulative?

Chevien explains that patients are often beset by fears and false hopes. To simply provide information in a detached manner is to abrogate the responsibility for acting in the patient's best interest. T. Ackerman agrees, warning that a legalistic view of patient autonomy has taken hold which he characterizes as "noninterference."[5] He goes on to explain that this view stems from a view of the physician–patient interaction as "a typical commodity exchange—the provision of technically competent medical care in return for financial compensation." Ackerman states that respecting a patient's refusal of treatment respects the patient's autonomy only if a thorough deliberation precedes the decision. Health professionals must do their best to understand patients' views of their illnesses and treatment options, and work to place patients in the best position to act for their own good.

Virtues of the Caregiver

The predisposition of health professionals to act for the good of the patient is the measure of their virtue. In *Nicomachean Ethics*, Aristotle defined virtue as the habit of acting for the good.[6] The cardinal virtues, fortitude, temperance, justice, and wisdom (i.e., prudence), were first described by Plato and then critiqued by Aristotle, who held that a virtuous character was developed by acting well. St. Thomas Aquinas was a central figure in developing a theology of the virtues, including both the cardinal and the theological virtues faith, hope, and charity. Romanus Cessario, O.P., points out that although development of the virtues requires self-reflection, the virtuous life is relational rather than self-absorbed. "For theological ethics, there exists a general, but real sense in which every virtue remains ordered to the kind of social communication which befits the unity of believers in Christ."[7]

Exploring the virtues helps to clarify what it is to be a virtuous physician, nurse, social worker, or other health professional. Prudence orients both the intellect and the appetites to actions which promote human flourishing. This virtue can guide decisions of health care professionals in the midst of difficult conflicts regarding end-of-life treatment. Institutional, family, and staff disagreements on how to proceed in a particular case can lead to confusion about which course of treatment is best. The virtue of prudence will help the caregiver to act for the good of the patient.

Charity and patience are needed to care for some patients who by their defiance or hostility may evoke anger in the caregiver. The number of patients admitted to hospitals with a primary or secondary diagnosis of substance abuse has increased dramatically in the past decade. Staff injuries caused by patients who are intoxicated or experiencing withdrawal have become common. Mother Teresa's counsel to see Christ in the distressing disguise of the poor requires the supreme charity and submissiveness that Jesus Himself demonstrated in his life on earth.[8]

The virtue of fortitude, or courage, is required by caregivers as they practice and interact with colleagues within their specialty. Physicians within the fields of gynecology and obstetrics who will not prescribe contraceptive agents and refuse to perform or refer for abortion may struggle to maintain their practice and have difficulty in obtaining staff privileges at secular hospitals. Nurses who decline to assist in abortions and patient teaching regarding contraception and pharmacists who decline to dispense contraceptives and abortifacients are accused of forcing their personal values on patients. In the face of this type of pressure within the professions, caregivers need the virtue of fortitude as their guide.

In contrast to the study of virtues, a study of the common vices in man may help one to recognize and avoid these vices in the health professions. In the *Divine Comedy*, Dante describes a journey through the circles of hell.[9] The outer circles featured those guilty of sins of paganism, gluttony, and avarice, while the darkest and innermost circle featured those guilty of Dante's most serious sin, betrayal. The three sufferers in the innermost circle of hell were Judas Iscariot, Brutus, and Cassius. What *kinds* of actions might place the health professional in Dante's innermost circle of hell? Objectively speaking, examples are the caregiver who performs or promotes abortion, the nurse who intentionally gives too much pain medication to a dying patient because his suffering seems senseless, the physician who provides what he knows to be useless treatment because of the profit involved, the social worker who sends an abused child back to his home because she is unwilling to take on the enormous amount of paperwork and effort required to retain the child in protective custody.

Evidence-Based Medicine

Evidence-based medicine refers to the process of integrating the best research evidence with clinical expertise and patient values to obtain the best clinical outcomes.[10] On its face, this seems to be common sense, but Pellegrino notes that the virtue of prudence is still required to distinguish the best available evidence from the best possible evidence and again to decide when evidence is strong enough to warrant taking action.[11]

Strengthening the virtue of health professions calls for open and honest appraisal of the members of these professions. This appraisal should be done within and among the various fields of health care. The use of hospital ethics committees is one way of attempting to promote virtues in health care. A group of persons representing not only members of the professions but also patients and family members can provide important insight by helping caregivers reflect on their actions. Including the study of the virtues in the education of health professionals is another way of promoting virtue. Perhaps the most important way to promote virtues in health care is by ensuring that virtuous persons serve as role models for those entering the professions. Senior physicians, nurses, social workers, and others who work within an institution should possess the virtues to which an institution is committed in patient care.

The special way in which Christian health professionals are called to view their vocation is described by Benedict Ashley, O.P., and Kevin O'Rourke O.P.: "Christians think of life as a gift of God and the body as a marvelous work of divine creation to be reverenced as a temple of God" (see 1 Cor 6:19; 2 Cor 6:16).[12] They explain that health professionals find a model in Jesus Christ the healer, and should recognize their dependence upon God who gives them the inspiration, insight, and courage to carry out their work.

Notes

[1] William Osler, *Aequanimitas* (Philadelphia: P. Blakiston's Son & Co, 1932), 159.

[2] Edmund D. Pellegrino, "The Four Principles and the Doctor–Patient Relationship: The Need for a Better Linkage," in *Principles of Health Care Ethics*, ed. Raanon Gillon (New York: John Wiley & Sons, 1994).

[3] Edmund D. Pellegrino and David C. Thomasma, *For the Patient's Good* (New York: Oxford University Press, 1988).

[4] E. M. Chevien, "Euthanasia Promises Marcus Welby, but Gives Us Jack Kevorkian," *Medical Economics* 72.1 (January 9, 1995): 25–26, 28.

[5] Terrence F. Ackerman, "Why Doctors Should Intervene," in *Biomedical Ethics* 3rd ed., ed, T. A. Mappes and J. Zembaty (New York: McGraw-Hill, 1991), 70; originally published in *Hastings Center Report* 12.4 (August 1982): 14–17.

[6] Aristotle, *Nicomachean Ethics*, trans. Martin Ostwald (Upper Saddle River, NJ: Prentice Hall, 1962).

[7] Romanus Cessario, *The Moral Virtues and Theological Ethics* (Notre Dame, IN: University of Notre Dame Press, 1992), 20.

[8] Malcolm Muggeridge, *Something Beautiful for God* (New York: HarperCollins Publishers, 1971).

[9] Dante Aligheiri, *Divine Comedy*, trans. John Ciardi (New York: New American Libray, 1982)

[10] Hans B. Kersten, E. Douglas Thompson, John G. Frohna, "The Use of Evidence-Based Medicine in Pediatrics: Past, Present, and Future," *Current Opinion in Pediatrics* 20.3 (2008) 326–331.

[11] Edmund D. Pellegrino, "Medical Evidence and Virtue Ethics: A Commentary on Zarkovich and Upshur," *Theoretical Medicine and Bioethics* 23.4–5 (July 2002): 397–402.

[12] Benedict M. Ashley and Kevin D. O'Rourke, *Health Care Ethics: A Theological Analysis*, 4th ed. (Washington, D.C.: Georgetown University Press, 1997), 80.(

✠

Editorial Summation: William Osler, one of the founders of the Johns Hopkins Hospital, taught that it is the role of the health professional—not of the hospital—provide care to the patients. He further held that this care is grounded in Christianity. It is the health professionals who are "agents of the Trust," of that trust which is at the core of the caregiver/patient relationship. According to Pellegrino the good of the patient includes at least four components: (1) the ultimate good of human life as perceived by the patient; 2) the good of the patient as a human person; (3) the patient's assessment of what is good; (4) the biomedical or clinical good. In obtaining informed consent for treatment from the patient, it is important that it be elicited from him or her in a manner and language which enables the patient to understand the nature of the treatment and its consequences as well as the consequences of treatment refusal. The physician, nurse, or other health-caregiver should be a virtuous person. The four cardinal virtues each have their own importance and contribution to make: prudence, justice, temperance, and fortitude. These need to be augmented by the theological virtues of faith, hope, and charity. Knowledge of the vices which may plague health-care workers is likewise useful in recognizing the *pitfalls* to avoid. Christian health professionals bring a special perspective to their work: life is a gift from God and the body is the temple of God. A model to emulate is Jesus Christ as He responded to the needs of the people.

PART VI

INSTITUTIONAL ISSUES

CHAPTER 24

Triage and the Duty to Care

Marie T. Hilliard, R.N.

A pandemic due to the avian flu virus (H5N1) is possible and, if it occurs, the event will not be unfamiliar to health care workers. History provides us with numerous examples. In the twentieth century alone, there were three pandemics, the largest being the 1918 "Spanish" influenza outbreak, in which forty to fifty million people died worldwide within one year.[1] Five hundred thousand persons died in the United States alone.[2] Such crises have generated heroic responses by health care workers. The question that arises today is whether such heroism will prevail in the face of varying perceptions concerning the duty of health care workers to care.

The World Health Organization has stated that a possible influenza pandemic is imminent.[3] In 1997, the first documented H5N1 infections in humans occurred; mortality rates in humans with the disease are over 50 percent.[4] As of September, 2008, 387 persons in fifteen countries contracted the disease. Of these, 245 persons in twelve countries have died from H5N1, demonstrating a mortality rate of over 63 percent.[5] It is estimated that in the United States alone such a pandemic could kill almost two million persons.[6] National preparedness plans are underway, involving health care workers and agencies.

Part of this preparedness includes surveying health care workers to determine their willingness to provide care during a pandemic. One study suggests that nearly half of local health department workers are likely not to report to duty; however, it showed that clinical staffers are more likely to report than technical and support staff.[7] In conjunction with an emergency preparedness training program for school health nurses, another study was conducted. Ninety percent of these nurses reported at least one barrier to reporting for duty in the event of such an emergency. Barriers frequently reported were family care responsibilities, transportation, and personal health issues.[8] A study of the nature of the catastrophic event and of the self-reported ability and willingness of health care workers to report to duty, indicates that health care workers were least willing to report to duty during a sudden acute respiratory distress syndrome (SARS) outbreak (48 percent). Concerns affecting willingness to report to duty include fear and concern for family and self and personal health problems.[9]

In fact, health care workers, including those who had recovered from SARS, have fears of infecting others, especially family members, which are equal to, if not greater than, fears for their own health.[10] Research indicates that providing treatment on site for family members increases the commitment to work of health care providers.[11] Furthermore, health care workers were perceived as a potential source of infection in the community.[12] Because of the similarities of the health impacts of an avian flu pandemic and the SARS coronavirus outbreak of 2003, such findings do not bode well for addressing public health needs in an avian flu pandemic.

Legal Perspectives

In examining the imperatives to care, analyses have been provided from legal, ethical, and moral perspectives. Legally, the issue of the duty to care is framed in the context of medical negligence and liability. The three-pronged analysis of liability is constructed in the framework preventing the occurrence of any damage. This analysis dictates that the damage must be a reasonable, foreseeable consequence of the negligence, there must be a proximate relationship of the health care provider to the victim, and the imposed liability must be just and convenient.[13] Duty to care is linked to a voluntary assumption of responsibility, including fiscal responsibility for claims of negligence.

Legally, in the absence of a physician–patient relationship, a physician can refuse to provide care. However, a physician has a duty to care for those with whom he or she has established a physician–patient relationship.[14] Furthermore, health care facilities accepting certain types of public funding may have obligations to treat certain categories of patients under certain conditions. Also, emergency rooms may be required to provide care to those presenting themselves with life-threatening conditions.[15]

Negligence is also addressed from a legal perspective in state practice acts. The National Council of State Boards of Nursing, in its model nursing practice act, does address negligence, but only in terms of reporting negligent behavior of the licensed professional. Moral turpitude is also addressed and is defined, in part, as "conduct that involves one or more of the following: intentional, knowing or reckless conduct that causes injury or places another in fear of imminent harm; conduct done knowingly contrary to justice or honesty; [or] conduct that is contrary to the accepted and customary rule of right and duty that a person owes to fellow human beings and society in general."[16] Of import is the last descriptor, which acknowledges that the nurse has a duty to "fellow human beings and society in general." However, nowhere does the model nursing practice act explicate this text.

"Essentials in a Modern Medical Practice Act," by the Federation of State Medical Boards of the United States, also contains a reference to negligence; however, negligence is to be defined by the state medical board. The guide does not contain the word "duty." It does reference moral turpitude, but only as an unlawful act as determined by a court of competent jurisdiction.[17] Therefore, the law provides us with little guidance, from a legal perspective, pursuant to a duty to care.

Ethical Standards of Care

In the absence of legal directions one can look toward ethical standards of care. There are those who hold that the duty to care in a pandemic is ethically obligatory for anyone who assumes the responsibilities of a chosen health care profession. Furthermore, duty of care can be used as a subtle instrument of intimidation of health care workers.[18] Society does have expectations of health care professionals, to whom they have provided special privileges, be it as simple as access to MD license plates for their cars. Signs of these societal expectations are obvious, as well as subtle. A daily calendar, usually given as a gift to a nurse, lists five reasons for becoming a nurse. Listed as number one of these reasons is "You can expose yourself to rare, exciting, and new diseases."[19] Although stated in jest, it clearly indicates societal expectations.

From an ethical perspective the term "duty of care" (used synonymously with "duty to care") refers to these special obligations; that is, doctors and nurses have a greater obligation of beneficence than most others. Beneficence is a foundational principle of the patient–provider relationship,[20] to further patient welfare and to advance patient well-being.[21] These special obligations exist for three reasons: health care professionals have a proportionally greater ability (than the public) to provide care; professionals, in choosing their professions, have assumed the risks of providing care; and the professions are legitimated by their contracts with society, resulting in the obligation of professionals to be available in times of emergency.[22] Furthermore, doctors give implicit consent to assuming the risks and responsibilities associated with the specialties in which they agree to practice. In a pandemic, the risks to health care workers are real: 30 percent of cases in the 2003 SARS outbreak were among health care professionals, some of whom died from the infection. In fact, Dr. Carlo Urbani of the World Health Organization succumbed to the virus, which he acquired while carrying out his professional duties.[23] One would hope to find direction in the professional codes of ethics in seeking guidance for responding to such dilemmas..

In examining statements from professional associations, one finds an ethical stance indicating that the duty of care is neither fixed nor absolute, but contextual. Factors to be considered are the risk level of the working environment (e.g., lack of protective equipment), the specialty of the health care worker, the likelihood of harm related to the benefits of care, and competing obligations of the health care worker as a member of a family and a community.[24] There are those who believe that health care workers have a right to resign from their positions when they believe their responsibilities to family outweigh those to the community.[25] In retrospect, one could ask whether, on September 11, 2001, New York City firefighters would have been justified in not attempting to ascend 110 flights of stairs in the World Trade Center.

In June 2004, in the aftermath of 9/11, the American Medical Association adopted an ethical policy statement, "Physician Obligation in Disaster Preparedness and Response." This policy states, in part:

National, regional, and local responses to epidemics, terrorist attacks, and other disasters require extensive involvement of physicians. Because of their commitment to care for the sick and injured, individual physicians have an obligation to provide urgent medical care during disasters. This ethical obligation holds even in the face of greater than usual risks to their own safety, health or life. The physician workforce, however, is not an unlimited resource; therefore, when participating in disaster responses, physicians should balance immediate benefits to individual patients with ability to care for patients in the future.[26]

As admirable as these words seem, they reflect a weakening from earlier policy statements, which, until 1970, included an admonition to alleviate suffering, even to the point of jeopardizing one's own life.[27]

The American Nurses Association *Code of Ethics for Nurses with Interpretive Statements* includes the word "duty" five times. Duty is discussed in relationship to confidentiality, protection of participants in research, addressing impaired practice, and preservation of integrity. Integrity is defined as, "an aspect of wholeness of character and is primarily a self concern of the individual nurse."[28] In terms of a duty to care, the focus is upon conscientious objection. In such circumstances the following statement is made: "The nurse who decides not to take part on the grounds of conscientious objection must communicate this decision in appropriate ways. Whenever possible, such a refusal should be made known in advance and in time for alternate arrangements to be made for patient care. The nurse is obliged to provide for the patient's safety, to avoid patient abandonment, and to withdraw only when assured that alternative sources of nursing care are available to the patient."[29] While, this section of the *Code* primarily deals with conscientious objection on moral or ethical grounds, an example reflecting the nurse's right to self protection is given pertaining to verbal abuse from co-workers or patients. No reference is made to negligence, epidemic, pandemic or disaster. However, the American Nurses Association has adopted a position statement which provides an ethical framework for nurses to determine if they have a duty to care in the face of personal risk. The statement recognizes the risks inherent in caring for those with communicable diseases:

> Even with the benefit of the recognition of risk and responsibility with guidelines for prevention, it is the nature of health problems such as acquired immunodeficiency syndrome (AIDS), cytomegalovirus

(CMV), hepatitis B or C, human immunodeficiency virus (HIV), severe acute respiratory syndrome (SARS), the threat of bioterrorism agents, including bubonic or pneumonic plague, smallpox, and viral hemorrhagic fever, and other newly diagnosed infectious diseases which may raise questions for the nurse regarding personal risk and responsibility for care of the patient.[30]

In the face of such risks, the nurse is to differentiate between a moral obligation or duty, and a moral option to care. Four fundamental criteria are presented to assist in determining whether a moral obligation to care exists for the nurse: the patient is at significant risk of harm, loss, or damage if the nurse does not assist; the nurse's intervention or care is directly relevant to preventing harm; the nurse's care will probably prevent harm, loss, or damage to the patient; and the benefit the patient will gain outweighs any harm the nurse might incur and does not present more than an acceptable risk to the nurse.[31] If all four are present, a duty to care exists. As with that of the American Medical Association, this position reflects a change in historical thinking on this matter. In 1926, a suggested code of ethics, which was published but never adopted, contained the following phrase: "The most precious possession of this profession is the ideal of service, extending even to the sacrifice of life itself."[32] Thus, there appears to be ambiguity in both the medical and nursing professions' understandings of the ethical duty to care in the face of personal risk.

Philosophical Approaches

Ethical frameworks have been developed to assist in resolving such ethical situations or dilemmas. "Ethical situations" are topics of current interest in applied bioethics which illustrate ethical concepts, such as allocation of resources.[33] In such situations, one usually finds two goods, such as justice and beneficence, in conflict. Ethical frameworks apply "ethical theories" to these situations or dilemmas. Ethical theories are the analytical methods or modes of philosophical reasoning (e.g., subjective and objective methods) utilized in ethical decision-making in these situations.[34] The problem is that these analytical methods vary greatly, potentially providing even less guidance than the previously mentioned legal frameworks and codes of ethics.

Subjective methods are relativistic in approach. No human act, in and of itself, is considered good or bad. The act is made good or bad relative to some other criterion. Relativist ethics include situationism, consequentialism, and utilitarianism. In situationism, an act is judged in the situation in which it is performed. The intent of the act is the criterion that determines the ethicalness of the act; for example, "I intend that my family remains healthy; therefore, I will not report to work in the event of a pandemic." In consequentialism, the end justifies the means; for example, "By not reporting to duty in a pandemic, I will not get sick." Thus, the ethicalness of the act is determined by the foreseen consequences, although some would hold that it is impossible to foresee all the consequences. In utilitarianism, the ethicalness is determined by the greatest good for the greatest number, as in triage. Utilitarian reasoning could lead a health care worker to conclude that it would be justified not to report to duty during a pandemic because, "If I report to duty and get sick, I cannot help numerous others in need *and* I could advance the spread of the disease by infecting others." From a utilitarian perspective, the "good" is determined by whatever maximizes pleasure and minimizes pain for the greatest number of persons. In fact, such an approach dictates the way in which many of our laws are promulgated. In such a case, recipients of these acts would hope to be in the majority. However, John Rawls holds that individuals have a duty to act according to the laws that they would propose if they were unaware of their present socioeconomic status; that is, in this case, access to health care providers would not be based on socioeconomic status. This is the foundation of John Rawls's rules by social contract.[35] Thus, his reasoning also is considered to be objective, as in deontological reasoning.

Objective methods dictate that some actions may never be done regardless of the circumstances. Actions are only hypothetically indifferent (e.g., speaking versus giving a verbal order for morphine administration). Included in these methods are principled reasoning, such as deontological reasoning, and law ethics. Kant's deontological reasoning dictates that one is to act only according to universal maxims; that is, one would will that those maxims would become universal laws.[36] Therefore, one always is to report to duty, in all circumstances. Deontological methods embrace duty and obligation, the substance of the question being addressed here. Duty and obligation are the very motives for action, regardless of the consequences. Acts are not performed to achieve happiness, but for duty's sake. This reasoning can lead to a form of legal positivism, that is, as long as the law dictates an action, it is ethical. The problem is that laws can change and may reflect the lowest common denominator. Reliance on the law by some physicians in Nazi Germany led to the Nuremberg Trials.

Ethic of the Good

Having examined legal imperatives and ethical reasoning, we move to a moral perspective, reflected in the "ethic of the good." The ethic of the good embraces the objective method of reasoning by the virtuous person. The concept of the virtuous person was proposed by Socrates, developed by Plato, and advanced by Aristotle. Aristotle held that the soul of the person is fitted by nature for virtue, but that virtue has to be acquired through sound choice. The virtuous person acts reasonably, by acting on behalf of ends rightly perceived as goods in pursuit of happiness. This is consistent with natural moral law. From St. Thomas Aquinas's perspective, God, the Creator of human nature, is the ultimate source of this happiness.[37] Whether from a theological or an Aristotelian perspective, natural moral law is part of the natural order, and thus is consistent with reasoning. The virtuous person would report to duty in a pandemic because it is virtuous to serve others in need. The "golden rule" fosters the good of society, leading to happiness. This same virtuous person also would act reasonably in assuming duties. For example, a nurse with an immunosuppressed family member in his or her household would not take on the responsibilities of a direct care giver to those who have contracted a pandemic flu.

The health care professional is not the only one with a moral duty; society has the duty to protect the health care worker by providing protective equipment, antiviral medications, and available vaccines. Furthermore, the provision of sufficient health care workers, through aids and incentives for preparation as well as recruitment and retention programs, is a societal responsibility. Thus, beneficence is not the only ethical principle at issue; justice also is, as it pertains to allocation of resources, particularly the allocation of health care providers. In earlier research, this author defined justice, pursuant to the obligations of the health care worker, as the equal distribution of rights and resources to all patients.[38] However, it became apparent through that research that all patients do not have equal needs. Equal distribution of resources to every person is inappropriate when one considers individual health needs, autonomy, and total societal needs and resources. Thus, in terms of societal resources, this definition must be refined to refer to the equitable distribution of resources to all patients. By this is meant that all persons should have an equal opportunity to access resources which they rightly perceive as goods in pursuit of happiness. In other words, it is reasonable for persons in our communities, when experiencing illness or the threat of illness, to expect to have access to health care workers.

Faith-Based Care and Triage

The U.S. Department of Health and Human Services estimates that a pandemic could cause illness in ninety million Americans, and that ten million of them could require hospitalization. The department also estimates that in the first year of a pandemic, less than 10 percent of the population will receive an effective vaccine. Shortages of vaccines, antivirals, equipment, and supplies will be inevitable, necessitating rationing of health care.[39] Most important, the strain on health care workers will be significant. It is well documented that the nursing shortage will take years to reverse.[40] Also, between 1970 and 1999, the number of public health workers in every federal health district declined.[41] It is important to identify, in advance, the providers of nongovernmental health care services. The largest such provider in the United States is the Catholic Church. In response to societal obligations, each Roman Catholic diocese in the United States has adopted the *Ethical and Religious Directives for Catholic Health Care Services* (2001). These directives state, "Catholic health care ministry seeks to contribute to the common good. The common good is realized when economic, political, and social conditions ensure protection for the fundamental rights of all individuals and enable all to fulfill their common purpose and reach their common goals."[42] This means protecting the fundamental rights of all persons, including employees.

Faith-based providers have obligations within a society. In the event of an anticipated pandemic, faith-based providers must be prepared for the following realities: (1) staff shortages due to the tensions between the need of health care workers to work to support their families and their need to protect their families from the virus; (2) staff refusals to report to duty either out of indolence or legitimate concerns, such as fear, real sickness, or governmental policy; (3) the need to create work opportunities such as working from home, provision of protective equipment, and child care if schools are closed; (4) staff who report to work showing signs of illness, and staff refusal of medical treatment for fear of getting sicker; (5) provision of supplies like food and water; and (6) the possibility of quarantines or forced social distancing.[43] However, these realities must be anticipated by all providers, not just faith-based providers. Furthermore, these realities will be compounded by the fact that studies indicate that a substantial number of health care workers will not come to work during a pandemic. Thus, the rationing of personnel also is inevitable.

Triage, the concept of determining who will live when not all can live, involves the rationing of scarce resources, including health care workers.[44] Options for such rationing in a pandemic that have been proposed as ethical include (1) prioritizing to prevent new infections (reserving vaccines and antiviral drugs); (2) prioritizing to protect essential medical and scientific personnel (with specialized training and a duty to care); (3) prioritizing the health and safety infrastructure (delineating the obligations of those workers who have been prioritized); (4) prioritizing patients or populations with the greatest medical needs, including use of age-based criteria (a controversial determinant that is not accepted by this author, although an overall-health criterion, based on a patient's ability to benefit from care, is accepted);[45] (5) prioritizing patients or populations who are chronically underserved (reflecting fairness in the application of actions); (6) prioritizing early detection and global response methods (cognizant that a new pandemic will have a disproportionate effect on the poorest of the world); and (7) prioritizing provisions for transparency and public cooperation (fostering trust and compliance with allocation plans).[46] Options 2 and 3 are the heart of the matter in this essay. While health care workers can claim a right to access scarce resources such as vaccines and antiviral drugs to minimize an acknowledged risk to their own health, at the same time they have an obligation to provide services to the community that justify their access to these limited resources. Thus, professional codes of ethics that provide for a subjective analysis of such risks would appear to provide for rights without corresponding obligations.

There is the question of the moral liceity of prioritizing patients or populations, either by those with the greatest medical needs, including use of age-based criteria, or by identifying those who have been chronically underserved. Clearly age-based triage immorally assigns a worth or dignity to those deemed to be more valuable to society. Triaging in relationship to medical needs can be used to discriminate against those who will consume the greatest resources, either in personnel or medical resources, or to serve those first, who are in life threatening situations. When health care personnel and medical resources are plentiful, the latter criterion meets the ethical standard of beneficence. However, when resources are scarce such an approach could violate the principle of nonmaleficence (to do not harm). Triage on the basis of the greatest good for the greatest number (utilitarianism) may be justified. However, decisions to treat or not to treat are not based on the subjective standard of individual worth, or even on an attempt to redress the injustices to the chronically underserved, but on the objective standard of who can benefit from the limited resources available. The availability of resources is one criterion of determining whether such resources are ordinary or extraordinary means. Thus this age-old criterion can be invoked. Limited resources, such as ventilators, dialysis, or even the services of limited health care personnel can be allocated licitly to those who have the best chance of benefiting from these resources.

Heroism and Virtue

The question that remains is whether historic professional heroism will prevail in the face of varying perceptions concerning the duty of health care workers to care. Legal liability provisions are framed in the context of an existing professional–patient relationship, which is not the usual preexisting scenario in a pandemic. Legal mandates in state practice acts are vague at best. As stated earlier, professional codes of ethics provide for subjective analyses of rights and obligations by the professional. Ethical theories, the analytical methods of philosophical reasoning, vary greatly in their approaches. Therefore, one is left with the natural moral law, either of Aristotle or Aquinas, also known as the "ethic of the good": "The grasping of the fundamental precepts of the natural moral law, whether undertaken theologically within the realm of faith, or outside it, comes about through the intuition of the *instinctus rationis* that perceives the ordering of nature toward that which is most appropriate to it."[47] The virtuous person acts reasonably by acting on behalf of ends perceived as goods in pursuit of happiness.

The virtuous person would report to duty in a pandemic because it is virtuous to serve others in need. He or she would be acting on behalf of an end, which is the health of the community, perceived as a good in pursuit of happiness. This good is a function of happiness, because we are members of this same community whose health we are protecting. This same virtuous person also would act reasonably in assuming duties. Thus, while the health care worker has an obligation to report to duty, allocation of responsibilities while on duty is to be consistent with the abilities and other obligations of the health care worker. At the same time, the reasoning person would recognize that all of society is at risk, including themselves and their loved ones, if the pandemic is not contained. A reasonable person would also recognize that in serving society one is serving oneself and one's family. Thus, there is one duty throughout: a duty to care for oneself, one's family, and society.

Notes

[1] Colin Lowry, "Last Chance to Stop Avian Flu Pandemic," *21st Century Science and Technology* 18.3 (Fall 2005): 32.

[2] Channing Bete Company, "How You Can Be Prepared for a Flu Pandemic: An Individual and Family Handbook" (Deerfield, MA: Channing Bete, 2006), 5, distributed by the State of Connecticut Comptroller's Office and Anthem Blue Cross and Blue Shield of Connecticut.

[3] Pan American Health Organization and World Health Organization, Subcommittee on Planning and Programming of the Executive Committee, Fortieth Session, "Influenza Epidemic: Progress Report," February 16, 2006 (SPP40/5), 6, http://www.ops-oms.org/english/gov/ce/spp/spp40-05-e.pdf.

[4] Lowry, "Last Chance," 27, 29.

[5] World Health Organization, "Cumulative Number of Confirmed Human Cases of Avian Influenza A/(H5N1) Reported to WHO," September 10, 2008, http://www.who.int/csr/disease/avian_influenza/country/cases_table_2008_09_10/en/index.html.

[6] Channing Bete, "How You Can Be Prepared," 5.

[7] R. D. Balicer et al., "Local Public Health Workers' Perceptions toward Responding to an Influenza Pandemic," *BMC Public Health* 6 (April 18, 2006): 99, http://www.astho.org/pubs/Pandemic/Flu/Workforce2.pdf.

[8] K. A. Qureshi et al., "Emergency Preparedness Training for Public Health Nurses: A Pilot Study," *Journal of Urban Health* 79.3 (September 2002): 413–416.

[9] K. A. Qureshi et al., "Health Care Workers' Ability and Willingness to Report to Duty during Catastrophic Disasters," *Journal of Urban Health* 82.3 (September 2005): 378–388.

[10] S. M. Ho et al., "Fear of Severe Acute Respiratory Syndrome (SARS) among Health Care Workers," *Journal of Consulting and Clinical Psychology* 73.2 (April 2005): 344–349.

[11] J. I. Syrett et al., "Will Emergency Health Care Providers Respond to Mass Casualty Incidents?" *Prehospital Emergency Care* 11.1 (January–March 2007): 49–54.

[12] Dessmon Y. H. Tai, "SARS Plague: Duty of Care or Medical Heroism," *Annals of the Academy of Medicine, Singapore* 35.5 (May 2006) 374–378.

[13] Suresh Nair, "Medical Negligence: Duty of Care," abridged, *SMA News* (1992):1, http://www.sma.org.sg/sma_news/3307/duty_of_care.pdf.

[14] Ibid., 2.

[15] "Establishing a Duty of Medical Care," Buchanan & Beckering P.L.C. Web site, accessed November 18, 2008, http://www.michiganpatient.com/michigan_medical_malpractice_duty_of_care.php.

[16] National Council of State Boards of Nursing (NCSBN), "Model Nursing Practice Act" (2004), III.4Z, https://www.ncsbn.org/Chapter3.pdf.

[17] Federation of State Medical Boards of the United States, "Essentials of a Modern Medical Practice Act," 11th ed. (2006), www.fsmb.org/pdf/GPROL_essentials_eleventh_edition.pdf.

[18] Daniel K. Sokol, "Virulent Epidemics and Scope of Healthcare Workers' Duty of Care," *Emerging Infectious Diseases* 12.8 (August 2006): 1238, http://www.cdc.gov/ncidod/EID/vol12no08/pdfs/06-0360.pdf.

[19]"Five Reasons to Become a Nurse," *Nurses 2007 Desk Calendar*, January 17, 2007 (Kansas City, MO: Andrews McMeel Publishing, 2006).

[20]P. Entralgo, S. Bloom, R. Purtilo, "Professional-Patient Relationship," in *Encyclopedia of Bioethics*, ed. Warren T. Reich (New York: Simon & Schuster, 1995).

[21]Carly Ruderman et al., "On Pandemics and the Duty to Care: Whose Duty? Who Cares?" *BMC Medical Ethics* 7.5 (April 20, 2006): 3.

[22]Ibid., 3.

[23]Ibid., 1–3.

[24]Sokol, "Virulent Epidemics," 1238–1239.

[25]Tai, "SARS Plague," 374–378.

[26]American Medical Association, "Physician Obligation in Disaster Preparedness and Response" in *Code of Medical Ethics: Current Opinions with Annotations*, 2006–2007 ed., (USA: AMWA, 2006): 286, https://catalog.ama-assn.org/Catalog/product/product_detail.jsp?productId=prod710108?checkXwho=done#

[27]Ruderman, "On Pandemics," 5.

[28]American Nurses Association, *Code of Ethics for Nurses with Interpretive Statements* (Silver Spring, MD: ANA, 2005), http://nursingworld.org/ethics/code/protected_nwcoe813.htm.

[29]Ibid.

[30]American Nurses Association, "Risk and Responsibility" position statement, June 21, 2006, 3, available from the ANA.

[31]Ibid.

[32]American Nurses Association, "A Suggested Code," *American Journal of Nursing*, August 1926. See also K. G. Hook and G. B. White, "Code of Ethics for Nurses with Interpretive Statements," ANA continuing education module, 2001, 3, http://nursingworld.org/mods/mod580/code.pdf, for a time line of the development of nursing's code of ethics.

[33]Rita Jean Payton, "A Bioethical Program for Baccalaureate Nursing Students" in *Ethics in Nursing Practice and Education*, ed. American Nurses Association Committee on Ethics (Kansas City, MO: ANA, 1980), 57–59.

[34]Ibid., 57–58.

[35]John Rawls, *A Theory of Justice*, rev. ed. (Oxford: Oxford University Press, 1999).

[36]Immanuel Kant, *The Metaphysics of Morals*, trans. and ed. Mary J. Gregor (Cambridge, U.K..: Cambridge University Press, 1996).

[37]Thomas Aquinas, *Summa theologiae*, trans. Fathers of the English Dominican Province (New York: Benziger, 1947).

[38]Marie T. Hilliard, "The Identification of Nursing Ethics Content and Teaching Strategies for Baccalaureate Nursing Curriculum through Policy Delphi" (Ph.D. diss., University of Connecticut, 1986), 174.

[39]Hastings Center, "Flu Pandemic and the Fair Allocation of Scarce Life-Saving Resources," bioethics background paper, September 12, 2006, 1, 2, http://www.thehastingscenter.org/pdf/flu_pandemic_and_the_fair_allocation_of_scarce_life_saving_resources.pdf.

[40]Tri-Council Members for Nursing, "Strategies to Reverse the New Nursing Shortage," American Association of Colleges of Nursing position statement, January 2001, http://www.aacn.nche.edu/Publications/positions/tricshortage.htm.

[41]Center for Health Policy, Columbia University School of Nursing, "The Public Health Workforce Enumeration 2000," Bureau of Health Professions, National Center for Health Workforce Information and Analysis, December 2000, ftp://ftp.hrsa.gov//bhpr/nationalcenter/phworkforce2000.pdf.

[42]U. S Conference of Catholic Bishops, *Ethical and Religious Directives for Catholic Health Care Services*, 4th ed. (Washington, D.C.: USCCB, 2001), 8–9.

[43]Hamilton County Pandemic Influenza Faith Advisory Committee, "Pandemic Flu Planning for Faith Communities" (Hamilton County, OH: General Health District, October 2006), available from Hamilton County Public Health.

[44]Hastings Center, "Flu Pandemic," 2.

[45]In fact, some hold that priority might be given to older persons and children, due to their higher risk of developing complications. See Channing Bete, "How You Can Be Prepared," 11.

[46]Lawrence O. Gostin, "Medical Countermeasures for Pandemic Influenza: Ethics and the Law," *Journal of the American Medical Association* 295.5 (February 1, 2006): 554–556.

[47]Wojciech Giertych, O.P., "New Prospects for the Application of the Natural Moral Law," address at the International Congress on the Natural Moral Law, Rome, February 14, 2007, in "Address of Papal Theologian on Natural Moral Law," ZENIT, February 24, 2007, http://www.zenit.org/article-19001?1=english.

✛

Editorial Summation: Will health care workers be willing to provide care during a pandemic, such as a potential avian flu outbreak? Some studies suggest that a significant percentage would be unwilling because of fear of provider or family member contracting disease, family care responsibilities, transportation problems, or personal health issues. The law provides us with little guidance on the correct approach to the duty to care, and the ethical standards of care adopted by the American Medical Association and the American Nurses Association appear flexible and less rigorous than those of the past, abandoning the ideal of heroism. Philosophical approaches to the question include the subjective methods of consequentialism and utilitarianism, and the objective methods of deontology and virtue ethics. The ethic of the good sees virtuous action as the key to happiness, both personal and social, and encourages right conduct under the guidance of reason. When faced with shortages of supplies, such as vaccines, antivirals, and even medical personnel, triage decisions must be based on who will most benefit from the receipt of these goods, and for whom they would be ordinary or proportionate means of conserving life, based upon criteria that include societal availability of such resources. The virtuous health care worker, acting in accord with the obligations to the patient, society, and the profession, will report to duty on behalf of the larger aim of benefiting the whole of society.

CHAPTER 25

Cooperating with Non-Catholic Partners

NCBC Ethicists

Replacement of traditional fee-for-service health care with capitation, the rising costs of new medical technologies, the duplication of health services among competitors, and the need to attract physician networks and managed care contracts are some of the factors that necessitate collaborative efforts among health care facilities. Because of the financial realities of health care delivery such as these, Catholic health care providers often enter into business agreements with non-Catholic providers in order to secure their ability to preserve the Catholic health care mission. Although the *Ethical and Religious Directives for Catholic Health Care Services* (*ERDs*) state that Catholic facilities should seek alliances with other Catholic institutions first, that is not, unfortunately, always possible.[a] The aim of this chapter is to set forth, in as clear a manner as possible, how the principle of cooperation may be used to assess whether or not a Catholic provider engages in immoral cooperation through a collaborative venture with a non-Catholic partner.

Not infrequently, the Catholic partner in a collaborative venture is accused of trying to impose Catholic values or teachings on the non-Catholic partner. However, every health care provider—individual or institutional—necessarily provides care consistent with its vision of what is ultimately good for the patient as a human being. This fact about health care delivery is inescapable whether or not the provider explicitly acknowledges the fact. Catholic health care holds to a view of the human good that is incompatible with certain actions such as abortion, euthanasia, and contraception. Non-Catholic providers in some cases deliver health care with a view of the patient's good as being compatible with choices for these same actions. The fact that a Catholic health care provider insists on preserving its mission in collaborative arrangements is not an imposition of Catholic values. It is rather an action in accord with the goal of every health care provider to deliver care consistent with a particular vision of the human good of the patient. The way in which a Catholic provider is able to limit collaboration with a partner who engages in procedures or activities that violate the dignity of human persons according to Catholic moral teaching is to structure the relationship consistent with the principle of cooperation. Proper adherence to this principle enables the Catholic provider to avoid immoral participation in what it views as contrary to human dignity.

There are five important prefatory points that need to be made for a correct understanding of the principle of cooperation. First, it is important to be clear about the meaning of "cooperation" as it functions in the principle. Cooperation means any free and knowing assistance of an individual or institution (the cooperator) in an immoral act performed by another individual or institution (the principal agent). The cooperator's assistance or contribution must be linked to the act of the principal agent in some identifiable way.

Second, cooperation in the immoral action of another is possible even if the principal agent does not acknowledge that the act is immoral. The moral status of actions is part of an objective moral order and not something determined by the subjective intention of the person.

Third, the term "evil" is not restricted only to what society views as heinous acts, but encompasses any act that lacks the moral goodness it ought to have. Thus, evil acts range from those that are morally less significant to those that are gravely immoral.

Fourth, cooperation in an act completed in the past is not possible, but is possible only for contemporaneous or future acts of a principal agent. Nonetheless, past completed actions (such as abortions used to obtain "biological material" for research) may contribute to legal and moral situations from which the Church has urged its members to withdraw in order "to affirm with clarity the value of human life."[b]

Finally, cooperation in evil must be distinguished from theological scandal. Scandal is any action, word, or deed that leads another to sin. Although they are sometimes related in concrete circumstances, cooperation is not, but scandal is a cause of an immoral will of another. "Scandal is an attitude or behavior which leads another to sin."[c] By way of advice, command, or example, the one who gives scandal helps to form the immoral will of another that did not previously exist. Cooperation, however, presupposes the immoral will of the principal agent. The assessment of institutional scandal is a pastoral one made by the local ordinary. The potential for scandal in a particular case may be such that it prohibits a collaborative arrangement that otherwise avoids immoral cooperation.[d]

The operative directive from the *ERDs* governing cooperation between Catholic and non-Catholic partners is n. 69, which states that:

> If a Catholic health care institution is considering entering into an arrangement with another organization that may be involved in activities judged morally wrong by the Church, participation in such activities must be limited to what is in accord with the moral principles governing cooperation.

The tradition holds that even justifiable cooperation in the immoral action of another is something that should be avoided, if this can be reasonably accomplished. If tolerable cooperation cannot be reasonably avoided, any cooperation that does exist should be limited. Therefore, this directive states that Catholic institutions should use the principle of cooperation in order to *limit* involvement in evil with non-Catholic providers, rather than to expand the ways in which the Catholic provider contributes to the procedures and activities in question.

Some may question whether a moral principle that developed as a guide for individuals can legitimately apply to institutions. This issue cannot be adequately addressed here. However, it is important to note these facts: the *ERDs* do employ the principle to evaluate and guide institutional relationships; the Congregation for the Doctrine of the Faith has allowed use of the principle for institutions; and many Catholic ethicists and theologians have successfully applied the principle to institutional relationships. The central reason why the principle of cooperation successfully applies to institutional relationships is that what pertains to individuals applies analogously to institutions. This fact about the institutional use of the principle parallels the function of the corporate person at law.[e]

Types of Cooperation: Formal and Material

Formal Cooperation

The designation of "cooperator" does not mean that the cooperation is morally justified. The cooperator is not immune from becoming a wrongdoer. Some types of cooperation cross the line into the actual doing of evil so that there are two wrongdoers: the original wrongdoer (the principal agent) and the cooperator. The principle of cooperation presumes that we know the different kinds of wrongdoing in the objective moral order. What needs articulation are the different sorts of cooperation which can serve as a guide for the cooperator to avoid evil while doing and pursuing good and to avoid becoming a wrongdoer as well.

Formal cooperation is any contribution to the principal agent's act in which the evil act is intended by the cooperator and this contribution is itself immoral. The formal cooperator contributes to one or more aspects of the act and intends that contribution in support of the act's immoral nature, either as an end or as a means to some other end of the cooperator. Formal cooperation can be either explicit or implicit. A Catholic health care provider who establishes the specific conditions under which direct sterilizations may be performed by a non-Catholic partner in a policy commits explicit formal cooperation in the immoral act of direct sterilization. In this instance the Catholic provider contributes to the way direct sterilization procedures are obtained and explicitly intends the immoral act by expressly establishing the conditions by which the procedure is done. To expressly state how a direct sterilization may be obtained is to intend what the procedure does.

An agent who performs implicit formal cooperation intentionally contributes to the principal agent's act not for the sake of the evil act itself, but as a means to some other end of the cooperator. The Catholic health care institution is especially susceptible to implicit formal cooperation because it can negotiate and adopt agreements that either establish or continue the provision of immoral procedures at the non-Catholic facility, not for its own sake, but as a means to achieve the good ends of Catholic health care.

What is done in the name of an institution consistent with its corporate documents, agreements, and policies is inescapably intentional. For example, a Catholic hospital may explicitly reject the immoral procedures and activities of a potential non-Catholic partner and yet negotiate and approve a legally binding agreement by means of which the non-Catholic partner is able to continue to engage in the immoral practices. The result is that the collaborative agreement simply enables them to be performed in a venue other than the Catholic facility.

It should be noted that mere physical distance of the immoral practices from the Catholic hospital is morally irrelevant if the Catholic institution is contractually committed to enabling the non-Catholic institution to continue the immoral practices through the provision of such things as space, personnel, management, and financing. When such collaboration occurs it is invariably provided by the Catholic institution not to bring about the immoral procedures, to be sure, but ultimately to seek other ends such as financial stability or the continuing provision of health care to the poor. Nonetheless, the immoral procedures would not be taking place but for the efforts of the Catholic partner to establish the conditions under which they are performed. To establish the enabling conditions for an immoral procedure or activity in this manner is to approve that which the conditions enable. This is implicit formal cooperation in evil and is immoral.

Therefore, as applied to health care collaboration agreements, implicit formal cooperation would include such things as negotiating, writing, or consenting to agreements which establish the governance, management, or financing of the immoral procedures of a non-Catholic entity or any institutional participation in those procedures and activities. More specifically, if the Catholic entity agrees in writing to assist in setting up a new facility or make use of an old one, or to provide personnel or equipment for the performance of immoral procedures or any institutional participation in those procedures and activities, then the Catholic institution is engaged in, at least, implicit formal cooperation. Implicit and explicit formal cooperation are both wrong under any circumstances and are not allowed by the *ERDs*.

Material Cooperation: Mediate and Immediate

If a cooperator does not intend the immoral act of a principal agent, but by an act that is in itself morally good or indifferent, contributes only to the circumstances associated with the principal agent's act without intending it, then the cooperator's action is called material cooperation. What distinguishes material from formal cooperation is that the material cooperator does not intend the evil of the principal agent. Some circumstances "touch upon" the evil act of the principal, meaning they contribute to bringing about the evil act. This can be understood as an essential circumstance of the immoral act. Some circumstances are more loosely connected with the evil act and are said to merely make possible the evil. This would be understood as a nonessential circumstance. For example, suppose an anesthesiologist is scheduled to provide anesthesia services to a patient undergoing a direct sterilization and does not intend that the patient be sterilized. Since anesthesia services assist in bringing about the sterilization, the anesthesiologist would be providing what is called an essential circumstance of the evil act. In contrast, consider building services personnel who clean the operating room (OR). Cleaning the OR only makes possible a direct sterilization. If one merely makes possible the evil act of another then the cooperator is said to contribute a nonessential circumstance.

Given these distinctions, material cooperation comes in two different sorts: mediate and immediate. Mediate material cooperation occurs when the cooperator assists in or contributes to the nonessential circumstances of the immoral act. A nonessential circumstance of an immoral act *makes possible* that act. Immediate material cooperation occurs when the cooperator assists in or contributes to the essential circumstances of the immoral act. An essential circumstance contributes to *bringing about* the immoral act of another.

Care must be exercised, however, in order to apply these terms correctly. When the immediate material cooperator is said to assist in bringing about the act of the principal agent, this should not be understood to mean that the cooperator is the principal cause of the immoral act, for then the cooperator would actually be a co-principal agent. The principal agent is the principal cause of the act and the immediate material cooperator helps to bring it about by contributing an essential circumstance associated with the principal agent's act. To clarify, the anesthesiologist does not bring about the act of sterilization himself, but helps bring it about by contributing those essential circumstances which are causally efficacious for *the principal* to perform the act of sterilization. Depending on the degree of institutional integration in a collaborative arrangement between Catholic and non-Catholic partners, the assessment of whether a circumstance is essential or nonessential can be more or less difficult.

Take the example of the provision of materials or instruments utilized for immoral procedures. Providing such instruments assists in or contributes to bringing about the immoral act since such instruments are the means by which the act is performed. This would be an example of institutional immediate material cooperation.

Now take the example of transportation, security, parking, and linen services at an institution where immoral procedures were taking place. These would be examples of institutional mediate material cooperation.

It is important to note for the question of cooperation (apart from scandal) that the physical remoteness or proximity of contributed services to an immoral act does not determine their moral status, but rather the *causal* relationship these services have to the act. Bringing about and making possible are different kinds of causal relation, and immediate and mediate cooperation relate to these two kinds of causal relation respectively. Also, even mediate material cooperation requires some justifying reason in order to take place. The more grave the evil being performed by the principal agent the more "remote" must be the mediate material cooperation. The more grave the evil, the more "remote" the action of the cooperator must be in terms of its being causally related to the action of the principal agent. It may justifiably be more "proximate" if the evil of the principal agent is less grave. Being a custodian in a Planned Parenthood facility would indeed be remote to the evils being performed. However, since the direct killing of the innocent is so grave, it is doubtful even this remote mediate material cooperation could be justified.

Immoral Cooperation, Culpability, and Duress

Immediate material cooperation in an intrinsic evil is itself an evil act. The reason is that by assisting in bringing about an immoral act (i.e., by contributing an essential circumstance) one is, in a derivative sense, responsible for that immoral act. In the case of immediate material cooperation the cooperator assists in bringing about the immoral act of the principal agent. This is enough to ground partial responsibility for that act. The ERDs are clear that immediate material cooperation by a Catholic health care institution in intrinsically evil acts is not permitted. "Catholic health care organizations are not permitted to engage in immediate material cooperation in actions that are intrinsically immoral, such as abortion, euthanasia, assisted suicide, and direct sterilization."[f] (We can add to this list several other intrinsically evil acts such as in vitro fertilization, artificial insemination by donor, the use of donor eggs, the cryopreservation of embryos, and embryonic destructive research.)

Even mediate material cooperation cannot always be justified. Mediate moral cooperation may be morally justified if there is a good to be preserved or evil that may

be avoided that is proportionate to the nonessential circumstances associated with the principal agent's act and the gravity of the evil of the principal agent's act. Historically, theologians have determined this proportionality of goods and evils in mediate material cooperation by applying the principle of double effect (see chapter 3D) to the cooperator. In the context of the principle of the double effect, the act in question is the cooperator's act; the good effect is the good achieved by the cooperator's act; the bad effect is the appropriation of the cooperator's act by the principal agent. In terms of the conditions of the principle of double effect,

- The cooperator's act is itself morally good or indifferent
- The cooperator does not intend the evil of the principal agent's act or the appropriation of his assistance
- The good effect is not achieved by means of the bad effect (the principal agent is the primary cause of the evil act and of the appropriation of the assistance of the cooperator)
- The good effect of the cooperator's act is proportionate to the bad effect

As can be determined from this, not all cases of mediate material cooperation in evil are permissible. For example, providing janitorial services to Planned Parenthood may be impermissible even though one is only contributing to the nonessential circumstances of the evil of abortion (i.e., one is only making possible those activities) taking place at the Planned Parenthood site. In particular, such cooperation may not satisfy condition of the good effect of the cooperator's act being proportionate to the bad effect (d) since there probably is not a *proportionate* reason for providing such services. In general, the graver the evil, such as the direct killing of the innocent in abortion, the more the cooperator needs to be causally distant from the evil act.

Some situations exist where the Catholic health care provider looks to negotiate an arrangement with a non-Catholic partner in order to maintain the presence and viability of the Catholic hospital, or even to survive. In order to preserve this great good, the Catholic institution may negotiate an arrangement that would involve immoral cooperation. An attempt is then made to justify this as an instance of "institutional duress": in the interest of preserving a good, a "moral sacrifice" has to be made.

Institutional duress associated with illicit cooperation does not justify such cooperation because duress does not change the *kind* of action being performed by the institution. There is an important difference here between institutional and individual cooperation though. For individual cooperators the fear that results from duress is a circumstance that substantially alters the subjective culpability of the individual cooperator, diminishing it or eliminating it altogether. For example, a clerk held at gunpoint is told to open the store safe. The clerk opens that safe and thus appears to cooperate immediately in the act of theft. The clerk does this in order to preserve the great good of his own life. But the clerk's cooperation may be justified for two reasons. First, the good of life is preferable to the loss of property and thus he cannot be blamed or held culpable for cooperating in the theft. Second, the clerk's actions may not even be an act of cooperation at all since the clerk does not knowingly *and freely* assist in an evil act of the principal agent (the thief).

Neither line of reasoning, however, can be applied to health care institutions. No human life is in jeopardy or under threat when a Catholic hospital closes down or is sold to a non-Catholic buyer, as regrettable and as tragic as that may be. There could be diminished access to quality health care in a given community, but this is not a specifically Catholic health care problem nor is it one for which the Catholic entity would be held morally culpable. Adequate access to quality health care is a great social concern for everyone and is beyond the capabilities of Catholic health care alone to address. Therefore, it is not a Catholic problem as such. It is certainly true that financial health and even the life of the Catholic institution may be at stake, but the loss of the health care facility is not equivalent to the loss of human life. This is why it is difficult to apply the notion of duress to issues concerning institutional cooperation. Because a Catholic health care institution freely chooses to collaborate in a way that implicates it in immoral cooperation, even though its survival is threatened by not collaborating, the cooperation is not justified.

Another reason why the notion of duress may not directly apply to institutions concerns the institutionalization of the immoral cooperation on a continual basis. This is what happens to a Catholic health care facility when it agrees, because of "duress," to immediate material cooperation in the provision of contraceptive sterilization, for example, or any other intrinsically evil act. After the agreement is signed—and the potential financial or other disaster has been averted—the Catholic partner finds itself contractually committed to continued immoral cooperation in immoral procedures. Such institutional cooperation in non-death-dealing immoral acts *might* be possible under duress on a one-time basis (for example,

if a court injunction should order a Catholic hospital to allow the performance of a direct sterilization by outside personnel), but it cannot become an integral part of the daily, ongoing operations of the Catholic facility. It would be strange indeed if the clerk who opened the safe to save his life continued to collaborate with the robber even after the threat of force was over. But this is exactly what sometimes happens to a Catholic health care facility when it agrees, because of duress, to illicit cooperation in evil. In such cases, the duress that was originally used to justify cooperation has passed, but the immoral cooperation has not.

There are, to be clear, cases of institutional duress which justify apparent immoral cooperation. The point has been to show that duress applied to individuals and to institutions is quite different. In addition to the issue of duress, the principle of cooperation itself applies in a different way to individuals versus institutions. Catholic institutions are bound to a more rigorous application of the principles of cooperation because of their public apostolic status. Catholic health care institutions are there not only to serve the sick but to give moral witness and to evangelize the culture. Recent Popes have repeatedly spoken of evangelizing culture and of the importance of giving public witness of Catholic teaching. Such a witness can provide an impetus for positive social change and attainment of a more socially just society.

We must remember that the fundamental purpose of any Catholic apostolate is to bear witness to Jesus Christ and the salvation which He won for all. Jesus cured the man crippled from birth, not primarily to allow him to walk, but to provide proof that He, Jesus Christ, had the power to transfigure the human person into His likeness. Jesus healed physically in order to give witness to a greater healing which He and His Church offer, namely, healing from moral evil. Catholic institutions, then, can do nothing that would contribute to the advancement of evil in the world, nor can they do anything that would lead to confusion in people's minds about what constitutes sin. Therefore, given the apostolic mission of the Catholic institution the application of the principle of cooperation is more strict for Catholic institutions than for individuals.

Terms of the Operating Agreement

Collaborative arrangements with a non-Catholic entity that wishes to engage in immoral activities must specify that the non-Catholic entity carry out the immoral procedures entirely through its own agency, on its own premises, and that it be the sole cause of any facility or practice which is established specifically for their provision. For legal purposes, the operating agreement may acknowledge the kinds of activities in which the non-Catholic entity will be engaged and that the Catholic entity will not be party to them because of its moral convictions. Such acknowledgments do not have the effect of making the Catholic partner implicitly intend the performance of these immoral procedures or activities since they are strictly acknowledgements and not a contractual agreement to assist in or formally establish such acts.

The collaborative agreement should also specify the procedures that the Catholic entity will not be engaged in; for example, it should not simply reference "procedures incompatible with the *ERDs*" but stipulate the procedures in question, such as tubal ligations and in vitro fertilization. In addition to specifying those acts which do violence to the dignity of the human person, the agreement should also note that the Catholic hospital will not involve itself in procedures which the magisterium of the Church would *in the future* judge to be immoral. The local ordinary should act as the final arbiter on such matters and as the ultimate interpreter of the *ERDs* and their application within his jurisdiction. Finally, because

a joint operating company formed by Catholic and non-Catholic entities represents the identity of the Catholic institution, the operations of the joint operating company must also be consistent with the *ERDs*.[g]

Notes

[1] U.S. Conference of Catholic Bishops, *Ethical and Religious Directives for Catholic Health Care Services*, 4th ed. (Washington, D.C.: USCCB, 2001).

[2] Congregation for the Doctrine of the Faith, *Instruction Dignitas personae on Certain Bioethical Questions* (December 8, 2008), n. 35.

[3] *Catechism of the Catholic Church*, 2nd ed., trans. U.S. Conference of Catholic Bishops (Vatican City: Libreria Editrice Vaticana, 1997), n. 2284.

[4] See USCCB, *Ethical and Religious Directives*, n. 71.

[5] Peter J. Cataldo, "State Mandated Immoral Procedures in Catholic Facilities: How Is Licit Compliance Possible?" in *Live the Truth: The Moral Legacy of John Paul II in Catholic Health Care*, ed. Edward J. Furton (Philadelphia: National Catholic Bioethics Center, 2006), 258–261.

[6] USCCB, *Ethical and Religious Directives*, n. 70.

[7] See chapter 26, "Models of Health Care Collaboration."

✠

Editorial Summation: Economic realities have forced many Catholic health care institutions to form some sort of alliance with non-Catholic institutions. When the non-Catholic institution requires that certain medical procedures be done which objectively are considered to be morally evil by the Catholic partner, the principle of cooperation with evil contained in the Church's moral tradition comes into play. Directive 69 of the ERDs is especially applicable and is directed to limiting such collaboration. The principle of cooperation in evil was developed historically to guide individual persons but may be applied analogously to corporate persons. The principle assumes that there is a distinction between the actions of the cooperator and those of the principal agent committing the wrongdoing, although the cooperator could also become a wrongdoer. Three components morally define the wrongdoer's act: (1) the moral object, namely, the precise good or evil which characterizes that act and which is freely chosen by the principal agent, the wrongdoer; (2) the intention (or purpose) for which the act is done; and (3) the circumstances associated with that act. The cooperator can participate in any or all of these components. If the cooperator intends any component of the evildoer's act, he is guilty of formal cooperation. Implicit formal cooperation occurs when the cooperator does not intend the wrongdoer's act as an end in itself but does intend the act as a means to some other objective. Catholic health care institutions can be susceptible to this type of formal cooperation. Both types are impermissible. Material cooperation, as distinct from formal, refers to the situation in which the cooperator does not intend the principal agent's act but is involved only with the circumstances of the act. If the material cooperation is with a morally licit circumstance, not essential to the principal agent's morally evil action, the material cooperation may be considered morally acceptable. Collaborative arrangements under the proper conditions can be limited to justified mediate material cooperation in any procedures or activities viewed as immoral in Catholic moral teaching.

CHAPTER 26

Models of Health Care Collaboration

Peter J. Cataldo

Presuming the approach explained in the preceding chapter, I will outline some models of collaboration that the National Catholic Bioethics Center has found to be conducive to licit cooperation and others that, in our opinion, commit the Catholic institution to implicit formal cooperation.

Cooperation and Collaboration

The initial efforts at constructing collaboration proposals are significantly aided by a *prima facie* principle for evaluating the risk of immoral cooperation: the risk of immoral cooperation in a health care collaboration is proportionate to the level of institutional integration present in the collaboration. Consequently, the greater the integration, the greater the risk of unacceptable cooperation in what Catholic moral teaching regards as morally objectionable procedures. Consistent with the principle, this analysis will proceed by examining collaboration models with minimal institutional integration (limited affiliations) and move to a model with maximal institutional integration (joint operating company). It is important to note that while these models are conducive to morally acceptable cooperation, they cannot by themselves legitimate any particular collaboration arrangement, nor do they necessarily overcome possible scandal.

Models of Licit Collaboration

Each limited affiliation model includes these essential characteristics: (1) there is no institutional integration of governance, management, or finances; (2) there are certain reserved powers critical to the preservation of institutional independence; (3) each institution retains its own assets and liabilities; (4) any and all joint activities are in compliance with the *Ethical and Religious Directives for Catholic Health Care Services* (*ERDs*), or with a morally equivalent "common-values statement" that prohibits specific procedures. This fourth common characteristic is established by a "mission" or "values" section in the joint agreement. It is also secured by sections in the agreement that provide for conflict resolution and exit strategies that both preserve the business purposes of the affiliation and protect the Catholic partner from illicit cooperation.

Joint Venture Agreement

In a joint venture agreement, two health care institutions jointly operate or provide one or a limited number of functions or services. For example, hospital A and hospital B might jointly operate pathology services.

Master Affiliation Agreement

A master affiliation agreement creates a "preferred status" between two or more health care institutions (the affiliates) for collaboration on a range of services and functions. Examples of what could be included are behavioral health, extended care, ambulatory care, physician networks, rehabilitation services, managed care contracting, academic affiliation, acute care services, clinical laboratories, diagnostic services, and administrative and support services. (These examples also apply to the limited management company and the joint management company below.) The master affiliation agreement includes provisions that exclude the same relationships with nonaffiliating institutions and identifies existing and potential geographical areas and organizations for possible affiliations. The agreement also stipulates that the terms and conditions for collaborative arrangements on individual services will be set forth in "separate agreements" that comply with the master affiliation agreement. Management of individual collaborative arrangements is not provided by a joint company but by the institutions that have established a separate agreement.

Limited Management Company

The purpose of a limited management company is to facilitate joint ventures between the collaborating institutions. The limited management company operating agreement provides for a board of managers that is responsible for strategic planning, program development for joint ventures, a business plan, and an annual budget. The operating agreement also establishes rights of first refusal and rights of participation in new transactions of the collaborating institutions. The joint venture participants capitalize, own, operate, and manage the joint ventures apart from the limited management company.

Joint Management Company

The operating agreement of a joint management company provides for a board with the same responsibilities as those for a limited management company. The essential difference between a limited management company and a joint management company is that the joint management company has the added function of actually managing and being a profit center for the joint ventures.

The limited affiliation models carry little or no risk of formal cooperation in the morally objectionable procedures of a non-Catholic partner as long as their corporate structures retain the four characteristics mentioned above. The models do not present any mechanism (either governance, management, or financing) by which the morally objectionable procedures of a non-Catholic partner are made possible. The only collaboration between the institutions is for specific joint ventures and programs that must comply with the *ERDs* or a morally equivalent common-values statement. This fact leaves only licit material cooperation (if any at all), because the collaboration either does not contribute or only remotely contributes to circumstances associated with the procedures in question.

Joint Operating Company

The purpose of a joint operating company is to create a centralized management authority over the collaborating institutions, which otherwise retain their independence in some important ways, e.g., separate governance, identities, assets and liabilities, and medical staffs. The scope of the joint operating company's authority extends from day-to-day operations of the system to managed care contracting and approval of capital expenditures. The high level of management integration between the collaborating institutions creates an increased risk of formal cooperation in any morally objectionable procedures provided by the non-Catholic partner. If the non-Catholic partner provides morally objectionable procedures, their governance, management, and financing must be completely segregated from the joint operating company. This segregation cannot be established through the joint operating agreement or by any representatives of the Catholic partner, although the fact of who will provide the procedures can be recognized in the agreement. As with the limited affiliation models, the activities of the joint operating company must comply with the *ERDs* or a morally equivalent common-values statement.

Merger and Consolidation

Mergers and consolidations are not collaborations, but they can radically affect the identity of a Catholic health care institution. In a merger, one hospital is subsumed into another "surviving corporation," which retains its identity. In a health care consolidation, two or more entities join and lose their corporate identities to a new corporation.

A consolidation or a merger has a single corporate identity. This fact means that what each member institution does, it does in the name of the whole system. Therefore, each member must comply with the *ERDs* or a morally equivalent common-values statement in order for a consolidation or a merger to fulfill its Catholic identity. If in the case of a merger the removal of the procedures from the non-Catholic facility must be delayed for financial or logistical reasons, the assets of the non-Catholic hospital can be acquired by a nonprofit community-based group on a temporary basis with certain powers being reserved to the Catholic institution so that control and ownership can be transferred to the Catholic institution once the morally objectionable procedures are removed.

Models of Illicit Collaboration

Models of collaboration in which the operating agreement provides the structure and mechanisms that enable morally objectionable procedures to take place at the non-Catholic facility implicate the Catholic institution in implicit formal cooperation. There are different ways in which this can occur. It can happen if the management of the morally objectionable procedures is linked to the executives of the joint entity, for example, if the CEO of the joint entity appoints the CEO of the non-Catholic partner who has management responsibility over the morally objectionable procedures. On the financial side, if an accounting mechanism is agreed to whereby the revenues from morally objectionable procedures are accounted for together with all other revenues from joint operations and then are separated out, the Catholic institution would still be illicitly cooperating in the collection of revenue from the procedures.

Implicit formal cooperation is also possible if the agreement establishes morally objectionable procedures at a former non-Catholic facility now owned and operated by a Catholic institution. Some of the ways in which this can occur is for the Catholic institution to lease space, utilities, ancillary services, and personnel for the purpose of providing morally objectionable procedures; lease or sell equipment and supplies for the same purpose; ensure that all policies, protocols, procedures, and standards associated with the morally objectionable procedures are consistent with those of the Catholic institution; or assist with the temporary transfer of patients so that the patients may receive morally objectionable procedures. These same illicit arrangements can also occur with an independent non-Catholic partner.

The NCBC recognizes the critical importance of collaborative arrangements between Catholic and non-Catholic health care institutions for the continuation of the Catholic health care ministry. What this and the preceding chapter have shown is that the Catholic moral tradition can be faithfully brought to bear on the question to produce concrete models of morally acceptable collaboration.

✠

Editorial Summation: Catholic health care ethics committees may be asked to evaluate proposals for collaboration with non-Catholic institutions. One of most important aspects of evaluating a collaborative arrangement is to determine whether the collaboration commits the Catholic institution to formal cooperation in any immoral procedures or actions. Formal cooperation must always be avoided. The greater the integration of governance, management, and finances as a result of the collaboration, the greater the chances are that the Catholic institution will be engaged in formal cooperation. This is because governance, management, and finances entail the intentions of the institution. Care must be taken to ensure that the governance, management, finances, and other institutional actions of the Catholic institution are completely segregated from the immoral actions. Limited affiliations do not involve institutional integration and therefore generally avoid formal cooperation. Because a collaborative arrangement like a joint operating company represents a high level of institutional integration, it is more difficult to segregate the immoral actions from the Catholic entity. Another benchmark for a committee to consider is material cooperation. Even if a Catholic institution has avoided formal cooperation in a collaborative arrangement, the institution might still be materially cooperating in the immoral procedures of the non-Catholic partner. Depending on the type of material cooperation, this can be acceptable. Finally, mergers and consolidations, though they are not collaborative arrangements, nevertheless represent complete institutional integration. Therefore, immoral procedures that are provided at a particular non-Catholic facility are necessarily also provided in the name of the participating Catholic institution(s). Unless the procedures have been properly segregated, this situation is likely to entail formal cooperation.

CHAPTER 27

Contraceptive Mandates and Immoral Cooperation

Marie T. Hilliard, R.N.

As the largest provider of nongovernmental, non-profit health care in the United States, Catholic health care is susceptible to being viewed as just another secular institution engaged in the welfare of the larger society, and at its behest. Those who wish to deny the ministerial nature of Catholic health care have capitalized on this misperception for their own political agendas. Advocates for abolishing sexual mores, for providing abortion on demand, and for redefining the human being as a bearer of rights have engaged political structures in their pursuit of reshaping Catholic health care in their own image. They have made some subtle and some blatantly obvious attempts at changing the public perception of the purposes of Catholic health care. These have escalated into legislative initiatives that attempt to force Catholic health care to violate the tenets of the Catholic Church in the delivery of health care.

First, there is a need to correct the misperception that the delivery of health care is a secular endeavor. The Christian woman Fabiola, who established a hospital in Rome around the year 390, was the earliest forerunner of today's nurse. Her decision to dedicate her wealth and her life to the care of the sick poor was grounded in her Christian faith. St. Benedict founded the Benedictine nursing order, based on the Christian ethic, around the year 500. The very names of the oldest foundations of health care, which continue to exist today—including the Hotel-Dieu in Paris, founded in 660—reflect the religious tradition of health care delivery. A structure for the delivery of nursing care was created by the Christian religious order the Hospitallers of Saint John of Jerusalem in 1113. This historically is considered to be the first organized structure for the delivery of health care. The first identified nurse

in the territory that was to become the United States was Catholic friar Juan de Mena, from Santo Domingo of Mexico. He arrived on the shores of the southern Texas coast in 1554. The friar was known for his humility and his charity toward the sick.

The second oldest public hospital in continuous existence in the United States, Charity Hospital in New Orleans (1736), despite being a public hospital, was under the administration of the Daughters of Charity from 1834 to 1970. The oldest hospital west of the Mississippi was established in St. Louis, Missouri, in 1828 by St. Elizabeth Seton's Sisters of Charity. Today, through the centuries of initiatives to apply the Gospel imperatives in the service of neighbor, Catholic health care is the largest provider of nongovernmental, nonprofit health care in the United States. With this stunning history of health care ministry in the Catholic tradition, it is disingenuous to identify Catholic health care as a secular function of society. Yet, state by state, there have been legislative initiatives to define Catholic health care ministries as secular endeavors, not protected by the free exercise clause of the First Amendment of the United States Constitution.

The Secular Redefinition of Catholic Health Care

The escalation of legislated health care mandates illustrates this trend to secularize Catholic health care. (See the regularly updated "Table of Legal Mandates State by State" at www. ncbcenter.org.) The majority of states mandate that contraceptive coverage, including prescription drugs and devices, be included in employee insurance plans that offer prescription coverage. Of these mandating states, few provide a true religious or conscience exemption. Increasingly states are mandating the administration of emergency contraception in emergency departments to victims of sexual assault, even when there is an indication that the medication would function as an abortifacient. Only in rare cases are states providing conscience exemptions for the health care agency. Pharmacists have been more successful in securing refusal provisions that protect them from having to violate their consciences in the dispensing of emergency contraception. Increasingly, however, they have had to seek court injunctions to protect their rights of conscience.

Of significant concern is the redefinition, in statutes or through the courts, of a religious employer. Arizona, Arkansas, California, Hawaii, New York, North Carolina, and Oregon are examples of states which have narrowly defined a religious employer to include only nonprofit agencies (which would include Church ministries) that serve or employ primarily members of their own faith (which would not include the majority of Church ministries). Here rests the example of a revisionist's view of the role of religion in society and the protections that should be provided to religious entities.

To define a religious employer as primarily hiring or serving its own members is the antithesis of the historical role of a religious ministry. The classic example of this can be seen in the parable of the Good Samaritan (Luke 10: 29–37). In defining who is one's neighbor, whom we are to love as we love ourselves, Jesus tells a young legal scholar the story of the compassionate Samaritan who, unlike a priest and Levite, stopped and ministered to a man who was beaten and robbed along the road to Jericho. The Samaritans were despised by the Jews. Jesus asks, "Which of these three, in your opinion, was neighbor to the robbers' victim?" The scholar answers, "The one who treated him with mercy," and Jesus tells him to "go and do likewise." Church ministries answer this call. They are not created to be self-serving and self-employing, but to care mercifully for those in need, regardless of their religion, ethnicity, gender, social status, vocational or marital status, or ability to pay. History supports this purpose of Church ministry.

Furthermore, Church hiring practices are based on the ministry being provided. In a Catholic school, where beliefs are imparted to the next generation, teachers of certain disciplines may be required to be Catholic. For the majority of ministries, competence in and adherence to the mission of the ministry are the usual criteria for employment. Finally, there are no client eligibility conditions (such as conversion to the Catholic faith) applied to recipients of Church ministry. However, states such as New York and California require that to be considered a religious employer one must have as a purpose the inculcation of religious values. It would be very interesting to see the response of state legislatures if Church ministries attempted to apply the very criteria that these legislatures have stated define a religious ministry: that is, for a Catholic hospital to hire only Catholic workers and to treat only Catholic patients, or those willing to be evangelized in the faith.

Not only have state legislatures redefined Church ministries, but so have the courts. In 2006, the New York State Court of Appeals, by a unanimous vote, upheld two lower court decisions requiring the Church to include contraceptive drugs and devices (including abortifacients) in their employee prescription drug plans. Religious or faith-based ministries may be exempted only if they evangelize, and employ and provide services primarily to their own members. Thus, while employers of Catholic schools and chanceries may be exempted, most other ministries may not be. In the decision, it was evident that what was viewed as the need to remedy a bias against women took precedence over the rights of people of faith. In considering the constitutionality of the narrow legal definition of a "religious employer," the justices acknowledged the reasoning of the New York legislature: "Those favoring a narrower exemption asserted that the broader one would deprive tens of thousands of women employed by church-affiliated organizations of contraceptive coverage. Their view prevailed."[1] In other words, the pro-contraception/pro-abortion agenda prevailed over religious freedom. This agenda was supported by the New York State Court of Appeals: "Finally, we must weigh against plaintiffs' interest in adhering to the tenets of their faith the State's substantial interest in fostering equality between the sexes, and in providing women with better health care."[2]

A similar bias was demonstrated by the Supreme Court of California. This court concluded that the California legislature did not violate the "free exercise [of religion] clause" of the California Constitution when mandating that Catholic Charities of Sacramento include contraceptive drugs and devices in its employee prescription coverage plan. The justices found that it is within the legislature's competence to identify subtle forms of gender discrimination, by which they referenced discrimination based on pregnancy, childbirth, or related medical conditions: "Certainly the interest in eradicating gender discrimination is compelling. We long ago concluded that discrimination based on gender violates the equal protection clause of the California Constitution ... and ... triggers the highest level of scrutiny."[3] Again, the pro-contraception/pro-abortion agenda prevailed over religious freedom.

The First Amendment of the U.S. Constitution states that Congress will make no law respecting a religious establishment. However, it immediately follows with a prohibition against violations of the free exercise of religion. These provisions have been described as the separation of church and state. However, no other concept of constitutional protections has been more misunderstood, or misused by those with their own political agendas. The constitutional scholar Stephen Carter addresses this misperception: "For the most significant aspect of the separation of church and state is not, as some seem to think, the shielding of the secular world from too strong a religious influence; the principal task of the separation of church and state is to secure religious freedom."[4]

Clearly, there has been a redefinition by the courts of the meaning of the First Amendment since its adoption in 1791. The mandate for demonstrating a prevailing state interest before passing a law that infringes on a religious freedom has been marginalized. When rights conflict (as in this case), the balance has tragically shifted from religious freedom to "reproductive rights." In the *Oregon v. Smith* decision in 1990, public employees who smoked peyote as part of a religious ritual were held to not be protected by the free exercise clause of the First Amendment.[5] The impact of the decision is that the state has no obligation to demonstrate a prevailing state interest if a legal mandate or prohibition is applied to all persons. This negates the very purpose of the free exercise of religion clause. As Carter states, "If the state bears no special burden to justify its infringement on religious practice, as long as the challenged statute is a neutral one, then the only protection a religious group receives is against legislation directed at that group. But legislation directed at a particular religious group, even in the absence of the free exercise clause, presumably would be prohibited by the equal protection clause."[6]

In response to the *Oregon v. Smith* decision, advocates for religious freedom succeeded in securing passage of the federal Religious Freedom Restoration Act of 1993. This legislation prohibited the government from limiting religious freedom in the absence of a compelling government interest, and even then the limitation had to be the least restrictive. In 1997, however, in the decision *Boerne v. Flores*, the U.S. Supreme Court overturned the law on the basis that it interfered with states' rights.[7]

In his analysis of the changing perception of the First Amendment, Carter cites the legal scholar Harold Berman, who asserts that contemporary thinking on the First Amendment is sharply discontinuous with that of the Founding Fathers. Berman further asserts that the establishment clause of the First Amendment should be understood to allow "government support of theistic and deistic belief systems more nearly comparable to the government support which is permitted to be given to agnostic and atheist belief systems."[8] While Berman's analysis addresses government support for faith-based endeavors, he identifies a phenomenon which some would consider to be a bias against religions by the very state(s) charged with protecting religious rights. Clearly, recent actions of legislatures and the courts have demonstrated this phenomenon. To fail in vigorously opposing such actions can have long-term and catastrophic implications for people of faith. Carter forecasts, "The potential transformation of the Establishment Clause from a guardian of religious freedom into a guarantor of public secularism raises prospects at once dismal and dreadful."[9] All one has to do is analyze the burgeoning list of mandates against religious freedom to understand the proportions of this very real threat. (See "Table of Legal Mandates" at www. ncbcenter.org.)

It will not end there. Ever-increasing threats exist, such as mandated assisted suicide and the recognition of same-sex unions, to name two examples. The question is, can the Church acquiesce under the misnomer of "the greater good?" Analyses of this conundrum have centered on proportionality of evil to good. There is a risk in refusing to comply with the legislative mandates (refusing to be complicit with evil) of losing one's right to engage in the social and health care ministries of Church. There is also the real concern that if the Church responds to the only morally tenable option—given the rulings in New York and California, for example—it would have to discontinue all prescription benefit coverage for employees. However, providing coverage for contraceptives and abortifacients may, in canonical terms, cause representatives of the Church to commit gravely imputable acts by cooperating with evil.

Grave Imputability

The concept of grave imputability relates to external violations of Church law. Canon 1321 §1 provides an insight into the nature of grave imputability: "No one is punished unless the external violation of a law or precept, committed by the person, is gravely imputable by reason of malice or negligence." Thus, one is accountable for violations of the law through both intentional commissions (malice) and omissions for which they are culpable (negligence).[10] The question is, could representatives of the Church be committing gravely imputable acts by allowing their employee benefit plans to pay for contraceptive drugs and devices, including abortifacients? Specifically, could they be considered in violation of canon 1282, which states, "All clerics or lay persons who take part in the administration of ecclesiastical goods by a legitimate title are bound to fulfill their functions in the name of the Church according to the norm of law?"

There is no question that the use of contraceptives, even by married couples, is gravely and intrinsically evil. Pope Paul VI states, "It is a serious error to think that a whole married life of otherwise normal relations can justify sexual intercourse which is deliberately contraceptive and so intrinsically wrong."[11] The *Catechism of the Catholic Church* states that contraception, even to regulate births, is morally unacceptable: "The regulation of births represents one of the aspects of responsible fatherhood and motherhood. Legitimate intentions on the part of the spouses do not justify recourse to morally unacceptable means (for example, direct sterilization or contraception)."[12]

What accountability, then, is borne by those who facilitate such use of morally unacceptable means? Pope Paul VI states that to make it easy for another to commit this intrinsic evil also is "an evil thing": "Not much experience is needed to be fully aware of human weakness and to understand that human beings—and especially the young, who are so exposed to temptation—need incentives to keep the moral law, and it is an evil thing to make it easy for them to break that law."[13] Causing another to break the law is, in and of itself, scandal, which is morally illicit.[14] Furthermore, the scandal is grave when it is caused by a representative of the Church, "who by nature or office [is] obliged to teach and educate others."[15]

This grave nature of the matter is compounded by the fact that almost all state contraceptive mandates include insurance coverage for "devices" such as intrauterine abortifacient devices. Abortion is one of the most serious violations of the law. "A person who procures a completed abortion incurs a *latae sententiae* excommunication" (can. 1398). A *latae sententiae* penalty is one that is incurred ipso facto when the specific external violation of the law is committed (can. 1314). Abortion includes the destruction of the embryo or fetus any time after conception (fertilization).[16] The *Ethical and Religious Directives for Catholic Health Care Services* are consistent with this interpretation of the meaning of abortion. Directive 36 states, in part, "It is not permissible, however, to initiate or to recommend treatments that have as their purpose or direct effect the removal, destruction, or interference with the implantation of a fertilized ovum."[17] Therefore, initiating or recommending the use of abortifacient drugs or devices is also prohibited.

Canon 1329 addresses the imputability as it pertains to accomplices without whose assistance the delict (external violation of the law) would not have been committed:

§1. If *ferendae sententiae* [imposed, not *latae sententiae*] penalties are established for the principal perpetrator, those who conspire together to commit a delict and are not expressly named in a law or precept are subject to the same penalties or to others of the same or lesser gravity.

§2. Accomplices who are not named in a law or precept incur a *latae sententiae* penalty attached to a delict if without their assistance the delict would not have been committed, and the penalty is of such a nature that it can affect them; otherwise, they can be punished by *ferendae sententiae* penalties.

Given these laws, are representatives of the Church accomplices when, under legal mandate, they allow their employees to receive contraceptive coverage, including coverage for abortifacient devices, through the Church's employee benefit plans? A relevant factor that exempts one from a penalty for a delict is coercion. However, there are provisions to this exemption. One relevant exemption pertains to "a person who acted coerced by grave fear, even if only relatively grave, or due to necessity or grave inconvenience unless the act is intrinsically evil or tends to the harm of souls" (can. 1323, 4°). The presence of legal coercion is a fact in contraceptive mandate laws, but the act of facilitating contraception and the use of abortifacients is "intrinsically evil" and "tends to harm souls." The bishops of the United States have issued a statement addressing the harm done to couples, in *Married Love and the Gift of Life*: "Suppressing fertility by using contraception denies part of the inherent meaning of married sexuality and does harm to the couple's unity."[18] Thus, this exemption from imputability does not apply.

One also can look at the meaning of "malice" in canon 1321 §1: the Latin text uses the word *dolo,* meaning "deliberate intent to violate the law."[19] One can also examine factors in cooperation with evil: "The term 'cooperation' refers to any specific assistance knowingly and freely given, either as a means or an end, to a morally evil act principally performed by another individual or institution."[20] In formal cooperation in evil, the cooperators in the evil act have the same intent as the principal agents of the act. For the representatives of the Church to engage in explicit formal cooperation in providing contraceptives and abortifacient devices to their employees, they must have the same intent as the medical professionals who provide these prescriptions or services. The intent could also be implicit, in giving assistance for a specific portion of the immoral act or in providing prerequisite assistance to enable the immoral act to occur.

There is much evidence to support the fact that bishops and other representatives of the Church have opposed contraceptive mandates as a violation of the moral teachings of the Church. Thus, there is no malice or deliberate attempt to violate Church law by complying with contraceptive mandates.

Ethicists have examined the other levels of cooperation pursuant to adhering to contraceptive mandates. Peter Cataldo differentiates these levels as follows:

> Cooperation is material if the act of the principal agent is not intended. The act of the cooperator in material cooperation is itself good or morally indifferent. Material cooperation can be either immediate or mediate. Immediate material cooperation contributes to the essential circumstances, and mediate material to the nonessential circumstances, of the principal agent's act. Mediate material cooperation can be either proximate through a direct causal influence, or remote through an indirect causal influence, upon the act of the principal agent. Immediate material cooperation by an institution in an intrinsically evil act such as contraception is never morally permissible. Mediate material cooperation can be morally tolerated if there is a great good to be preserved or a grave evil to be avoided.[21]

The question is whether enabling payment for the prescription constitutes an essential circumstance, making the immoral act possible.

There are numerous permutations of employee benefit plans used by Church corporations. Employee benefit plans are funded, in part, by the employer and in part by all of the employees participating in the plan. There is nothing more essential to the completion of an act than the payment for the act, which would not be completed without such payment, thus, making the material cooperation immediate. Even if one did not agree with this premise, and held that cooperation with contraceptive mandates constitutes mediate material cooperation, one would have to analyze the good being preserved and the grave evil to be avoided in determining whether the cooperation is licit. As state earlier, there are goods to be preserved: the continuance of the health care and social ministries of the Church, and the continued employment of thousands of persons provided with prescription coverage. However, to preserve these goods requires cooperation in the intrinsically evil acts of contraception and abortion (through abortifacient

devices). While canon 1324 §1, 5° provides for a tempering of a penalty if a violation is perpetrated under coercion, and 1324 §3 precludes a *latae sententiae* penalty under such circumstance, canon 1323, 4° states that one is still subject to a penalty for violating a law, even if coerced, if the act is intrinsically evil or tends to harm souls.

The evil of cooperating in contraception and abortion is not the only evil to be averted. By cooperating with contraceptive mandate laws, Church employers are forcing their employees to contribute to the insurance pools that pay for the immoral prescriptions and services. There is a third evil to be averted, and it is that which was predicted by Paul VI in *Humanae vitae*. He predicted that government would impose its will in the area of contraception:

> Who will prevent public authorities from favoring those contraceptive methods which they consider more effective? Should they regard this as necessary, they may even impose their use on everyone. It could well happen, therefore, that when people, either individually or in family or social life, experience the inherent difficulties of the divine law and are determined to avoid them, they may give into the hands of public authorities the power to intervene in the most personal and intimate responsibility of husband and wife.[22]

By collaborating, even under protest, with contraceptive and abortifacient mandates, the Church is paving the way for further government intrusions. This is a grave evil to be avoided. The Church has made every legal attempt to overturn the contraceptive mandate laws. To date, all efforts to secure judicial recourse have failed. To continue to comply with such mandates can only lead to a further erosion of religious freedom. Furthermore, to acquiesce to a redefinition of our ministries as secular entities not only is historically inaccurate but also has significant implications for the future of religion in the United States. To comply now would appear to be akin to negligence.

The second criterion of grave imputability for a violation of the law, culpable negligence, is also addressed in canon 1321 §1: "No one is punished unless the external violation of a law or precept, committed by the person, is gravely imputable by reason of malice or negligence [*culpa*]." To comply with contraceptive and abortifacient mandates could constitute ecclesiastical negligence pursuant to canon 1389 §2: "A person who through culpable negligence illegitimately places or omits an act of ecclesiastical power, ministry, or function with harm to another is to be punished with a just penalty." Canon 1321

§2 states that ordinary negligence due to the omission of necessary diligence is not punishable by law: "A penalty established by a law or precept binds the person who has deliberately violated the law or precept; however, a person who violated a law or precept by omitting necessary diligence is not punished unless the law or precept provides otherwise." However, canon 1321 continues, "when an external violation has occurred, imputability is presumed unless it is otherwise apparent" (can. 1321 §3).

Need for Decisive Action

Concerning culpable negligence, no one could accuse the Church of not performing due diligence on the matter. Extensive legal resources have been expended in the pursuit of religious freedom. Now that legal remedies are being exhausted, the issue is how will the Church act in accord with its due diligence? Now is the time to act: to refuse to comply, so that no further harm can be done to the ministries of the Church, her employees, and the future of religious freedom. The history of Catholic health care is being rewritten by legislatures and courts, who are denying the ministerial nature that is its foundation. The essential meaning of religion is being redefined to deny its very essence. Furthermore, for the Church not to act will fulfill the prophesies of Paul VI, as well as those of Carter: "The potential transformation of the Establishment Clause from a guardian of religious freedom into a guarantor of public secularism raises prospects at once dismal and dreadful."[23]

Since the U.S. Supreme Court declared the federal Religious Freedom Restoration Act of 1993 unconstitutional, efforts to remedy this in Congress have stalled. In 2000, Congress passed a limited version of an RFRA, the Religious Land Use and Institutional Persons Act. This legislation restricts government intrusion into the use of religious land, and protects religious freedom of institutionalized persons. The final recourse to redress the contraceptive mandate laws and rulings of New York and California is the U.S. Supreme Court. However, in October 2004 the U.S. Supreme Court refused to hear the challenge to the decision of the Supreme Court of California; and in October 2007 the U.S. Supreme Court refused to hear a challenge to the New York Court of Appeals decision. Now what should be done?

Eventually the Church will have to say, "Enough. We will not be complicit in the violation of moral law." This will require significant employee relations and public relations campaigns to demonstrate the source of the problem: violation by the government of religious freedoms that the drafters of the U.S. Constitution intended to

protect. Sufficient notice of the intent to no longer comply, perhaps by no longer offering prescription coverage to employees, will be needed. Then the very secular society that depends on the services of the Church, which is the largest provider of nongovernmental, nonprofit health care, social services, human services, and education in the United States, will be responsible for the outcome.

Notes

This article is based on a presentation by the author at the Twenty-first NCBC Workshop for Bishops in Dallas, Texas, February 2007. An earlier version appeared under the title "Contraceptive Mandates and the Avoidance of Culpable Negligence" in the proceedings of that workshop, *Urged On by Christ: Catholic Health Care in Tension with Contemporary Culture*, ed. Edward J. Furton (Philadelphia: NCBC, 2007), 127–141.

[1] *Catholic Charities of the Diocese of Albany v. Gregory V. Serio*, New York Court of Appeals, no. 110 (October 19, 2006), 4.

[2] Ibid., 16.

[3] *Catholic Charities of Sacramento v. Superior Court (Dept. of Managed Care)*, Supreme Court of California, no. S099822 (March 1, 2004), 41–42.

[4] Stephen L. Carter, *The Culture of Disbelief: How American Law and Politics Trivialize Religious Devotion* (New York: Basic Books, 1993), 107.

[5] *Employment Division, Dept. of Human Resources of Oregon v. Smith*, 494 U.S. 872 (1990).

[6] Carter, *Culture of Disbelief*, 127.

[7] *City of Boerne v. Flores, Archbishop of San Antonio*, 521 U.S. 507 (1997). Interestingly, this case involved the Archdiocese of San Antonio, which challenged a town historic property ordinance that prevented the archdiocese from demolishing part of a church in Boerne, Texas. The challenge was based on the federal Religious Freedom Restoration Act of 1993, which this decision overturned.

[8] Harold J. Berman, "The Religious Clauses of the First Amendment in Historical Perspective," in *Religion and Politics*, ed. W. Laswon Taitte (Dallas: University of Texas Press, 1989), 72, cited in Carter, *Culture of Disbelief*, 119–120.

[9] Carter, *Culture of Disbelief*, 122–123.

[10] Canon Law Society of America, *Code of Canon Law: Latin–English Edition, New English Translation* (Washington, D.C.: CLSA, 1999).

[11] Paul VI, *Humanae vitae* (July 25, 1968), n. 14.

[12] U.S. Conference of Catholic Bishops, *Catechism of the Catholic Church*, 2nd ed. (Washington, D.C.: USCCB, 1997), n. 2399.

[13] Paul VI, *Humanae vitae*, n. 17.

[14] *Catechism*, n. 2284.

[15] Ibid., n. 2285.

[16] Pontifical Council for Legislative Texts, *Interpretationes*

Authenticae (can. 1398), *AAS* 80 (1988), 1818.

[17] U.S. Conference of Catholic Bishops, *Ethical and Religious Directives for Catholic Health Care Services*, 4th ed. (Washington, D.C.: USCCB, 2001), n. 36.

[18] U.S. Conference of Catholic Bishops, *Married Love and the Gift of Life* (Washington, D.C: USCCB, Nov. 14, 2006), 3.

[19] Thomas J. Green, "Sanctions in the Church," in *New Commentary on the Code of Canon Law,* eds. John P. Beal, James A. Coriden, and Thomas J. Green (Mahwah, NJ: Paulist Press, 2000), 1540.

[20] Peter Cataldo, "Compliance with Contraceptive Insurance Mandates: Licit or Illicit Cooperation in Evil?" *National Catholic Bioethics Quarterly* 4.1 (Spring 2004): 106.

[21] Ibid., 110.

[22] Paul VI, *Humanae vitae*, n. 17.

[23] Carter, *Culture of Disbelief*, 122–123.

Editorial Summation: The hospital, as a health care ministry, was founded by Catholics in response to Christ's call to go out and heal the sick. This remains the essence of the Catholic health care mission. A number of states have nonetheless enacted laws affirming that religious employers are those that hire and minister solely to their own members, thus stripping Catholic health care ministries of their religious identity. Contraceptive and other mandates have then been levied on these newly "secularized" institutions. The courts have joined in this effort, arguing that the "right" to contraception takes precedence over religious freedom. At the same time, there has been a significant change in the meaning of the First Amendment. What was designed to protect religious ministries from government intrusions has become a means of secularizing religious institutions against their will. Future government mandates are likely to include assisted suicide and recognition of same-sex marriages. By agreeing to these mandates, representatives of the Church risk grave imputability in the wrongs of others, as defined by canon law. Cooperative actions are imputable either through malice of will or through negligence. Sponsors of employee benefit plans which include contraceptive coverage risk canonical penalties because payment contributions indicate immediate material cooperation with an intrinsic evil. Furthermore, by collaborating, even under protest, the Church encourages further government intrusions on religious freedom. There is a need for a decisive response from the Church to these violations of its liberty.

CHAPTER 28

Legal Issues for Ethics Committees

Nicholas P. Cafardi

A Dual Reality: Civil and Canon Law

Catholic health care facilities must function under a dual reality. They are creatures of both the civil law and the canon law. Civilly, they exist as nonprofit corporations under the laws of the various states. Canonically, they exist as the incorporated apostolates of the religious institute, diocese, or other public juridic person in the Church that is their founder, sustainer, and sponsor.[1] As a result of operating under this dual reality, where allegiance is owed to both the civil law and canon law, Catholic health care facilities in all of their parts, including their ethics committees, must be conscious of the obligations imposed on them by both legal systems. This chapter will first consider the civil-law obligations of these ethics committees and then will turn to their canonical obligations.

Civil Law Liability of Ethics Committees

There is no one uniform type of ethics committee in use in all Catholic health care facilities, nor is there one uniform civil law statute in use throughout the United States that describes, limits, or circumscribes the civil law rights and liabilities of such committees. The potential civil law liability of an ethics committee and its individual members will depend on the functions that the committee exercises and how it exercises them. The more deeply involved an ethics committee is in the actual delivery of patient care, as opposed to performing a primarily educational function or an after-the-fact, reviewing function to determine whether ethical standards were met in the care of an individual patient, then the more likely it is that civil law liability for committee actions may exist.

Protective Statutes

Many states have laws that protect health care facility peer review committees from civil and even criminal liability for their actions, and some state statutes are so broadly drawn that an argument could be made that the actions of all committees, including ethics committees, are immunized by these types of statutes. Of course, interpretation of state statutes is a matter for the courts of each state. In recent years, there has been a movement in some states to adopt statutes that specifically immunize ethics committees from legal (civil and criminal) liability for their deliberations and decisions. By far, however, in the majority of states, the existence of a statute which creates a clear immunity for the actions of a health care facility ethics committee is not the case. Since the laws among the states on the immunity of health care facility ethics committees from the civil or criminal consequences of their actions differ greatly, it is critical that health care facility counsel should evaluate and communicate to members of the ethics committee what their potential liability might be. In the case of civil liability, as opposed to criminal liability, the individual exposure of ethics committee members is a risk that should be allocated to one or another of the health care facility's insurance policies.

Liability through Negligence

The potential civil law liability of a health care facility ethics committee for its actions can occur in a number of ways. First, it is the common law of all the states that a person is liable to an injured party if that person's negligence was the foreseeable cause of the harm to the injured party. If the health care facility ethics committee in a consultation confirms the prior diagnosis of the treating physician in rendering its ethical opinion, for example that a fetus was anencephalic, with no ability to sustain independent life apart from the mother, then the committee is in effect rendering a second medical opinion and could be held liable if that opinion was improperly arrived at through the use of insufficient facts or through the improper interpretation of the facts at hand with consequent harm to the patient. If a health care facility ethics committee is functioning at least in part in the nature of a consulting physician, then the committee and its members can expect to bear the liability of a consulting physician. There are, of course, other ways that the negligent conduct of an ethics committee could be the source of a foreseeable harm to an injured party, but the confirmation of an incorrect diagnosis is certainly a primary example. The general rule of civil law liability is as stated above: a person is liable to an injured party when that person's misconduct or negligence was the cause of a foreseeable harm to the injured party.

Liability through Respondeat Superior

A second way in which a health care facility ethics committee might be civilly liable for harm to a patient is in situations where the health care facility rules require deference to the decisions of the ethics committee in certain sensitive areas of patient care. Where it is mandatory to consult the ethics committee and where it is mandatory to follow their advice, then it is reasonable to expect that if following their advice leads to a civil law injury or tort to the patient, the ethics committee shares legal responsibility for the harm. For example, suppose that an elderly parent, when competent, had signed an advance directive (living will) that indicated a desire to continue all reasonable means of treatment in the event that the parent became unconscious in hospital care. The parent, when competent, also signed a legal document identifying a son as being the proxy in such circumstances. Now the parent is hospitalized in a terminal condition, unconscious, imminently dying, and relying on a ventilator as well as artificial feeding. The son asserts his proxy rights asking to withdraw his parent from both the ventilator and artificial feeding to let death occur naturally, explaining that his parent did not intend or foresee these circumstances in the signed advance directive. The ethics committee is consulted and supports the son's request, finding that, in the circumstances, it does not violate Catholic ethical principles. The ventilator and artificial feeding are then withdrawn and the parent dies. Afterward, however, a daughter sues both the hospital and its ethics committee, claiming that the ethics committee knowingly ignored the previously signed living will, thereby helping to cause the death of her parent.[2]

Liability as a Joint Tortfeasor

A third way in which a health care facility ethics committee could be civilly liable is in the nature of what the civil law refers to as joint tortfeasors. This concept is also basic to the common law. A person who assists or furthers the wrongful actions of another shares the legal responsibility for any harm that ensues to a third party. This is a bit different from the second case above, inasmuch as in this case, following the decision of the ethics committee is not mandatory, but discretionary with the physician. Should a physician, relying on the advice of a health care facility ethics committee, commit an act or omission that ends up harming a patient, the ethics committee could be as responsible as the physician for the injury, not as the master ordering the servant to do a tortious act, but as a co-performer of the act.

Liability for Malpractice

A fourth way in which civil law liability might attach to the health care facility ethics committee is by way of a direct malpractice claim against the committee and its members. This would require the patient to argue and the court to accept the characterization that the ethics committee and the patient had a professional relationship, not just that the patient was the patient of the treating physician but that, when the ethics committee was consulted, the patient became the patient of the ethics committee as well. If such a professional relationship could be established between the patient and the ethics committee, then any harm that ensued to the patient as a result of the committee's failure to give competent advice creates a pathway for liability to flow back to the ethics committee. Under the common law, a professional, whether legal, medical, or otherwise, owes a duty of care to those on whose behalf the professional is consulted, even if the person does not consult the professional directly. In these circumstances it is assumed that the ethics committee was consulted by the treating physician on behalf of the patient. So it could be said that the ethics committee, in its professional capacity as a health care facility reviewing body, had a duty of care toward that patient. If the duty is not properly carried out (according to prevailing standards of professionalism) and the patient is thereby harmed, liability of the committee to the patient results.

Liability for Invasion of Privacy

A fifth way in which a health care facility ethics committee might have civil law exposure is in the area of privacy. Medical records might need to be reviewed in the course of the ethics committee's consultation. These could be the records of the patient involved in the case, or they could be the records of other patients to which the ethics committee refers in an attempt to be consistent in its advice or rulings. Health care facility patients have a reasonable expectation of privacy as to their files, and normally no one outside the treating or consulting physician should be expected to see the patient's file. If the health care facility ethics committee is composed solely of physicians on the health care facility staff, then arguably there is a limited privilege on their behalf to review all patient files for the appropriate medical reasons. In an attempt to obtain a balanced view of the issues facing the committee, most health care facility ethics committees have non-physician members, such as professional ethicists and even members of the public. There is a serious question whether such individuals should have automatic access to patient files without some type of disclosure to the patient and consent from him or her. Without more consent, the examination of a patient's files by parties not directly giving care to the patient, or those not on the health care facility's medical staff who do not enjoy a limited privilege to examine patient records, could result in liability to the patient for an invasion of privacy. Also, rules promulgated by the federal government under HIPAA (the Health Insurance Portability and Accountability Act) impose serious penalties on health care facilities themselves for the "knowing misuse of individually indentifiable health information."

Liability through Breach of Confidentiality

Hand in hand with privacy concerns goes the obligation to treat patient file information with confidentiality. Every member of the health care facility ethics committee owes this duty of confidentiality to the patients whose files they might have access to in the course of performing their committee duties. Breach of this duty of confidentiality, by discussing patient file information outside the confines of the committee's deliberations, is a sixth way in which legal liability of committee members toward the patient can be incurred. Information obtained in confidence must be kept in confidence, and its improper disclosure to unrelated third parties could expose committee members to legal responsibility to the patient whose file information they have revealed.

Liability through Discriminatory Activity

A seventh way in which a health care facility ethics committee might have civil law exposure is in the area of discriminatory activity. A number of jurisdictions across the United States, primarily municipalities but also some states, have adopted laws that prohibit discrimination based on gender, gender identity, or sexual orientation. If a Catholic health care facility ethics committee were to be consulted on whether or not transgender surgery was an available option at the Catholic facility, and were it to advise that such surgery is not available because it offends Catholic ethical principles, the prospective patient could argue that the committee had discriminated against him or her on a basis prohibited by law. Sometimes such laws have exceptions for religious organizations, but more often they do not. Such discrimination, if it were proved, could result in civil law fines imposed by the local or state human relations commission, or in locales where the anti-discrimination law allows private suits, a verdict of damages in favor of the discriminated-against person. Depending on its level of involvement in such decision making at the hospital level, there is potential civil law liability for the ethics committee in such situations.

Protection through Insurance

It should be emphasized that these seven possible ways in which health care facility ethics committees could be civilly liable for their actions as committee members are only legal theories. All of these exist in the literature discussing the rights and duties of ethics committees. To date, while there have been a small number of lawsuits filed on behalf of patients alleging wrongdoing by an ethics committee (and always in conjunction with others, i.e., the health care facility itself and the treating physicians), none has been successful in convincing a court to hold the committee or its individual members as wrongdoers. But the theories do exist, and lawyers are certainly able to use them in crafting creative complaints seeking to produce the largest possible pool of defendants. The real answer to the potential civil law liability of a health care facility ethics committee is, of course, to see that ethics committees act with the highest degree of professionalism and to see that their activities are adequately covered by the health care facility's insurance policies. In a paraphrase of St. Anselm, insure and act professionally.

Criminal Liability

Criminal liability of ethics committees and their members will be an exceedingly rare event, much more rare than civil law liability, which itself is a rare occurrence. Nonetheless, the world is changing, and it is important to be aware that some of the seven areas of civil law liability discussed above, could, in some jurisdictions, have a criminal component. When an action is covered by a criminal statute, assisting in the performance of the criminal act by providing advice, by actively participating, or by directing the action, can submit the advising, assisting, or participating party to criminal liability *in pari passu* with the person who actually does the act. To use an example based on the discriminatory activity described above, should an anti-discrimination statute go beyond civil fines and sanctions and actually criminalize conduct that discriminates on the basis of gender, gender identity, or sexual orientation, then the members of the ethics committee who have advised a Catholic hospital not to perform transgender surgery may have advised it to commit a criminal act. While this example seems removed from reality, the fact is that Catholic hospitals have been sued civilly (although not prosecuted criminally) for refusing breast augmentation surgery to a transgendered person on ethical grounds.

Canonical Principles

It was stated at the beginning of this chapter that Catholic health care facilities are subject to a dual reality. As creatures of both the civil and canon law, they have obligations under both legal systems. We have just examined the civil law principles that affect the ethics committees of Catholic health care facilities. Now we turn to the canonical principles. All of these canonical rules derive from one basic perception: Catholic health care facilities, founded, sustained, or sponsored by a public juridic person within the Church (a religious institute, a society of apostolic life, a diocese, and so forth), remain a canonical part of the sponsoring public juridic person, even when the juridic person has taken civil law steps to create a separate civil law identity for the health care facility. Such facilities are the incorporated apostolates of their sponsoring public juridic person, and as such they are bound to follow the canon law of the Church.

The Sponsored Activities of
Public Juridic Persons

Perhaps the area in which the canon law of the Church influences Catholic health care facilities most directly is in the nature of the health care that they deliver. When public juridic persons sponsor health care institutions, they are obliged to see that the delivery of health care in those institutions conforms to the teachings of the Church. Just as the juridic person itself is bound by the canon law to act in accordance with the Church's teachings, so too are all its sponsored activities, even when those activities have been separately incorporated in the civil law. This is the case because the sponsored activities of a public juridic person are identified in the canon law with the public juridic person itself. As a matter of fact, the *Code of Canon Law*, in establishing the criteria for the creation of public

juridic persons, requires that every public juridic person have a specific apostolic activity ("a purpose congruent with the mission of the Church," can. 114) in order to qualify for recognition under the Church's law.

The Ethical and Religious Directives

In the field of health care, bishops of the United States have established the *Ethical and Religious Directives for Catholic Health Care Services* (*ERDs*).[3] These directives were approved most recently in 2001 by the U.S. Conference of Catholic Bishops. They set forth the standards that a health care facility must follow to operate as a *Catholic* health care facility. As directive 5 specifies:

> Catholic health services must adopt these directives as policy, require adherence to them within the institution as a condition for medical privileges and employment, and provide appropriate instruction regarding the directives for administration, medical and nursing staff, and other personnel.

These *ERDs*, then, are of the essence in Catholic health care. The public juridic persons who sponsor health care facilities and their lay collaborators in this ministry are obliged, under the canon law, to see that these facilities operate according to the directives.

Use of Corporate Mechanisms to
Guarantee Catholic Identity

Obviously the sponsoring public juridic person cannot do this directly. It must be done through the appropriate corporate structures and organs within the health care corporation. Typically, the mission statement, the corporate articles and bylaws, and the medical staff bylaws of the health care corporation all commit the Catholic health care facility to follow the *ERDs*. This is one reason why it is crucial that the sponsoring public juridic person have the ultimate approval over these corporate documents, to ascertain that they contain the appropriate civil law language to give life to the canonical obligations that the sponsor has in regard to its incorporated apostolic activities, primary among which is the obligation to see that the sponsored activity is performed in conformity with the Church's law and teachings.

The Ethics Committee
and Its Canonical Role

A major corporate organ for the implementation of the *ERDs* in a Catholic health care facility will, of course, be the ethics committee. In fact, the *ERDs* foresee this method of implementation in directive 37:

An ethics committee or some alternate form of ethical consultation should be available to assist by advising on particular ethical situations, by offering educational opportunities, and by reviewing and recommending policies. To these ends, there should be appropriate standards for medical ethical consultation within a particular diocese that will respect the diocesan bishop's pastoral responsibility as well as assist members of ethics committees to be familiar with Catholic medical ethics and, in particular, these directives.

The ethics committee has an important role to play in guaranteeing the health care facility's Catholic identity. Since the protection of this identity is a canonical obligation of the sponsoring public juridic person, the sponsor should view the ethics committee as a key collaborator in this task. The members of the ethics committee at a Catholic health care facility should understand that, in giving life to the *ERDs*, they are assisting the sponsor, be it the religious institute, diocese, or other juridic person, in carrying out one of the juridic person's key canonical duties in regard to the health care facility. That obligation is the maintenance of the facility's Catholic identity through the assurance that all health care provided by the facility will be provided in conformity with the law and teachings of the Church.

Ethics Committee as Collaborator in Catholic Identity

As a collaborator in Catholic identity, following the *ERDs* in its deliberations and its results is not a matter of mere preference for ethics committees at Catholic health care facilities. It is essential to their task, which is not simply to see that patients are ethically treated, although that of course is critical, but also to see that in the treatment of its patients the Catholic health care facility is true to its Catholic nature and true to the obligations imposed on the sponsoring public juridic person under the canon law to conduct all of its sponsored activities in accordance

with the laws and teachings of the Church. Members of ethics committees at Catholic health care facilities should understand this important dual role that they play as collaborators with the sponsoring public juridic person in the operation of a Catholic health care facility. They must assist the sponsor both in assuring that the health care facility provides ethical treatment to its patients and that the treatment that is provided meets Catholic ethical norms. A health care facility could not fail to follow the *ERDs* and still call itself Catholic in any meaningful sense. Since the sponsoring public juridic person is required by the canon law to conduct all of its apostolic activities in harmony with the Church's law and teachings, the role of the ethics committee in assuring that all health care services provided by the Catholic health care facility are in compliance with the *ERDs* really helps the sponsor meet its canonical obligations in regard to the activity of its incorporated health care apostolates.

Notes

[1] *"Public juridic person.* An aggregate of persons or aggregate of things constituted by operation of law or by an act of competent ecclesiastical authority as its own legal person, existing independently of other persons, endowed with its own rights and duties, which are fitting to its own nature; previously referred to as a *moral person."* Adam J. Maida and Nicholas P. Cafardi, *Church Property, Church Finances, and Church-Related Corporations* (St. Louis, MO: Catholic Health Association, 1984), 324.

[2] The author is indebted for this example, and its phrasing, to Gerard Magill, Ph.D., Vernon Gallagher Chair for the Integration of Science, Theology, Philosophy and Law at Duquesne University. This is a basic concept in the common law: the party who directs a harmful action shares legal responsibility for it. This is sometimes referred to as the principle of master–servant or *respondeat superior.* The master or person in superior authority is responsible for the wrongful acts that the servant or person in a subsidiary position does at the master's direction.

[3] 4th ed., Washington, D.C.: USCCB, 2001.

✠

Editorial Summation: Catholic health care ethics committees are under civil law obligations and canon law obligations. Civil law obligations will differ according to the degree to which the committee is involved in patient care and the applicable state statutes. They include liability through negligence, as a result of a mandate to comply with the decisions of an ethics committee (*respondeat superior*), as a co-performer of a wrongful act (joint tortfeasor), through malpractice brought directly against the committee or its members, and through invasion of privacy or breach of confidentiality. While these are potential areas of civil-law liability, no lawsuits against ethics committees have yet been successful. Criminal liability is a possibility if the action in question is covered by a criminal statute. Both civil and criminal liability remain a source of concern at Catholic health care facilities because of conflicts between Catholic identity and the wider culture's changing moral values. Catholic health care institutions that are founded, sustained, or sponsored by a "public juridic person" (e.g., a diocese, religious order, or religious congregation) are bound by the canon law of the Church. This is true even if the health care institution also has a separate civil law identity. As a work of the public juridic person, the Catholic health care institution is bound to carry out its activities in accordance with the teachings of the Church. One of the important ways in which this is accomplished is compliance with the *ERDs*, and one of the important vehicles by which the institution brings the *ERDs* to life is the ethics committee. Members of the committee should understand and accept their role in assisting the institution and its sponsor to fulfill their respective canon law responsibilities. A health care facility could not fail to follow the *ERDs* and still call itself Catholic in any meaningful sense.

CHAPTER 29

Organizational Ethics and Catholic Health Care

Joseph J. Piccione

In the 1990s, the term "organizational ethics" rapidly entered the health care vocabulary. It represents both long-standing concerns about the conduct of institutions such as hospitals and health systems, and new insights regarding the culture of these entities.

Culture is the inner life of the institution, where the organization's professed and accepted values are embedded and transmitted to its everyday operation. Attentiveness to this inner life of health care institutions regards the way persons in these entities (both as individuals and in management processes) translate values into actions.

This chapter examines organizational ethics in contemporary health care and its application to Catholic health care institutions in the United States. Obviously, many of the norms of this ethic will be common to all health care entities, as health care providers work within a common legal framework.

For example, one immediate practical application for health care organizational ethics is that managerial decisions that seek to avoid necessary cost or maximize profit run the risk of compromising patient care; managers and leaders must be aware of this in an ethical culture and make decisions that affirm the institution's care ethic.

It should be expected that the leadership and the internal culture of Catholic health care services will support ethical decision making by individuals at every level of the facility or service and provide the environment for good organizational decision making. As part of their unique presence within the national health care sector, Catholic health care entities should have a characteristic self-understanding as works of the Church that carry a unique perspective on organizational ethics and a specific conceptual framework based on the Catholic moral and social justice tradition that addresses and extends beyond operational issues.

At times, Catholic identity will also take the institution beyond its service area to assist in meeting international health care needs. The Catholic social justice tradition is one that is attuned to global responsiveness.

The energy for self-understanding and ethical reflection in Catholic health care is rooted in the Holy Spirit and the charism of service given to the work, reflected in the mission identity, internal education, and culture of the ministry. Pope Benedict XVI teaches that that the Church is a living force of love in a particular time and place, with other entities to address the suffering present at all times and places; "she is alive with the love enkindled by the Spirit of Christ."[1]

At the very heart of the Catholic health care ministry is its self-understanding, prompted by the Holy Spirit for recognition by every generation. The American Bishops provide a foundational element for an interpretive framework for this ministry: "The mystery of Christ casts light on every facet of Catholic health care: to see Christian love as the animating principle of health care."[2] Pope Benedict XVI identifies this ministry of service as a ministry of charity/love/*diakonia* and locates it within the foundational understanding of the Church:

> The Church's deepest nature is expressed in her three-fold responsibility: of proclaiming the word of God (*kerygma-martyria*), celebrating the sacraments (*leitourgia*), and exercising the ministry of charity (*diakonia*). These duties presuppose each other and are inseparable. For the Church, charity is not a kind of welfare activity that could equally be left to others, but is a part of her nature, an indispensable expression of her very being.[3]

Ethics and mission are necessarily related; a robust mission culture should facilitate internal conversation and development of asking probing questions *within* the organizational culture.

Canonical sponsors and boards also have a unique opportunity for practical example and responsibility for the internal organizational culture. This deeper perspective that ethics is a manifestation of the life *within* the ministry should also provide a continuing impetus to self-understanding and self-renewal under the guidance and support of the Holy Spirit. This chapter proposes that the present formative period of organizational ethics provides a unique opportunity for its development within Catholic health care.

Organizational Ethics Today

Organizational ethics may have started as a focus on particular behaviors or actions taken under the identity of a health care institution. Where it is more mature it would examine actions that are possible due to the lived culture within institutions rather than the actions of discrete individuals, as would business ethics. At the same time, the culture (understood as lived values) does have an effect on the individual as moral agent, as supportive or corruptive. Culture is emerging as a key to understanding the actions of individuals and their decision making within institutions.

With respect to individuals in a general view, we understand the meaning of particular actions by examining the action itself as well as the person. What did this person intend or understand about the act or the situation? What good or goal was sought? What is the particular role or office of the individual person that may have suggested particular obligations or courses of action? Or even more deeply, what is the person's self-understanding in the light of faith and personal reflection? As actions need a context to be properly understood, so do the values that guide human actions, so that there is not a purely external perspective.

Considering organizations as such, the question remains whether it can be properly said that organizations and corporations perform moral acts. However, there is an increasingly common expectation that they do display ethical behaviors. Common sense recognizes that human persons control the actions of the organization, and their actions as persons have ethical import in themselves and through the organization.

Persons acting in concert can form corporations under civil law to pursue specific goals. The legal fiction of "person" given to corporations permits a range of actions by the entity, creates expectations, and provides protection for the corporate person and the individuals who own an interest in the corporations.

Similarly, the *Code of Canon Law* (1983) views an institutional work of the Church (parish, hospital, university) as a "juridic person" (see cann. 113–123). Previous compilations referred to the institution as a "moral person." These entities have their own identity and purpose in respective areas of the Church's life and ministry. The canonical stewards of the ministries of the Church, such as religious institutes and boards, are responsible for the actions of their organizations as well as the internal culture and unique sense of ministry and mission, which should permeate the organization and support its ethical culture.

Organizational ethics in contemporary American culture appeared in the wake of highly publicized corporate misconduct. In the 1980s, defense-industry contractors drew attention with news reports about grossly overpriced wrenches and scores of other common items that cost hundreds of taxpayer dollars each.

After the media attention moved on, the work of government oversight committees began. Among the requirements the industry met as a condition for future federal contracts was development of internal ethics programs and the voluntary reporting of violations. Voluntarily reported violations would be treated more favorably than those discovered by government review programs. Federal government experience in defense industry contracting provided a basis of experience which is now applied in fraud and abuse in the health care sector. In the 1990s, the retail entity Sears experienced several jolting revelations of unethical conduct that led to new internal ethics initiatives. Companies with ethics-and-values initiatives usually provide guidance and materials to each worker. These initiatives present ethics in a positive light and contribute to the success of the companies.

Bioethics and Organizational Ethics

The 1990s saw a review of the phenomenon of bioethics, including the development of bioethics as a profession within the health care delivery system, as well as charting the next steps of the movement.

In a 1998 essay in the *Kennedy Institute of Ethics Journal*, Edmund Pellegrino charted the recent history of bioethics since the early 1970s.[4] At a time of ever-increasing technological interventions, bioethics in the United States had developed a national presence with goals of influencing medical education and humanizing the experience of patients in health care settings.

With a focus on the patient—a human being at a time of unique, personal vulnerability—bioethics advocated fundamental respect for the person and the individual's meaningful participation in health care decision making. This decision making necessarily requires a relationship among persons——the patient and professional caregivers—providing the context for the patient's reflection and decision making.

Clinical bioethics remains a work in progress, which finds new roots in ancient values. Pellegrino remains a leading and dynamic voice for awareness of these values, especially that of love-based human solidarity, which is a foundational contribution of the religious health care tradition. A personalized vision of health care decision making views the decisions made by patients or surrogates at a time of vulnerability to be of a higher order than typical consumer transactions. According to Pellegrino, the bioethics movement has made great contributions to clinical encounters, although many of the goals have not yet been attained.[5]

During the first decades of its historical development, the bioethics movement has focused its attention first on the clinical environment, usually for a specific individual in a particular case. Organizational ethics in health care has been seen as the next wave of the bioethics movement and is the natural development of clinical ethics. This new emphasis in bioethics recognizes that clinical encounters are located in a particular health care organization and culture, with its own embedded values-discernment and values-application processes.

For those approaching organizational ethics in health care from the bioethics movement, there is the hope that organizational ethics will provide support for decision making in case-specific situations. Given the complexity of the contemporary health care delivery system, organizational ethics can align organizational and "business" decisions with the stated values of the health care organization, resulting in an improvement of the environment of care, caregivers' interrelationships, and patient care. Much of the literature in organizational ethics is quite practical in orientation. It presents principles for application by health care leadership: physician, nursing, and managerial decision makers.

Pellegrino and others expressed hope in the 1990s that the organizational ethics application would lead to health care organizational ethics committees which would run parallel to institutional clinical ethics committees. This has not yet occurred on a widespread basis. The next section will suggest that the fraud and abuse initiatives of the federal government shifted much internal attention in health care to the compliance model. The section after that will suggest that patient safety and quality are providing a new focus for health care organizational purpose, ethics, and response to social expectations.

In a way, the new attention to patient safety and quality fulfills the early hopes and vision of organizational ethics. An early leader of health care organizational ethics, Robert Lyman Potter, had the prophetic vision that the ethics movement and the quality movement will find the opportunity to collaborate on the common ground of organizational ethics. He presents a definition of organizational ethics as "the discernment of values for guiding managerial decisions that affect patient care."[6]

Another reference in the practical application of ethics is John Abbot Worthley's *Organizational Ethics in the Compliance Context*, essays on ethical dynamics in corporate cultures.[7] Not all the essays are specific to health care organizations, but they support of the goals of the volume, and case studies illustrate the topics of Worthley's chapters.

The case study for a chapter titled "Ethics of Information Privacy and Confidentiality," for example, clearly illustrates the belief that organizational ethics influences patient care. In this case, an eighty-four-year-old patient who becomes disoriented and confused in strange settings presents in a hospital emergency room following a fall. An abnormal heart rhythm leads to his admission to the hospital. It is not known at the time of this admission, however, that this abnormal heart rhythm had been detected a month earlier during another procedure in the same hospital. This second hospitalization was preventable and was caused by a series of issues: the medical records had not yet been updated as a cost-saving measure, and his son's telephone number was incorrect. Later, billing and other confidentiality issues emerged. This type of case scenario is a very effective way of demonstrating that the operational and clinical are not "separate worlds" within the same institution. Business decisions are not merely business decisions when they affect human persons.

The Joint Commission, the Federal Government, and Other Prompts of Organizational Ethics

The mission and purpose of a health care organization and its ethical obligations arising from the care of persons at a time of unique vulnerability should command the organization's attention, from sponsor and board leadership through to the entire organization. Mission statements and codes of ethical behavior for the conduct of their relationships with patients as well as with physicians, insurance companies, and suppliers are widespread but require application to decision-making processes and their alignment with professed ethical values, as well as legal provisions to assure that they are operational and normative.

In the 1990s, initiatives from the Joint Commission, then known as the Joint Commission on Accreditation of Healthcare Organizations (JCAHO), the national credentialing organization for health care organizations, and the federal government took significant steps to draw new attention to organizational ethics. These initiatives will be treated in turn.

Prior to the mid-1990s, the JCAHO manual for the accreditation process wove ethics through all its chapters; there was a shift beginning with the 1996 *Accreditation Manual for Hospitals*, when ethics was aggregated into a new first chapter "Patient Rights and Organization Ethics," with a certain prominence by this location.

The overview section of this chapter in the JCAHO manual begins with a bold vision for ethics, which offers a powerful redefinition of the "good outcome" from a solely clinical perspective: "The goal of the patient rights and organizational ethics function is to help improve patient outcomes by respecting each patient's rights and conducting business relationships with patients and the public in an ethical manner."[8] The Joint Commission, in addition to its survey and credentialing functions, seems to have the interest, expressed by the reformatting and ongoing emphasis on ethics which has continued since the mid-1990s, to help its further development within the American health care community.

Federal government initiatives quickly were able to extend beyond the "carrots and sticks" of the Joint Commission; the government could impose fines and pursue criminal actions against health care administrators and individual practitioners. Fines and imprisonment got the attention of health care leaders. The Joint Commission may have its carrots and sticks, but the federal government has a system of prisons.

In 1991, the Federal Sentencing Commission issued guidelines dealing with health care billing fraud and abuse that have, according to John Worthley, "resulted in the concept of 'compliance' becoming one of the most visible and 'buzz word' notions in corporate America."[9] In addition, the Health Insurance Portability and Accountability Act of 1997 (HIPAA) has its own requirements, with particular concern for confidentiality and privacy standards, that are spelled out by regulation and implementation.

Analogous to the government oversight of the defense industry, the Federal Sentencing Guidelines provide a

compliance "carrot" to hospitals. Those institutions which have internal codes of ethics, training, monitoring, and enforcement in place can hope for lessened penalties assessed for future infractions.

The analogy between defense contractors and healthcare is a sound one in the sense that defense expenditures are made by the federal government and about half of health care expenditures are federal government funds.

If the first phase of new federal involvement was represented by fraud and abuse (with an abiding presence), the next phase is the recognition by the federal government that it can be a "smart purchaser" of health care services through regulatory expectations that procedures and services be medically necessary and beneficial for the patient. This new phase has already been sustained by the federal courts. While this brings a certain legal "threat" to health care providers, it more importantly provides a significant new support for the patient safety movement, which is the most important engine of change within the American health care delivery system.

Processes and Organizational Commitment in Organizational Ethics

What internal resources will health care institutions bring to the cause of organizational ethics? In a 1996 article in *Bioethics Forum,* Paul Schyve, M.D., senior vice-president of JCAHO, wrote that as no particular mechanism is required for clinical ethics consultation, none is specified for organizational ethics:

> This deliberate reticence acknowledges that different mechanisms may best meet the needs of different organizations and that innovation in developing more effective mechanisms is to be encouraged. The common mechanisms currently in use—ethics committees and consultation services—have generally focused on issues in clinical ethics, often involving the care of an individual patient. While not required by Joint Commission standards, it is suggested that existing mechanisms, such as ethics committees and consultation services, be expanded to provide services to those facing challenges in the area of business ethics.[10]

Since the mid-1990s, patient safety and quality have ascended as primary indicators of the core mission and underlying culture of health care organizations. Writing ten years after the 1996 article, Schyve, now of the Joint Commission, states that patient safety and quality are entering the "hard" phase after initial advances in safety and quality, because the next stage is building the organizational culture for safety and quality.

Organizational ethics in health care, in addition to the business, legal, and regulatory dimensions, is increasingly being defined by the demands of health care's core identity: safe and effective treatment and care.

In one way, this is both a return to the foundational Hippocratic ethical value of "do no harm" and, at the same time, application of the foundational value to the future, by means of an ongoing convergence within the health care delivery system, a convergence of (1) national studies and movements for patient *safety* and quality, (2) federal *government regulation* and payment that will be increasingly keyed to safety and quality, and (3) the next step within clinical *ethics*, which can turn to safety and quality in health care processes and traditional ethics issues, such as informed consent, within these processes.

Application of the Vision, Concerns, and Processes of Organizational Ethics to Catholic Health Care

The lived experience of organizational ethics is not new in the health care sector in the nation or the Catholic health care ministry. Much of the Catholic reflection is rooted in the traditional identity of Catholic health care entities as the apostolic works of the Church entrusted to particular religious institutes (orders and congregations) and their diverse charisms.

In the era when religious institutes (mostly institutes of women religious) were identified with the hospitals and nursing homes they operated, the vowed religious sisters and brothers brought the unique culture and spirituality of their respective institutes to their health care work. It was often hard to separate the religious and their spirit from the identity of the hospital, because the religious often lived on the hospital grounds. The work was simply an extension of their religious lives and commitments. There was no question of congruence of values in their daily health care ministry. Of course, the vowed religious would occasionally fall short of their own ideal of discipleship, but they had an ideal and it was known.

The external environment of health care, however, which is one of continuing transformation and upheaval, presents unique threats to the self-understanding of the Catholic institution and its mission. In *Helping and Healing*, Edmund Pellegrino and David Thomasma provide an overview of the inner risks to mission presented by this environment:

> Christian churches and Christian communities have never been so directly challenged as they are today

by fiscal expediency to compromise the Christian call to love and justice. For the last two decades, and especially in the last five years, the tendency has been to translate a legitimate concern for the rising costs of health care into a justification to commercialize and monetarize the care of the sick. The thesis is advanced that subjecting health care to market forces—competition, advertising, consumer choice—will control costs and demand and assure quality as well.[11]

These external pressures can lead to an erosion of the religious vision of service, self-identity, and mission in health care.

The compliance mentality of some nonreligious health care organizations may not seem to vary markedly from that of defense industry corporations. For these entities, external legal threats and risks seem to be the factors that drive their response and shape their internal cultures. Yet the compliance effort has created good new tools and many effective internal safeguards.

Should external legal sanction be the most important force of motivation for Catholic health care entities? Certainly the rapid response to government regulations is prudent; the government expects a rapid response.

But perhaps further theoretical work on the nature of the good health care institution is needed. Theological reflection begins with attentiveness and listening to the goals of the health care system and the professions within it, particularly to the vision of the humanization of the world the delivery system and professions propose. These sometimes anguished professional responses to the challenges of health care safety and quality appeal to our natural law tradition, which takes account of common human values and their demands. Writing to the Romans, St. Paul noted that the Gentiles, who, without the law and through their innate sense, would act as the law would have them, and "show that the demands of the law are written in their hearts, while their conscience also bears witness" (Rom. 2:15).

Theological reflection can appreciate the demands and response to a sense of the "inwardness" of law, which has a deep appreciation in the Catholic moral tradition. For example, Rev. Jean Tonneau, O.P., states that in the theology of St. Thomas Aquinas, law and grace become inner prompts to the Christian for a life characterized by virtue, reflectiveness, and spiritual joy.[12]

It would seem that the vibrant Catholic health care ministry of the future would also possess this reflective capacity. Perhaps this competency is yet another issue and challenge to the ministry stemming from the significant decline in the number of vowed religious, who were naturally inclined to this inwardness of law through their charisms of their community. In many Catholic health care systems much of the attention of the remaining vowed religious is on the sponsor level; thus, a significant amount of the operational reflective process must be taken up by lay leaders if it is to continue in the ministry.

Similarly, a virtue model of organizational ethics seems most appropriate to Catholic health care. The teaching of Scripture, the experience of our moral tradition, and the examples of the religious foundresses and founders of Catholic hospitals encourage a robust response which encompasses compliance.

Philip Boyle presents a definition of organizational ethics with a natural-law basis that seems very compatible with the inner life and understanding of religious institutions, although it can speak to all organizations:

> The medieval theologian Thomas Aquinas summarized human moral obligation in this way: "Good is to be done and promoted, and evil is to be avoided." [*ST* I-II, q. 91, a. 2.] With the possible exception of Catholic health care providers, however, it is unlikely that people in modern health care organizations or those who lead them would turn to St. Thomas for counsel on organizational ethics. From an organizational perspective, however, his formulation is noteworthy because it highlights the need to *support* the good. Good is to be not only done but *promoted*. By this reckoning, a health care organization should act to support the staff in doing good on its behalf. It also seems that the organization should act to discourage employees from conduct that is wrong.[13]

Toward a Catholic Health Care Model of Organizational Ethics

At various points in their histories, leaders of institutions can ask themselves these questions, which should also apply to ecclesial ministries: Why are we here? What are we about? What does it mean to be a ministry of service? What will characterize a good institutional ministry of service? Clearly, the Church does not view her sponsorship of health care institutions as business ventures, although there are very real business dimensions of any institutional presence. Pellegrino and Thomasma make a very strong ratification of the Gospel-based mandate and *need* for Catholic institutional health care in our time, despite the risks of providing health care in the current environment:

> The institutional Church must, as it has for centuries, remain involved in sponsoring health care institutions

today for several very good reasons. First, hospitals and health care institutions, as we know them today, were born under the aegis of the Church. The reasons for them are as cogent today as they were then. Second, the Church-sponsored institution is increasingly the last resort of the poor in a community and the only safety net available. Third, the religious hospital is the only place in which religious medical moral principles can be exemplified and applied daily in medical decisions. This option in medical models must be available to anyone so committed. Fourth, hospital and health care agencies provide concrete examples of what being a Christian means. To be a Christian is to infuse everything we do with the message of love and justice Christ gave to us, a message that forever changes the way we are expected to live with each other.[14]

The personalism of Pellegrino and Thomasma also suggests that the fourth reason for the Catholic hospital, Christian solidarity, also includes meeting the spiritual needs of patients as part of the overall understanding of its identity. Pastoral care, then, is a significant indicator of Catholic health care. It cannot stand as an "add-on" to clinical services but must provide an integrated response to the needs of the human person encountered in the concrete. Pope Benedict writes that Christian "love does not simply offer people material help, but refreshment and care for their souls, something which is even more necessary than material support."[15]

Given the issues addressed in this chapter, some parameters for a model of Catholic organizational ethics can illustrate the nature of Catholic health care. This is especially useful when many are asking if there is any distinctiveness in Church-sponsored health care services:

1. *Catholic health care should be a work of the Church; a ministry of loving service.* In an address to the assembly of the Catholic Health Association in Phoenix in 1987, Pope John Paul II stated that health care was one of the principal forms of outreach and service of the Church offered to humanity in the name of Jesus.[16] Pope Benedict XVI stated the person-centered focus of the ministries of service:

> Yet while professional competence is a primary, fundamental requirement, it is not of itself sufficient. We are dealing with human beings, and human beings always need something more than technically proper care. They need humanity. They need heartfelt concern. Those who work for the Church's charitable organizations must be distinguished by the fact that they do not merely meet the needs of the moment, but

that they dedicate themselves to others with heartfelt concern, enabling them to experience the richness of their humanity.[17]

Do we see our health care organization through the vision of faith as a work manifesting love to persons as the Holy Spirit prompts and supports the Church in the charisms of service? Does our internal reflection support this identity? Do we sufficiently form leadership, management, and co-workers in our mission of service? Are our specific clinical services safe and effective?

2. *Catholic health care should be characterized by virtue ethics and the Christian vision of law and grace as means of responding to God and moving toward human fulfillment.* Do we look for God's transforming grace in our institutions and in their inner organizational lives? Do our managerial and decision-making processes reflect our mission and identity? Do our clinical services meet the test of the virtue of justice: that they are safe and effective, and that our clinical processes support good patient decision making and true informed consent?

3. *Catholic health care should have a clear inner awareness of its mission to give an institutional response to the Gospel.* Mission and value statements provide a substantive basis for alignment of all the actions and decision-making processes of the hospital or system. Do we utilize these statements for these operational ends? Do our current mission or values statements reflect our inner hearts and discipleship? Would our founders recognize the charism of the religious institute(s) in the contemporary statements? In a culture that has a hard time confronting the reality of death, do our treatment and care processes support this in a codependency or do we support palliative and hospice care?

4. *Catholic health care should be aligned with Catholic moral teaching and the teaching authority of the Church.* The *Ethical and Religious Directives for Catholic Health Care Services* (*ERDs*), issued and revised from time to time by the United States Conference of Catholic Bishops, is a policy document for our ministry. How thoroughly do we use it and teach it? Do we use it only as a reference for sex and death issues? Have we read the significance the Catholic tradition attaches to prudential discernment and its demands for a meaningful and demanding clinical informed consent? Do we use the *ERDs* as a guide for Catholic social justice issues for the persons we serve, advocacy for the poor and marginalized, and as an internal guide for development of a community of caregivers? In light of concern about organizational ethics, might not a rereading of the *ERDs* be a good place to begin?

5. *Catholic health care should personalize its health care services and encounters.* The health care encounter is a privileged one of trust in a relationship of persons as well as a meeting with the wonders of medical technology. This encounter, under the virtues of charity and justice, is extended to all persons, affirming the creation of all persons by God. Do we promote this personal vision of health care?[18] Do we value nurses and other direct caregivers as the "front line" of care, and as being among the greatest representatives of our vision of personalized caring? Do we promote a culture and community of mutual respect and caring?

6. *Catholic health care should provide opportunities for renewal in our ministry of service.* Health care in the United States has lost a significant measure of the public trust it was once accorded. Could the example of Pope John Paul II in his Jubilee Year 2000 acknowledgment of the shortcomings and failures of the members of the Church over history give a good example to our ministry as well? A *mea culpa* is good for the soul, and only institutions that freely admit the gaps between their ideals and their performance experience renewal and hope. Renewal by God's grace is most proper to the Christian soul and for organized Christian activity. Do we see societal expectations for patient safety and quality as a challenge and an opportunity for renewal?

7. *Catholic health care ministry should witness to human dignity and justice, particularly in access of all persons to basic health care services in the United States.* The Sermon on the Mount, the Matthew 25 discourse on the Last Judgment in which our Lord identifies with the sick and marginalized, and the parable of the Good Samaritan (Luke 10:25–37) are Gospel challenges for response to persons in their time of vulnerability defining a religious sense of service. As Pope John Paul II wrote in *Evangelium vitae* (The Gospel of Life), "In our service of charity, *we must be inspired and distinguished by a specific attitude*: we must care for the other as a person for whom God has made us responsible."[19] Do we advocate for health care access for all persons to the legislative process? Do we educate about and advocate for the ministry and its legitimate conscience rights?

American health care is experiencing challenges, ongoing financial restructuring and a new paradigm of patient safety and quality, not previously encountered. A return to an original vision of Christian service can provide Catholic institutions with the necessary interpretive framework so that it may progress into the future.

General societal discussion of, and expectations for, organizational ethics in health care institutions can be the opportunity for Catholic health care to embrace contemporary insights, to build on our core values, and to recommit to those values. We have the occasion to understand ourselves and our institutions and engage in a reflective process toward renewed foundations for our work. This process is one that is proper to discipleship and gives a unique gift to the disciple—renewal in the response to the Gospel call.

Notes

¹Benedict XVI, *Deus caritas est* (December 25, 2005), n. 28b.

²U.S. Conference of Catholic Bishops, *Ethical and Religious Directives for Catholic Health Care Services*, 4th ed. (Washington, D.C.: USCCB, 2001), general introduction.

³*Deus caritas est*, n. 25a.

⁴Edmund D. Pellegrino, "The Origins and Evolution of Bioethics: Some Personal Reflections," *Kennedy Institute of Ethics Journal* 9.1 (Winter 1998): 73–88.

⁵See Pellegrino, "Origins."

⁶Robert Lyman Potter, "On Our Way to Integrated Bioethics: Clinical/Organizational/ Communal," *Journal of Clinical Ethics* 10.3 (Fall 1999): 173.

⁷John Abbot Worthley, *Organizational Ethics in the Compliance Context* (Chicago: Health Administration Press, 1999).

⁸Joint Commission for Accreditation of Healthcare Organizations (JCAHO), *Comprehensive Accreditation Manual for Hospitals* (Oakbrook Terrace, IL: JCAHO, 1996), RI-1. Annual editions with updates are published by the Joint Commission.

⁹Worthley, *Organizational Ethics*, 18.

¹⁰Paul M. Schyve, "Patient Rights and Organizational Ethics: The Joint Commission Perspective," *Bioethics Forum* 12.2 (Summer 1996): 16.

¹¹Edmund D. Pellegrino and David C. Thomasma, *Helping and Healing: Religious Commitment in Health Care* (Washington, D.C.: Georgetown University Press, 1997), 127–128.

¹²Jean Tonneau, "The Teaching of the Thomist Tract on Law," *The Thomist* 34.1 (1970): 13–83.

¹³Philip Boyle et al., *Organizational Ethics in Health Care: Principles, Cases, and Practical Solutions* (San Francisco: Jossey-Bass, 2001), 52.

¹⁴Pellegrino and Thomasma, *Helping and Healing*, 157.

¹⁵*Deus caritas est*, n. 28b.

¹⁶John Paul II, "The Church's Teaching in the Biomedical Field Defends the Dignity and Fundamental Rights of the Human Person" (September 14, 1987), in *L'Osservatore Romano* (English), September 21, 1987, 19–20.

¹⁷Benedict XVI, *Deus caritas est*, n. 31a.

¹⁸See *Ethical and Religious Directives*, part 3, intro.

¹⁹John Paul II, *Evangelium vitae* (March 25, 1995), n. 87 (original emphasis).

Editorial Summation: Culture is the inner life of the institution, where the organization's values are embedded and transmitted to its everyday operation. The leadership and internal culture of Catholic health care services should support ethical decision making by individuals at every level of the facility or service and provide the environment for good organizational decision making. Ethics and mission are necessarily related; a robust mission culture should facilitate internal conversation and probing questions within the organizational culture. Culture is a key to understanding the actions of individuals and their decision making within institutions. For those approaching organizational ethics in health care from the bioethics movement, there is the hope that organizational ethics will provide support for decision making in case-specific situations. Given the complexity of the contemporary health care delivery system, organizational ethics can align organizational and business decisions with the stated values of the health care organization, resulting in improvements in the environment of care, caregivers' interrelationships, and patient care. Much of the Catholic reflection on organizational ethics is rooted in the traditional identity of Catholic health care entities as the apostolic works of the Church entrusted to particular religious institutes (orders and congregations) and their diverse charisms. However, the external environment of health care, which is one of continuing transformation and upheaval, presents unique threats to the self-understanding of the Catholic institution and its mission. These external pressures can lead to an erosion of the religious vision of service, self-identity, and mission in health care. Catholic institutions would do well to recollect the natural law tradition and the role of virtue ethics. The Catholic hospital also includes meeting the spiritual needs of patients as part of the overall understanding of its identity. Pastoral care, then, is a significant indicator of Catholic health care.

SELECTED CHURCH DOCUMENTS

Pope Pius XII

The Prolongation of Life

Address to an International Congress of Anesthesiologists

November 24, 1957

Dr. Bruno Haid, chief of the anesthesia section at the surgery clinic of the University of Innsbruck, has submitted to Us three questions on medical morals treating the subject known as "resuscitation" [*la réanimation*].

We are pleased, gentlemen, to grant this request, which shows your great awareness of professional duties, and your will to solve in the light of the principles of the Gospel the delicate problems that confront you.

Problems of Anesthesiology

According to Dr. Haid's statement, modern anesthesiology deals not only with problems of analgesia and anesthesia properly so-called, but also with those of "resuscitation." This is the name given in medicine, and especially in anesthesiology, to the technique which makes possible the remedying of certain occurrences which seriously threaten human life, especially asphyxia, which formerly, when modern anesthetizing equipment was not yet available, would stop the heartbeat and bring about death in a few minutes. The task of the anesthesiologist has therefore extended to acute respiratory difficulties, provoked by strangulation or by open wounds of the chest. The anesthesiologist intervenes to prevent asphyxia resulting from the internal obstruction of breathing passages by the contents of the stomach or by drowning, to remedy total or partial respiratory paralysis in cases of serious tetanus, of poliomyelitis, of poisoning by gas, sedatives, or alcoholic intoxication, or even in cases of paralysis of the central respiratory apparatus caused by serious trauma of the brain.

The Practice of "Resuscitation"

In the practice of resuscitation and in the treatment of persons who have suffered head wounds, and sometimes in the case of persons who have undergone brain surgery or of those who have suffered trauma of the brain through anoxia and remain in a state of deep unconsciousness, there arise

---

English version originally published in *The Pope Speaks* 4.4 (Spring 1958): 393–398, based on the French text reported in *L'Osservatore Romano*, November 25–26, 1957. Translation based on one released by the NCWC News Service.

a number of questions that concern medical morality and involve the principles of the philosophy of nature even more than those of analgesia.

It happens at times—as in the aforementioned cases of accidents and illnesses, the treatment of which offers reasonable hope of success—that the anesthesiologist can improve the general condition of patients who suffer from a serious lesion of the brain and whose situation at first might seem desperate. He restores breathing either through manual intervention or with the help of special instruments, clears the breathing passages, and provides for the artificial feeding of the patient.

Thanks to this treatment, and especially through the administration of oxygen by means of artificial respiration, a failing blood circulation picks up again and the appearance of the patient improves, sometimes very quickly, to such an extent that the anesthesiologist himself, or any other doctor who, trusting his experience, would have given up all hope, maintains a slight hope that spontaneous breathing will be restored. The family usually considers this improvement an astonishing result and is grateful to the doctor.

If the lesion of the brain is so serious that the patient will very probably, and even most certainly, not survive, the anesthesiologist is then led to ask himself the distressing question as to the value and meaning of the resuscitation processes. As an immediate measure he will apply artificial respiration by intubation and by aspiration of the respiratory tract; he is then in a safer position and has more time to decide what further must be done. But he can find himself in a delicate position, if the family considers that the efforts he has taken are improper and opposes them. In most cases this situation arises, not at the beginning of resuscitation attempts, but when the patient's condition, after a slight improvement at first, remains stationary and it becomes clear that only automatic artificial respiration is keeping him alive. The question then arises if one must, or if one can, continue the resuscitation process despite the fact that the soul may already have left the body.

The solution to this problem, already difficult in itself, becomes even more difficult when the family—themselves Catholic perhaps—insist that the doctor in charge, especially the anesthesiologist, remove the artificial respiration apparatus in order to allow the patient, who is already virtually dead, to pass away in peace.

A Fundamental Problem

Out of this situation there arises a question that is fundamental from the point of view of religion and the philosophy of nature. When, according to Christian faith, has death occurred in patients on whom modern methods of resuscitation have been used? Is Extreme Unction valid, at least as long as one can perceive heartbeats, even if the vital functions properly so-called have already disappeared, and if life depends only on the functioning of the artificial respiration apparatus?

Three Questions

The problems that arise in the modern practice of resuscitation can therefore be formulated in three questions:

First, does one have the right, or is one even under the obligation, to use modern artificial-respiration equipment in all cases, even those which, in the doctor's judgment, are completely hopeless?

Second, does one have the right, or is one under obligation, to remove the artificial-respiration apparatus when, after several days, the state of deep unconsciousness does not improve if, when it is removed, blood circulation will stop within a few minutes? What must be done in this case if the family of the patient, who has already received the last sacraments, urges the doctor to remove the apparatus? Is Extreme Unction still valid at this time?

Third, must a patient plunged into unconsciousness through central paralysis, but whose life—that is to say, blood circulation—is maintained through artificial respiration, and in whom there is no improvement after several days, be considered *de facto* or even *de jure* dead? Must one not wait for blood circulation to stop, in spite of the artificial respiration, before considering him dead?

Basic Principles

We shall willingly answer these three questions. But before examining them, We would like to set forth the principles that will allow formulation of the answer.

Natural reason and Christian morals say that man (and whoever is entrusted with the task of taking care of his fellowman) has the right and the duty in case of serious illness to take the necessary treatment for the preservation of life and health. This duty that one has toward himself, toward God, toward the human community, and in most cases toward certain determined persons, derives from well-ordered charity, from submission to the Creator, from social justice and even from strict justice, as well as from devotion toward one's family.

But normally one is held to use only ordinary means—according to circumstances of persons, places, times, and culture—that is to say, means that do not involve any grave burden for oneself or another. A more strict obligation would be too burdensome for most men and would render the attainment of the higher, more important good too difficult. Life, health, all temporal activities are in fact subordinated to spiritual ends.

On the other hand, one is not forbidden to take more than the strictly necessary steps to preserve life and health, as long as he does not fail in some more serious duty.

Administration of the Sacraments

Where the administration of sacraments to an unconscious man is concerned, the answer is drawn from the doctrine and practice of the Church which, for its part, follows the Lord's will as its rule of action. Sacraments are meant, by virtue of divine institution, for men of this world who are in the course of their earthly life, and, except for baptism itself, presupposed prior baptism of the recipient. He who is not a man, who is not yet a man, or is no longer a man, cannot receive the sacraments. Furthermore, if someone expresses his refusal, the sacraments cannot be administered to him against his will. God compels no one to accept sacramental grace.

When it is not known whether a person fulfills the necessary conditions for valid reception of the sacraments, an effort must be made to solve the doubt. If this effort fails, the sacrament will be conferred under at least a tacit condition (with the phrase *Si capax est*, "If you are capable," which is the broadest condition). Sacraments are instituted by Christ for men in order to save their souls. Therefore, in cases of extreme necessity, the Church tries extreme solutions in order to give man sacramental grace and assistance.

The Fact of Death

The question of the fact of death and that of verifying the fact itself (*de facto*) or its legal authenticity (*de jure*) have, because of their consequences, even in the field of morals and of religion, an even greater importance. What We have just said about the presupposed essential elements for the valid reception of a sacrament has shown this. But the importance of the question extends also to effects in matters of inheritance, marriage and matrimonial processes, benefices (vacancy of a benefice), and to many other questions of private and social life.

It remains for the doctor, and especially the anesthesiologist, to give a clear and precise definition of "death" and the "moment of death" of a patient who passes away in a state of unconsciousness. Here one can accept the usual concept of complete and final separation of the soul from the body; but in practice one must take into account the lack of precision of the terms "body" and "separation." One can put aside the possibility of a person being buried alive, for removal of the artificial respiration apparatus must necessarily bring about stoppage of blood circulation and therefore death within a few minutes.

In case of insoluble doubt, one can resort to presumptions of law and of fact. In general, it will be necessary to presume that life remains, because there is involved here a fundamental right received from the Creator, and it is necessary to prove with certainty that it has been lost.

We shall now pass to the solution of the particular questions.

A Doctor's Rights and Duties

1. Does the anesthesiologist have the right, or is he bound, in all cases of deep unconsciousness, even in those that are considered to be completely hopeless in the opinion of the competent doctor, to use modern artificial respiration apparatus, even against the will of the family?

In ordinary cases one will grant that the anesthesiologist has the right to act in this manner, but he is not bound to do so, unless this becomes the only way of fulfilling another certain moral duty.

The rights and duties of the doctor are correlative to those of the patient. The doctor, in fact, has no separate or independent right where the patient is concerned. In general he can take action only if the patient explicitly or implicitly, directly or indirectly, gives him permission. The technique of resuscitation which concerns us here does not contain anything immoral in itself. Therefore the patient, if he were capable of making a personal decision, could lawfully use it and, consequently, give the doctor permission to use it. On the other hand, since these forms of treatment go beyond the ordinary means to which one is bound, it cannot be held that there is an obligation to use them nor, consequently, that one is bound to give the doctor permission to use them.

The rights and duties of the family depend in general upon the presumed will of the unconscious patient if he is of age and *sui juris*. Where the proper and independent duty of the family is concerned, they are usually bound only to the use of ordinary means.

Consequently, if it appears that the attempt at resuscitation constitutes in reality such a burden for the family that one cannot in all conscience impose it upon them, they can lawfully insist that the doctor should discontinue these attempts, and the doctor can lawfully comply. There is not involved here a case of direct disposal of the life of the patient, nor of euthanasia in any way: this would never be licit. Even when it causes the arrest of circulation, the interruption of attempts at resuscitation is never more than an indirect cause of the cessation of life, and one must apply in this case the principle of double effect and of "*voluntarium in causa.*"

Extreme Unction

2. We have, therefore, already answered the second question in essence: "Can the doctor remove the artificial respiration apparatus before the blood circulation has come to a complete stop? Can he do this, at least, when the patient has already received Extreme Unction? Is this Extreme Unction valid when it is administered at the moment when circulation ceases, or even after?"

We must give an affirmative answer to the first part of this question, as We have already explained. If Extreme Unction has not yet been administered, one must seek to prolong respiration until this has been done. But as far as concerns the validity of Extreme Unction at the moment when blood circulation stops completely or even after this moment, it is impossible to answer "yes" or "no."

If, as in the opinion of doctors, this complete cessation of circulation means a sure separation of the soul from the body, even if particular organs go on functioning, Extreme Unction would certainly not be valid, for the recipient would certainly not be a man anymore. And this is an indispensable condition for the reception of the sacraments.

If, on the other hand, doctors are of the opinion that the separation of the soul from the body is doubtful, and that this doubt cannot be solved, the validity of Extreme Unction is also doubtful. But, applying her usual rules: "The sacraments are for men" and "In case of extreme measures" the Church allows the sacrament to be administered conditionally in respect to the sacramental sign.

When Is One "Dead"?

3. "When the blood circulation and the life of a patient who is deeply unconscious because of a central paralysis are maintained only through artificial respiration, and no improvement is noted after a few days, at what time does the Catholic Church consider the patient 'dead' or when must he be declared dead according to natural law (questions *de facto* and *de jure*)?"

(Has death already occurred after grave trauma of the brain, which has provoked deep unconsciousness and central breathing paralysis, the fatal consequences of which have nevertheless been retarded by artificial respiration? Or does it occur, according to the present opinion of doctors, only when there is complete arrest of circulation despite prolonged artificial respiration?)

Where the verification of the fact in particular cases is concerned, the answer cannot be deduced from any religious and moral principle and, under this aspect, does not fall within the competence of the Church. Until an answer can be given, the question must remain open. But considerations of a general nature allow us to believe that human life continues for as long as its vital functions—distinguished from the simple life of organs—manifest themselves spontaneously or even with the help of artificial processes. A great number of these cases are the object of insoluble doubt, and must be dealt with according to the presumptions of law and of fact of which We have spoken.

May these explanations guide you and enlighten you when you must solve delicate questions arising in the practice of your profession. As a token of divine favors which We call upon you and all those who are dear to you, We heartily grant you Our Apostolic Blessing.

APPENDIX II

Pope Paul VI

Encyclical Letter *Humanae vitae*

On the Regulation of Birth

July 25, 1968

The Transmission of Life

1. The transmission of human life is a most serious role in which married people collaborate freely and responsibly with God the Creator. It has always been a source of great joy to them, even though it sometimes entails many difficulties and hardships.

The fulfillment of this duty has always posed problems to the conscience of married people, but the recent course of human society and the concomitant changes have provoked new questions. The Church cannot ignore these questions, for they concern matters intimately connected with the life and happiness of human beings.

I. The Problem and the Competency of the Magisterium

New Formulation of the Problem

2. The changes that have taken place are of considerable importance and varied in nature. In the first place there is the rapid increase in population which has made many fear that world population is going to grow faster than available resources, with the consequence that many families and developing countries would be faced with greater hardships. This can easily induce public authorities to be tempted to take even harsher measures to avert this danger. There is also the fact that not only working and housing conditions but the greater demands made both in the economic and educational field pose a living situation in which it is frequently difficult these days to provide properly for a large family. Also noteworthy is a new understanding of the dignity of woman and her place in society, of the value of conjugal love in marriage and the relationship of conjugal acts to this love.

But the most remarkable development of all is to be seen in man's stupendous progress in the domination and rational organization of the forces of nature to the point that he is endeavoring to extend this control over every aspect of his

own life—over his body, over his mind and emotions, over his social life, and even over the laws that regulate the transmission of life.

New Questions

3. This new state of things gives rise to new questions. Granted the conditions of life today and taking into account the relevance of married love to the harmony and mutual fidelity of husband and wife, would it not be right to review the moral norms in force till now, especially when it is felt that these can be observed only with the gravest difficulty, sometimes only by heroic effort?

Moreover, if one were to apply here the so-called principle of totality, could it not be accepted that the intention to have a less prolific but more rationally planned family might transform an action which renders natural processes infertile into a licit and provident control of birth? Could it not be admitted, in other words, that procreative finality applies to the totality of married life rather than to each single act? A further question is whether, because people are more conscious today of their responsibilities, the time has not come when the transmission of life should be regulated by their intelligence and will rather than through the specific rhythms of their own bodies.

Interpreting the Moral Law

4. This kind of question requires from the teaching authority of the Church a new and deeper reflection on the principles of the moral teaching on marriage—a teaching which is based on the natural law as illuminated and enriched by Divine Revelation.

No member of the faithful could possibly deny that the Church is competent in her magisterium to interpret the natural moral law. It is in fact indisputable, as Our predecessors have many times declared,[1] that Jesus Christ, when He communicated his divine power to Peter and the other apostles and sent them to teach all nations his commandments,[2] constituted them as the authentic guardians and interpreters of the whole moral law, not only, that is, of the law of the Gospel but also of the natural law. For the natural law, too, declares the will of God, and its faithful observance is necessary for men's eternal salvation.[3]

Vatican edition. Latin text: *Acta Apostolicae Sedis* 60 (1968): 481–503; English translation: *The Pope Speaks* 13 (Fall 1969): 329–346.

In carrying out this mandate, the Church has always issued appropriate documents on the nature of marriage, the correct use of conjugal rights, and the duties of spouses. These documents have been more copious in recent times.[4]

Special Studies

5. The consciousness of the same responsibility induced Us to confirm and expand the commission set up by Our predecessor Pope John XXIII, of happy memory, in March 1963. This commission included married couples as well as many experts in the various fields pertinent to these questions. Its task was to examine views and opinions concerning married life, and especially on the correct regulation of births; and it was also to provide the teaching authority of the Church with such evidence as would enable it to give an apt reply in this matter, which not only the faithful but also the rest of the world were waiting for.[5]

When the evidence of the experts had been received, as well as the opinions and advice of a considerable number of Our brethren in the episcopate—some of whom sent their views spontaneously, while others were requested by Us to do so—We were in a position to weigh with more precision all the aspects of this complex subject. Hence We are deeply grateful to all those concerned.

The Magisterium's Reply

6. However, the conclusions arrived at by the commission could not be considered by Us as definitive and absolutely certain, dispensing Us from the duty of examining personally this serious question. This was all the more necessary because, within the commission itself, there was not complete agreement concerning the moral norms to be proposed, and especially because certain approaches and criteria for a solution to this question had emerged which were at variance with the moral doctrine on marriage constantly taught by the magisterium of the Church.

Consequently, now that We have sifted carefully the evidence sent to Us and intently studied the whole matter, as well as prayed constantly to God, We, by virtue of the mandate entrusted to Us by Christ, intend to give Our reply to this series of grave questions.

II. Doctrinal Principles

A Total Vision of Man

7. The question of human procreation, like every other question which touches human life, involves more than the limited aspects specific to such disciplines as biology, psychology, demography, or sociology. It is the whole man and the whole mission to which he is called that must be considered: both its natural, earthly aspects and its supernatural, eternal aspects. And since in the attempt to justify artificial methods of birth control many appeal to the demands of married love or of responsible parenthood, these two important realities of married life must be accurately defined and analyzed. This is what We mean to do, with special reference to what the Second Vatican Council taught with the highest authority in its Pastoral Constitution on the Church in the World of Today.

God's Loving Design

8. Married love particularly reveals its true nature and nobility when we realize that it takes its origin from God, who is love,[6] "the Father from whom every family in heaven and on earth is named."[7]

Marriage, then, is far from being the effect of chance or the result of the blind evolution of natural forces. It is in reality the wise and provident institution of God the Creator whose purpose was to effect in man his loving design. As a consequence, husband and wife, through that mutual gift of themselves, which is specific and exclusive to them alone, develop that union of two persons in which they perfect one another, cooperating with God in the generation and rearing of new lives.

The marriage of those who have been baptized is, in addition, invested with the dignity of a sacramental sign of grace, for it represents the union of Christ and his Church.

Married Love

9. In the light of these facts, the characteristic features and exigencies of married love are clearly indicated, and it is of the highest importance to evaluate them exactly.

This love is above all fully human, a compound of sense and spirit. It is not, then, merely a question of natural instinct or emotional drive. It is also, and above all, an act of the free will, whose trust is such that it is meant not only to survive the joys and sorrows of daily life, but also to grow, so that husband and wife become in a way one heart and one soul, and together attain their human fulfillment.

It is a love which is total—that very special form of personal friendship in which husband and wife generously share everything, allowing no unreasonable exceptions and not thinking solely of their own convenience. Whoever really loves his partner loves not only for what he receives, but loves that partner for the partner's own sake, content to be able to enrich the other with the gift of himself.

Married love is also faithful and exclusive of all other, and this until death. This is how husband and wife understood it on the day on which, fully aware of what they were doing, they freely vowed themselves to one another in marriage. Though this fidelity of husband and wife sometimes presents difficulties, no one has the right to assert that it is impossible; it is, on the contrary, always honorable and meritorious. The example of countless married couples proves not only that fidelity is in accord with the nature of marriage, but also that it is the source of profound and enduring happiness.

Finally, this love is fecund. It is not confined wholly to the loving interchange of husband and wife; it also contrives to go beyond this to bring new life into being. "Marriage and conjugal love are by their nature ordained toward the procreation and education of children. Children are really the supreme gift of marriage and contribute in the highest degree to their parents' welfare."[8]

Responsible Parenthood

10. Married love, therefore, requires of husband and wife the full awareness of their obligations in the matter of responsible parenthood, which today, rightly enough, is much insisted upon, but which at the same time should be rightly understood. Thus, we do well to consider responsible parenthood in the light of its varied legitimate and interrelated aspects.

With regard to the biological processes, responsible parenthood means an awareness of, and respect for, their proper functions. In the procreative faculty the human mind discerns biological laws that apply to the human person.[9]

With regard to man's innate drives and emotions, responsible parenthood means that man's reason and will must exert control over them.

With regard to physical, economic, psychological, and social conditions, responsible parenthood is exercised by those who prudently and generously decide to have more children, and by those who, for serious reasons and with due respect to moral precepts, decide not to have additional children for either a certain or an indefinite period of time.

Responsible parenthood, as we use the term here, has one further essential aspect of paramount importance. It concerns the objective moral order which was established by God, and of which a right conscience is the true interpreter. In a word, the exercise of responsible parenthood requires that husband and wife, keeping a right order of priorities, recognize their own duties toward God, themselves, their family, and human society.

From this it follows that they are not free to act as they choose in the service of transmitting life, as if it were wholly up to them to decide what is the right course to follow. On the contrary, they are bound to ensure that what they do corresponds to the will of God the Creator. The very nature of marriage and its use makes his will clear, while the constant teaching of the Church spells it out.[10]

Observing the Natural Law

11. The sexual activity, in which husband and wife are intimately and chastely united with one another, through which human life is transmitted, is, as the recent council recalled, "noble and worthy."[11] It does not, moreover, cease to be legitimate even when, for reasons independent of their will, it is foreseen to be infertile. For its natural adaptation to the expression and strengthening of the union of husband and wife is not thereby suppressed. The fact is, as experience shows, that new life is not the result of each and every act of sexual intercourse. God has wisely ordered laws of nature and the incidence of fertility in such a way that successive births are already naturally spaced through the inherent operation of these laws. The Church, nevertheless, in urging men to the observance of the precepts of the natural law, which it interprets by its constant doctrine, teaches that each and every marital act must of necessity retain its intrinsic relationship to the procreation of human life.[12]

Union and Procreation

12. This particular doctrine, often expounded by the magisterium of the Church, is based on the inseparable connection, established by God, which man on his own initiative may not break, between the unitive significance and the procreative significance which are both inherent to the marriage act.

The reason is that the fundamental nature of the marriage act, while uniting husband and wife in the closest intimacy, also renders them capable of generating new life—and this as a result of laws written into the actual nature of man and of woman. And if each of these essential qualities, the unitive and the procreative, is preserved, the use of marriage fully retains its sense of true mutual love and its ordination to the supreme responsibility of parenthood to which man is called. We believe that our contemporaries are particularly capable of seeing that this teaching is in harmony with human reason.

Faithfulness to God's Design

13. Men rightly observe that a conjugal act imposed on one's partner without regard to his or her condition or personal and reasonable wishes in the matter is no true act of love, and therefore offends the moral order in its particular application to the intimate relationship of husband and wife. If they further reflect, they must also recognize that an act of mutual love which impairs the capacity to transmit life which God the Creator, through specific laws, has built into it, frustrates his design which constitutes the norm of marriage, and contradicts the will of the Author of life. Hence to use this divine gift while depriving it, even if only partially, of its meaning and purpose, is equally repugnant to the nature of man and of woman, and is consequently in opposition to the plan of God and his holy will. But to experience the gift of married love while respecting the laws of conception is to acknowledge that one is not the master of the sources of life but rather the minister of the design established by the Creator. Just as man does not have unlimited dominion over his body in general, so also, and with more particular reason, he has no such dominion over his specifically sexual faculties, for these are concerned by their very nature with the generation of life, of which God is the source. "Human life is sacred—all men must recognize that fact," Our predecessor Pope John XXIII recalled. "From its very inception it reveals the creating hand of God."[13]

Unlawful Birth-Control Methods

14. Therefore We base Our words on the first principles of a human and Christian doctrine of marriage when We are obliged once more to declare that the direct interruption of the generative process already begun and, above all, all direct abortion, even for therapeutic reasons, are to be absolutely excluded as lawful means of regulating the number of children.[14]

Equally to be condemned, as the magisterium of the Church has affirmed on many occasions, is direct sterilization, whether of the man or of the woman, whether permanent or temporary.[15] Similarly excluded is any action which either before, at the moment of, or after sexual intercourse, is specifically intended to prevent procreation—whether as an end or as a means.[16]

Neither is it valid to argue, as a justification for sexual intercourse which is deliberately contraceptive, that a lesser evil is to be preferred to a greater one, or that such intercourse would merge with procreative acts of past and future to form a single entity and so be qualified by exactly the same moral goodness as these. Though it is true that sometimes it is lawful to tolerate a lesser moral evil in order to avoid a greater evil or in order to promote a greater good,[17] it is never lawful, even for the gravest reasons, to do evil that good may come of it[18]—in other words, to intend directly something which of its very nature contradicts the moral order and which must therefore be judged unworthy of man, even though the intention is to protect or promote the welfare of an individual, of a family or of society in general. Consequently, it is a serious error to think that a whole married life of otherwise normal relations can justify sexual intercourse which is deliberately contraceptive and so intrinsically wrong.

Lawful Therapeutic Means

15. On the other hand, the Church does not consider at all illicit the use of those therapeutic means necessary to cure bodily diseases, even if a foreseeable impediment to procreation should result therefrom—provided such impediment is not directly intended for any motive whatsoever.[19]

Recourse to Infertile Periods

16. Now as We noted earlier (n. 3 above), some people today raise the objection against this particular doctrine of the Church concerning the moral laws governing marriage, that human intelligence has both the right and responsibility to control those forces of irrational nature which come within its ambit and to direct them toward ends beneficial to man. Others ask on the same point whether it is not reasonable in so many cases to use artificial birth control if by so doing the harmony and peace of a family are better served and more suitable conditions are provided for the education of children already born. To this question We must give a clear reply. The Church is the first to praise and commend the application of human intelligence to an activity in which a rational creature such as man is so closely associated with his Creator. But she affirms that this must be done within the limits of the order of reality established by God.

If therefore there are well-grounded reasons for spacing births, arising from the physical or psychological condition of husband or wife, or from external circumstances, the Church teaches that married people may then take advantage of the natural cycles immanent in the reproductive system and engage in marital intercourse only during those times that are infertile, thus controlling birth in a way which does not in the least offend the moral principles which We have just explained.[20]

Neither the Church nor her doctrine is inconsistent when she considers it lawful for married people to take advantage of the infertile period but condemns as always unlawful the use of means which directly prevent conception, even when the reasons given for the latter practice may appear to be upright and serious. In reality, these two cases are completely different. In the former the married couple rightly use a faculty provided them by nature. In the latter they obstruct the natural development of the generative process. It cannot be denied that in each case the married couple, for acceptable reasons, are both perfectly clear in their intention to avoid children and wish to make sure that none will result. But it is equally true that it is exclusively in the former case that husband and wife are ready to abstain from intercourse during the fertile period as often as, for reasonable motives, the birth of another child is not desirable. And when the infertile period recurs, they use their married intimacy to express their mutual love and safeguard their fidelity toward one another. In doing this they certainly give proof of a true and authentic love.

Consequences of Artificial Methods

17. Responsible men can become more deeply convinced of the truth of the doctrine laid down by the Church on this issue if they reflect on the consequences of methods and plans for artificial birth control. Let them first consider how easily this course of action could open wide the way for marital infidelity and a general lowering of moral standards. Not much experience is needed to be fully aware of human weakness and to understand that human beings—and especially the young, who are so exposed to temptation—need incentives to keep the moral law, and it is an evil thing to make it easy for them to break that law. Another effect that gives cause for alarm is that a man who grows accustomed to the use of contraceptive methods may forget the reverence due to a woman, and, disregarding her physical and emotional equilibrium, reduce her to being a mere instrument for the satisfaction of his own desires, no longer considering her as his partner whom he should surround with care and affection.

Finally, careful consideration should be given to the danger of this power passing into the hands of those public authorities who care little for the precepts of the moral law. Who will blame a government which in its attempt to resolve the problems affecting an entire country resorts to the same measures as are regarded as lawful by married people in the solution of a particular family difficulty? Who will prevent public authorities from favoring those contraceptive methods which they consider more effective? Should they regard this as necessary, they may even impose their use on everyone. It could well happen, therefore, that when people, either individually or in family or social life, experience the inherent difficulties of the divine law and are determined to avoid them, they may give into the hands of public authorities the power to intervene in the most personal and intimate responsibility of husband and wife.

Limits to Man's Power

Consequently, unless we are willing that the responsibility of procreating life should be left to the arbitrary decision of men, we must accept that there are certain limits, beyond which it is wrong to go, to the power of man over his own body and its natural functions—limits, let it be said, which no one, whether as a private individual or as a public authority, can lawfully exceed. These limits are expressly imposed because of the reverence due to the whole human organism and its natural functions, in the light of the principles We stated earlier, and in accordance with a correct understanding of the "principle of totality" enunciated by Our predecessor Pope Pius XII.[21]

Concern of the Church

18. It is to be anticipated that perhaps not everyone will easily accept this particular teaching. There is too much clamorous outcry against the voice of the Church, and this is intensified by modern means of communication. But it comes as no surprise to the Church that she, no less than her divine Founder, is destined to be a "sign of contradiction."[22] She does not, because of this, evade the duty imposed on her of proclaiming humbly but firmly the entire moral law, both natural and evangelical. Since the Church did not make either of these laws, she cannot be their arbiter—only their guardian and interpreter. It could never be right for her to declare lawful what is in fact unlawful, since that, by its very nature, is always opposed to the true good of man.

In preserving intact the whole moral law of marriage, the Church is convinced that she is contributing to the creation of a truly human civilization. She urges man not to betray his personal responsibilities by putting all his faith in technical expedients. In this way she defends the dignity of husband and wife. This course of action shows that the Church, loyal to the example and teaching of the divine Savior, is sincere and unselfish in her regard for men whom she strives to help even now during this earthly pilgrimage "to share God's life as sons of the living God, the Father of all men."[23]

III. Pastoral Directives

The Church, Mater et Magistra

19. Our words would not be an adequate expression of the thought and solicitude of the Church, Mother and Teacher of all peoples, if, after having recalled men to the observance and respect of the divine law regarding matrimony, they did not also support mankind in the honest regulation of birth amid the difficult conditions which today afflict families and peoples. The Church, in fact, cannot act differently toward men than did the Redeemer. She knows their weaknesses, she has compassion on the multitude, she welcomes sinners. But at the same time she cannot do otherwise than teach the law. For it is in fact the law of human life restored to its native truth and guided by the Spirit of God.[24]

Observing the Divine Law

20. The teaching of the Church regarding the proper regulation of birth is a promulgation of the law of God himself. And yet there is no doubt that to many it will appear not merely difficult but even impossible to observe. Now it is true that like all good things which are outstanding for their nobility and for the benefits which they confer on men, so this law demands from individual men and women, from families and from human society, a resolute purpose and great endurance. Indeed it cannot be observed unless God comes to their help with the grace by which the good will of men is sustained and strengthened. But to those who consider this matter diligently it will indeed be evident that this endurance enhances man's dignity and confers benefits on human society.

Value of Self-Discipline

21. The right and lawful ordering of birth demands, first of all, that spouses fully recognize and value the true blessings of family life and that they acquire complete mastery over themselves and their emotions. For if with the aid of reason and of free will they are to control their natural drives, there can be no doubt at all of the need for self-denial. Only then will the expression of love, essential to married life, conform to right order. This is especially clear in the practice of periodic continence. Self-discipline of this kind is a shining witness to the chastity of husband and wife and, far from being a hindrance to their love of one another, transforms it by giving it a more truly human character. And if this self-discipline does demand that they persevere in their purpose and efforts, it has at the same time the salutary effect of enabling husband and wife to develop their personalities and to be enriched with spiritual blessings. For it brings to family life abundant fruits of tranquillity and peace. It helps in solving difficulties of other kinds. It fosters in husband and wife thoughtfulness and loving consideration for one another. It helps them to repel inordinate self-love, which is the opposite of charity. It arouses

in them a consciousness of their responsibilities. And finally, it confers upon parents a deeper and more effective influence in the education of their children. As their children grow up, they develop a right sense of values and achieve a serene and harmonious use of their mental and physical powers.

Promotion of Chastity

22. We take this opportunity to address those who are engaged in education and all those whose right and duty it is to provide for the common good of human society. We would call their attention to the need to create an atmosphere favorable to the growth of chastity so that true liberty may prevail over license and the norms of the moral law may be fully safeguarded.

Everything therefore in the modern means of social communication which arouses men's baser passions and encourages low moral standards, as well as every obscenity in the written word and every form of indecency on the stage and screen, should be condemned publicly and unanimously by all those who have at heart the advance of civilization and the safeguarding of the outstanding values of the human spirit. It is quite absurd to defend this kind of depravity in the name of art or culture [25] or by pleading the liberty which may be allowed in this field by the public authorities.

Appeal to Public Authorities

23. And now We wish to speak to rulers of nations. To you most of all is committed the responsibility of safeguarding the common good. You can contribute so much to the preservation of morals. We beg of you, never allow the morals of your peoples to be undermined. The family is the primary unit in the state; do not tolerate any legislation which would introduce into the family those practices which are opposed to the natural law of God. For there are other ways by which a government can and should solve the population problem—that is to say by enacting laws which will assist families and by educating the people wisely so that the moral law and the freedom of the citizens are both safeguarded.

Seeking True Solutions

We are fully aware of the difficulties confronting the public authorities in this matter, especially in the developing countries. In fact, We had in mind the justifiable anxieties which weigh upon them when We published Our encyclical letter *Populorum Progressio*. But now We join Our voice to that of Our predecessor John XXIII of venerable memory, and We make Our own his words: "No statement of the problem and no solution to it is acceptable which does violence to man's essential dignity; those who propose such solutions base them on an utterly materialistic conception of man himself and his life. The only possible solution to this question is one which envisages the social and economic progress both of individuals and of the whole of human society, and which respects and promotes true human values." [26] No one can, without being grossly unfair, make Divine Providence responsible for what clearly seems to be the result of misguided governmental policies, of an insufficient sense of social justice, of a selfish accumulation of material goods, and finally of a culpable failure to undertake those initiatives and responsibilities which would raise the standard of living of peoples and their children. [27] If only all governments which were able would do what some are already doing so nobly, and bestir themselves to renew their efforts and their undertakings! There must be no relaxation in the programs of mutual aid between all the branches of the great human family. Here We believe an almost limitless field lies open for the activities of the great international institutions.

To Scientists

24. Our next appeal is to men of science. These can "considerably advance the welfare of marriage and the family and also peace of conscience, if by pooling their efforts they strive to elucidate more thoroughly the conditions favorable to a proper regulation of births." [28] It is supremely desirable, and this was also the mind of Pius XII, that medical science should by the study of natural rhythms succeed in determining a sufficiently secure basis for the chaste limitation of offspring. [29] In this way scientists, especially those who are Catholics, will by their research establish the truth of the Church's claim that "there can be no contradiction between two divine laws—that which governs the transmitting of life and that which governs the fostering of married love." [30]

To Christian Couples

25. And now We turn in a special way to Our own sons and daughters, to those most of all whom God calls to serve Him in the state of marriage. While the Church does indeed hand on to her children the inviolable conditions laid down by God's law, she is also the herald of salvation and through the sacraments she flings wide open the channels of grace through which man is made a new creature responding in charity and true freedom to the design of his Creator and Savior, experiencing too the sweetness of the yoke of Christ. [31]

In humble obedience then to her voice, let Christian husbands and wives be mindful of their vocation to the Christian life, a vocation which, deriving from their Baptism, has been confirmed anew and made more explicit by the Sacrament of Matrimony. For by this sacrament they are strengthened and, one might almost say, consecrated to the faithful fulfillment of their duties. Thus will they realize to the full their calling and bear witness as becomes them, to Christ before the world. [32] For the Lord has entrusted to them the task of making visible to men and women the holiness and joy of the law which united inseparably their love for one another and the cooperation they give to God's love, God who is the Author of human life.

We have no wish at all to pass over in silence the difficulties, at times very great, which beset the lives of Christian married couples. For them, as indeed for every one of us, "the gate is narrow and the way is hard, that leads to life."[33] Nevertheless it is precisely the hope of that life which, like a brightly burning torch, lights up their journey, as, strong in spirit, they strive to live "sober, upright, and godly lives in this world,"[34] knowing for sure that "the form of this world is passing away."[35]

Recourse to God

For this reason husbands and wives should take up the burden appointed to them, willingly, in the strength of faith and of that hope which "does not disappoint us, because God's love has been poured into our hearts through the Holy Spirit who has been given to us."[36] Then let them implore the help of God with unremitting prayer and, most of all, let them draw grace and charity from that unfailing font which is the Eucharist. If, however, sin still exercises its hold over them, they are not to lose heart. Rather must they, humble and persevering, have recourse to the mercy of God, abundantly bestowed in the Sacrament of Penance. In this way, for sure, they will be able to reach that perfection of married life which the Apostle sets out in these words: "Husbands, love your wives, as Christ loved the Church.... Even so husbands should love their wives as their own bodies. He who loves his wife loves himself. For no man ever hates his own flesh, but nourishes and cherishes it, as Christ does the Church.... This is a great mystery, and I mean in reference to Christ and the Church; however, let each one of you love his wife as himself, and let the wife see that she respects her husband."[37]

Family Apostolate

26. Among the fruits that ripen if the law of God be resolutely obeyed, the most precious is certainly this, that married couples themselves will often desire to communicate their own experience to others. Thus it comes about that in the fullness of the lay vocation will be included a novel and outstanding form of the apostolate by which, like ministering to like, married couples themselves, by the leadership they offer, will become apostles to other married couples. And surely among all the forms of the Christian apostolate it is hard to think of one more opportune for the present time.[38]

To Doctors and Nurses

27. Likewise we hold in the highest esteem those doctors and members of the nursing profession who, in the exercise of their calling, endeavor to fulfill the demands of their Christian vocation before any merely human interest. Let them therefore continue constant in their resolution always to support those lines of action which accord with faith and with right reason. And let them strive to win agreement and support for these policies among their professional colleagues. Moreover, they should regard it as an essential part of their skill to make themselves fully proficient in this difficult field of medical knowledge. For then, when married couples ask for their advice, they may be in a position to give them right counsel and to point them in the proper direction. Married couples have a right to expect this much from them.

To Priests

28. And now, beloved sons, you who are priests, you who in virtue of your sacred office act as counselors and spiritual leaders both of individual men and women and of families—We turn to you filled with great confidence. For it is your principal duty—We are speaking especially to you who teach moral theology—to spell out clearly and completely the Church's teaching on marriage. In the performance of your ministry you must be the first to give an example of that sincere obedience, inward as well as outward, which is due to the magisterium of the Church. For, as you know, the pastors of the Church enjoy a special light of the Holy Spirit in teaching the truth.[39] And this, rather than the arguments they put forward, is why you are bound to such obedience. Nor will it escape you that if men's peace of soul and the unity of the Christian people are to be preserved, then it is of the utmost importance that in moral as well as in dogmatic theology all should obey the magisterium of the Church and should speak as with one voice. Therefore We make Our own the anxious words of the great Apostle Paul and with all Our heart We renew Our appeal to you: "I appeal to you, brethren, by the name of our Lord Jesus Christ, that all of you agree and that there be no dissensions among you, but that you be united in the same mind and the same judgment."[40]

Christian Compassion

29. Now it is an outstanding manifestation of charity toward souls to omit nothing from the saving doctrine of Christ; but this must always be joined with tolerance and charity, as Christ himself showed in his conversations and dealings with men. For when He came, not to judge, but to save the world,[41] was He not bitterly severe toward sin, but patient and abounding in mercy toward sinners?

Husbands and wives, therefore, when deeply distressed by reason of the difficulties of their life, must find stamped in the heart and voice of their priest the likeness of the voice and the love of our Redeemer. So speak with full confidence, beloved sons, convinced that while the Holy Spirit of God is present to the magisterium proclaiming sound doctrine, He also illumines from within the hearts of the faithful and invites their assent. Teach married couples the necessary way of prayer and prepare them to approach more often with great faith the Sacraments of the Eucharist and of Penance. Let them never lose heart because of their weakness.

To Bishops

30. And now as We come to the end of this encyclical letter, We turn Our mind to you, reverently and lovingly, beloved and venerable brothers in the episcopate, with whom We share more closely the care of the spiritual good of the People of God. For We invite all of you, We implore you, to give a lead to your priests who assist you in the sacred ministry, and to the faithful of your dioceses, and to devote yourselves with all zeal and without delay to safeguarding the holiness of marriage, in order to guide married life to its full human and Christian perfection. Consider this mission as one of your most urgent responsibilities at the present time.

As you well know, it calls for concerted pastoral action in every field of human diligence, economic, cultural, and social. If simultaneous progress is made in these various fields, then the intimate life of parents and children in the family will be rendered not only more tolerable, but easier and more joyful. And life together in human society will be enriched with fraternal charity and made more stable with true peace when God's design which He conceived for the world is faithfully followed.

A Great Work

31. Venerable brothers, beloved sons, all men of good will, great indeed is the work of education, of progress, and of charity to which We now summon all of you. And this We do relying on the unshakable teaching of the Church, which teaching Peter's successor together with his brothers in the Catholic episcopate faithfully guards and interprets. And We are convinced that this truly great work will bring blessings both on the world and on the Church. For man cannot attain that true happiness for which he yearns with all the strength of his spirit, unless he keeps the laws which the Most High God has engraved in his very nature. These laws must be wisely and lovingly observed. On this great work, on all of you and especially on married couples, We implore from the God of all holiness and pity an abundance of heavenly grace as a pledge of which We gladly bestow Our Apostolic blessing.

Given at St. Peter's, Rome, on the 25th day of July,
the feast of St. James the Apostle,
in the year 1968, the sixth of Our pontificate.

Notes

[1] See Pius IX, encyclical letter *Qui pluribus, Pii IX P.M. Acta*, 1, pp. 9–10; St. Pius X, encyclical letter *Singulari quadam*, AAS 4 (1912): 658; Pius XI, encyclical letter *Casti connubii*, AAS 22 (1930): 579–581; Pius XII, address *Magnificate Dominum* to the episcopate of the Catholic World, AAS 46 (1954): 671–672; John XXIII, encyclical letter *Mater et Magistra, AAS* 53 (1961): 457.

[2] See Matt. 28:18–19.

[3] See Matt. 7:21.

[4] See Council of Trent, Roman Catechism, pt. II, ch. 8; Leo XIII, encyclical letter *Arcanum, Acta Leonis XIII*, 2 (1880), 26–29; Pius XI, encyclical letter *Divini illius Magistri*, AAS 22 (1930): 58–61; idem, encyclical letter *Casti connubii*, AAS 22 (1930): 545–546; Pius XII, Address to Italian Medico-Biological Union of St. Luke, *Discorsi e radiomessaggi di Pio XII*, VI, 191–192; idem, to Italian Association of Catholic Midwives, AAS 43 (1951): 835–854; idem, to the association known as the Family Campaign, and other family associations, AAS 43 (1951): 857–859; idem, to the Seventh Congress of the International Society of Hematology, AAS 50 (1958): 734–735 [TPS 6: 394–395]; John XXIII, encyclical letter *Mater et Magistra*, AAS 53 (1961): 446–447 [TPS 7: 330–331]; Second Vatican Council, *Pastoral Constitution on the Church in the World of Today* (*Gaudium et spes*), nn. 47–52, AAS 58 (1966): 1067–1074 [TPS 11: 289–295]; Code of Canon Law, canons 1067, 1068 §1, canon 1076, §§1–2.

[5] See Paul VI, Address to Sacred College of Cardinals, AAS 56 (1964): 588 [TPS 9: 355–356]; idem, to Commission for the Study of Problems of Population, Family and Birth, AAS 57 (1965): 388 [TPS 10: 225]; idem, to National Congress of the Italian Society of Obstetrics and Gynecology, AAS 58 (1966): 1168 [TPS 11: 401–403].

[6] See 1 John 4:8.

[7] Eph. 3:15.

[8] Second Vatican Council, *Pastoral Constitution on the Church in the World of Today*, n. 50, AAS 58 (1966): 1070–1072 [TPS 11: 292–293].

[9] See St. Thomas, *Summa theologiae*, III, q. 94.2.

[10] See Second Vatican Council, *Pastoral Constitution on the Church in the World of Today*, nn. 50–51, AAS 58 (1966): 1070–1073 [TPS 11: 292–293].

[11] Ibid., n. 49, AAS 58 (1966): 1070 [TPS 11: 291–292].

[12] See Pius XI, *Casti connubi*, AAS 22 (1930): 560; Pius XII, Address to Midwives, AAS 43 (1951): 843.

[13] See John XXIII, *Mater et Magistra*, AAS 53 (1961): 447 [TPS 7I: 331].

[14] See Council of Trent, Roman Catechism, pt. II, ch. 8; Pius XI, *Casti connubii*, AAS 22 (1930): 562–564; Pius XII, Address to Medico-Biological Union of St. Luke, *Discorsi eradiomessaggi*, VI, 191–192; idem, Address to Midwives, AAS 43 (1951): 842–843; idem, Address to Family Campaign and other family associations, AAS 43 (1951): 857–859; John XXIII, encyclical letter *Pacem in terris*, AAS 55 (1963): 259–260 [TPS 9: 15–16]; Second Vatican Council, *Pastoral Constitution on the Church in the World of Today*, n. 51, AAS 58 (1966): 1072 [TPS 11: 293].

[15] See Pius XI, *Casti connubii*, AAS 22 (1930): 565; Decree of the Holy Office (February 22, 1940), AAS 32 (1940): 73; Pius XII, Address to Midwives, AAS 43 (1951): 843–844; idem, to the Society of Hematology, AAS 50 (1958): 734–735 [TPS 6: 394–395].

[16] See Council of Trent, Roman Catechism, pt. II, ch. 8; Pius XI, *Casti connubii*, AAS 22 (1930): 559–561; Pius XII, Address to Midwives, AAS 43 (1951): 843; idem, to the Society of Hematology, AAS 50 (1958): 734–735 [TPS 6: 394–395]; John XXIII, *Mater et Magistra*, AAS 53 (1961): 447 [TPS 7: 331].

[17] See Pius XII, Address to National Congress of Italian Society of the Union of Catholic Jurists, AAS 45 (1953): 798–799 [TPS 1, 67–69].

[18] See Rom. 3:8.

[19] See Pius XII, Address to Twenty-Sixth Congress of Italian Association of Urology, AAS 45 (1953):, 674–675; idem, to Society of Hematology, AAS 50 (1958): 734–735 [TPS 6: 394–395].

[20] See Pius XII, Address to Midwives, AAS 43 (1951): 846.

[21] See Pius XII, Address to Association of Urology, AAS 45 (1953): 674–675; idem, to leaders and members of Italian Association of Cornea Donors and Italian Association for the Blind, AAS 48 (1956): 461–462 [TPS 3: 200–201].

[22] Luke 2:34.

[23] See Paul VI, encyclical letter *Populorum progressio*, AAS 59 (1967): 268 [TPS 12: 151].

[24] See Rom. 8.

[25] See Second Vatican Council, *Decree on the Media of Social Communication*, nn. 6–7, AAS 56 (1964): 147 [TPS 9: 340–341].

[26] *Mater et Magistra*, AAS 53 (1961): 447 [TPS 7: 331].

[27] See *Populorum progressio*, nn. 48–55, AAS 59 (1967): 281–284 [TPS 12: 160–162].

[28] Second Vatican Council, *Pastoral Constitution on the Church in the World of Today*, n. 52, AAS 58 (1966): 1074 [TPS 11: 294].

[29] Address to Family Campaign and other family associations, AAS 43 (1951): 859.

[30] Second Vatican Council, *Pastoral Constitution on the Church in the World of Today*, n. 51, AAS 58 (1966): 1072 [TPS 11: 293].

[31] See Matt. 11:30.

[32] See Second Vatican Council, *Pastoral Constitution on the Church in the World of Today*, n. 48, AAS 58 (1966): 1067–1069 [TPS 11: 290–291]; idem, *Dogmatic Constitution on the Church*, n. 35, AAS 57 (1965): 40–41 [TPS 10: 382–383].

[33] Matt.7:14; see Heb. 12:11.

[34] See Titus 2:12.

[35] See 1 Cor. 7:31.

[36] Rom. 5:5.

[37] Eph. 5:25, 28–29, 32–33.

[38] See Second Vatican Council, *Dogmatic Constitution on the Church*, nn. 35, 41, AAS 57 (1965): 40–45 [TPS 10: 382–383, 386–387; idem, *Pastoral Constitution on the Church in the World of Today*, nn. 48–49, AAS 58 (1966): 1067–1070 [TPS 11: 290–292]; idem, *Decree on the Apostolate of the Laity*, n. 11, AAS 58 (1966): 847–849 [TPS 11: 128–129].

[39] See Second Vatican Council, *Dogmatic Constitution on the Church*, n. 25, AAS 57 (1965): 29–31 [TPS 10: 375–376].

[40] 1 Cor. 1:10.

[41] See John 3:17.

APPENDIX III

Congregation for the Doctrine of the Faith

Declaration on Procured Abortion

November 18, 1974

1. The problem of procured abortion and of its possible legal liberalization has become more or less everywhere the subject of impassioned discussions. These debates would be less grave were it not a question of human life, a primordial value, which must be protected and promoted. Everyone understands this, although many look for reasons, even against all evidence, to promote the use of abortion. One cannot but be astonished to see a simultaneous increase of unqualified protests against the death penalty and every form of war and the vindication of the liberalization of abortion, either in its entirety or in ever broader indications. The Church is too conscious of the fact that it belongs to her vocation to defend man against everything that could disintegrate or lessen his dignity to remain silent on such a topic. Because the Son of God became man, there is no man who is not his brother in humanity and who is not called to become a Christian in order to receive salvation from Him.

2. In many countries the public authorities which resist the liberalization of abortion laws are the object of powerful pressures aimed at leading them to this goal. This, it is said, would violate no one's conscience, for each individual would be left free to follow his own opinion, while being prevented from imposing it on others. Ethical pluralism is claimed to be a normal consequence of ideological pluralism. There is, however, a great difference between the one and the other, for action affects the interests of others more quickly than does mere opinion. Moreover, one can never claim freedom of opinion as a pretext for attacking the rights of others, most especially the right to life.

3. Numerous Christian lay people, especially doctors, but also parents' associations, statesmen, or leading figures in posts of responsibility have vigorously reacted against this propaganda campaign. Above all, many episcopal conferences and many bishops acting in their own name have judged it opportune to recall very strongly the traditional doctrine of the Church.[1] With a striking convergence, these documents admirably emphasize an attitude of respect for life which is at the same time human and Christian. Nevertheless, it has happened that several of these documents here or there have encountered reservation or even opposition.

4. Charged with the promotion and the defense of faith and morals in the universal Church,[2] the Sacred Congregation for the Doctrine of the Faith proposes to recall this teaching in its essential aspects to all the faithful. Thus in showing the unity of the Church, it will confirm by the authority proper to the Holy See what the bishops have opportunely undertaken. It hopes that all the faithful, including those who might have been unsettled by the controversies and new opinions, will understand that it is not a question of opposing one opinion to another, but of transmitting to the faithful a constant teaching of the supreme magisterium, which teaches moral norms in the light of faith.[3] It is therefore clear that this declaration necessarily entails a grave obligation for Christian consciences.[4] May God deign to enlighten also all men who strive with their whole heart to "act in truth" (John 3:21).

5. "Death was not God's doing, he takes no pleasure in the extinction of the living" (Wisd. 1:13). Certainly God has created beings who have only one lifetime, and physical death cannot be absent from the world of those with a bodily existence. But what is immediately willed is life, and in the visible universe everything has been made for man who is the image of God and the world's crowning glory (cf. Gen. 1:26–28). On the human level, "it was the devil's envy that brought death into the world" (Wisd. 2:24). Introduced by sin, death remains bound up with it: death is the sign and fruit of sin. But there is no final triumph for death. Confirming faith in the Resurrection, the Lord proclaims in the Gospel: "God is God, not of the dead, but of the living" (Matt. 22:32). And death like sin will be definitively defeated by resurrection in Christ (cf. 1 Cor. 15:20–27). Thus we understand that human life, even on this earth, is precious. Infused by the Creator,[5] life is again taken back by Him (cf. Gen. 2:7; Wisd. 15:11). It remains under his protection: man's blood cries out to Him (cf. Gen. 4:10), and He will demand an account of it, "for in the image of God man was made" (Gen. 9:5–6). The commandment of God is formal: "You shall not kill" (Exod. 20:13). Life is at the same time a gift and a responsibility. It is received as a "talent" (cf. Matt. 25:14–30); it must be put to proper use. In order that life may bring forth fruit, many tasks are offered to man in this world, and he must not shirk them. More important still, the Christian knows that eternal life depends on what, with the grace of God, he does with his life on earth.

6. The tradition of the Church has always held that human life must be protected and favored from the beginning, just as at the various stages of its development. Opposing the morals

of the Greco-Roman world, the Church of the first centuries insisted on the difference that exists on this point between those morals and Christian morals. In the *Didache* it is clearly said: "You shall not kill by abortion the fruit of the womb and you shall not murder the infant already born."[6] Athenagoras emphasizes that Christians consider as murderers those women who take medicines to procure an abortion; he condemns the killers of children, including those still living in their mother's womb, "where they are already the object of the care of Divine Providence."[7] Tertullian did not always perhaps use the same language; he nevertheless clearly affirms the essential principle: "To prevent birth is anticipated murder; it makes little difference whether one destroys a life already born or does away with it in its nascent stage. The one who will be a man is already one."[8]

7. In the course of history, the Fathers of the Church, her pastors, and her Doctors have taught the same doctrine—the various opinions on the infusion of the spiritual soul did not introduce any doubt about the illicitness of abortion. It is true that in the Middle Ages, when the opinion was generally held that the spiritual soul was not present until after the first few weeks, a distinction was made in the evaluation of the sin and the gravity of penal sanctions. Excellent authors allowed for this first period more lenient case solutions which they rejected for following periods. But it was never denied at that time that procured abortion, even during the first days, was objectively grave fault. This condemnation was in fact unanimous. Among the many documents it is sufficient to recall certain ones. The first Council of Mainz in 847 reconsidered the penalties against abortion which had been established by preceding councils. It decided that the most rigorous penance would be imposed "on women who procure the elimination of the fruit conceived in their womb."[9] The Decree of Gratian reported the following words of Pope Stephen V: "That person is a murderer who causes to perish by abortion what has been conceived."[10] St. Thomas, the Common Doctor of the Church, teaches that abortion is a grave sin against the natural law.[11] At the time of the Renaissance, Pope Sixtus V condemned abortion with the greatest severity.[12] A century later, Innocent XI rejected the propositions of certain lax canonists who sought to excuse an abortion procured before the moment accepted by some as the moment of the spiritual animation of the new being.[13] In our days the recent Roman pontiffs have proclaimed the same doctrine with the greatest clarity. Pius XI explicitly answered the most serious objections.[14] Pius XII clearly excluded all direct abortion, that is, abortion which is either an end or a means.[15] John XXIII recalled the teaching of the Fathers on the sacred character of life "which from its beginning demands the action of God the Creator."[16] Most recently, the Second Vatican Council, presided over by Paul VI, has most severely condemned abortion: "Life must be safeguarded with extreme care from conception; abortion and infanticide are abominable crimes."[17] The same Paul VI, speaking on this subject on many occasions, has not been afraid to declare that this teaching of the Church "has not changed and is unchangeable."[18]

8. Respect for human life is not just a Christian obligation. Human reason is sufficient to impose it on the basis of the analysis of what a human person is and should be. Constituted by a rational nature, man is a personal subject capable of reflecting on himself and of determining his acts and hence his own destiny: he is free. He is consequently master of himself; or rather, because this takes place in the course of time, he has the means of becoming so: this is his task. Created immediately by God, man's soul is spiritual and therefore immortal. Hence man is open to God, he finds his fulfillment only in Him. But man lives in the community of his equals; he is nourished by interpersonal communication with men in the indispensable social setting. In the face of society and other men, each human person possesses himself, he possesses life and different goods, he has these as a right. It is this that strict justice demands from all in his regard.

9. Nevertheless, temporal life lived in this world is not identified with the person. The person possesses as his own a level of life that is more profound and that cannot end. Bodily life is a fundamental good, here below it is the condition for all other goods. But there are higher values for which it could be legitimate or even necessary to be willing to expose oneself to the risk of losing bodily life. In a society of persons the common good is for each individual an end which he must serve and to which he must subordinate his particular interest. But it is not his last end and, from this point of view, it is society which is at the service of the person, because the person will not fulfill his destiny except in God. The person can be definitively subordinated only to God. Man can never be treated simply as a means to be disposed of in order to obtain a higher end.

10. In regard to the mutual rights and duties of the person and of society, it belongs to moral teaching to enlighten consciences; it belongs to the law to specify and organize external behavior. There is precisely a certain number of rights which society is not in a position to grant since these rights precede society; but society has the function to preserve and to enforce them. These are the greater part of those which are today called "human rights" and which our age boasts of having formulated.

11. The first right of the human person is his life. He has other goods, and some are more precious, but this one is fundamental—the condition of all the others. Hence it must be protected above all others. It does not belong to society, nor does it belong to public authority in any form to recognize this right for some and not for others: all discrimination is evil, whether it be founded on race, sex, color, or religion. It is not recognition by another that constitutes this right. This right is antecedent to its recognition; it demands recognition, and it is strictly unjust to refuse it.

12. Any discrimination based on the various stages of life is no more justified than any other discrimination. The right to life remains complete in an old person, even one greatly weakened; it is not lost by one who is incurably sick. The right to life is no less to be respected in the small infant just born than in the mature person. In reality, respect for human life is called for from the time that the process of generation begins. From the time that the ovum is fertilized, a life is begun which is neither that of the father nor of the mother, it is rather the life of a new human being with his own growth. It would never be made human if it were not human already.

13. To this perpetual evidence—perfectly independent of the discussions on the moment of animation [19]—modern genetic science brings valuable confirmation. It has demonstrated that, from the first instant, there is established the program of what this living being will be: a man, this individual man with his characteristic aspects already well-determined. Right from fertilization is begun the adventure of a human life, and each of its capacities requires time—a rather lengthy time—to find its place and to be in a position to act. The least that can be said is that present science, in its most evolved state, does not give any substantial support to those who defend abortion. Moreover, it is not up to biological sciences to make a definitive judgment on questions which are properly philosophical and moral such as the moment when a human person is constituted or the legitimacy of abortion. From a moral point of view this is certain: even if a doubt existed concerning whether the fruit of conception is already a human person, it is objectively a grave sin to dare to risk murder. "The one who will be a man is already one." [20]

14. Divine law and natural reason, therefore, exclude all right to the direct killing of an innocent man. However, if the reasons given to justify an abortion were always manifestly evil and valueless the problem would not be so dramatic. The gravity of the problem comes from the fact that in certain cases, perhaps in quite a considerable number of cases, by denying abortion one endangers important values to which it is normal to attach great value, and which may sometimes even seem to have priority. We do not deny these very great difficulties. It may be a serious question of health, sometimes of life or death, for the mother; it may be the burden represented by an additional child, especially if there are good reasons to fear that the child will be abnormal or retarded; it may be the importance attributed in different classes of society to considerations of honor or dishonor, of loss of social standing, and so forth. We proclaim only that none of these reasons can ever objectively confer the right to dispose of another's life, even when that life is only beginning. With regard to the future unhappiness of the child, no one, not even the father or mother, can act as its substitute—even if it is still in the embryonic stage—to choose in the child's name, life or death. The child itself, when grown up, will never have the right to choose suicide; no more

may his parents choose death for the child while it is not of an age to decide for itself. Life is too fundamental a value to be weighed against even very serious disadvantages. [21]

15. The movement for the emancipation of women, insofar as it seeks essentially to free them from all unjust discrimination, is on perfectly sound ground. [22] In the different forms of cultural background, there is a great deal to be done in this regard. But one cannot change nature. Nor can one exempt women, any more than men, from what nature demands of them. Furthermore, all publicly recognized freedom is always limited by the certain rights of others.

16. The same must be said of the claim to sexual freedom. If by this expression one is to understand the mastery progressively acquired by reason and by authentic love over instinctive impulse, without diminishing pleasure but keeping it in its proper place—and in this sphere this is the only authentic freedom—then there is nothing to object to. But this kind of freedom will always be careful not to violate justice. If, on the contrary, one is to understand that men and women are "free" to seek sexual pleasure to the point of satiety, without taking into account any law or the essential orientation of sexual life to its fruits of fertility, [23] then this idea has nothing Christian in it. It is even unworthy of man. In any case it does not confer any right to dispose of human life—even if embryonic—or to suppress it on the pretext that it is burdensome.

17. Scientific progress is opening to technology—and will open still more—the possibility of delicate interventions, the consequences of which can be very serious, for good as well as for evil. These are achievements of the human spirit which in themselves are admirable. But technology can never be independent of the criterion of morality, since technology exists for man and must respect his finality. Just as there is no right to use nuclear energy for every possible purpose, so there is no right to manipulate human life in every possible direction. Technology must be at the service of man, so as better to ensure the functioning of his normal abilities, to prevent or to cure his illnesses, and to contribute to his better human development. It is true that the evolution of technology makes early abortion more and more easy, but the moral evaluation is in no way modified because of this.

18. We know what seriousness the problem of birth control can assume for some families and for some countries. That is why the last council and subsequently the encyclical *Humanae vitae* of July 25, 1968, spoke of "responsible parenthood." [24] What we wish to say again with emphasis, as was pointed out in the conciliar constitution *Gaudium et spes*, in the encyclical *Populorum progressio*, and in other papal documents, is that never, under any pretext, may abortion be resorted to, either by a family or by the political authority, as a legitimate means of regulating births. [25] The damage to moral values is always a greater evil for the common good than any disadvantage in the economic or demographic order.

19. The moral discussion is being accompanied more or less everywhere by serious juridical debates. There is no country where legislation does not forbid and punish murder. Furthermore, many countries had specifically applied this condemnation and these penalties to the particular case of procured abortion. In these days a vast body of opinion petitions the liberalization of this latter prohibition. There already exists a fairly general tendency which seeks to limit, as far as possible, all restrictive legislation, especially when it seems to touch upon private life. The argument of pluralism is also used. Although many citizens, in particular the Catholic faithful, condemn abortion, many others hold that it is licit, at least as a lesser evil. Why force them to follow an opinion which is not theirs, especially in a country where they are in the majority? In addition it is apparent that, where they still exist, the laws condemning abortion appear difficult to apply. The crime has become too common for it to be punished every time, and the public authorities often find that it is wiser to close their eyes to it. But the preservation of a law which is not applied is always to the detriment of authority and of all the other laws. It must be added that clandestine abortion puts women, who resign themselves to it and have recourse to it, in the most serious dangers for future pregnancies and also in many cases for their lives. Even if the legislator continues to regard abortion as an evil, may he not propose to restrict its damage?

20. These arguments and others in addition that are heard from varying quarters are not conclusive. It is true that civil law cannot expect to cover the whole field of morality or to punish all faults. No one expects it to do so. It must often tolerate what is in fact a lesser evil, in order to avoid a greater one. One must, however, be attentive to what a change in legislation can represent. Many will take as authorization what is perhaps only the abstention from punishment. Even more, in the present case, this very renunciation seems at the very least to admit that the legislator no longer considers abortion a crime against human life, since murder is still always severely punished. It is true that it is not the task of the law to choose between points of view or to impose one rather than another. But the life of the child takes precedence over all opinions. One cannot invoke freedom of thought to destroy this life.

21. The role of law is not to record what is done, but to help in promoting improvement. It is at all times the task of the State to preserve each person's rights and to protect the weakest. In order to do so the State will have to right many wrongs. The law is not obliged to sanction everything, but it cannot act contrary to a law which is deeper and more majestic than any human law: the natural law engraved in men's hearts by the Creator as a norm which reason clarifies and strives to formulate properly, and which one must always struggle to understand better, but which it is always wrong to contradict. Human law can abstain from punishment, but it cannot declare to be right what would be opposed to the natural law,

for this opposition suffices to give the assurance that a law is not a law at all.

22. It must in any case be clearly understood that whatever may be laid down by civil law in this matter, man can never obey a law which is in itself immoral, and such is the case of a law which would admit in principle the lawfulness of abortion. Nor can he take part in a propaganda campaign in favor of such a law, or vote for it. Moreover, he may not collaborate in its application. It is, for instance, inadmissible that doctors or nurses should find themselves obliged to cooperate closely in abortions and have to choose between the law of God and their professional situation.

23. On the contrary, it is the task of law to pursue a reform of society and of conditions of life in all milieux, starting with the most deprived, so that always and everywhere it may be possible to give every child coming into this world a welcome worthy of a person. Help for families and for unmarried mothers, assured grants for children, a statute for illegitimate children and reasonable arrangements for adoption—a whole positive policy must be put into force so that there will always be a concrete, honorable, and possible alternative to abortion.

24. Following one's conscience in obedience to the law of God is not always the easy way. One must not fail to recognize the weight of the sacrifices and the burdens which it can impose. Heroism is sometimes called for in order to remain faithful to the requirements of the divine law. Therefore, we must emphasize that the path of true progress of the human person passes through this constant fidelity to a conscience maintained in uprightness and truth; and we must exhort all those who are able to do so to lighten the burdens still crushing so many men and women, families and children, who are placed in situations to which, in human terms, there is no solution.

25. A Christian's outlook cannot be limited to the horizon of life in this world. He knows that during the present life another one is being prepared, one of such importance that it is in its light that judgments must be made.[26] From this viewpoint there is no absolute misfortune here below, not even the terrible sorrow of bringing up a handicapped child. This is the contradiction proclaimed by the Lord: "Happy those who mourn: they shall be comforted" (Matt. 5:5). To measure happiness by the absence of sorrow and misery in this world is to turn one's back on the Gospel.

26. But this does not mean that one can remain indifferent to these sorrows and miseries. Every man and woman with feeling, and certainly every Christian, must be ready to do what he can to remedy them. This is the law of charity, of which the first preoccupation must always be the establishment of justice. One can never approve of abortion; but it is above all necessary to combat its causes. This includes political action, which will be in particular the task of the law. But it is necessary at the same time to influence morality and to do

everything possible to help families, mothers, and children. Considerable progress in the service of life has been accomplished by medicine. One can hope that such progress will continue, in accordance with the vocation of doctors, which is not to suppress life but to care for it and favor it as much as possible. It is equally desirable that, in suitable institutions, or, in their absence, in the outpouring of Christian generosity and charity every form of assistance should be developed.

27. There will be no effective action on the level of morality unless at the same time an effort is made on the level of ideas. A point of view—or even more, perhaps a way of thinking—which considers fertility as an evil cannot be allowed to spread without contradiction. It is true that not all forms of culture are equally in favor of large families. Such families come up against much greater difficulties in an industrial and urban civilization. Thus in recent times the Church has insisted on the idea of responsible parenthood, the exercise of true human and Christian prudence. Such prudence would not be authentic if it did not include generosity. It must preserve awareness of the grandeur of the task of cooperating with the Creator in the transmission of life, which gives new members to society and new children to the Church. Christ's Church has the fundamental solicitude of protecting and favoring life. She certainly thinks before all else of the life which Christ came to bring: "I have come so that they may have life and have it to the full" (John 10:10). But life at all its levels comes from God, and bodily life is for man the indispensable beginning. In this life on earth sin has introduced, multiplied, and made harder to bear suffering and death. But in taking their burden upon himself, Jesus Christ has transformed them: for whoever believes in Him, suffering and death itself become instruments of resurrection. Hence Saint Paul can say: "I think that what we suffer in this life can never be compared to the glory, as yet unrevealed, which is waiting for us" (Rom. 8:18). And, if we make this comparison we shall add with him: "Yes, the troubles which are soon over, though they weigh little, train us for the carrying of a weight of eternal glory which is out of all proportion to them" (2 Cor. 4:17).

The Supreme Pontiff Pope Paul VI, in an audience granted to the undersigned Secretary of the Sacred Congregation for the Doctrine of the Faith on June 28, 1974, has ratified this Declaration on Procured Abortion and has confirmed it and ordered it to be promulgated.

Given at Rome, at the Sacred Congregation
for the Doctrine of the Faith,
on November 18, the Commemoration of the
Dedication of the Basilicas of Saints Peter and Paul,
in the year 1974.

Franciscus Card. Seper
Prefect
Hieronymus Hamer
Titular Archbishop of Lorium
Secretary

Notes

[1] A certain number of bishops' documents are to be found in Gr. Caprile, *Non Uccidere, Il Magistero della Chiesa sull'aborto* (Rome: 1973), pt. II, 47–300.

[2] *Regimini Ecclesiae Universae*, III, 1, 29. Cf. ibid., 31, *AAS* 59 (1967): 897. On the Sacred Congregation for the Doctrine of the Faith depend all the questions which are related to faith and morals or which are bound up with the faith.

[3] Second Vatican Council, *Lumen gentium*, n. 12, *AAS* 57 (1965): 16–17. The present declaration does not envisage all the questions which can arise in connection with abortion: it is for theologians to examine and discuss them. Only certain basic principles are here recalled which must be for the theologians themselves a guide and a rule, and confirm certain fundamental truths of Catholic doctrine for all Christians.

[4] Second Vatican Council, *Lumen gentium*, n. 25, *AAS* 57 (1965): 29–31.

[5] The authors of Scripture do not make any philosophical observations on when life begins, but they speak of the period of life which precedes birth as being the object of God's attention: He creates and forms the human being, like that which is molded by his hand (cf. Ps. 118:73). It would seem that this theme finds expression for the first time in Jer. 1:5. It appears later in many other texts. Cf. Isa. 49:1–5; 46:3; Job 10:8–12; Ps. 22:10; 71:6; 139:13. In the Gospels we read in Luke 1:44: "For the moment your greeting reached my ears, the child in my womb leapt for joy."

[6] *Didache apostolorum*, Funk edition, *Patres apostolici*, V, 2. *The Epistle of Barnabas*, IX, 5, uses the same expressions (cf. Funk, *Patres apostolici*, 91–93).

[7] Athenagoras, *A Plea on Behalf of Christians*, 35 (cf. *PG* 6, 970: *S.C.* 3, 166–167). One may also consult the *Epistle to Diogentus* (V, 6, Funk, *Patres apostolici*, I 399: S.C. 33), where it says of Christians: "They procreate children, but they do not reject the fetus."

[8] Tertullian, *Apologeticum* (IX. 8, *PL* 1, 371–372, *Corp. Christ.* I, p. 103, 1, 31–36).

[9] Canon 21 (Mansi, 14, p. 909). Cf. Council of Elvira, canon 63 (Mansi, 2, p. 16); and the Council of Ancyra, canon 21 (ibid., 519). See also the decree of Gregory III regarding the penance to be imposed upon those who are culpable of this crime (Mansi 13, 292, c. 17).

[10] Gratian, *Concordantia discordantium canonum*, c. 20, C. 2, q. [2]. During the Middle Ages appeal was often made to the authority of St. Augustine who wrote as follows in regard to this matter in *De nuptiis et concupiscentiis*, c. 15: "Sometimes this sexually indulgent cruelty or this cruel sexual indulgence goes so far as to procure potions which produce sterility. If the desired result is not achieved, the mother terminates the life and expels the fetus which was in her womb in such a way that the child dies before having lived, or, if the baby was living already in its mother's womb, it is killed before being born." *PL* 44, 423–424, *CSEL* 33, 619. Cf. the *Decree of Gratian*, q. 2, C. 32, c. 7.

[11] *Commentary on the Sentences*, bk. IV, dist. 31, exposition of the text.

[12] Constitution *Effraenatum* in 1588, *Bullarium Romanum*, V, 1, pp. 25–27; *Fontes iuris canonici*, I, no. 165, pp. 308–311.

[13] Dz-Sch. 1184. Cf. also the constitution *Apostolicae sedis* of Pius IX, *Acta Pii IX*, V, 5572; *AAS* 5 [1869]: 305–331; *Fontes iuris canonici*, III, no. 552, pp. 24–31.

[14] Encyclical *Casti connubii*, *AAS* 22 (1930): 562–565; DzSch. 3719–3721.

[15] The statements of Pius XII are express, precise, and numerous; they would require a whole study on their own. We quote only this one from the Discourse to the Saint Luke Union of Italian Doctors of November 12, 1944, because it formulates the principle in all its universality: "As long as a man is not guilty, his life is untouchable, and therefore any act directly tending to destroy it is illicit, whether such destruction is intended as an end in itself or only as a means to an end, whether it is a question of life in the embryonic stage or in a stage of full development or already in its final stages." *Discourses and Radiomessages*, VI, 183ff.

[16] Encyclical *Mater et magistra*, *AAS* 53 (1961): 447.

[17] *Gaudium et spes*, n. 51. Cf. n. 27, *AAS* 58 (1966): 1072; cf. 1047.

[18] The speech *Salutiamo con paterna effusione* (December 9, 1972), *AAS* 64 (1972): 737. Among the witnesses of this unchangeable doctrine one will recall the declaration of the Holy Office, condemning direct abortion. Denzinger 1890, *AAS* 17 (1884): 556; *AAS* 22 (1888–1890), 748; Dz-Sch 3258.

[19] This declaration expressly leaves aside the question of the moment when the spiritual soul is infused. There is not a unanimous tradition on this point, and authors are as yet in disagreement. For some it dates from the first instant; for others it could not at least precede nidation. It is not within the competence of science to decide between these views, because the existence of an immortal soul is not a question in its field. It is a philosophical problem from which our moral affirmation remains independent for two reasons: 1) supposing a belated animation, there is still nothing less than a human life, preparing for and calling for a soul in which the nature received from parents is completed; 2) on the other hand, it suffices that this presence of the soul be probable (and one can never prove the contrary) in order that the taking of life involve accepting the risk of killing a man, not only waiting for, but already in possession of his soul.

[20] Tertullian, *Apologeticum*.

[21] Cardinal Villot, Secretary of State, wrote on October 19, 1973, to Cardinal Döpfner, regarding the protection of human life: "(Die Kirche) kann jedoch sur Behebung solcher Notsituationen weder empfängnisverhütende Mittel noch erst recht nicht die Abtreibung als sittlich erlaubt erkennen."(*L'Osservatore Romano* (German), October 26, 1973, 3.

[22] John XXIII, encyclical *Pacem in terris*, *AAS* 55 (1963): 267. Second Vatican Council, constitution *Gaudium et spes*, n. 29. Speech of Paul VI, *Salutiamo*, *AAS* 64 (1972): 779.

[23] *Gaudium et spes*, n. 48: "Indole autem sua naturali, ipsum institutum matrimonii amorque coniugalis ad procreationem et educationem prolis ordinantur, iisque veluti suo fastigio coronantur." Also n. 50: "Matrimonium et amor coniugalis indole sua ad prolem procreandam et educandam ordinantur."

[24] *Gaudium et spes*, nn. 50–51. Paul VI, encyclical *Humanae vitae*, n. 10, *AAS* 60, (1968): 487.

[25] *Gaudium et spes*, n. 87. Paul VI, encyclical *Populorum progressio*, n. 31; Address to the United Nations, *AAS* 57 (1965): 883. John XXIII, *Mater et magistra*, *AAS* 53 (1961): 445–448. Responsible parenthood supposes the use of only morally licit methods of birth regulation. Cf. *Humanae vitae*, n. 14 (ibid., p. 490).

[26] Cardinal Villot, Secretary of State, wrote to the World Congress of Catholic Doctors held in Barcelona, May 26, 1974: "Por lo que a la vida humana se refiere, esta non es ciertamente univoca, más bien se podría decir que es un haz de vidas. No se puede reducir, sin mutilarlas gravemente, las zonas de su ser, que, en su estrecha dependencia e interaccíon están ordenadas las unas a las otras: zona corporal, zona afectiva, zona mental, y ese transfondo del alma donde la vida divina, recibida por la gracia, puede desplegarse mediante los dones del Espíritu Santo." *L'Osservatore Romano*, May 29, 1974.

APPENDIX IV

Congregation for the Doctrine of the Faith

Quaecumque sterilizatio
Responses on Sterilization in Catholic Hospitals

March 13, 1975

This sacred congregation has diligently considered not only the problem of contraceptive sterilization for therapeutic purposes but also the opinions indicated by different people toward a solution, and the conflicts relative to requests for cooperation in such sterilizations in Catholic hospitals. The congregation has resolved to respond to these questions in this way:

1. Any sterilization which of itself, that is, of its own nature and condition, has the sole immediate effect of rendering the generative faculty incapable of procreation, is to be considered direct sterilization, as the term is understood in the declarations of the pontifical magisterium, especially of Pius XII.[1] Therefore, notwithstanding any subjectively right intention of those whose actions are prompted by the care or prevention of physical or mental illness which is foreseen or feared as a result of pregnancy, such sterilization remains absolutely forbidden according to the doctrine of the Church. And indeed the sterilization of the faculty itself is forbidden for an even graver reason than the sterilization of individual acts, since it induces a state of sterility in the person which is almost always irreversible.

Neither can any mandate of public authority, which would seek to impose direct sterilization as necessary for the common good, be invoked, for such sterilization damages the dignity and inviolability of the human person.[2] Likewise, neither can one invoke the principle of totality in this case, in virtue of which principal interference with organs is justified for the greater good of the person; sterility intended in itself is not oriented to the integral good of the person as rightly pursued, "the proper order of goods being preserved,"[3] inasmuch as it damages the ethical good of the person, which is the highest good, since it deliberately deprives foreseen and freely chosen sexual activity of an essential element. Thus article 20 of the medical-ethics code promulgated by the conference in 1971 faithfully reflects the doctrine which is to be held, and its observance should be urged.

2. The congregation, while it confirms this traditional doctrine of the Church, is not unaware of the dissent against this teaching from many theologians. The congregation, however, denies that doctrinal significance can be attributed to this fact as such, so as to constitute a "theological source" which the faithful might invoke and thereby abandon the authentic magisterium and follow the opinions of private theologians which dissent from it.[4]

3. Insofar as the management of Catholic hospitals is concerned:

a. Any cooperation institutionally approved or tolerated in actions which are in themselves, that is, by their nature and condition, directed to a contraceptive end, namely, that the natural effects of sexual actions deliberately performed by the sterilized subject be impeded, is absolutely forbidden. For the official approbation of direct sterilization and, *a fortiori*, its management and execution in accord with hospital regulations, is a matter which, in the objective order, is by its very nature (or intrinsically) evil. The Catholic hospital cannot cooperate with this for any reason. Any cooperation so supplied is totally unbecoming the mission entrusted to this type of institution and would be contrary to the necessary proclamation and defense of the moral order.

b. The traditional doctrine regarding material cooperation, with the proper distinctions between necessary and free, proximate and remote, remains valid, to be applied with the utmost prudence, if the case warrants.

c. In the application of the principle of material cooperation, if the case warrants, great care must be taken against scandal and the danger of any misunderstanding by an appropriate explanation of what is really being done.

This sacred congregation hopes that the criteria recalled in this letter will satisfy the expectations of that episcopate, in order that, with the uncertainties of the faithful cleared up, the bishops might more easily respond to their pastoral duty.

Notes

[1]Cf. esp. the two allocutions to the Catholic Union of Obstetricians and to the International Society of Hematology; in *AAS* 43 (1951): 843–844; *AAS* 50 (1958): 734–737; and in the encyclical of Paul VI *Humanae vitae*, n. 14, cf. *AAS* 60 (1968): 490–491.

[2]Cf. Pius XI, encyclical *Casti Connubii*, *AAS* 22 (1930): 565.

[3]Paul VI, *Humanae vitae*, *AAS* 60 (1968): 487.

[4]Cf. Vatican Council II, constitution *Lumen gentium*, n. 25, 1, *AAS* 57 (1965): 29–30; Pius XII, Allocution to the Most Reverend Cardinals, *AAS* 46 (1954): 672; idem, encyclical *Humani generis*, *AAS* 42 (1950): 568; Paul VI, Allocution to the meeting regarding the theology of Vatican Council II, *AAS* 58 (1966): 889–896, esp. 890–894; idem, the Allocution to the Members of the Congregation of the Most Holy Redeemer, *AAS* 59 (1967): 960–963, esp. 962.

Congregation for the Doctrine of the Faith

Declaration on Euthanasia

May 5, 1980

The rights and values pertaining to the human person occupy an important place among the questions discussed today. In this regard, the Second Vatican Ecumenical Council solemnly reaffirmed the lofty dignity of the human person, and in a special way his or her right to life. The council therefore condemned crimes against life "such as any type of murder, genocide, abortion, euthanasia, or willful suicide" (Pastoral Constitution Gaudium et spes, n. 27).

More recently, the Sacred Congregation for the Doctrine of the Faith has reminded all the faithful of Catholic teaching on procured abortion.[1] The congregation now considers it opportune to set forth the Church's teaching on euthanasia.

It is indeed true that, in this sphere of teaching, the recent popes have explained the principles, and these retain their full force[2]; but the progress of medical science in recent years has brought to the fore new aspects of the question of euthanasia, and these aspects call for further elucidation on the ethical level.

In modern society, in which even the fundamental values of human life are often called into question, cultural change exercises an influence upon the way of looking at suffering and death; moreover, medicine has increased its capacity to cure and to prolong life in particular circumstances, which sometimes give rise to moral problems.

Thus people living in this situation experience no little anxiety about the meaning of advanced old age and death. They also begin to wonder whether they have the right to obtain for themselves or their fellow men an "easy death," which would shorten suffering and which seems to them more in harmony with human dignity.

A number of episcopal conferences have raised questions on this subject with the Sacred Congregation for the Doctrine of the Faith.

The congregation, having sought the opinion of experts on the various aspects of euthanasia, now wishes to respond to the bishops' questions with the present declaration, in order to help them to give correct teaching to the faithful entrusted to their care, and to offer them elements for reflection that they can present to the civil authorities with regard to this very serious matter.

The considerations set forth in the present document concern in the first place all those who place their faith and hope in Christ, who, through his life, death, and resurrection, has given a new meaning to existence and especially to the death of the Christian, as St. Paul says: "If we live, we live to the Lord; and if we die, we die to the Lord" (Rom. 14:8; cf. Phil. 1:20).

As for those who profess other religions, many will agree with us that faith in God the Creator, Provider, and Lord of life—if they share this belief—confers a lofty dignity upon every human person and guarantees respect for him or her.

It is hoped that this declaration will meet with the approval of many people of good will, who, philosophical or ideological differences notwithstanding, have nevertheless a lively awareness of the rights of the human person. These rights have often, in fact, been proclaimed in recent years through declarations issued by international congresses[3]; and since it is a question here of fundamental rights inherent in every human person, it is obviously wrong to have recourse to arguments from political pluralism or religious freedom in order to deny the universal value of those rights.

I. The Value of Human Life

Human life is the basis of all goods, and is the necessary source and condition of every human activity and of all society. Most people regard life as something sacred and hold that no one may dispose of it at will, but believers see in life something greater, namely, a gift of God's love, which they are called upon to preserve and make fruitful. And it is this latter consideration that gives rise to the following consequences:

1. No one can make an attempt on the life of an innocent person without opposing God's love for that person, without violating a fundamental right, and therefore without committing a crime of the utmost gravity.[4]

2. Everyone has the duty to lead his or her life in accordance with God's plan. That life is entrusted to the individual as a good that must bear fruit already here on earth, but that finds its full perfection only in eternal life.

3. Intentionally causing one's own death, or suicide, is therefore equally as wrong as murder; such an action on the part of a person is to be considered as a rejection of God's sovereignty and loving plan. Furthermore, suicide is also often a refusal of love for self, the denial of a natural instinct to live, a flight from the duties of justice and charity owed to one's neighbor, to various communities or to the whole of society although, as is generally recognized, at times there are

psychological factors present that can diminish responsibility or even completely remove it.

However, one must clearly distinguish suicide from that sacrifice of one's life whereby for a higher cause, such as God's glory, the salvation of souls, or the service of one's brethren, a person offers his or her own life or puts it in danger (cf. John 15:14).

II. Euthanasia

In order that the question of euthanasia can be properly dealt with, it is first necessary to define the words used.

Etymologically speaking, in ancient times *euthanasia* meant an *easy death* without severe suffering. Today one no longer thinks of this original meaning of the word, but rather of some intervention of medicine whereby the suffering of sickness or of the final agony are reduced, sometimes also with the danger of suppressing life prematurely. Ultimately, the word "euthanasia" is used in a more particular sense to mean "mercy killing," for the purpose of putting an end to extreme suffering, or having abnormal babies, the mentally ill, or the incurably sick from the prolongation, perhaps for many years, of a miserable life, which could impose too heavy a burden on their families or on society.

It is, therefore, necessary to state clearly in what sense the word is used in the present document.

By euthanasia is understood an action or an omission which of itself or by intention causes death, in order that all suffering may in this way be eliminated. Euthanasia's terms of reference, therefore, are to be found in the intention of the will and in the methods used. It is necessary to state firmly once more that nothing and no one can in any way permit the killing of an innocent human being, whether a fetus or an embryo, an infant or an adult, an old person, or one suffering from an incurable disease, or a person who is dying.

Furthermore, no one is permitted to ask for this act of killing, either for himself or herself or for another person entrusted to his or her care, nor can he or she consent to it, either explicitly or implicitly. Nor can any authority legitimately recommend or permit such an action.

For it is a question of the violation of the divine law, an offense against the dignity of the human person, a crime against life, and an attack on humanity.

It may happen that, by reason of prolonged and barely tolerable pain, for deeply personal or other reasons, people may be led to believe that they can legitimately ask for death or obtain it for others. Although in these cases the guilt of the individual may be reduced or completely absent, nevertheless the error of judgment into which the conscience falls, perhaps in good faith, does not change the nature of this act of killing, which will always be in itself something to be rejected. The pleas of gravely ill people who sometimes ask for death are not to be understood as implying a true desire for euthanasia;

in fact, it is almost always a case of an anguished plea for help and love. What a sick person needs, besides medical care, is love, the human and supernatural warmth with which the sick person can and ought to be surrounded by all those close to him or her, parents and children, doctors and nurses.

III. The Meaning of Suffering for Christians and the Use of Painkillers

Death does not always come in dramatic circumstances after barely tolerable sufferings. Nor do we have to think only of extreme cases. Numerous testimonies which confirm one another lead one to the conclusion that nature itself has made provision to render more bearable at the moment of death separations that would be terribly painful to a person in full health. Hence it is that a prolonged illness, advanced old age, or a state of loneliness or neglect can bring about psychological conditions that facilitate the acceptance of death.

Nevertheless the fact remains that death, often preceded or accompanied by severe and prolonged suffering, is something which naturally causes people anguish.

Physical suffering is certainly an unavoidable element of the human condition; on the biological level, it constitutes a warning of which no one denies the usefulness; but, since it affects the human psychological makeup, it often exceeds its own biological usefulness and so can become so severe as to cause the desire to remove it at any cost.

According to Christian teaching, however, suffering, especially suffering during the last moments of life, has a special place in God's saving plan; it is in fact a sharing in Christ's passion and a union with the redeeming sacrifice which He offered in obedience to the Father's will. Therefore, one must not be surprised if some Christians prefer to moderate their use of painkillers, in order to accept voluntarily at least a part of their sufferings and thus associate themselves in a conscious way with the sufferings of Christ crucified (cf. Matt. 27:34).

Nevertheless it would be imprudent to impose a heroic way of acting as a general rule. On the contrary, human and Christian prudence suggest for the majority of sick people the use of medicines capable of alleviating or suppressing pain, even though these may cause as a secondary effect semi-consciousness and reduced lucidity. As for those who are not in a state to express themselves, one can reasonably presume that they wish to take these painkillers, and have them administered according to the doctor's advice.

But the intensive use of painkillers is not without difficulties, because the phenomenon of habituation generally makes it necessary to increase their dosage in order to maintain their efficacy. At this point it is fitting to recall a declaration by Pius XII, which retains its full force; in answer to a group of doctors who had put the question: "Is the suppression of pain and consciousness by the use of narcotics ... permitted by religion and morality to the doctor and the patient (even at the approach of death and if one foresees that the use of narcotics will shorten life)?" the pope said: "If no other means exist, and if, in the given circumstances, this does not prevent the carrying out of other religious and moral duties: Yes." [5] In this case, of course, death is in no way intended or sought, even if the risk of it is reasonably taken; the intention is simply to relieve pain effectively, using for this purpose painkillers available to medicine.

However, painkillers that cause unconsciousness need special consideration. For a person not only has to be able to satisfy his or her moral duties and family obligations; he or she also has to prepare himself or herself with full consciousness for meeting Christ. Thus Pius XII warns: "It is not right to deprive the dying person of consciousness without a serious reason." [6]

IV. Due Proportion in the Use of Remedies

Today it is very important to protect, at the moment of death, both the dignity of the human person and the Christian concept of life, against a technological attitude that threatens to become an abuse.

Thus some people speak of a "right to die," which is an expression that does not mean the right to procure death either by one's own hand or by means of someone else, as one pleases, but rather the right to die peacefully with human and Christian dignity. From this point of view, the use of therapeutic means can sometimes pose problems.

In numerous cases, the complexity of the situation can be such as to cause doubts about the way ethical principles should be applied. In the final analysis, it pertains to the conscience either of the sick person, or of those qualified to speak in the sick person's name, or of the doctors, to decide, in the light of moral obligations and of the various aspects of the case.

Everyone has the duty to care for his or her own health or to seek such care from others. Those whose task it is to care for the sick must do so conscientiously and administer the remedies that seem necessary or useful.

However, is it necessary in all circumstances to have recourse to all possible remedies?

In the past, moralists replied that one is never obliged to use "extraordinary" means. This reply, which as a principle still holds good, is perhaps less clear today, by reason of the imprecision of the term and the rapid progress made in the treatment of sickness. Thus some people prefer to speak of "proportionate" and "disproportionate" means. In any case, it will be possible to make a correct judgment as to the means by studying the type of treatment to be used, its degree of complexity or risk, its cost and the possibilities of using it, and comparing these elements with the result that can be expected, taking into account the state of the sick person and his or her physical and moral resources.

In order to facilitate the application of these general principles, the following clarifications can be added:

• If there are no other sufficient remedies, it is permitted, with the patient's consent, to have recourse to the means provided by the most advanced medical techniques, even if these means are still at the experimental stage and are not without a certain risk. By accepting them, the patient can even show generosity in the service of humanity.

• It is also permitted, with the patient's consent, to interrupt these means, where the results fall short of expectations. But for such a decision to be made, account will have to be taken of the reasonable wishes of the patient and the patient's family, as also of the advice of the doctors who are specially competent in the matter. The latter may in particular judge that the investment in instruments and personnel is disproportionate to the results foreseen; they may also judge that the techniques applied impose on the patient strain or suffering out of proportion with the benefits which he or she may gain from such techniques.

• It is also permissible to make do with the normal means that medicine can offer. Therefore one cannot impose on anyone the obligation to have recourse to a technique which is already in use but which carries a risk or is burdensome. Such a refusal is not the equivalent of suicide; on the contrary, it should be considered as an acceptance of the human condition, or a wish to avoid the application of a medical procedure disproportionate to the results that can be expected, or a desire not to impose excessive expense on the family or the community.

• When inevitable death is imminent in spite of the means used, it is permitted in conscience to take the decision to refuse forms of treatment that would only secure a precarious and burdensome prolongation of life, so long as the normal care due to the sick person in similar cases is not interrupted. In such circumstances the doctor has no reason to reproach himself with failing to help the person in danger.

Conclusion

The norms contained in the present declaration are inspired by a profound desire to service people in accordance with the plan of the Creator. Life is a gift of God, and on the other hand death is unavoidable; it is necessary, therefore, that we, without in any way hastening the hour of death, should be able to accept it with full responsibility and dignity. It is true that death marks the end of our earthly existence, but at the same time it opens the door to immortal life. Therefore, all must prepare themselves for this event in the light of human values, and Christians even more so in the light of faith.

As for those who work in the medical profession, they ought to neglect no means of making all their skill available to the sick and dying; but they should also remember how much more necessary it is to provide them with the comfort of boundless kindness and heartfelt charity. Such service to people is also service to Christ the Lord, who said: "As you did it to one of the least of these my brethren, you did it to me" (Matt. 25:40).

At the audience granted to the undersigned prefect, his Holiness Pope John Paul II approved this declaration, adopted at the ordinary meeting of the Sacred Congregation for the Doctrine of the Faith, and ordered its publication.

Rome, the Sacred Congregation
for the Doctrine of the Faith,
May 5, 1980.

Franjo Cardinal Seper
Prefect
Jerome Hamer, O.P.
Tit. Archbishop of Lorium
Secretary

Notes

[1] Congregation for the Doctrine of the Faith, *Declaration On Procured Abortion* (November 18, 1974), *AAS* 66 (1974): 730–747.

[2] Pius XII, Address to those attending the Congress of the International Union of Catholic Women's Leagues (September 11, 1947), *AAS* 39 (1947): 483; idem, Address to the Italian Catholic Union Of Midwives (October 29, 1951), *AAS* 43 (1951): 835–854; idem, Speech to the Members of the International Office of Military Medicine Documentation (October 19, 1953), *AAS* 45 (1953): 744–754; idem, Address to those taking part in the IXth Congress of the Italian Anaesthesiological Society (February 24, 1957), *AAS* 49 (1957): 146; cf. also idem, Address on "Reanimation" (November 24, 1957), *AAS* 49 (1957): 1027–1033; Paul VI, Address to the members of The United National Special Committee on Apartheid (May 22, 1974), *AAS* 66 (1974): 346; John Paul II, Address to the Bishops of the United States of America (October 5, 1979), *AAS* 71 (1979): 1225.

[3] One thinks especially of recommendation 779 (1976) on the rights of the sick and dying, of the Parliamentary Assembly of the Council of Europe at its XXVIIth Ordinary Session; cf. Sipeca, no. 1, March 1977, 14–15.

[4] We leave aside completely the problems of the death penalty and of war, which involve specific considerations that do not concern the present subject.

[5] Pius XII, Address (February 24, 1957), *AAS* 49 (1957): 147.

[6] Ibid., 145; cf. idem, Address (September 9, 1958), *AAS* 50 (1958): 694.

Congregation for the Doctrine of the Faith

Donum Vitae

Instruction on Respect for Human Life in its Origin and on the Dignity of Procreation

February 22, 1987

Replies to Certain Questions of the Day

Foreword

The Congregation of the Doctrine of the Faith has been approached by various episcopal conferences or individual bishops, by theologians, doctors, and scientists, concerning biomedical techniques which make it possible to intervene in the initial phase of the life of a human being and in the very processes of procreation, and their conformity with the principles of Catholic morality. The present instruction, which is the result of wide consultation and in particular of a careful evaluation of the declarations made by episcopates, does not intend to repeat all the Church's teaching on the dignity of human life as it originates and on procreation, but to offer, in the light of the previous teaching of the magisterium, some specific replies to the main questions being asked in this regard.

The exposition is arranged as follows: an introduction will recall the fundamental principles, of an anthropological and moral character, which are necessary for a proper evaluation of the problems and for working out replies to those questions; the first part will have as its subject respect for the human being from the first moment of his or her existence; the second part will deal with the moral questions raised by technical interventions on human procreation; the third part will offer some orientations on the relationships between moral law and civil law in terms of the respect due to human embryos and fetuses* and as regards the legitimacy of techniques of artificial procreation.

---

*The terms "zygote," "pre-embryo," "embryo," and "fetus" can indicate in the vocabulary of biology successive stages of the development of a human being. The present Instruction makes free use of these terms, attributing to them an identical ethical relevance, in order to designate the result (whether visible or not) of human generation, from the first moment of its existence until birth. The reason for this usage is clarified by the text (cf I, n. 1).

Introduction

1. Biomedical Research and the Teaching of the Church

The gift of life which God the Creator and Father has entrusted to man calls him to appreciate the inestimable value of what he has been given and to take responsibility for it: this fundamental principle must be placed at the center of one's reflection in order to clarify and solve the moral problems raised by artificial interventions on life as it originates and on the processes of procreation.

Thanks to the progress of the biological and medical sciences, man has at his disposal ever more effective therapeutic resources; but he can also acquire new powers, with unforeseeable consequences, over human life at its very beginning and in its first stages. Various procedures now make it possible to intervene not only in order to assist but also to dominate the processes of procreation. These techniques can enable man to "take in hand his own destiny," but they also expose him "to the temptation to go beyond the limits of a reasonable dominion over nature."[1] They might constitute progress in the service of man, but they also involve serious risks. Many people are therefore expressing an urgent appeal that in interventions on procreation the values and rights of the human person be safeguarded. Requests for clarification and guidance are coming not only from the faithful but also from those who recognize the Church as "an expert in humanity"[2] with a mission to serve the "civilization of love"[3] and of life.

The Church's magisterium does not intervene on the basis of a particular competence in the area of the experimental sciences; but having taken account of the data of research and technology, it intends to put forward, by virtue of its evangelical mission and apostolic duty, the moral teaching corresponding to the dignity of the person and to his or her integral vocation. It intends to do so by expounding the criteria of moral judgment as regards the applications of scientific research and technology, especially in relation to human life and its beginnings. These criteria are the respect, defense, and promotion of man, his "primary and fundamental right" to life,[4] his dignity as a person who is endowed with a spiritual soul and with moral responsibility [5] and who is called to beatific communion with God.

The Church's intervention in this field is inspired also by the love which she owes to man, helping him to recognize and respect his rights and duties. This love draws from the font of Christ's love: as she contemplates the mystery of the Incarnate Word, the Church also comes to understand the "mystery of man" [6]; by proclaiming the Gospel of salvation, she reveals to man his dignity and invites him to discover fully the truth of his own being. Thus the Church once more puts forward the divine law in order to accomplish the work of truth and liberation.

For it is out of goodness—in order to indicate the path of life—that God gives human beings his commandments and the grace to observe them: and it is likewise out of goodness—in order to help them persevere along the same path—that God always offers to everyone his forgiveness. Christ has compassion on our weaknesses: He is our Creator and Redeemer. May his Spirit open men's hearts to the gift of God's peace and to an understanding of his precepts.

2. Science and Technology at the Service of the Human Person

God created man in his own image and likeness: "male and female he created them" (Gen. 1:27), entrusting to them the task of "having dominion over the earth" (Gen. 1:28). Basic scientific research and applied research constitute a significant expression of this dominion of man over creation. Science and technology are valuable resources for man when placed at his service and when they promote his integral development for the benefit of all; but they cannot of themselves show the meaning of existence and of human progress. Being ordered to man, who initiates and develops them, they draw from the person and his moral values the indication of their purpose and the awareness of their limits.

On the one hand, it would be illusory to claim that scientific research and its applications are morally neutral; on the other hand one cannot derive criteria for guidance from mere technical efficiency, from research's possible usefulness to some at the expense of others, or, worse still, from prevailing ideologies. Thus science and technology require, for their own intrinsic meaning, an unconditional respect for the fundamental criteria of the moral law: that is to say, they must be at the service of the human person, of his inalienable rights and his true and integral good according to the design and will of God. [7]

The rapid development of technological discoveries gives greater urgency to this need to respect the criteria just mentioned: science without conscience can only lead to man's ruin. "Our era needs such wisdom more than bygone ages if the discoveries made by man are to be further humanized. For the future of the world stands in peril unless wiser people are forthcoming." [8]

3. Anthropology and Procedures in the Biomedical Field

Which moral criteria must be applied in order to clarify the problems posed today in the field of biomedicine? The answer to this question presupposes a proper idea of the nature of the human person in his bodily dimension.

For it is only in keeping with his true nature that the human person can achieve self-realization as a "unified totality" [9]: and this nature is at the same time corporal and spiritual. By virtue of its substantial union with a spiritual soul, the human body cannot be considered as a mere complex of tissues, organs, and functions, nor can it be evaluated in the same way as the body of animals; rather it is a constitutive part of the person who manifests and expresses himself through it.

The natural moral law expresses and lays down the purposes, rights, and duties which are based upon the bodily and spiritual nature of the human person. Therefore this law cannot be thought of as simply a set of norms on the biological level; rather it must be defined as the rational order whereby man is called by the Creator to direct and regulate his life and actions and in particular to make use of his own body. [10]

A first consequence can be deduced from these principles: an intervention on the human body affects not only the tissues, the organs, and their functions but also involves the person himself on different levels. It involves, therefore, perhaps in an implicit but nonetheless real way, a moral significance and responsibility. Pope John Paul II forcefully reaffirmed this to the World Medical Association when he said: "Each human person in his absolutely unique singularity, is constituted not only by his spirit, but by his body as well. Thus, in the body and through the body, one touches the person himself in his concrete reality. To respect the dignity of man consequently amounts to safeguarding this identity of the man *corpore et anima unus*, as the Second Vatican Council says (*Gaudium et spes*, n. 14, par. 1). It is on the basis of this anthropological vision that one is to find the fundamental criteria for decision making in the case of procedures which are not strictly therapeutic, as, for example, those aimed at the improvement of the human biological condition." [11]

Applied biology and medicine work together for the integral good of human life when they come to the aid of a person stricken by illness and infirmity and when they respect his or her dignity as a creature of God. No biologist or doctor can reasonably claim, by virtue of his scientific competence, to be able to decide about people's origin and destiny. This norm must be applied in a particular way in the field of sexuality and procreation, in which man and woman actualize the fundamental values of love and life.

God, who is love and life, has inscribed in man and woman the vocation to share in a special way in his mystery of personal communion and in his work as Creator and Father. [12] For this reason marriage possesses specific goods and values in its union and in procreation which cannot be likened to those existing in lower forms of life. Such values and meanings are of the personal order and determine from the moral point of view the meaning and limits of artificial interventions regarding procreation and the origin of human life. These interventions are not to be rejected on the grounds that they are artificial. As such, they bear witness to the possibilities of the art of medicine. But they must be given a moral evaluation in reference to the dignity of the human person, who is called to realize his vocation from God to the gift of love and the gift of life.

4. Fundamental Criteria for a Moral Judgment

The fundamental values connected with the techniques of artificial human procreation are two: the life of the human being called into existence and the special nature of the transmission of human life in marriage. The moral judgment on such methods of artificial procreation must therefore be formulated in reference to these values.

Physical life, with which the course of human life in the world begins, certainly does not itself contain the whole of a person's value, nor does it represent the supreme good of man, who is called to eternal life. However, it does constitute in a certain way the "fundamental value of life, precisely because upon this physical life all the other values of the person are based and developed."[13] The inviolability of the innocent human being's right to life "from the moment of conception until death"[14] is a sign and requirement of the very inviolability of the person to whom the Creator has given the gift of life.

By comparison with the transmission of other forms of life in the universe, the transmission of human life has a special character of its own, which derives from the special nature of the human person. "The transmission of human life is entrusted by nature to a personal and conscious act and as such is subject to the all-holy laws of God: immutable and inviolable laws which must be recognized and observed. For this reason one cannot use means and follow methods which could be licit in the transmission of the life of plants and animals."[15]

Advances in technology have now made it possible to procreate apart from sexual relations through the meeting in vitro of the germ cells previously taken from the man and the woman. But what is technically possible is not for that very reason morally admissible. Rational reflection on the fundamental values of life and of human procreation is, therefore, indispensable for formulating a moral evaluation of such technological interventions on a human being from the first stages of his development.

5. Teachings of the Magisterium

On its part, the magisterium of the Church offers to human reason in this field too the light of Revelation: the doctrine concerning man taught by the magisterium contains many elements which throw light on the problems being faced here.

From the moment of conception, the life of every human being is to be respected in an absolute way because man is the only creature on earth that God has "wished for himself"[16] and the spiritual soul of each man is "immediately created" by God[17]; his whole being bears the image of the Creator. Human life is sacred because from its beginning it involves "the creative action of God"[18] and it remains forever in a special relationship with the Creator, who is its sole end.[19] God alone is the Lord of life from its beginning until its end: no one can, in any circumstance, claim for himself the right directly to destroy an innocent human being.[20]

Human procreation requires on the part of the spouses responsible collaboration with the fruitful love of God[21]; the gift of human life must be actualized in marriage through the specific and exclusive acts of husband and wife, in accordance with the laws inscribed in their persons and in their union.[22]

I. Respect for Human Embryos

Careful reflection on this teaching of the magisterium and on the evidence of reason, as mentioned above, enables us to respond to the numerous moral problems posed by technical interventions upon the human being in the first phases of his life and upon the processes of his conception.

1. What Respect Is Due to the Human Embryo, Taking into Account His Nature and Identity?

The human being must be respected as a person—from the very first instant of his existence.

The implementation of procedures of artificial fertilization has made possible various interventions upon embryos and human fetuses. The aims pursued are of various kinds: diagnostic and therapeutic, scientific and commercial. From all of this serious problems arise. Can one speak of a right to experimentation upon human embryos for the purpose of scientific research? What norms or laws should be worked out with regard to this matter? The response to these problems presupposes a detailed reflection on the nature and specific identity—the word "status" is used—of the human embryo itself.

At the Second Vatican Council, the Church for her part presented once again to modern man her constant and certain doctrine according to which: "Life, once conceived, must be protected with the utmost care; abortion and infanticide are abominable crimes."[23] More recently, the Charter of the Rights of the Family, published by the Holy See, confirmed that "Human life must be absolutely respected and protected from the moment of conception."[24]

This congregation is aware of the current debates concerning the beginning of human life, concerning the individuality of the human being and concerning the identity of the human person. The congregation recalls the teachings found in the *Declaration on Procured Abortion*: "From the time that the ovum is fertilized, a new life is begun which is neither that of the father nor of the mother; it is rather the life of a new human being with his own growth. It would never be made human if it were not human already. To this perpetual evidence ... modern genetic science brings valuable confirmation. It has demonstrated that, from the first instant, the program is fixed as to what this living being will be: a man, this individual man with his characteristic aspects already well-determined. Right from fertilization is begun the adventure of a human life, and each of its great capacities requires time ... to find its place and to be in a position to act."[25] This teaching remains valid and is further confirmed, if confirmation were needed, by recent findings of human biological science which recognize that in the zygote * resulting from fertilization the biological identity of a new human individual is already constituted.

Certainly no experimental datum can be in itself sufficient to bring us to the recognition of a spiritual soul; nevertheless, the conclusions of science regarding the human embryo provide a valuable indication for discerning by the use of reason a personal presence at the moment of this first appearance of a human life: how could a human individual not be a human person? The magisterium has not expressly committed itself to an affirmation of a philosophical nature, but it constantly reaffirms the moral condemnation of any kind of procured abortion. This teaching has not been changed and is unchangeable.[26]

Thus the fruit of human generation, from the first moment of its existence, that is to say from the moment the zygote has formed, demands the unconditional respect that is morally due to the human being in his bodily and spiritual totality. The human being is to be respected and treated as a person from the moment of conception; and therefore from that same moment his rights as a person must be recognized, among which in the first place is the inviolable right of every innocent human being to life.

This doctrinal reminder provides the fundamental criterion for the solution of the various problems posed by the development of the biomedical sciences in this field: since the embryo must be treated as a person, it must also be defended in its integrity, tended, and cared for, to the extent possible, in the same way as any other human being as far as medical assistance is concerned.

2. Is Prenatal Diagnosis Morally Licit?

If prenatal diagnosis respects the life and integrity of the embryo and the human fetus and is directed towards its safeguarding or healing as an individual, then the answer is affirmative.

For prenatal diagnosis makes it possible to know the condition of the embryo and of the fetus when still in the mother's womb. It permits, or makes it possible to anticipate earlier and more effectively, certain therapeutic, medical, or surgical procedures.

Such diagnosis is permissible, with the consent of the parents after they have been adequately informed, if the methods employed safeguard the life and integrity of the embryo and the mother, without subjecting them to disproportionate risks.[27] But this diagnosis is gravely opposed to the moral law when it is done with the thought of possibly inducing an abortion, depending upon the results: a diagnosis which shows the existence of a malformation or a hereditary illness must not be the equivalent of a death-sentence. Thus a woman would be committing a gravely illicit act if she were to request such a diagnosis with the deliberate intention of having an abortion should the results confirm the existence of a malformation or abnormality. The spouse or relatives or anyone else would similarly be acting in a manner contrary to the moral law if they were to counsel or impose such a diagnostic procedure on the expectant mother with the same intention of possibly proceeding to an abortion. So too the specialist would be guilty of illicit collaboration if, in conducting the diagnosis and in communicating its results, he were deliberately to contribute to establishing or favoring a link between prenatal diagnosis and abortion.

In conclusion, any directive or program of the civil and health authorities or of scientific organizations which in any way were to favor a link between prenatal diagnosis and abortion, or which were to go as far as directly to induce expectant mothers to submit to prenatal diagnosis planned for the purpose of eliminating fetuses which are affected by malformations or which are carriers of hereditary illness, is to be condemned as a violation of the unborn child's right to life and as an abuse of the prior rights and duties of the spouses.

3. Are Therapeutic Procedures Carried Out on the Human Embryo Licit?

As with all medical interventions on patients, *one must uphold as licit procedures carried out on the human embryo which respect the life and integrity of the embryo and do not involve disproportionate risks for it but are directed towards its healing, the improvement of its condition of health, or its individual survival.* Whatever the type of medical, surgical, or other therapy, the free and informed consent of the parents is required, according to the deontological rules followed in the case of children. The application of this moral principle may call for delicate and particular precautions in the case of embryonic or fetal life.

The legitimacy and criteria of such procedures have been clearly stated by Pope John Paul II: "A strictly therapeutic intervention whose explicit objective is the healing of various maladies such as those stemming from chromosomal defects will, in principle, be considered desirable, provided it

---

* The zygote is the cell produced when the nuclei of the two gametes have fused.

is directed to the true promotion of the personal well-being of the individual without doing harm to his integrity or worsening his conditions of life. Such an intervention would indeed fall within the logic of the Christian moral tradition." [28]

4. How Is One Morally To Evaluate Research and Experimentation * on Human Embryos and Fetuses?

Medical research must refrain from operations on live embryos, unless there is a moral certainty of not causing harm to the life or integrity of the unborn child and the mother, and on condition that the parents have given their free and informed consent to the procedure. It follows that all research, even when limited to the simple observation of the embryo, would become illicit were it to involve risk to the embryo's physical integrity or life by reason of the methods used or the effects induced.

As regards experimentation, and presupposing the general distinction between experimentation for purposes which are not directly therapeutic and experimentation which is clearly therapeutic for the subject himself, in the case in point one must also distinguish between experimentation carried out on embryos which are still alive and experimentation carried out on embryos which are dead. *If the embryos are living, whether viable or not, they must be respected just like any other human person; experimentation on embryos which is not directly therapeutic is illicit.*[29]

No objective, even though noble in itself, such as a foreseeable advantage to science, to other human beings or to society, can in any way justify experimentation on living human embryos or fetuses, whether viable or not, either inside or outside the mother's womb. The informed consent ordinarily required for clinical experimentation on adults cannot be granted by the parents, who may not freely dispose of the physical integrity or life of the unborn child. Moreover, experimentation on embryos and fetuses always involves risk, and indeed in most cases it involves the certain expectation of harm to their physical integrity or even their death.

To use human embryos or fetuses as the object or instrument of experimentation constitutes a crime against their

---

* Since the terms "research" and "experimentation" are often used equivalently and ambiguously, it is deemed necessary to specify the exact meaning given them in this document.

1) By *research* is meant any inductive-deductive process which aims at promoting the systematic observation of a given phenomenon in the human field or at verifying a hypothesis arising from previous observations.

2) By *experimentation* is meant any research in which the human being (in the various stages of his existence: embryo, fetus, child or adult) represents the object through which or upon which one intends to verify the effect, at present unknown or not sufficiently known, of a given treatment (e.g., pharmacological, teratogenic, surgical, etc.).

dignity as human beings having a right to the same respect that is due to the child already born and to every human person.

The *Charter of the Rights of the Family* published by the Holy See affirms: "Respect for the dignity of the human being excludes all experimental manipulation or exploitation of the human embryo." [30] The practice of keeping human embryos alive *in vivo* or *in vitro* for experimental or commercial purposes is totally opposed to human dignity.

In the case of experimentation that is clearly therapeutic, namely, when it is a matter of experimental forms of therapy used for the benefit of the embryo itself in a final attempt to save its life, and in the absence of other reliable forms of therapy, recourse to drugs or procedures not yet fully tested can be licit.[31]

The corpses of human embryos and fetuses, whether they have been deliberately aborted or not, must be respected just as the remains of other human beings. In particular, they cannot be subjected to mutilation or to autopsies if their death has not yet been verified and without the consent of the parents or of the mother. Furthermore, the moral requirements must be safeguarded, that there be no complicity in deliberate abortion and that the risk of scandal be avoided. Also, in the case of dead fetuses, as for the corpses of adult persons, all commercial trafficking must be considered illicit and should be prohibited.

5. How Is One Morally To Evaluate the Use for Research Purposes of Embryos Obtained by Fertilization in Vitro?

Human embryos obtained in vitro are human beings and subjects with rights: their dignity and right to life must be respected from the first moment of their existence. *It is immoral to produce human embryos destined to be exploited as disposable "biological material."*

In the usual practice of in vitro fertilization, not all of the embryos are transferred to the woman's body; some are destroyed. Just as the Church condemns induced abortion, so she also forbids acts against the life of these human beings. *It is a duty to condemn the particular gravity of the voluntary destruction of human embryos obtained in vitro for the sole purpose of research, either by means of artificial insemination or by means of "twin fission." By acting in this way the researcher usurps the place of God; and, even though he may be unaware of this, he sets himself up as the master of the destiny of others inasmuch as he arbitrarily chooses whom he will allow to live and whom he will send to death, and kills defenseless human beings.*

Methods of observation or experimentation which damage or impose grave and disproportionate risks upon embryos obtained in vitro are morally illicit for the same reasons. Every human being is to be respected for himself, and cannot be reduced in worth to a pure and simple instrument for the advantage of others. *It is therefore not in conformity with the moral law deliberately to expose to death human embryos obtained "in vitro."* In consequence of the fact that they have been produced in vitro, those embryos which are not transferred into the body of the mother and are called "spare" are exposed to an absurd fate, with no possibility of their being offered safe means of survival which can be licitly pursued.

6. What Judgment Should Be Made on Other Procedures of Manipulating Embryos Connected with the "Techniques of Human Reproduction"?

Techniques of fertilization in vitro can open the way to other forms of biological and genetic manipulation of human embryos, such as attempts or plans for fertilization between human and animal gametes and the gestation of human embryos in the uterus of animals, or the hypothesis or project of constructing artificial uteruses for the human embryo. *These procedures are contrary to the human dignity proper to the embryo, and at the same time they are contrary to the right of every person to be conceived and to be born within marriage and from marriage.*[32] *Also, attempts or hypotheses for obtaining a human being without any connection with sexuality through "twin fission," cloning or parthenogenesis are to be considered contrary to the moral law, since they are in opposition to the dignity both of human procreation and of the conjugal union.*

The freezing of embryos, even when carried out in order to preserve the life of an embryo—cryopreservation—*constitutes an offense against the respect due to human beings* by exposing them to grave risks of death or harm to their physical integrity, and depriving them, at least temporarily, of maternal shelter and gestation, thus placing them in a situation in which further offenses and manipulation are possible.

Certain attempts to influence chromosomic or genetic inheritance are not therapeutic but are aimed at producing human beings selected according to sex or other predetermined qualities. These manipulations are contrary to the personal dignity of the human being and his or her integrity and identity. Therefore, in no way can they be justified on the grounds of possible beneficial consequences for future humanity.[33] Every person must be respected for himself: in this consists the dignity and right of every human being from his or her beginning.

II. Interventions Upon Human Procreation

By "artificial procreation" or "artificial fertilization" are understood here the different technical procedures directed towards obtaining a human conception in a manner other than the sexual union of man and woman. This instruction deals with fertilization of an ovum in a test tube (in vitro fertilization) and artificial insemination through transfer into the woman's genital tracts of previously collected sperm.

A preliminary point for the moral evaluation of such technical procedures is constituted by the consideration of the circumstances and consequences which those procedures involve in relation to the respect due the human embryo. Development of the practice of in vitro fertilization has required innumerable fertilizations and destructions of human embryos. Even today, the usual practice presupposes a hyper-ovulation on the part of the woman: a number of ova are withdrawn, fertilized, and then cultivated in vitro for some days. Usually not all are transferred into the genital tracts of the woman; some embryos, generally called "spare," are destroyed or frozen. On occasion, some of the implanted embryos are sacrificed for various eugenic, economic, or psychological reasons. Such deliberate destruction of human beings or their utilization for different purposes to the detriment of their integrity and life is contrary to the doctrine on procured abortion already recalled.

The connection between in vitro fertilization and the voluntary destruction of human embryos occurs too often. This is significant: through these procedures, with apparently contrary purposes, life and death are subjected to the decision of man, who thus sets himself up as the giver of life and death by decree. This dynamic of violence and domination may remain unnoticed by those very individuals who, in wishing to utilize this procedure, become subject to it themselves. The facts recorded and the cold logic which links them must be taken into consideration for a moral judgment on IVF and ET (in vitro fertilization and embryo transfer): the abortion mentality which has made this procedure possible thus leads, whether one wants it or not, to man's domination over the life and death of his fellow human beings and can lead to a system of radical eugenics.

Nevertheless, such abuses do not exempt one from a further and thorough ethical study of the techniques of artificial procreation considered in themselves, abstracting as far as possible from the destruction of embryos produced in vitro.

The present instruction will therefore take into consideration in the first place the problems posed by heterologous artificial fertilization (II, nn. 1–3),* and subsequently those linked with

---

* By the term *heterologous artificial fertilization or procreation*, the Instruction means techniques used to obtain a human conception artificially by the use of gametes coming from at least one donor other than the spouses who are joined in marriage. Such techniques can be of two types

a) *Heterologous IVF and ET*: the technique used to obtain a human conception through the meeting in vitro of gametes taken from at least one donor other than the two spouses joined in marriage.

b) *Heterologous artificial insemination*: the technique used to obtain a human conception through the transfer into the genital tracts of the woman of the sperm previously collected from a donor other than the husband.

homologous artificial fertilization (II, nn. 4–6).* Before formulating an ethical judgment on each of these procedures, the principles and values which determine the moral evaluation of each of them will be considered.

A. Heterologous Artificial Fertilization

1. Why Must Human Procreation Take Place in Marriage?

Every human being is always to be accepted as a gift and blessing of God. However, from the moral point of view a truly responsible procreation vis-à-vis the unborn child must be the fruit of marriage.

For human procreation has specific characteristics by virtue of the personal dignity of the parents and of the children: the procreation of a new person, whereby the man and the woman collaborate with the power of the Creator, must be the fruit and the sign of the mutual self-giving of the spouses, of their love, and of their fidelity.[34] The fidelity of the spouses in the unity of marriage involves reciprocal respect of their right to become a father and a mother only through each other.

The child has the right to be conceived, carried in the womb, brought into the world, and brought up within marriage: it is through the secure and recognized relationship to his own parents that the child can discover his own identity and achieve his own proper human development.

The parents find in their child a confirmation and completion of their reciprocal self-giving: the child is the living image of their love, the permanent sign of their conjugal union, the living and indissoluble concrete expression of their paternity and maternity.[35]

By reason of the vocation and social responsibilities of the person, the good of the children and of the parents contributes to the good of civil society; the vitality and stability of society require that children come into the world within a family and that the family be firmly based on marriage.

---

*By *artificial homologous fertilization or procreation*, the Instruction means the technique used to obtain a human conception using the gametes of the two spouses joined in marriage. Homologous artificial fertilization can be carried out by two different methods:

a) *Homologous IVF and ET*: the technique used to obtain a human conception through the meeting in vitro of the gametes of the spouses joined in marriage.

b) *Homologous artificial insemination*: the technique used to obtain a human conception through the transfer into the genital tracts of a married woman of the sperm previously collected from her husband.

The tradition of the Church and anthropological reflection recognize in marriage and in its indissoluble unity the only setting worthy of truly responsible procreation.

2. Does Heterologous Artificial Fertilization Conform to the Dignity of the Couple and to the Truth of Marriage?

Through IVF and ET and heterologous artificial insemination, human conception is achieved through the fusion of gametes of at least one donor other than the spouses who are united in marriage. *Heterologous artificial fertilization is contrary to the unity of marriage, to the dignity of the spouses, to the vocation proper to parents, and to the child's right to be conceived and brought into the world in marriage and from marriage.*[36]

Respect for the unity of marriage and for conjugal fidelity demands that the child be conceived in marriage; the bond existing between husband and wife accords the spouses, in an objective and inalienable manner, the exclusive right to become father and mother solely through each other.[37] Recourse to the gametes of a third person, in order to have sperm or ovum available, constitutes a violation of the reciprocal commitment of the spouses and a grave lack in regard to that essential property of marriage which is its unity.

Heterologous artificial fertilization violates the rights of the child; it deprives him of his filial relationship with his parental origins and can hinder the maturing of his personal identity. Furthermore, it offends the common vocation of the spouses who are called to fatherhood and motherhood: it objectively deprives conjugal fruitfulness of its unity and integrity; it brings about and manifests a rupture between genetic parenthood, gestational parenthood, and responsibility for upbringing. Such damage to the personal relationships within the family has repercussions on civil society: what threatens the unity and stability of the family is a source of dissension, disorder, and injustice in the whole of social life.

These reasons lead to a negative moral judgment concerning heterologous artificial fertilization: consequently fertilization of a married woman with the sperm of a donor different from her husband and fertilization with the husband's sperm of an ovum not coming from his wife are morally illicit. Furthermore, the artificial fertilization of a woman who is unmarried or a widow, whoever the donor may be, cannot be morally justified.

The desire to have a child and the love between spouses who long to obviate a sterility which cannot be overcome in any other way constitute understandable motivations; but subjectively good intentions do not render heterologous artificial fertilization conformable to the objective and inalienable properties of marriage or respectful of the rights of the child and of the spouses.

3. Is "Surrogate" * Motherhood Morally Licit?

No, for the same reasons which lead one to reject heterologous artificial fertilization: for it is contrary to the unity of marriage and to the dignity of the procreation of the human person.

Surrogate motherhood represents an objective failure to meet the obligations of maternal love, of conjugal fidelity, and of responsible motherhood; it offends the dignity and the right of the child to be conceived, carried in the womb, brought into the world and brought up by his own parents; it sets up, to the detriment of families, a division between the physical, psychological, and moral elements which constitute those families.

B. Homologous Artificial Fertilization

Since heterologous artificial fertilization has been declared unacceptable, the question arises of how to evaluate morally the process of homologous artificial fertilization: IVF and ET and artificial insemination between husband and wife. First a question of principle must be clarified.

4. From the Moral Point of View What Connection Is Required Between Procreation and the Conjugal Act?

a) The Church's teaching on marriage and human procreation affirms the "inseparable connection, willed by God and unable to be broken by man on his own initiative, between the two meanings of the conjugal act: the unitive meaning and the procreative meaning. Indeed, by its intimate structure, the conjugal act, while most closely uniting husband and wife, makes them capable of the generation of new lives, according to laws inscribed in the very being of man and of woman."[38] This principle, which is based upon the nature of marriage and the intimate connection of the goods of marriage, has well-known consequences on the level of responsible fatherhood and motherhood. "By safeguarding both these essential aspects, the unitive and the procreative, the conjugal act preserves in its fullness the sense of true mutual love and its ordination toward man's exalted vocation to parenthood.[39]

---

* By "surrogate mother" the instruction means:

a) the woman who carries in pregnancy an embryo implanted in her uterus and who is genetically a stranger to the embryo because it has been obtained through the union of the gametes of "donors." She carries the pregnancy with a pledge to surrender the baby once it is born to the party who commissioned or made the agreement for the pregnancy.

b) the woman who carries in pregnancy an embryo to whose procreation she has contributed the donation of her own ovum, fertilized through insemination with the sperm of a man other than her husband. She carries the pregnancy with a pledge to surrender the child once it is born to the party who commissioned or made the agreement for the pregnancy.

The same doctrine concerning the link between the meanings of the conjugal act and between the goods of marriage throws light on the moral problem of homologous artificial fertilization, since "it is never permitted to separate these different aspects to such a degree as positively to exclude either the procreative intention or the conjugal relation."[40]

Contraception deliberately deprives the conjugal act of its openness to procreation and in this way brings about a voluntary dissociation of the ends of marriage. Homologous artificial fertilization, in seeking a procreation which is not the fruit of a specific act of conjugal union, objectively effects an analogous separation between the goods and the meanings of marriage.

Thus, *fertilization is licitly sought when it is the result of a "conjugal act which is per se suitable for the generation of children to which marriage is ordered by its nature and by which the spouses become one flesh."[41] But from the moral point of view procreation is deprived of its proper perfection when it is not desired as the fruit of the conjugal act, that is to say of the specific act of the spouses' union.*

b) The moral value of the intimate link between the goods of marriage and between the meanings of the conjugal act is based upon the unity of the human being, a unity involving body and spiritual soul.[42] Spouses mutually express their personal love in the "language of the body," which clearly involves both "spousal meanings" and parental ones.[43] The conjugal act by which the couple mutually express their self-gift at the same time expresses openness to the gift of life. It is an act that is inseparably corporal and spiritual. It is in their bodies and through their bodies that the spouses consummate their marriage and are able to become father and mother. In order to respect the language of their bodies and their natural generosity, the conjugal union must take place with respect for its openness to procreation; and the procreation of a person must be the fruit and the result of married love. The origin of the human being thus follows from a procreation that is "linked to the union, not only biological but also spiritual, of the parents, made one by the bond of marriage."[44] Fertilization achieved outside the bodies of the couple remains by this very fact deprived of the meanings and the values which are expressed in the language of the body and in the union of human persons.

c) Only respect for the link between the meanings of the conjugal act and respect for the unity of the human being make possible procreation in conformity with the dignity of the person. In his unique and unrepeatable origin, the child must be respected and recognized as equal in personal dignity to those who give him life. The human person must be accepted in his parents' act of union and love; the generation of a child must therefore be the fruit of that mutual giving[45] which is realized in the conjugal act wherein the spouses cooperate as servants and not as masters in the work of the Creator who is Love.[46]

In reality, the origin of a human person is the result of an act of giving. The one conceived must be the fruit of his parents' love. He cannot be desired or conceived as the product of an intervention of medical or biological techniques; that would be equivalent to reducing him to an object of scientific technology. No one may subject the coming of a child into the world to conditions of technical efficiency which are to be evaluated according to standards of control and dominion.

The moral relevance of the link between the meanings of the conjugal act and between the goods of marriage, as well as the unity of the human being and the dignity of his origin, demand that the procreation of a human person be brought about as the fruit of the conjugal act specific to the love between spouses. The link between procreation and the conjugal act is thus shown to be of great importance on the anthropological and moral planes, and it throws light on the positions of the magisterium with regard to homologous artificial fertilization.

5. Is Homologous in Vitro Fertilization Morally Licit?

The answer to this question is strictly dependent on the principles just mentioned. Certainly one cannot ignore the legitimate aspirations of sterile couples. For some, recourse to homologous IVF and ET appears to be the only way of fulfilling their sincere desire for a child. The question is asked whether the totality of conjugal life in such situations is not sufficient to ensure the dignity proper to human procreation. It is acknowledged that IVF and ET certainly cannot supply for the absence of sexual relations[47] and cannot be preferred to the specific acts of conjugal union, given the risks involved for the child and the difficulties of the procedure. But it is asked whether, when there is no other way of overcoming the sterility which is a source of suffering, homologous in vitro fertilization may not constitute an aid, if not a form of therapy, whereby its moral licitness could be admitted.

The desire for a child—or at the very least an openness to the transmission of life—is a necessary prerequisite from the moral point of view for responsible human procreation. But this good intention is not sufficient for making a positive moral evaluation of in vitro fertilization between spouses. The process of IVF and ET must be judged in itself and cannot borrow its definitive moral quality from the totality of conjugal life of which it becomes part nor from the conjugal acts which may precede or follow it.[48]

It has already been recalled that, in the circumstances in which it is regularly practiced, IVF and ET involves the destruction of human beings, which is something contrary to the doctrine on the illicitness of abortion previously mentioned.[49] But even in a situation in which every precaution were taken to avoid the death of human embryos, homologous IVF and ET dissociates from the conjugal act the actions which are directed to human fertilization. For this reason the very nature of homologous IVF and ET also must be taken into account, even abstracting from the link with procured abortion.

Homologous IVF and ET is brought about outside the bodies of the couple through actions of third parties whose competence and technical activity determine the success of the procedure. Such fertilization entrusts the life and identity of the embryo into the power of doctors and biologists and establishes the domination of technology over the origin and destiny of the human person. Such a relationship of domination is in itself contrary to the dignity and equality that must be common to parents and children.

Conception in vitro is the result of the technical action which presides over fertilization. *Such fertilization is neither in fact achieved nor positively willed as the expression and fruit of a specific act of the conjugal union. In homologous IVF and ET, therefore, even if it is considered in the context of de facto existing sexual relations, the generation of the human person is objectively deprived of its proper perfection: namely, that of being the result and fruit of a conjugal act* in which the spouses can become "cooperators with God for giving life to a new person."[50]

These reasons enable us to understand why the act of conjugal love is considered in the teaching of the Church as the only setting worthy of human procreation. For the same reasons the so-called "simple case," i.e., a homologous IVF and ET procedure that is free of any compromise with the abortive practice of destroying embryos and with masturbation, remains a technique which is morally illicit because it deprives human procreation of the dignity which is proper and connatural to it.

Certainly, homologous IVF and ET fertilization is not marked by all that ethical negativity found in extra-conjugal procreation; the family and marriage continue to constitute the setting for the birth and upbringing of the children. Nevertheless, in conformity with the traditional doctrine relating to the goods of marriage and the dignity of the person, *the Church remains opposed from the moral point of view to homologous in vitro fertilization. Such fertilization is in itself illicit and in opposition to the dignity of procreation and of the conjugal union, even when everything is done to avoid the death of the human embryo.*

Although the manner in which human conception is achieved with IVF and ET cannot be approved, every child which comes into the world must in any case be accepted as a living gift of the divine Goodness and must be brought up with love.

6. How Is Homologous Artificial Insemination to Be Evaluated from the Moral Point of View?

Homologous artificial insemination within marriage cannot be admitted except for those cases in which the technical means is not a substitute for the conjugal act but serves to facilitate and to help so that the act attains its natural purpose.

The teaching of the magisterium on this point has

already been stated.[51] This teaching is not just an expression of particular historical circumstances but is based on the Church's doctrine concerning the connection between the conjugal union and procreation and on a consideration of the personal nature of the conjugal act and of human procreation. "In its natural structure, the conjugal act is a personal action, a simultaneous and immediate cooperation on the part of the husband and wife, which by the very nature of the agents and the proper nature of the act is the expression of the mutual gift which, according to the words of Scripture, brings about union 'in one flesh.'"[52] Thus moral conscience "does not necessarily proscribe the use of certain artificial means destined solely either to the facilitating of the natural act or to ensuring that the natural act normally performed achieves its proper end."[53] If the technical means facilitates the conjugal act or helps it to reach its natural objectives, it can be morally acceptable. If, on the other hand, the procedure were to replace the conjugal act, it is morally illicit.

Artificial insemination as a substitute for the conjugal act is prohibited by reason of the voluntarily achieved dissociation of the two meanings of the conjugal act. Masturbation, through which the sperm is normally obtained, is another sign of this dissociation: even when it is done for the purpose of procreation, the act remains deprived of its unitive meaning: "It lacks the sexual relationship called for by the moral order, namely the relationship which realizes 'the full sense of mutual self-giving and human procreation in the context of true love.'"[54]

7. What Moral Criterion Can Be Proposed with regard to Medical Intervention in Human Procreation?

The medical act must be evaluated not only with reference to its technical dimension but also and above all in relation to its goal, which is the good of persons and their bodily and psychological health. The moral criteria for medical intervention in procreation are deduced from the dignity of human persons, of their sexuality, and of their origin.

Medicine which seeks to be ordered to the integral good of the person must respect the specifically human values of sexuality.[55] *The doctor is at the service of persons and of human procreation. He does not have the authority to dispose of them or to decide their fate.* "A medical intervention respects the dignity of persons when it seeks to assist the conjugal act either in order to facilitate its performance or in order to enable it to achieve its objective once it has been normally performed."[56]

On the other hand, it sometimes happens that a medical procedure technologically replaces the conjugal act in order to obtain a procreation which is neither its result nor its fruit. In this case the medical act is not, as it should be, at the service of conjugal union but rather appropriates to itself the procreative function and thus contradicts the dignity and the inalienable rights of the spouses and of the child to be born.

The humanization of medicine, which is insisted upon today by everyone, requires respect for the integral dignity of the human person first of all in the act and at the moment in which the spouses transmit life to a new person. It is only logical therefore to address an urgent appeal to Catholic doctors and scientists that they bear exemplary witness to the respect due to the human embryo and to the dignity of procreation. The medical and nursing staff of Catholic hospitals and clinics are in a special way urged to do justice to the moral obligations which they have assumed, frequently also as part of their contract. Those who are in charge of Catholic hospitals and clinics and who are often religious will take special care to safeguard and promote a diligent observance of the moral norms recalled in the present instruction.

8. The Suffering Caused by Infertility in Marriage

The suffering of spouses who cannot have children or who are afraid of bringing a handicapped child into the world is a suffering that everyone must understand and properly evaluate.

On the part of the spouses, the desire for a child is natural: it expresses the vocation to fatherhood and motherhood inscribed in conjugal love. This desire can be even stronger if the couple is affected by sterility which appears incurable. Nevertheless, marriage does not confer upon the spouses the right to have a child, but only the right to perform those natural acts which are per se ordered to procreation.[57]

A true and proper right to a child would be contrary to the child's dignity and nature. The child is not an object to which one has a right, nor can he be considered as an object of ownership: rather, a child is a gift, "the supreme gift"[58] *and the most gratuitous gift of marriage, and is a living testimony of the mutual giving of his parents. For this reason, the child has the right, as already mentioned, to be the fruit of the specific act of the conjugal love of his parents; and he also has the right to be respected as a person from the moment of his conception.*

Nevertheless, whatever its cause or prognosis, sterility is certainly a difficult trial. The community of believers is called to shed light upon and support the suffering of those who are unable to fulfill their legitimate aspiration to motherhood and fatherhood. Spouses who find themselves in this sad situation are called to find in it an opportunity for sharing in a particular way in the Lord's cross, the source of spiritual fruitfulness. Sterile couples must not forget that "even when procreation is not possible, conjugal life does not for this reason lose its value. Physical sterility in fact can be for spouses the occasion for other important services in the life of the human person, for example, adoption, various forms of educational work, and assistance to other families and to poor or handicapped children."[59]

Many researchers are engaged in the fight against sterility. While fully safeguarding the dignity of human procreation some have achieved results which previously seemed unattainable. Scientists therefore are to be encouraged to continue their research with the aim of preventing the causes of sterility and of being able to remedy them so that sterile couples will be able to procreate in full respect for their own personal dignity and that of the child to be born.

III. Moral and Civil Law

The Values and Moral Obligations That Civil Legislation Must Respect and Sanction in this Matter

The inviolable right to life of every innocent human individual and the rights of the family and of the institution of marriage constitute fundamental moral values, because they concern the natural condition and integral vocation of the human person; at the same time they are constitutive elements of civil society and its order.

For this reason the new technological possibilities which have opened up in the field of biomedicine require the intervention of the political authorities and of the legislator, since an uncontrolled application of such techniques could lead to unforeseeable and damaging consequences for civil society. Recourse to the conscience of each individual and to the self-regulation of researchers cannot be sufficient for ensuring respect for personal rights and public order. If the legislator responsible for the common good were not watchful, he could be deprived of his prerogatives by researchers claiming to govern humanity in the name of the biological discoveries and the alleged "improvement" processes which they would draw from those discoveries. "Eugenism" and forms of discrimination between human beings could come to be legitimized: this would constitute an act of violence and a serious offense to the equality, dignity, and fundamental rights of the human person.

The intervention of the public authority must be inspired by the rational principles which regulate the relationships between civil law and moral law. The task of the civil law is to ensure the common good of people through the recognition of and the defense of fundamental rights and through the promotion of peace and of public morality.[60] In no sphere of life can the civil law take the place of conscience or dictate norms concerning things which are outside its competence. It must sometimes tolerate, for the sake of public order, things which it cannot forbid without a greater evil resulting. However, the inalienable rights of the person must be recognized and respected by civil society and the political authority. These human rights depend neither on single individuals nor on parents; nor do they represent a concession made by society and the state: they pertain to human nature and are inherent in the person by virtue of the creative act from which the person took his or her origin.

Among such fundamental rights one should mention in this regard: a) every human being's right to life and physical integrity from the moment of conception until death; b) the rights of the family and of marriage as an institution and, in this area, the child's right to be conceived, brought into the world, and brought up by his parents. To each of these two themes it is necessary here to give some further consideration.

In various states certain laws have authorized the direct suppression of innocents: the moment a positive law deprives a category of human beings of the protection which civil legislation must accord them, the state is denying the equality of all before the law. When the state does not place its power at the service of the rights of each citizen, and in particular of the more vulnerable, the very foundations of a state based on law are undermined. The political authority consequently cannot give approval to the calling of human beings into existence through procedures which would expose them to those very grave risks noted previously. The possible recognition by positive law and the political authorities of techniques of artificial transmission of life and the experimentation connected with it would widen the breach already opened by the legalization of abortion.

As a consequence of the respect and protection which must be ensured for the unborn child from the moment of his conception, the law must provide appropriate penal sanctions for every deliberate violation of the child's rights. The law cannot tolerate—indeed it must expressly forbid—that human beings, even at the embryonic stage, should be treated as objects of experimentation, be mutilated or destroyed with the excuse that they are superfluous or incapable of developing normally.

The political authority is bound to guarantee to the institution of the family, upon which society is based, the juridical protection to which it has a right. From the very fact that it is at the service of people, the political authority must also be at the service of the family. Civil law cannot grant approval to techniques of artificial procreation which, for the benefit of third parties (doctors, biologists, economic or governmental powers), take away what is a right inherent in the relationship between spouses; and, therefore, civil law cannot legalize the donation of gametes between persons who are not legitimately united in marriage.

Legislation must also prohibit, by virtue of the support which is due to the family, embryo banks, post-mortem insemination and "surrogate motherhood."

It is part of the duty of the public authority to ensure that the civil law is regulated according to the fundamental norms of the moral law in matters concerning human rights, human life, and the institution of the family. Politicians must commit themselves, through their interventions upon public opinion, to securing in society the widest possible consensus on such essential points and to consolidating this consensus wherever it risks being weakened or is in danger of collapse.

In many countries, the legalization of abortion and juridical tolerance of unmarried couples makes it more difficult to secure respect for the fundamental rights recalled by this instruction. It is to be hoped that states will not become responsible for aggravating these socially damaging situations of injustice. It is rather to be hoped that nations and states will realize all the cultural, ideological, and political implications connected with the techniques of artificial procreation and will find the wisdom and courage necessary for issuing laws which are more just and more respectful of human life and the institution of the family.

The civil legislation of many states confers an undue legitimation upon certain practices in the eyes of many today; it is seen to be incapable of guaranteeing that morality which is in conformity with the natural exigencies of the human person and with the "unwritten laws" etched by the Creator upon the human heart. All men of good will must commit themselves, particularly within their professional field and in the exercise of their civil rights, to ensuring the reform of morally unacceptable civil laws and the correction of illicit practices. In addition, "conscientious objection" vis-à-vis such laws must be supported and recognized. A movement of passive resistance to the legitimation of practices contrary to human life and dignity is beginning to make an ever sharper impression upon the moral conscience of many, especially among specialists in the biomedical sciences.

Conclusion

The spread of technologies of intervention in the processes of human procreation raises very serious moral problems in relation to the respect due to the human being from the moment of conception, to the dignity of the person, of his or her sexuality, and of the transmission of life.

With this instruction the Congregation for the Doctrine of the Faith, in fulfilling its responsibility to promote and defend the Church's teaching in so serious a matter, addresses a new and heartfelt invitation to all those who, by reason of their role and their commitment, can exercise a positive influence and ensure that, in the family and in society, due respect is accorded to life and love. It addresses this invitation to those responsible for the formation of consciences and of public opinion, to scientists and medical professionals, to jurists and politicians. It hopes that all will understand the incompatibility between recognition of the dignity of the human person and contempt for life and love, between faith in the living God and the claim to decide arbitrarily the origin and fate of a human being.

In particular, the Congregation for the Doctrine of the Faith addresses an invitation with confidence and encouragement to theologians, and above all to moralists, that they study more deeply and make ever more accessible to the faithful the contents of the teaching of the Church's magisterium in the light of a valid anthropology in the matter of sexuality and marriage and in the context of the necessary interdisciplinary approach. Thus they will make it possible to understand ever

more clearly the reasons for and the validity of this teaching. By defending man against the excesses of his own power, the Church of God reminds him of the reasons for his true nobility; only in this way can the possibility of living and loving with that dignity and liberty which derive from respect for the truth be ensured for the men and women of tomorrow. The precise indications which are offered in the present instruction, therefore, are not meant to halt the effort of reflection but rather to give it a renewed impulse in unrenounceable fidelity to the teaching of the Church.

In the light of the truth about the gift of human life and in the light of the moral principles which flow from that truth, everyone is invited to act in the area of responsibility proper to each and, like the good Samaritan, to recognize as a neighbor even the littlest among the children of men (cf. Luke 10:29–37). Here Christ's words find a new and particular echo: "What you do to one of the least of my brethren, you do unto me" (Matt. 25:40).

During an audience granted to the undersigned prefect after the plenary session of the Congregation for the Doctrine of the Faith, the supreme pontiff, John Paul II, approved this instruction and ordered it to be published.

Given at Rome, from the
Congregation for the Doctrine of the Faith,
February 22, 1987, the Feast of the Chair of St. Peter,
the Apostle.

Joseph Cardinal Ratzinger
Prefect
Alberto Bovone
Titular Archbishop of Caesarea in Numidia
Secretary

Notes

[1] Pope John Paul II, Discourse to those taking part in the Eighty-first Congress of the Italian Society of Internal Medicine and the Eighty-second Congress of the Italian Society of General Surgery (October 27, 1980), *AAS* 72 (1980): 1126.

[2] Pope Paul VI, Discourse to the General Assembly of the United Nations Organization (October 4, 1965), *AAS* 57 (1965): 878; idem, encyclical *Populorum progressio*, n. 13, *AAS* 59 (1967): 263.

[3] Pope Paul VI, Homily during the Mass closing the Holy Year (December 25, 1975), *AAS* 68 (1976): 145; Pope John Paul II, encyclical *Dives in misericordia*, n. 30, *AAS* 72 (1980): 1224.

[4] Pope John Paul II, Discourse to those taking part in the Thirty-fifth General Assembly of the World Medical Association (October 29, 1983), *AAS* 76 (1984): 390.

[5] Cf. Second Vatican Council, declaration *Dignitatis humanae*, n. 2.

[6] Second Vatican Council, pastoral constitution *Gaudium et spes*, n. 22; Pope John Paul II, encyclical *Redemptor hominis*, n. 8, *AAS* 71 (1979): 270–272.

[7] Cf. Second Vatican Council, *Gaudium et spes*, n. 35.

[8] Second Vatican Council, *Gaudium et spes*, n. 15; cf. also Pope Paul VI, *Populorum progressio*, n. 20, *AAS* 59 (1967): 267; Pope John Paul II, *Redemptor hominis*, n. 15, *AAS* 71 (1979): 286–289; idem, apostolic exhortation *Familiaris consortio*, n. 8, *AAS* 74 (1982): 89.

[9] Pope John Paul II, *Familiaris consortio*, n. 11, *AAS* 74 (1982): 92.

[10] Cf. Pope Paul VI, encyclical *Humanae vitae*, n. 10, *AAS* 60 (1968): 487–488.

[11] Pope John Paul II, Thirty-fifth General Assembly, *AAS* 76 (1984): 393.

[12] Cf. Pope John Paul II, *Familiaris consortio*, n. 11, *AAS* 74 (1982): 91–92; cf also Second Vatican Council, *Gaudium et spes*, n. 50.

[13] Sacred Congregation for the Doctrine of the Faith, *Declaration on Procured Abortion*, n. 9, *AAS* 66 (1974): 736–737.

[14] Pope John Paul II, Thirty-fifth General Assembly, *AAS* 76 (1984): 390.

[15] Pope John XXIII, encyclical *Mater et magistra*, III, *AAS* 53 (1961): 447.

[16] Second Vatican Council, *Gaudium et spes*, n. 24.

[17] Cf. Pope Pius XII, encyclical *Humani generis*, *AAS* 42 (1950): 575; Pope Paul VI, *Professio fidei*, *AAS* 60 (1968): 436.

[18] Pope John XXIII, *Mater et magistra*, III, *AAS* 53 (1961): 447; cf. Pope John Paul II, Discourse to priests participating in a seminar on "Responsible Procreation," (September 17, 1983), *Insegnamenti di Giovanni Paolo II*, VI, 2 (1983): 562: "At the origin of each human person there is a creative act of God: no man comes into existence by chance; he is always the result of the creative love of God."

[19] Cf. Second Vatican Council, *Gaudium et spes*, n. 24.

[20] Cf. Pope Pius XII, Discourse to the Saint Luke Medical-Biological Union (November 12, 1944), *Discorsi e Radiomessaggi* VI (1944–1945), 191–192.

[21] Cf. Second Vatican Council, *Gaudium et spes*, n. 50.

[22] Cf. ibid., n. 51: "When it is a question of harmonizing married love with the responsible transmission of life, the moral character of one's behavior does not depend only on the good intention and the evaluation of the motives: the objective criteria must be used, criteria drawn from the nature of the human person and human acts, criteria which respect the total meaning of mutual self-giving and human procreation in the context of true love."

[23] Ibid.

[24] Holy See, *Charter of the Rights of the Family*, n. 4, *L'Osservatore Romano*, November 25, 1983.

[25] Sacred Congregation for the Doctrine of the Faith, *Declaration on Procured Abortion*, nn. 12–13, *AAS* 66 (1974): 738.

[26] Cf. Pope Paul VI, Discourse to participants in the Twenty-third National Congress of Italian Catholic Jurists (December 9, 1972), *AAS* 64 (1972): 777.

[27] "The obligation to avoid disproportionate risks involves an authentic respect for human beings and the uprightness of therapeutic intentions. It implies that the doctor above all … must carefully evaluate the possible negative consequences which the necessary use of a particular exploratory technique may have upon the unborn child and avoid recourse to diagnostic procedures which do not offer sufficient guarantees of their honest purpose and substantial harmlessness. And if, as often happens in human choices, a degree of risk must be undertaken, he will take care to assure that it is justified by a truly urgent need for the diagnosis and by the importance of the results that can be achieved by it for the benefit of the unborn child himself" (Pope John Paul II, Discourse to Participants in the Pro-life Movement Congress [December 3, 1982], *Insegnamenti di Giovanni Paolo* II, V, 3 [1982], 1512). This clarification concerning "proportionate risk" is also to be kept in mind in the following sections of the present instruction, whenever this term appears.

[28] Pope John Paul II, Thirty-fifth General Assembly, *AAS* 76 (1984): 392.

[29] Cf. Pope John Paul II, Address to a Meeting of the Pontifical Academy of Sciences (October 23, 1982), *AAS* 75 (1983): 37: "I condemn, in the most explicit and formal way, experimental manipulations of the human embryo since the human being, from conception to death, cannot be exploited for any purpose whatsoever."

[30] Holy See, *Charter of the Rights of the Family*, n. 4b.

[31] Cf. Pope John Paul II, Address to the Participants in the Convention of the Pro-Life Movement (December 3, 1982), *Insegnamenti di Giovanni Paolo* II, V, 3 (1982), 1511: "Any form of experimentation on the fetus that may damage its integrity or worsen its condition is unacceptable, except in the case of a final effort to save it from death." Sacred Congregation for the Doctrine of the Faith, *Declaration on Euthanasia*, n. 4, *AAS* 72 (1980): 550: "In the absence of other sufficient remedies, it is permitted, with the patient's consent, to have recourse to the means provided by the most advanced medical techniques, even if these means are still at the experimental stage and are not without a certain risk."

[32] No one, before coming into existence, can claim a subjective right to begin to exist; nevertheless, it is legitimate to affirm the right of the child to have a fully human origin through conception in conformity with the personal nature of the human being. Life is a gift that must be bestowed in a manner worthy both of the subject receiving it and of the subjects transmitting it. This statement is to be borne in mind also for what will be explained concerning artificial human procreation.

[33] Cf. Pope John Paul II, Thirty-fifth General Assembly, *AAS* 76 (1984): 391.

[34] Cf. Second Vatican Council, *Gaudium et spes*, n. 50.

[35] Cf. Pope John Paul II, *Familiaris consortio*, n. 14, *AAS* 74 (1982): 96.

[36] Cf. Pope Pius XII, Discourse to those taking part in the Fourth International Congress of Catholic Doctors, (September 29, 1949), *AAS* 41 (1949): 559. According to the plan of the Creator, "A man leaves his father and his mother and cleaves to his wife, and they become one flesh" (Gen. 2:24). The unity of marriage, bound to the order of creation, is a truth accessible to natural reason. The Church's Tradition and Magisterium

frequently make reference to the book of Genesis, both directly and through the passages of the New Testament that refer to it: Matt. 19:4–6; Mark 10:5–8; Eph. 5:31. Cf. Athenagoras, *Legatio por christianis*, 33, *PG* 6, 965–967; St. Chrysostom, *In Matthaeum homiliae*, LXII, 19, 1, *PG* 58, 597; St. Leo the Great, *Epist. ad Rusticum*, 4, *PL* 54, 1204; Innocent III, *Epist. Gaudemus in Domino*, DS 778; Council of Lyons II, IV Session, DS 860; Council of Trent, XXIV Session, DS 1798, 1802; Pope Leo XIII, encyclical *Arcanum divinae sapientiae*, *AAS* 12 (1879–1880): 388–391; Pope Pius XI, *Casti connubii*, *AAS* 22 (1930): 546–547; Second Vatican Council, *Gaudium et spes*, n. 48; Pope John Paul II, *Familiaris consortio*, n. 19, *AAS* 74 (1982): 101–102; Code of Canon Law, can. 1056.

[37] Cf. Pope Pius XII, Fourth International Congress, *AAS* 41 (1949): 560; Discourse to those taking part in the Congress of the Italian Catholic Union of Midwives (October 29, 1951), *AAS* 43 (1951): 850; Code of Canon Law, can. 1134.

[38] Pope Paul VI, *Humanae vitae*, n. 12, *AAS* 60 (1968): 488–489.

[39] Ibid.

[40] Pope Pius XII, Discourse to those taking part in the Second Naples World Congress on Fertility and Human Sterility (May 19, 1956), *AAS* 48 (1956), 470.

[41] Code of Canon Law, can. 1061. According to this canon, the conjugal act is that by which the marriage is consummated if the couple "have performed (it) between themselves in a human manner."

[42] Cf. Second Vatican Council, *Gaudium et spes*, n. 14.

[43] Cf. Pope John Paul II, General Audience (January 16, 1980), *Insegnamenti di Giovanni Paolo II*, III, 1 (1980), 148–152.

[44] Pope John Paul II, Thirty-fifth General Assembly, *AAS* 76 (1984): 393.

[45] Cf. Second Vatican Council, *Gaudium et spes*, n. 51.

[46] Cf. ibid., n. 50.

[47] Cf. Pope Pius XII, Fourth International Congress, *AAS* 41 (1949): 560: "It would be erroneous . . . to think that the possibility of resorting to this means (artificial fertilization) might render valid a marriage between persons unable to contract it because of the impedimentum inpotentiae."

[48] A similar question was dealt with by Pope Paul VI, *Humanae vitae*, n. 14, *AAS* 60 (1968): 490–491.

[49] Cf. I, 1ff above.

[50] Pope John Paul II, *Familiaris consortio*, n. 14, *AAS* 74 (1982): 96.

[51] Cf. Response of the Holy Office (March 17, 1897), DS 3323; Pope Pius XII, Fourth International Congress, *AAS* 41 (1949): 560; Italian Catholic Union of Midwives, *AAS* 43 (1951): 850; Second Naples World Congress, *AAS* 48 (1956): 471–473; Discourse to those taking part in the Seventh International Congress of the International Society of Hematology (September 12, 1958), *AAS* 50 (1958): 733; Pope John XXIII, *Mater et magistra*, III, *AAS* 53 (1961): 447.

[52] Pope Pius XII, Italian Catholic Union of Midwives, *AAS* 43 (1951): 850.

[53] Pope Pius XII, Fourth International Congress, *AAS* 41 (1949): 560.

[54] Sacred Congregation for the Doctrine of the Faith, *Declaration on Certain Questions Concerning Sexual Ethics*, n. 9, *AAS* 68 (1976): 86, which quotes *Gaudium et spes*, n. 51. Cf. Decree of the Holy Office (August 2, 1929), *AAS* 21 (1929): 490; Pope Pius XII, Discourse to those taking part in the Twenty-sixth Congress of the Italian Society of Urology (October 8, 1953), *AAS* 45 (1953): 678.

[55] Cf. Pope John XXIII, *Mater et magistra*, III, *AAS* 53 (1961): 447.

[56] Cf. Pope Pius XII, Fourth International Congress, *AAS* 41 (1949): 560.

[57] Cf. Pope Pius XII, Second Naples World Congress, *AAS* 48 (1956): 471–473.

[58] Second Vatican Council, *Gaudium et spes*, n. 50.

[59] Pope John Paul II, *Familiaris consortio*, n. 14, *AAS* 74 (1982): 97.

[60] Cf. Second Vatican Council, *Dignitatis humanae*, n. 7.

APPENDIX VII

Committee for Pro-life Activities
National Conference of Catholic Bishops (*U.S.*)

Nutrition and Hydration: Moral and Pastoral Reflections

1992

Modern medical technology seems to confront us with many questions not faced even a decade ago. Corresponding changes in medical practice have benefited many, but have also prompted fears by some that they will be aggressively treated against their will or denied the kind of care that is their due as human persons with inherent dignity. Current debates about life-sustaining treatment suggest that our society's moral reflection is having difficulty keeping pace with its technological progress.

A religious view of life has an important contribution to make to these modern debates. Our Catholic tradition has developed a rich body of thought on these questions, which affirms a duty to preserve human life but recognizes limits to that duty.

Our first goal in making this statement is to reaffirm some basic principles of our moral tradition, to assist Catholics and others in making treatment decisions in accord with respect for God's gift of life.

These principles do not provide clear and final answers to all moral questions that arise as individuals make difficult decisions. Catholic theologians may differ on how best to apply moral principles to some questions not explicitly resolved by the Church's teaching authority. Likewise, we understand that those who must make serious health-care decisions for themselves or for others face a complexity of issues, circumstances, thoughts, and emotions in each unique case.

This is the case with some questions involving the medically assisted provision of nutrition and hydration to helpless patients—those who are seriously ill, disabled or persistently unconscious. These questions have been made more urgent by widely publicized court cases and the public debate to which they have given rise.

Our second purpose in issuing this statement, then, is to provide some clarification of the moral issues involved in decisions about medically assisted nutrition and hydration. We are fully aware that such guidance is not necessarily final, because there are many unresolved medical and ethical questions related to these issues and the continuing development of medical technology will necessitate ongoing reflection. But these decisions already confront patients, families, and health-care personnel every day. They arise whenever competent patients make decisions about medically assisted nutrition and hydration for their own present situation, when they consider signing an advance directive such as a "living will" or health-care proxy document, and when families or other proxy decision makers make decisions about those entrusted to their care. We offer guidance to those who, facing these issues, might be confused by opinions that at times threaten to deny the inherent dignity of human life. We therefore address our reflections first to those who share our Judeo-Christian traditions, and second to others concerned about the dignity and value of human life who seek guidance in making their own moral decisions.

Moral Principles

The Judeo-Christian moral tradition celebrates life as the gift of a loving God, and respects the life of each human being because each is made in the image and likeness of God. As Christians we also believe we are redeemed by Christ and called to share eternal life with Him. From these roots the Catholic tradition has developed a distinctive approach to fostering and sustaining human life. Our Church views life as a sacred trust, a gift over which we are given stewardship and not absolute dominion. The Church thus opposes all direct attacks on innocent life. As conscientious stewards we have a duty to preserve life, while recognizing certain limits to that duty:

1. Because human life is the foundation for all other human goods, it has a special value and significance. Life is "the first right of the human person" and "the condition of all the others."[1]

2. All crimes against life, including "euthanasia or willful suicide," must be opposed.[2] Euthanasia is "an action or an omission which of itself or by intention causes death, in order that all suffering may in this way be eliminated." Its terms of reference are to be found "in the intention of the will and in the methods used."[3] Thus defined, euthanasia is an attack on life which no one has a right to make or request, and which no government or other human authority can legitimately recommend or permit. Although individual guilt may be reduced or absent because of suffering or emotional factors that cloud the conscience, this does not change the objective

wrongfulness of the act. It should also be recognized that an apparent plea for death may really be a plea for help and love.

3. Suffering is a fact of human life, and has special significance for the Christian as an opportunity to share in Christ's redemptive suffering. Nevertheless there is nothing wrong in trying to relieve someone's suffering; in fact, it is a positive good to do so, as long as one does not intentionally cause death or interfere with other moral and religious duties.[4]

4. Everyone has the duty to care for his or her own life and health and to seek necessary medical care from others, but this does not mean that all possible remedies must be used in all circumstances. One is not obliged to use either "extraordinary" means or "disproportionate" means of preserving life—that is, means which are understood as offering no reasonable hope of benefit or as involving excessive burdens. Decisions regarding such means are complex and should ordinarily be made by the patient in consultation with his or her family, chaplain or pastor, and physician when that is possible.[5]

5. In the final stage of dying one is not obliged to prolong the life of a patient by every possible means: "When inevitable death is imminent in spite of the means used, it is permitted in conscience to take the decision to refuse forms of treatment that would only secure a precarious and burdensome prolongation of life, so long as the normal care due to the sick person in similar cases is not interrupted."[6]

6. While affirming life as a gift of God, the Church recognizes that death is unavoidable and that it can open the door to eternal life. Thus, "without in any way hastening the hour of death," the dying person should accept its reality and prepare for it emotionally and spiritually.[7]

7. Decisions regarding human life must respect the demands of justice, viewing each human being as our neighbor and avoiding all discrimination based on age or dependency.[8] A human being has "a unique dignity and an independent value, from the moment of conception and in every stage of development, whatever his or her physical condition." In particular, "the disabled person (whether the disability be the result of a congenital handicap, chronic illness or accident, or from mental or physical deficiency, and whatever the severity of the disability) is a fully human subject, with the corresponding innate, sacred, and inviolable rights." First among these is "the fundamental and inalienable right to life."[9]

8. The dignity and value of the human person, which lie at the foundation of the Church's teaching on the right to life, also provide a basis for any just social order. Not only to become more Christian, but to become more truly human, society should protect the right to life through its laws and other policies.[10]

While these principles grow out of a specific religious tradition, they appeal to a common respect for the dignity of the human person. We commend them to all people of good will.

Questions About Medically Assisted Nutrition and Hydration

In what follows we apply these well-established moral principles to the difficult issue of providing medically assisted nutrition and hydration to persons who are seriously ill, disabled, or persistently unconscious. We recognize the complexity involved in applying these principles to individual cases and acknowledge that, at this time and on this particular issue, our applications do not have the same authority as the principles themselves.

1. Is the withholding or withdrawing of medically assisted nutrition and hydration always a direct killing?

In answering this question one should avoid two extremes.

First, it is wrong to say that this could not be a matter of killing simply because it involves an omission rather than a positive action. In fact a deliberate omission may be an effective and certain way to kill, especially to kill someone weakened by illness. Catholic teaching condemns as euthanasia "an action *or an omission* which of itself or by intention causes death, in order that all suffering may in this way be eliminated." Thus "euthanasia includes not only active mercy killing, but also the omission of treatment when the purpose of the omission is to kill the patient."[11]

Second, we should not assume that all or most decisions to withhold or withdraw medically assisted nutrition and hydration are attempts to cause death. To be sure, any patient will die if all nutrition and hydration are withheld.[12] But sometimes other causes are at work—for example, the patient may be imminently dying, whether feeding takes place or not, from an already existing terminal condition. At other times, although the shortening of the patient's life is one foreseeable result of an omission, the real *purpose* of the omission was to relieve the patient of a particular procedure that was of limited usefulness to the patient or unreasonably burdensome for the patient and the patient's family or caregivers. This kind of decision should not be equated with a decision to kill or with suicide.

The harsh reality is that some who propose withdrawal of nutrition and hydration from certain patients do directly *intend* to bring about a patient's death, and would even prefer a change in the law to allow for what they see as more "quick and painless" means to cause death.[13] In other words, nutrition and hydration (whether orally administered or medically assisted) are sometimes withdrawn not because a patient is dying, but precisely because a patient is not dying (or not dying quickly) and someone believes it would be better if he or she did, generally because the patient is perceived as having an unacceptably low "quality of life" or as imposing burdens on others.[14]

When deciding whether to withhold or withdraw medically assisted nutrition and hydration, or other forms of life support, we are called by our moral tradition to ask ourselves: What will my decision do for this patient? And what am I trying to achieve by doing it? We must be sure that it is not our intent to cause the patient's death—either for its own sake or as a means to achieving some other goal such as the relief of suffering.

2. Is medically assisted nutrition and hydration a form of "treatment" or "care"?

Catholic teaching provides that a person in the final stages of dying need not accept "forms of treatment that would only secure a precarious and burdensome prolongation of life," but should still receive "the normal care due to the sick person in similar cases."[15] All patients deserve to receive normal care out of respect for their inherent dignity as persons. As Pope John Paul II has said, a decision to forgo "purely experimental or ineffective interventions" does not "dispense from the valid therapeutic task of sustaining life or from assistance with the normal means of sustaining life. Science, even when it is unable to heal, can and should care for and assist the sick."[16] But the teaching of the Church has not resolved the question whether medically assisted nutrition and hydration should always be seen as a form of normal care.[17]

Almost everyone agrees that oral feeding, when it can be accepted and assimilated by a patient, is a form of care owed to all helpless people. Christians should be especially sensitive to this obligation, because giving food and drink to those in need is an important expression of Christian love and concern (Matt. 10:42 and 25:35; Mark 9:41). But our obligations become less clear when adequate nutrition and hydration require the skills of trained medical personnel and the use of technologies that may be perceived as very burdensome—that is, as intrusive, painful or repugnant. Such factors vary from one type of feeding procedure to another, and from one patient to another, making it difficult to classify all feeding procedures as either "care" or "treatment."

Perhaps this dilemma should be viewed in a broader context. Even medical "treatments" are morally obligatory when they are "ordinary" means—that is, if they provide a reasonable hope of benefit and do not involve excessive burdens. Therefore, we believe people should make decisions in light of a simple and fundamental insight: *Out of respect for the dignity of the human person, we are obliged to preserve our own lives, and help others preserve theirs, by the use of means that have a reasonable hope of sustaining life without imposing unreasonable burdens on those we seek to help, that is, on the patient and his or her family and community.*

We must therefore address the question of benefits and burdens next, recognizing that a full moral analysis is only possible when one knows the effects of a given procedure on a particular patient.

3. What are the benefits of medically assisted nutrition and hydration?

According to international codes of medical ethics, a physician will see a medical procedure as appropriate "if in his or her judgment it offers hope of saving life, reestablishing health or alleviating suffering."[18]

Nutrition and hydration, whether provided in the usual way or with medical assistance, do not by themselves remedy pathological conditions, except those caused by dietary deficiencies. But patients benefit from them in several ways. First, for all patients who can assimilate them, suitable food and fluids sustain life, and providing them normally expresses loving concern and solidarity with the helpless. Second, for patients being treated with the hope of a cure, appropriate food and fluids are an important element of sound health care. Third, even for patients who are imminently dying and incurable, food and fluids can prevent the suffering that may arise from dehydration, hunger, and thirst.

The benefit of sustaining and fostering life is fundamental, because life is our first gift from a loving God and the condition for receiving his other gifts. But sometimes even food and fluids are no longer effective in providing this benefit, because a patient has entered the final stage of a terminal condition. At such times we should make the dying person as comfortable as possible and provide nursing care and proper hygiene as well as companionship and appropriate spiritual aid. Such a person may lose all desire for food and drink and even be unable to ingest them. Initiating medically assisted feeding or intravenous fluids in this case may increase the patient's discomfort while providing no real benefit; ice chips or sips of water may instead be appropriate to provide comfort and counteract the adverse effects of dehydration.[19] Even in the case of the imminently dying patient, of course, any action or omission that of itself or by intention causes death is to be absolutely rejected.

As Christians who trust in the promise of eternal life, we recognize that death does not have the final word. Accordingly we need not always prevent death until the last possible moment; but we should never intentionally cause death or abandon the dying person as though he or she were unworthy of care and respect.

4. What are the burdens of medically assisted nutrition and hydration?

Our tradition does not demand heroic measures in fulfilling the obligation to sustain life. A person may legitimately refuse even procedures that effectively prolong life, if he or she believes they would impose excessively grave burdens on himself or herself, or on his or her family and community. Catholic theologians have traditionally viewed medical treatment as excessively burdensome if it is "too painful, too damaging to the patient's bodily self and functioning, too psychologically repugnant to the patient, too restrictive of the patient's liberty and preferred activities, too suppressive of the patient's mental life, or too expensive."[20]

Because assessment of these burdens necessarily involves some subjective judgments, a conscious and competent patient is generally the best judge of whether a particular burden or risk is too grave to be tolerated in his or her own case. But because of the serious consequences of withdrawing all nutrition and hydration, patients and those helping them make decisions should assess such burdens or risks with special care.

Here we offer some brief reflections and cautions regarding the kinds of burdens sometimes associated with medically assisted nutrition and hydration.

Physical Risks and Burdens

The risks and objective complications of medically assisted nutrition and hydration will depend on the procedure used and the condition of the patient. In a given case a feeding procedure may become harmful or even life-threatening. (These medical data are discussed at length in an appendix to this paper.)

If the risks and burdens of a particular feeding procedure are deemed serious enough to warrant withdrawing it, we should not automatically deprive the patient of all nutrition and hydration but should ask whether another procedure is feasible that would be less burdensome. We say this because some helpless patients, including some in a "persistent vegetative state," receive tube feedings not because they cannot swallow food at all but because tube feeding is less costly and difficult for health-care personnel.[21]

Moreover, because burdens are assessed in relation to benefits, we should ask whether the risks and discomfort of a feeding procedure are really excessive as compared with the adverse effects of dehydration or malnutrition.

Psychological Burdens on the Patient

Many people see feeding tubes as frightening or even as bodily violations. Assessments of such burdens are necessarily subjective; they should not be dismissed on that account, but we offer some practical cautions to help prevent abuse.

First, in keeping with our moral teaching against the intentional causing of death by omission, one should distinguish between repugnance to a particular procedure and repugnance to life itself. The latter may occur when a patient views a life of helplessness and dependency on others as itself a heavy burden, leading him or her to wish or even to pray for death. Especially in our achievement-oriented society, the burden of living in such a condition may seem to outweigh any possible benefit of medical treatment and even lead a person to despair. But we should not assume that the burdens in such a case always outweigh the benefits; for the sufferer, given good counseling and spiritual support, may be brought again to appreciate the precious gift of life.

Second, our tradition recognizes that when treatment decisions are made, "account will have to be taken of the *reasonable* wishes of the patient and the patient's family, as also of the advice of the doctors who are specially competent in the matter."[22] The word "reasonable" is important here. Good health-care providers will try to help patients assess psychological burdens with full information and without undue fear of unfamiliar procedures.[23] A well-trained and compassionate hospital chaplain can provide valuable personal and spiritual support to patients and families facing these difficult situations.

Third, we should not assume that a feeding procedure is inherently repugnant to all patients without specific evidence. In contrast to Americans' general distaste for the idea of being supported by "tubes and machines," some studies indicate surprisingly favorable views of medically assisted nutrition and hydration among patients and families with actual experience of such procedures.[24]

Economic and Other Burdens on Caregivers

While some balk at the idea, in principle cost can be a valid factor in decisions about life support. For example, money spent on expensive treatment for one family member may be money otherwise needed for food, housing, and other necessities for the rest of the family. Here, also, we offer some cautions.

First, particularly when a form of treatment "carries a risk or is burdensome" on other grounds, a critically ill person may have a legitimate and altruistic desire "not to impose excessive expense on the family or the community."[25] Even for altruistic reasons a patient should not directly intend his or her own death by malnutrition or dehydration, but may accept an earlier death as a consequence of his or her refusal of an unreasonably expensive treatment. Decisions *by others* to deny an incompetent patient medically assisted nutrition and hydration for reasons of cost raise additional concerns about justice to the individual patient, who could wrongly be deprived of life itself to serve the less fundamental needs of others.

Second, we do not think individual decisions about medically assisted nutrition and hydration should be determined by macro-economic concerns such as national budget priorities and the high cost of health care. These social problems are serious, but it is by no means established that they require depriving chronically ill and helpless patients of effective and easily tolerated measures that they need to survive.[26]

Third, tube feeding alone is generally not very expensive and may cost no more than oral feeding.[27] What is seen by many as a grave financial and emotional burden on caregivers is the total long-term care of severely debilitated patients, who may survive for many years with no life support except medically assisted nutrition and hydration and nursing care.

The difficulties families may face in this regard, and their need for improved financial and other assistance from the rest of society, should not be underestimated. While caring for a helpless loved one can provide many intangible benefits to family members and bring them closer together, the responsibilities of care can also strain even close and loving family relationships; complex medical decisions must be made under emotionally difficult circumstances not easily appreciated by those who have never faced such situations.

Even here, however, we must try to think through carefully what we intend by withdrawing medically assisted nutrition and hydration. Are we deliberately trying to make sure that the patient dies, in order to relieve caregivers of the financial and emotional burdens that will fall upon them if the patient survives? Are we really implementing a decision to withdraw all other forms of care, precisely because the patient offers so little response to the efforts of caregivers? Decisions like these seem to reach beyond the weighing of burdens and benefits of medically assisted nutrition and hydration as such.

In the context of official Church teaching, it is not yet clear to what extent we may assess the burden of a patient's total care rather than the burden of a particular treatment when we seek to refuse "burdensome" life support. On a practical level, those seeking to make good decisions might assure themselves of their own intentions by asking: Does my decision aim at relieving the patient of a particularly grave burden imposed by medically assisted nutrition and hydration? Or does it aim to avoid the total burden of caring for the patient? If so, does it achieve this aim by deliberately bringing about his or her death?

Rather than leaving families to confront such dilemmas alone, society and government should improve their assistance to families whose financial and emotional resources are strained by long-term care of loved ones.[28]

5. What role should "quality of life" play in our decisions?

Financial and emotional burdens are willingly endured by most families to raise their children or to care for mentally aware but weak and elderly family members. It is sometimes argued that we need not endure comparable burdens to feed and care for persons with severe mental and physical disabilities, because their low "quality of life" makes it unnecessary or pointless to preserve their lives.[29]

But this argument—even when it seems motivated by a humanitarian concern to reduce suffering and hardship—ignores the equal dignity and sanctity of all human life. Its key assumption—that people with disabilities necessarily enjoy life less than others or lack the potential to lead meaningful lives—is also mistaken.[30] Where suffering does exist, society's response should not be to neglect or eliminate the lives of people with disabilities, but to help correct their inadequate

living conditions.[31] Very often the worst threat to a good "quality of life" for these people is not the disability itself, but the prejudicial attitudes of others—attitudes based on the idea that a life with serious disabilities is not worth living.[32]

This being said, our moral tradition allows for three ways in which the "quality of life" of a seriously ill patient is relevant to treatment decisions.

1. Consistent with respect for the inherent sanctity of life, we should relieve needless suffering and support morally acceptable ways of improving each patient's quality of life.[33]

2. One may legitimately refuse a treatment because it would itself create an impairment imposing new serious burdens or risks on the patient. This decision to avoid the new burdens or risks created by a treatment is not the same as directly intending to end life in order to avoid the burden of living in a disabled state.[34]

3. Sometimes a disabling condition may directly influence the benefits and burdens of a specific treatment for a particular patient. For example, a confused or demented patient may find medically assisted nutrition and hydration more frightening and burdensome than other patients do because he or she cannot understand what it is. The patient may even repeatedly pull out feeding tubes, requiring burdensome physical restraints if this form of feeding is to be continued. In such cases, ways of alleviating such special burdens should be explored before concluding that they justify withholding all food and fluids needed to sustain life.

These humane considerations are quite different from a "quality of life" ethic that would judge individuals with disabilities or limited potential as not worthy of care or respect. It is one thing to withhold a procedure because it would impose new disabilities on a patient, and quite another thing to say that patients who already have such disabilities should not have their lives preserved. A means considered ordinary or proportionate for other patients should not be considered extraordinary or disproportionate for severely impaired patients solely because of a judgment that their lives are not worth living.

In short, while considerations regarding a person's quality of life have some validity in weighing the burdens and benefits of medical treatment, at the present time in our society judgments about the quality of life are sometimes used to promote euthanasia. The Church must emphasize the sanctity of life of each person as a fundamental principle in all moral decision making.

6. Do persistently unconscious patients represent a special case?

Even Catholics who accept the same basic moral principles may strongly disagree on how to apply them to patients who appear to be persistently unconscious—that is, those who are in a permanent coma or a "persistent vegetative state" (PVS).[35]

Some moral questions in this area have not been explicitly resolved by the Church's teaching authority.

On some points there is wide agreement among Catholic theologians.

1. An unconscious patient must be treated as a living human person with inherent dignity and value. Direct killing of such a patient is as morally reprehensible as the direct killing of anyone else. Even the medical terminology used to describe these patients as "vegetative" unfortunately tends to obscure this vitally important point, inviting speculation that a patient in this state is a "vegetable" or a subhuman animal.[36]

2. The area of legitimate controversy does not concern patients with conditions like mental retardation, senility, dementia, or even temporary unconsciousness.

Where serious disagreement begins is with the patient who has been diagnosed as completely and permanently unconscious after careful testing over a period of weeks or months.

Some moral theologians argue that a particular form of care or treatment is morally obligatory only when its benefits outweigh its burdens to a patient or the care providers. In weighing burdens, they say, the total burden of a procedure and the consequent requirements of care must be taken into account. If no benefit can be demonstrated, the procedure, whatever its burdens, cannot be obligatory. These moralists also hold that the chief criterion to determinate benefit of a procedure cannot be merely that it prolongs physical life, since physical life is not an absolute good but is relative to the spiritual good of the person. They assert that the spiritual good of the person is union with God, which can be advanced only by human acts, i.e., conscious, free acts. Since the best current medical opinion holds that persons in the persistent vegetative state (PVS) are incapable now or in the future of conscious, free human acts, these moralists conclude that, when careful diagnosis verifies this condition, it is not obligatory to prolong life by such interventions as a respirator, antibiotics, or medically assisted hydration and nutrition. To decide to omit non-obligatory care, therefore, is not to intend the patient's death, but only to avoid the burden of the procedure. Hence, though foreseen, the patient's death is to be attributed to the patient's pathological condition and not to the omission of care. Therefore, these theologians conclude, while it is always wrong directly to intend or cause the death of such patients, the natural dying process which would have occurred without these interventions may be permitted to proceed.

While this rationale is convincing to some, it is not theologically conclusive and we are not persuaded by it. In fact, other theologians argue cogently that theological inquiry could lead one to a more carefully limited conclusion.

These moral theologians argue that while particular treatments can be judged useless or burdensome, it is morally questionable and would create a dangerous precedent to imply that any human life is not a positive good or "benefit." They emphasize that while life is not the highest good, it is always and everywhere a basic good of the human person and not merely a means to other goods. They further assert that if the "burden" one is trying to relieve by discontinuing medically assisted nutrition and hydration is the burden of remaining alive in the allegedly undignified condition of PVS, such a decision is unacceptable, because one's intent is only achieved by deliberately ensuring the patient's death from malnutrition or dehydration. Finally, these moralists suggest that PVS is best seen as an extreme form of mental and physical disability—one whose causes, nature, and prognosis are as yet imperfectly understood—and not as a terminal illness or fatal pathology from which patients should generally be allowed to die. Because the patient's life can often be sustained indefinitely by medically assisted nutrition and hydration that is not unreasonably risky or burdensome for that patient, they say, we are not dealing here with a case where "inevitable death is imminent in spite of the means used."[37] Rather, because the patient will die in a few days if medically assisted nutrition and hydration are discontinued,[38] but can often live a long time if they are provided, the inherent dignity and worth of the human person obligates us to provide this patient with care and support.

Further complicating this debate is a disagreement over what responsible Catholics should do in the absence of a final resolution of this question. Some point to our moral tradition of probabilism, which would allow individuals to follow the appropriate moral analysis that they find persuasive. Others point to the principle that in cases where one might risk unjustly depriving someone of life, we should take the safer course.

In the face of the uncertainties and unresolved medical and theological issues, it is important to defend and preserve important values. On the one hand, there is a concern that patients and families should not be subjected to unnecessary burdens, ineffective treatments, and indignities when death is approaching. On the other hand, it is important to ensure that the inherent dignity of human persons, even those who are persistently unconscious, is respected, and that no one is deprived of nutrition and hydration with the intent of bringing on his or her death.

It is not easy to arrive at a single answer to some of the real and personal dilemmas involved in this issue. In study, prayer, and compassion, we continue to reflect on this issue and hope to discover additional information that will lead to its ultimate resolution.

In the meantime, at a practical level, we are concerned that withdrawal of all life support, including nutrition and hydration, not be viewed as appropriate or automatically indicated for the entire class of PVS patients simply because of a judgment that they are beyond the reach of medical treatment that would restore consciousness. We note the current absence of conclusive scientific data on the causes and implications of different degrees of brain damage, on the PVS patient's ability to experience pain, and on the reliability of prognoses for many such patients.[39] We do know that many of these patients have a good prognosis for long-term survival when given medically assisted nutrition and hydration, and a certain prognosis for death otherwise—and we know that many in our society view such an early death as a positive good for a patient in this condition. Therefore we are gravely concerned about current attitudes and policy trends in our society that would too easily dismiss patients without apparent mental faculties as non-persons or as undeserving of human care and concern. In this climate, even legitimate moral arguments intended to have a careful and limited application can easily be misinterpreted, broadened, and abused by others to erode respect for the lives of some of our society's most helpless members.

In light of these concerns, it is our considered judgment that while legitimate Catholic moral debate continues, decisions about these patients should be guided by a presumption in favor of medically assisted nutrition and hydration. A decision to discontinue such measures should be made in light of a careful assessment of the burdens and benefits of nutrition and hydration for the individual patient and his or her family and community. Such measures must not be withdrawn in order to cause death, but they may be withdrawn if they offer no reasonable hope of sustaining life or pose excessive risks or burdens. We also believe that social and health-care policies should be carefully framed so that these patients are not routinely classified as "terminal" or as prime candidates for the discontinuance of even minimal means of life support.

7. Who should make decisions about medically assisted nutrition and hydration?

"Who decides?" In our society many believe this is the most important or even the only important question regarding this issue, and many understand it in terms of who has *legal* status to decide. Our Catholic tradition is more concerned with the principles for good *moral* decision making, which apply to everyone involved in a decision. Some general observations are appropriate here.

A competent patient is the primary decision maker about his or her own health care and is in the best situation to judge how the benefits and burdens of a particular procedure will be experienced. Ideally the patient will act with the advice of loved ones, of health-care personnel who have expert knowledge of medical aspects of the case, and of pastoral counselors who can help explore the moral issues and spiritual values involved. A patient may wish to make known his or her general wishes about life support in advance; such expressions cannot have the weight of a fully informed decision made in the actual circumstances of an illness, but can help guide others

in the event of a later state of incompetency.[40] Morally even the patient making decisions for himself or herself is bound by norms that prohibit the directly intended causing of death through action or omission and by the distinction between ordinary and extraordinary means.

When a patient is not competent to make his or her own decisions, a proxy decision maker who shares the patient's moral convictions, such as a family member or guardian, may be designated to represent the patient's interests and interpret his or her wishes. Here, too, moral limits remain relevant—that is, morally the proxy may not deliberately cause a patient's death or refuse what is clearly ordinary means, even if he or she believes the patient would have made such a decision.

Health-care personnel should generally follow the reasonable wishes of patient or family, but must also consult their own consciences when participating in these decisions. A physician or nurse told to participate in a course of action that he or she views as clearly immoral has a right and responsibility either to refuse to participate in this course of action or to withdraw from the case, and he or she should be given the opportunity to express the reasons for such refusal in the appropriate forum. Social and legal policies must protect such rights of conscience.

Finally, because these are matters of life and death for human persons, society as a whole has a legitimate interest in responsible decision making.[41]

Conclusion

In this document we reaffirm moral principles that provide a basis for responsible discussion of the morality of life support. We also offer tentative guidance on how to apply these principles to the difficult issue of medically assisted nutrition and hydration.

We reject any omission of nutrition and hydration intended to cause a patient's death. We hold for a presumption in favor of providing medically assisted nutrition and hydration to patients who need it, which presumption would yield in cases where such procedures have no medically reasonable hope of sustaining life or pose excessive risks or burdens. Recognizing that judgments about the benefits and burdens of medically assisted nutrition and hydration in individual cases have a subjective element and are generally best made by the patient directly involved, we also affirm a legitimate role for families' love and guidance, health-care professionals' ethical concerns, and society's interest in preserving life and protecting the helpless. In rejecting broadly permissive policies on withdrawal of nutrition and hydration from vulnerable patients, we must also help ensure that the burdens of caring for the helpless are more equitably shared throughout our society.

We recognize that this document is our first word, not our last word, on some of the complex questions involved in this subject. We urge Catholics and others concerned about the dignity of the human person to study these reflections and participate in the continuing public discussion of how best to address the needs of the helpless in our society.

Appendix

Technical Aspects of Medically Assisted Nutrition and Hydration

Procedures for providing nourishment and fluids to patients who cannot swallow food orally are either "parenteral" (bypassing the digestive tract) or "enteral" (using the digestive tract).

Parenteral or intravenous feeding is generally considered "more hazardous and more expensive" than enteral feeding.[42] It can be subdivided into peripheral intravenous feeding (using a needle inserted into a peripheral vein) and central intravenous feeding, also known as total parenteral feeding or hyperalimentation (using a larger needle inserted into a central vein near the heart). Peripheral intravenous lines can provide fluids and electrolytes as well as some nutrients; they can maintain fluid balance and prevent dehydration, but cannot provide adequate nutrition in the long term.[43] Total parenteral feeding can provide a more adequate nutritional balance, but poses significant risks to the patient and may involve costs an order of magnitude higher than other methods of tube feeding. It is no longer considered experimental and has become "a mainstay for helping critically ill patients to survive acute illnesses where the prognosis had previously been nearly hopeless," but its feasibility for life-long maintenance of patients without a functioning gastrointestinal tract has been questioned.[44]

Because of the limited usefulness of peripheral intravenous feeding and the special burdens of total parenteral feeding— and because few patients so completely lack a digestive system that they must depend on these measures for their sole source of nutrition—enteral tube feeding is the focus of the current debate over medically assisted nutrition and hydration. Such methods are used when a patient has a functioning digestive system but is unable or unwilling to ingest food orally and/or to swallow. The most common routes for enteral tube feeding are nasogastric (introducing a thin plastic tube through the nasal cavity to reach into the stomach), gastrostomy (surgical insertion of a tube through the abdominal wall into the stomach), and jejunostomy (surgical insertion of a tube through the abdominal wall into the small intestine).[45] These methods are the primary focus of this document.

Each method of enteral tube feeding has potential side effects. For example, nasogastric tubes must be inserted and monitored carefully so that they will not introduce food or fluids into the lungs. They may also irritate sensitive tissues and create discomfort; confused or angry patients may sometimes try to remove them; and efforts to restrain a patient to prevent this can impose additional discomfort and other

burdens. On the positive side, insertion of these tubes requires no surgery and only a modicum of training.[46]

Gastrostomy and jejunostomy tubes are better tolerated by many patients in need of long-term feeding. Their most serious physical burdens arise from the fact that their insertion requires surgery using local or general anesthesia, which involves some risk of infection and other complications. Once the surgical procedure is completed, these tubes can often be maintained without serious pain or medical complications, and confused patients do not often attempt to remove them.[47]

Notes

[1] Congregation for the Doctrine of the Faith (CDF), *Declaration on Procured Abortion* (1974), n. 11.

[2] Second Vatican Council, *Gaudium et spes*, n. 27. Suicide must be distinguished from "that sacrifice of one's life whereby for a higher cause, such as God's glory, the salvation of souls or the service of one's brethren, a person offers his or her own life or puts it in danger." Congregation for the Doctrine of the Faith, *Declaration on Euthanasia* (1980), pt. I.

[3] CDF, *Declaration on Euthanasia*, pt. II.

[4] See ibid., pt. III; United States Catholic Conference, *Ethical and Religious Directives for Catholic Health Facilities* (1971), n. 29.

[5] CDF, *Declaration on Euthanasia*, pt. IV.

[6] Ibid.

[7] Ibid., conclusion.

[8] Vatican Council II, *Gaudium et spes*, n. 27; CDF, *Declaration on Procured Abortion*, n. 12.

[9] Document of the Holy See for the International Year of Disabled Persons (March 4, 1981), I.1, II.1, *Origins* 10 (1981): 747–748.

[10] CDF, *Declaration on Euthanasia*, intro.; CDF, *Declaration on Procured Abortion*, nn. 10–11, 21; Sacred Congregation for the Doctrine of the Faith, *Instruction on Respect for Human Life in Its Origin* (1987), pt. III.

[11] Archbishop John Roach, "Life-Support Removal: No Easy Answers," *Catholic Bulletin* (March 7, 1991): 1, citing Bio/medical Ethics Commission of the Archdiocese of St. Paul -Minneapolis.

[12] "If all fluids and nutrition are withdrawn from any patient, regardless of the condition, he or she will die—inevitably and invariably. Death may come in a few days or take up to two weeks. Rarely in medicine is an earlier death for the patient so certain." Ronald E. Cranford, M.D., "Patients with Permanent Loss of Consciousness," in *By No Extraordinary Means*, ed. Joanne Lynn (Indiana University Press, 1986), 191.

[13] See the arguments made by a judge in the Elizabeth Bouvia case and by the attorneys in the Hector Rodas case, among others. See *Bouvia v. Superior Court*, 225 *Cal. Rptr.* 297, 307–308 (1986) (Compton, J., concurring); "Complaint for the Declaratory Relief in Rodas Case," *Issues in Law and Medicine* 2 (1987): 499–501, quoted verbatim from *Rodas v. Erkenbrack*, no. 87 ev 142 (Mesa County, CO, filed January 30, 1987).

[14]As one medical ethicist observes, interest in a broadly permissive policy for removing nutrition and hydration has grown "because a denial of nutrition may in a long run become the only effective way to make certain that a large number of biologically tenacious patients actually die." Daniel Callahan, "On Feeding the Dying," *Hastings Center Report* 13 (October 1983): 22.

[15]Alfred O'Rahilly, *Moral Principles* (Cork, Ireland: Cork University Press, 1948), no. 5.

[16]Address to a Human Pre-Leukemia Conference (November 15, 1985), *AAS* 78 (1986): 361. Also see his October 21, 1985, address to a study group of the Pontifical Academy of Sciences: "Even when the sick are incurable, they are never untreatable; whatever their condition, appropriate care should be provided for them." *AAS* 78 (1986): 314; *Origins* 15 (December 5, 1985): 416.

[17]Some groups advising the Holy See have ventured opinions on this point, but these do not have the force of official Church teaching. For example, in 1985 a study group of the Pontifical Academy of Sciences concluded: "If a patient is in a permanent, irreversible coma, as far as can be foreseen, treatment is not required, but all care should be lavished on him, including feeding." Pontifical Academy of Sciences, "The Artificial Prolongation of Life," *Origins* 15 (December 5, 1985): 415. Since comatose patients cannot generally take food orally, the statement evidently refers to medically assisted feeding. Similar statements are found in: Pontifical Council *Cor Unum, Question of Ethics Regarding the Fatally Ill and the Dying* (1981), 9; "Ne Eutanasia Ne Accanimento Terapeutico," *La Civilta Cattolica* 3280 (February 21, 1987): 324.

[18]World Medical Association, *Declaration of Helsinki* (1975), II.1.

[19]See Joyce V. Zerwekh, "The Dehydration Question," *Nursing* (January 1983): 47–51.

[20]See William E. May et al., "Feeding and Hydrating the Permanently Unconscious and Other Vulnerable Persons," *Issues in Law and Medicine* 3 (Winter 1987): 208.

[21]Ronald E. Cranford, "The Persistent Vegetative State: The Medical Reality (Getting the Facts Straight)," *Hastings Center Report* 18 (February/March 1988): 31.

[22]CDF, *Declaration on Euthanasia*, pt. IV, emphasis added.

[23]Current ethical guidelines for nurses, while generally defending patient autonomy, reflect this concern: "Obligations to prevent harm and bring benefit ... require that nurses seek to understand the patient's reasons for refusal. ... Nurses should make every effort to correct inaccurate views, to modify superficially held beliefs and overly dramatic gestures, and to restore hope where there is reason to hope." American Nurses' Association Committee on Ethics, "Guidelines on Withdrawing or Withholding Food and Fluid," *BioLaw* 2 (October 1988): U1124–1125.

[24]In one such study, "70 percent of patients and families were 100 percent willing to undergo intensive care again to achieve even one month of survival"; "age, severity of critical illness, length of stay, and charges for intensive care did not influence willingness to undergo intensive care." Danis et al., "Patients' and Families' Preferences for Medical Intensive Care," *Journal of the American Medical Association* 260 (August 12, 1988): 797. In another study, out of thirty-three people who had close relatives in a "persistent vegetative state," twenty-nine agreed with the initial decision to initiate tube feeding and twenty-five strongly agreed that such feeding should be continued, although none of those surveyed had made the decision to initiate it. Tresch et al., "Patients in a Persistent Vegetative State: Attitudes and Reactions of Family Members," *Journal of the American Geriatrics Society* 39 (January 1991): 17–21.

[25]CDF, *Declaration on Euthanasia*, pt. IV.

[26]"In striving to contain medical care costs, it is important to avoid discriminating against the critically ill and dying, to shun invidious comparisons of the economic value of various individuals to society, and to refuse to abandon patients and hasten death to save money." Hastings Center, *Guidelines on the Termination of Life-Sustaining Treatment and Care of the Dying* (Briar Cliff Manor, N.Y.: Hastings Center, 1987), 120.

[27]A possible exception is total parenteral feeding, which requires carefully prepared sterile formulas and more intensive daily monitoring. Ironically, some current health-care policies may exert economic pressure in favor of TPN because it is easier to obtain third-party reimbursement. Families may pay more for other forms of feeding because some insurance companies do not see them as "medical treatment." See U.S. Congress, Office of Technology Assessment, *Life-Sustaining Technologies and the Elderly*, OTA-BA-306 (Washington, D.C.: July 1987), 286.

[28]"One can never claim that one wishes to bring comfort to a family by suppressing one of its members. The respect, the dedication, the time, and the means required for the care of handicapped persons, even of those whose mental faculties are gravely affected, is the price that a society should generously pay in order to remain truly human." Document of the Holy See for the International Year of Disabled Persons, II.1, p. 748. The Holy See acknowledges that society as a whole should willingly assume these burdens, not leave them on the shoulders of individuals and families.

[29]E.g., see P. Singer, "Sanctity of Life or Quality of Life?" *Pediatrics* 72 (July 1983): 128–129. On the use and misuse of the term "quality of life" see John Cardinal O'Connor, "Who Will Care for the AIDS Victims?" *Origins* 19 (January 18, 1990): 544–548. Some Catholic theologians agree that a low "quality of life" justifies withdrawal of medically assisted feeding only from patients diagnosed as permanently unconscious. This argument is discussed separately in section 6 below.

[30]See David Milne, "Urges MDs to Get Birth-Defects Patient's Own Story," *Medical Tribune* (December 12, 1979): 6.

[31]National Conference of Catholic Bishops, *Pastoral Statement of the United States Catholic Bishops on Persons with Disabilities* (Washington, D.C.: United States Catholic Conference, 1978).

[32]Some patients with disabilities ask for death because all their efforts to build a life of self-respect are thwarted; a "right to die" is the first right for which they receive enthusiastic support from the able-bodied. See Paul K. Longmore, "Elizabeth

Bouvia, Assisted Suicide, and Social Prejudice," *Issues in Law and Medicine* 3 (Fall 1987): 141–168.

[33]"Quality of life must be sought, in so far as it is possible, by proportionate and appropriate treatment, but it presupposes life and the right to life for everyone, without discrimination and abandonment." Pope John Paul II, Address to the Eleventh European Congress of Perinatal Medicine (April 14, 1988), *AAS* 80 (1988): 1426; *The Pope Speaks* 33 (1988): 264–265.

[34]See Archbishop Roger Mahony, "Two Statements on the Bouvia Case," *Linacre Quarterly* 55 (February 1988): 85–87.

[35]Coma and persistent vegetative state are not the same. Coma, strictly speaking, is generally not a long-term condition, for within a few weeks a comatose patient usually dies, recovers, or reaches the plateau of a persistent vegetative state. "Coma implies the absence of both arousal and content. In terms of observable behavior, the comatose patient appears to be asleep, but unlike the sleeping patient, he cannot be aroused from this state. ... The patient in the vegetative state appears awake but shows no evidence of content, either confused or appropriate. He often has sleep-wake cycles but cannot demonstrate an awareness either of himself or his environment." Levy, "The Comatose Patient," in *The Clinical Neurosciences*, ed. Rosenberg, vol. I (New York: Churchill Livingstone, 1983), 956.

[36]While this pejorative connotation was surely not intended by those coining the phrase, we invite the medical profession to consider a less discriminatory term for this diagnostic state.

[37]See O'Rahilly, *Moral Principles*, n. 5.

[38]Because patients need nutritional support to live during the weeks or months of observation required for responsible assessment of PVS, the cases discussed here involve decisions about discontinuing such support rather than initiating it.

[39]One recent scientific study of recovery rates followed up eighty-four patients with a firm diagnosis of PVS. Of these patients, "41 percent became conscious by six months, 52 percent regained consciousness by one year, and 58 percent recovered consciousness within the three-year follow-up interval." The study was unable to identify "predictors of recovery from the vegetative state," that is, there is no established test by which physicians can tell in advance which PVS patients will ultimately wake up. The data "do not exclude the possibility of vegetative patients regaining consciousness after the second year," though this "must be regarded as a rare event." Levin, Saydjari et al., "Vegetative State After Closed-Head Injury: A Traumatic Coma Data Bank Report," *Archives of Neurology* 48 (June 1991): 580–585.

[40]Some Catholic moralists, using the concept of a "virtual intention," note that a person may give spiritual significance to his or her later suffering during incompetency, by deciding in advance to join these sufferings with those of Christ for the redemption of others.

[41]See: NCCB, Committee for Pro-Life Activities, "Guidelines for Legislation on Life-Sustaining Treatment" (November 10, 1984), *Origins* 14 (January 24, 1985); "The Rights of the Terminally Ill" (July 2, 1986), *Origins* 16.12 (September 4, 1986): 222–224; United States Catholic Conference, Brief as *Amicus Curiae* in Support of Petitioners, *Cruzan v. Director of Missouri Department of Health v. McCanse*, U.S. Supreme Court, No. 88-1503, published in *Origins* 19 (October 26, 1989): 345–351.

[42]David Major, M.D., "The Medical Procedures for Providing Food and Water: Indications and Effects," in *By No Extraordinary Means*, ed. Joanne Lynn (Bloomington, IN: Indiana University Press, 1986), 27.

[43]Peripheral veins (e.g., those found in an arm or leg) will eventually collapse after a period of intravenous feeding and will collapse much faster if complex nutrients such as proteins are included in the formula. See U.S. Congress, Office of Technology Assessment (OTA), *Life-Sustaining Technologies and the Elderly*, OTA-BA-3 16 (Washington, D.C.: U.S. Government Printing Office, July 1987), 283–284.

[44]Major, "The Medical Procedures for Providing Food and Water," 22, 24–25. Also see OTA, *Life-Sustaining Technologies*, 284–286.

[45]See Major, "The Medical Procedures for Providing Food and Water," 22, 25–26.

[46]Major, "The Medical Procedures for Providing Food and Water," 22; OTA, *Life-Sustaining Technologies*, 282–283; Ross Laboratories, *Tube Feedings: Clinical Application* (1982), 28–30.

[47]Major, "The Medical Procedures for Providing Food and Water," 22; OTA, *Life-Sustaining Technologies*, 282. Many ethicists observe that there is no morally significant difference in principle between withdrawing a life-sustaining procedure and failing to initiate it. However, surgically implanting a feeding tube and maintaining it once implanted may involve a different proportion of benefit to burden, because the transient risks of the initial surgical procedure will not continue or recur during routine maintenance of the tube.

Congregation for the Doctrine of the Faith

Responses to Questions Proposed concerning "Uterine Isolation" and Related Matters

July 31, 1993

The cardinal members of the Congregation for the Doctrine of the Faith in answer to the questions examined in ordinary session decreed the following replies:

Q. 1. When the uterus becomes so seriously injured (e.g., during a delivery of a Caesarian section) so as to render medically indicated even its total removal (hysterectomy) in order to counter an immediate serious threat to the life or health of the mother, is it licit to perform such a procedure notwithstanding the permanent sterility which will result for the woman?

R. AFFIRMATIVE.

Q. 2. When the uterus (e.g., as a result of previous Caesarian sections) is in a state such that, while not constituting in itself a present risk to the life or health of the woman, nevertheless is foreseeably incapable of carrying a future pregnancy to term without danger to the mother, danger which in some cases could be serious, is it licit to remove the uterus (hysterectomy) in order to prevent a possible future danger deriving from conception?

R. NEGATIVE.

Q. 3. In the same situation as in number 2, is it licit to substitute tubal ligation, also called "uterine isolation," for the hysterectomy, since the same end would be attained of averting the risks of a possible pregnancy by means of a procedure which is much simpler for the doctor and less serious for the woman, and since in addition, in some cases, the ensuing sterility might be reversible?

R. NEGATIVE.

Explanation

In the first case, the hysterectomy is licit because it has a directly therapeutic character, even though it may be foreseen that permanent sterility will result. In fact, it is the pathological condition of the uterus (e.g., a hemorrhage which cannot be stopped by other means), which makes its removal medically indicated. The removal of the organ has as its aim, therefore, the curtailing of a serious present danger to the woman independent of a possible future pregnancy.

From the moral point of view, the cases of hysterectomy and "uterine isolation" in the circumstances described in numbers 2 and 3 are different. These fall into the moral category of direct sterilization which in the Congregation of the Doctrine of the Faith's document *Quaecumque Sterilizatio* (AAS 68 [1976]: 738–740, n. 1) is defined as an action "whose sole, immediate effect is to render the generative faculty incapable of procreation." And the same document continues: "It [direct sterilization] is absolutely forbidden ... according to the teaching of the Church, even when it is motivated by a subjectively right intention of curing or preventing a physical or psychological ill-effect which is foreseen or feared as a result of pregnancy."

In point of fact, the uterus as described in number 2 does not constitute in and of itself any present danger to the woman. Indeed the proposal to substitute "uterine isolation" for hysterectomy under the same conditions shows precisely that the uterus in and of itself does not pose a pathological problem for the woman. Therefore, the described procedures do not have a properly therapeutic character but are aimed in themselves at rendering sterile future sexual acts freely chosen. The end of avoiding risks to the mother, deriving from a possible pregnancy, is thus pursued by means of a direct sterilization, in itself always morally illicit, while other ways, which are morally licit, remain open to free choice.

The contrary opinion which considers the interventions described in numbers 2 and 3 as indirect sterilizations, licit under certain conditions, cannot be regarded as valid and may not be followed in Catholic hospitals.

During an audience granted to the undersigned prefect, the Sovereign Pontiff John Paul II approved these responses adopted in an ordinary session of the Congregation for the Doctrine of the Faith, and ordered them to be published.

Rome, at the Congregation for the Doctrine of the Faith, the 31st of July 1993.

Joseph Cardinal Ratzinger
Prefect
+ Alberto Bovone
Titular Archbishop of Caesarea in Numidia
Secretary

APPENDIX IX

Pope John Paul II

Selections from Encyclical Letter *Evangelium vitae*
"The Gospel of Life"

March 25, 1995

1. The Gospel of life is at the heart of Jesus' message. Lovingly received day after day by the Church, it is to be preached with dauntless fidelity as "good news" to the people of every age and culture.

At the dawn of salvation, it is the birth of a child which is proclaimed as joyful news: "I bring you good news of a great joy which will come to all the people; for to you is born this day in the city of David a Savior, who is Christ the Lord" (Luke 2:10–11). The source of this "great joy" is the birth of the Savior; but Christmas also reveals the full meaning of every human birth, and the joy which accompanies the birth of the Messiah is thus seen to be the foundation and fulfillment of joy at every child born into the world (cf. John 16:21).

When he presents the heart of his redemptive mission, Jesus says: "I came that they may have life, and have it abundantly" (John 10:10). In truth, he is referring to that "new" and "eternal" life which consists in communion with the Father, to which every person is freely called in the Son by the power of the sanctifying Spirit. It is precisely in this "life" that all the aspects and stages of human life achieve their full significance.

The Incomparable Worth of the Human Person

2. Man is called to a fullness of life which far exceeds the dimensions of his earthly existence, because it consists in sharing the very life of God. The loftiness of this supernatural vocation reveals *the greatness* and *the inestimable* value of human life even in its temporal phase. Life in time, in fact, is the fundamental condition, the initial stage and an integral part of the entire unified process of human existence. It is a process which, unexpectedly and undeservedly, is enlightened by the promise and renewed by the gift of divine life, which will reach its full realization in eternity (cf. 1 John 3:1–2). At the same time, it is precisely this supernatural calling which highlights the *relative character* of each individual's earthly life. After all, life on earth is not an "ultimate" but a "penultimate" reality; even so, it remains *a sacred reality* entrusted to us, to be preserved with a sense of responsibility and brought to perfection in love and in the gift of ourselves to God and to our brothers and sisters.

The Church knows that this *Gospel of life*, which she has received from her Lord,[1] has a profound and persuasive echo in the heart of every person—believer and non-believer alike—because it marvelously fulfills all the heart's expectations while infinitely surpassing them. Even in the midst of difficulties and uncertainties, every person sincerely open to truth and goodness can, by the light of reason and the hidden action of grace, come to recognize in the natural law written in the heart (cf. Rom. 2:14–15) the sacred value of human life from its very beginning until its end, and can affirm the right of every human being to have this primary good respected to the highest degree. Upon the recognition of this right, every human community and the political community itself are founded.

In a special way, believers in Christ must defend and promote this right, aware as they are of the wonderful truth recalled by the Second Vatican Council: "By his incarnation the Son of God has united himself in some fashion with every human being."[2] This saving event reveals to humanity not only the boundless love of God who "so loved the world that he gave his only Son" (John 3:16), but also the *incomparable value of every human person.*

The Church, faithfully contemplating the mystery of the Redemption, acknowledges this value with ever new wonder.[3] She feels called to proclaim to the people of all times this "Gospel," the source of invincible hope and true joy for every period of history. *The Gospel of God's love for man, the Gospel of the dignity of the person, and the Gospel of life are a single and indivisible Gospel.*

For this reason, man—living man—represents the primary and fundamental way for the Church.[4]

New Threats to Human Life

3. Every individual, precisely by reason of the mystery of the Word of God who was made flesh (cf. John 1:14), is entrusted to the maternal care of the Church. Therefore every threat to human dignity and life must necessarily be felt in the Church's very heart; it cannot but affect her at the core of her faith in the Redemptive Incarnation of the Son of God, and engage her in her mission of proclaiming the Gospel of life in all the world and to every creature (cf. Mark 16:15).

Today this proclamation is especially pressing because of the extraordinary increase and gravity of threats to the life of individuals and peoples, especially where life is weak and defenseless. In addition to the ancient scourges of poverty, hunger, endemic diseases, violence, and war, new threats are emerging on an alarmingly vast scale.

The Second Vatican Council, in a passage which retains all its relevance today, forcefully condemned a number of crimes and attacks against human life. Thirty years later, taking up the words of the council and with the same forcefulness I repeat that condemnation in the name of the whole Church, certain that I am interpreting the genuine sentiment of every upright conscience: "Whatever is opposed to life itself, such as any type of murder, genocide, abortion, euthanasia, or willful self-destruction, whatever violates the integrity of the human person, such as mutilation, torments inflicted on body or mind, attempts to coerce the will itself; whatever insults human dignity, such as subhuman living conditions, arbitrary imprisonment, deportation, slavery, prostitution, the selling of women and children; as well as disgraceful working conditions, where people are treated as mere instruments of gain rather than as free and responsible persons; all these things and others like them are infamies indeed. They poison human society, and they do more harm to those who practice them than to those who suffer from the injury. Moreover, they are a supreme dishonor to the Creator."[5]

4. Unfortunately, this disturbing state of affairs, far from decreasing, is expanding: with the new prospects opened up by scientific and technological progress there arise new forms of attacks on the dignity of the human being. At the same time a new cultural climate is developing and taking hold, which gives crimes against life *a new and—if possible—even more sinister character*, giving rise to further grave concern: broad sectors of public opinion justify certain crimes against life in the name of the rights of individual freedom, and on this basis they claim not only exemption from punishment but even authorization by the state, so that these things can be done with total freedom and indeed with the free assistance of health care systems.

All this is causing a profound change in the way in which life and relationships between people are considered. The fact that legislation in many countries, perhaps even departing from basic principles of their Constitutions, has determined not to punish these practices against life, and even to make them altogether legal, is both a disturbing symptom and a significant cause of grave moral decline. Choices once unanimously considered criminal and rejected by the common moral sense are gradually becoming socially acceptable. Even certain sectors of the medical profession, which by its calling is directed to the defense and care of human life, are increasingly willing to carry out these acts against the person. In this way the very nature of the medical profession is distorted and contradicted, and the dignity of those who practice it is degraded. In such a cultural and legislative situation, the serious demographic, social, and family problems which weigh upon many of the world's peoples and which require responsible and effective attention from national and international bodies, are left open

to false and deceptive solutions, opposed to the truth and the good of persons and nations.

The end result of this is tragic: not only is the fact of the destruction of so many human lives still to be born or in their final stage extremely grave and disturbing, but no less grave and disturbing is the fact that conscience itself, darkened as it were by such widespread conditioning, is finding it increasingly difficult to distinguish between good and evil in what concerns the basic value of human life. . . .

Chapter I
The Voice of Your Brother's Blood
Cries to Me from the Ground:
Present-Day Threats to Human Life

. . . "What have you done?" (Gen 4:10):
The Eclipse of the Value of Life

11. Here though we shall concentrate particular attention on *another category of attacks*, affecting life in its earliest and in its final stages, attacks which present *new characteristics with respect to the past and which raise questions of extraordinary seriousness*. It is not only that in generalized opinion these attacks tend no longer to be considered as "crimes"; paradoxically they assume the nature of "rights," to the point that the state is called upon to give them *legal recognition and to make them available through the free services of health care personnel*. Such attacks strike human life at the time of its greatest frailty, when it lacks any means of self-defense. Even more serious is the fact that, most often, those attacks are carried out in the very heart of and with the complicity of the family—the family which by its nature is called to be the "sanctuary of life."

How did such a situation come about? Many different factors have to be taken into account. In the background there is the profound crisis of culture, which generates skepticism in relation to the very foundations of knowledge and ethics, and which makes it increasingly difficult to grasp clearly the meaning of what man is, the meaning of his rights and his duties. Then there are all kinds of existential and interpersonal difficulties, made worse by the complexity of a society in which individuals, couples, and families are often left alone with their problems. There are situations of acute poverty, anxiety, or frustration in which the struggle to make ends meet, the presence of unbearable pain, or instances of violence, especially against women, make the choice to defend and promote life so demanding as sometimes to reach the point of heroism.

All this explains, at least in part, how the value of life can today undergo a kind of "eclipse," even though conscience does not cease to point to it as a sacred and inviolable value, as is evident in the tendency to disguise certain crimes against life in its early or final stages by using innocuous medical terms which distract attention from the fact that what is involved is the right to life of an actual human person.

12. In fact, while the climate of widespread moral uncertainty can in some way be explained by the multiplicity and gravity of today's social problems, and these can sometimes mitigate the subjective responsibility of individuals, it is no less true that we are confronted by an even larger reality, which can be described as a *veritable structure of sin*. This reality is characterized by the emergence of a culture which denies solidarity and in many cases takes the form of a veritable "culture of death." This culture is actively fostered by powerful cultural, economic, and political currents which encourage an idea of society excessively concerned with efficiency. Looking at the situation from this point of view, it is possible to speak in a certain sense of a *war of the powerful against the weak*: a life which would require greater acceptance, love, and care is considered useless, or held to be an intolerable burden, and is therefore rejected in one way or another. A person who, because of illness, handicap, or, more simply, just by existing, compromises the well-being or life-style of those who are more favored tends to be looked upon as an enemy to be resisted or eliminated. In this way a kind of *"conspiracy against life"* is unleashed. This conspiracy involves not only individuals in their personal, family, or group relationships, but goes far beyond, to the point of damaging and distorting, at the international level, relations between peoples and states.

13. In order to facilitate the spread of *abortion*, enormous sums of money have been invested and continue to be invested in the production of pharmaceutical products which make it possible to kill the fetus in the mother's womb without recourse to medical assistance. On this point, scientific research itself seems to be almost exclusively preoccupied with developing products which are ever more simple and effective in suppressing life and which at the same time are capable of removing abortion from any kind of control or social responsibility.

It is frequently asserted that *contraception*, if made safe and available to all, is the most effective remedy against abortion. The Catholic Church is then accused of actually promoting abortion, because she obstinately continues to teach the moral unlawfulness of contraception. When looked at carefully, this objection is clearly unfounded. It may be that many people use contraception with a view to excluding the subsequent temptation of abortion. But the negative values inherent in the "contraceptive mentality"—which is very different from responsible parenthood, lived in respect for the full truth of the conjugal act—are such that they in fact strengthen this temptation when an unwanted life is conceived. Indeed, the pro-abortion culture is especially strong precisely where the Church's teaching on contraception is rejected. Certainly, from the moral point of view contraception and abortion are *specifically different* evils: the former contradicts the full truth of the sexual act as the proper expression of conjugal love, while the latter destroys the life of a human being; the former is opposed to the virtue of chastity in marriage, the

latter is opposed to the virtue of justice and directly violates the divine commandment "You shall not kill."

But despite their differences of nature and moral gravity, contraception and abortion are often closely connected, as fruits of the same tree. It is true that in many cases, contraception and even abortion are practiced under the pressure of real-life difficulties, which nonetheless can never exonerate from striving to observe God's law fully. Still, in very many other instances such practices are rooted in a hedonistic mentality unwilling to accept responsibility in matters of sexuality, and they imply a self-centered concept of freedom which regards procreation as an obstacle to personal fulfillment. The life which could result from a sexual encounter thus becomes an enemy to be avoided at all costs, and abortion becomes the only possible decisive response to failed contraception.

The close connection which exists, in mentality, between the practice of contraception and that of abortion is becoming increasingly obvious. It is being demonstrated in an alarming way by the development of chemical products, intrauterine devices, and vaccines which, distributed with the same ease as contraceptives, really act as abortifacients in the very early stages of the development of the life of the new human being.

14. The various *techniques of artificial reproduction*, which would seem to be at the service of life and which are frequently used with this intention, actually open the door to new threats against life. Apart from the fact that they are morally unacceptable, since they separate procreation from the fully human context of the conjugal act,[14] these techniques have a high rate of failure: not just failure in relation to fertilization but with regard to the subsequent development of the embryo, which is exposed to the risk of death, generally within a very short space of time. Furthermore, the number of embryos produced is often greater than that needed for implantation in the woman's womb, and these so-called "spare embryos" are then destroyed or used for research which, under the pretext of scientific or medical progress, in fact reduces human life to the level of simple "biological material" to be freely disposed of.

Prenatal diagnosis, which presents no moral objections if carried out in order to identify the medical treatment which may be needed by the child in the womb, all too often becomes an opportunity for proposing and procuring an abortion. This is eugenic abortion, justified in public opinion on the basis of a mentality—mistakenly held to be consistent with the demands of "therapeutic interventions"—which accepts life only under certain conditions and rejects it when it is affected by any limitation, handicap, or illness.

Following this same logic, the point has been reached where the most basic care, even nourishment, is denied to babies born with serious handicaps or illnesses. The contemporary scene, moreover, is becoming even more alarming by reason of the proposals, advanced here and there, to justify even infanticide, following the same arguments used to justify the right to abortion. In this way, we revert to a state of barbarism which one hoped had been left behind forever.

15. Threats which are no less serious hang over the *incurably ill* and the *dying*. In a social and cultural context which makes it more difficult to face and accept suffering, the *temptation* becomes all the greater *to resolve the problem of suffering by eliminating it at the root*, by hastening death so that it occurs at the moment considered most suitable.

Various considerations usually contribute to such a decision, all of which converge in the same terrible outcome. In the sick person, the sense of anguish, of severe discomfort, and even of desperation brought on by intense and prolonged suffering can be a decisive factor. Such a situation can threaten the already fragile equilibrium of an individual's personal and family life, with the result that, on the one hand, the sick person, despite the help of increasingly effective medical and social assistance, risks feeling overwhelmed by his or her own frailty; and on the other hand, those close to the sick person can be moved by an understandable even if misplaced compassion. All this is aggravated by a cultural climate which fails to perceive any meaning or value in suffering, but rather considers suffering the epitome of evil, to be eliminated at all costs. This is especially the case in the absence of a religious outlook which could help to provide a positive understanding of the mystery of suffering.

On a more general level, there exists in contemporary culture a certain Promethean attitude which leads people to think that they can control life and death by taking the decisions about them into their own hands. What really happens in this case is that the individual is overcome and crushed by a death deprived of any prospect of meaning or hope. We see a tragic expression of all this in the spread of *euthanasia—disguised* and surreptitious, or practiced openly and even legally. As well as for reasons of a misguided pity at the sight of the patient's suffering, euthanasia is sometimes justified by the utilitarian motive of avoiding costs which bring no return and which weigh heavily on society. Thus it is proposed to eliminate malformed babies, the severely handicapped, the disabled, the elderly, especially when they are not self-sufficient, and the terminally ill. Nor can we remain silent in the face of other more furtive, but no less serious and real, forms of euthanasia. These could occur for example when, in order to increase the availability of organs for transplants, organs are removed without respecting objective and adequate criteria which verify the death of the donor.

16. Another present-day phenomenon, frequently used to justify threats and attacks against life, is the *demographic* question. This question arises in different ways in different parts of the world. In the rich and developed countries there is a disturbing decline or collapse of the birthrate. The poorer countries, on the other hand, generally have a high rate of population growth, difficult to sustain in the context of low economic and social development, and especially where there is extreme underdevelopment. In the face of overpopulation in the poorer countries, instead of forms of global intervention at the international level—serious family and social policies, programs of cultural development and of fair production and distribution of resources—anti-birth policies continue to be enacted.

Contraception, sterilization, and abortion are certainly part of the reason why, in some cases, there is a sharp decline in the birthrate. It is not difficult to be tempted to use the same methods and attacks against life also where there is a situation of "demographic explosion."

The Pharaoh of old, haunted by the presence and increase of the children of Israel, submitted them to every kind of oppression and ordered that every male child born of the Hebrew women was to be killed (cf. Exod. 1:7–22). Today not a few of the powerful of the earth act in the same way. They too are haunted by the current demographic growth and fear that the most prolific and poorest peoples represent a threat for the well-being and peace of their own countries. Consequently, rather than wishing to face and solve these serious problems with respect for the dignity of individuals and families and for every person's inviolable right to life, they prefer to promote and impose by whatever means a massive program of birth control. Even the economic help which they would be ready to give is unjustly made conditional on the acceptance of an anti-birth policy.

17. Humanity today offers us a truly alarming spectacle, if we consider not only how extensively attacks on life are spreading but also their unheard-of numerical proportion and the fact that they receive widespread and powerful support from a broad consensus on the part of society, from widespread legal approval and the involvement of certain sectors of health-care personnel.

As I emphatically stated at Denver, on the occasion of the Eighth World Youth Day, "with time the threats against life have not grown weaker. They are taking on vast proportions. They are not only threats coming from the outside, from the forces of nature or the 'Cains' who kill the 'Abels'; no, they are *scientifically and systematically programmed threats*. The twentieth century will have been an era of massive attacks on life, an endless series of wars and a continual taking of innocent human life. False prophets and false teachers have had the greatest success."[15] Aside from intentions, which can be varied and perhaps can seem convincing at times, especially if presented in the name of solidarity, we are in fact faced by an objective "*conspiracy against life*," involving even international institutions, engaged in encouraging and carrying out actual campaigns to make contraception, sterilization, and abortion widely available. Nor can it be denied that the mass media are often implicated in this conspiracy, by lending credit to that culture which presents recourse to contraception, sterilization, abortion, and even euthanasia as a mark of progress and a victory of freedom, while depicting as enemies of freedom and progress those positions which are unreservedly pro-life.

"Am I my brother's keeper?" (Gen. 4:9):
A Perverse Idea of Freedom

18. The panorama described needs to be understood not only in terms of the phenomena of death which characterize it but also in the *variety of causes* which determine it. The Lord's question: "What have you done?" (Gen. 4:10), seems almost like an invitation addressed to Cain to go beyond the material dimension of his murderous gesture, in order to recognize in it all the gravity of the *motives* which occasioned it and the *consequences* which result from it.

Decisions that go against life sometimes arise from difficult or even tragic situations of profound suffering, loneliness, a total lack of economic prospects, depression, and anxiety about the future. Such circumstances can mitigate even to a notable degree subjective responsibility and the consequent culpability of those who make these choices which in themselves are evil. But today the problem goes far beyond the necessary recognition of these personal situations. It is a problem which exists at the cultural, social, and political level, where it reveals its more sinister and disturbing aspect in the tendency, ever more widely shared, to interpret the above crimes against life as *legitimate expressions of individual freedom, to be acknowledged and protected as actual rights.*

In this way, and with tragic consequences, a long historical process is reaching a turning-point. The process which once led to discovering the idea of "human rights"—rights inherent in every person and prior to any Constitution and State legislation—is today marked by a *surprising contradiction.* Precisely in an age when the inviolable rights of the person are solemnly proclaimed and the value of life is publicly affirmed, the very right to life is being denied or trampled upon, especially at the more significant moments of existence: the moment of birth and the moment of death.

On the one hand, the various declarations of human rights and the many initiatives inspired by these declarations show that at the global level there is a growing moral sensitivity, more alert to acknowledging the value and dignity of every individual as a human being, without any distinction of race, nationality, religion, political opinion, or social class.

On the other hand, these noble proclamations are unfortunately contradicted by a tragic repudiation of them in practice. This denial is still more distressing, indeed more scandalous, precisely because it is occurring in a society which makes the affirmation and protection of human rights its primary objective and its boast. How can these repeated affirmations of principle be reconciled with the continual increase and widespread justification of attacks on human life? How can we reconcile these declarations with the refusal to accept those who are weak and needy, or elderly, or those who have just been conceived? These attacks go directly against respect for life and they *represent a direct threat to the entire culture of human rights*. It is a threat capable, in the end, of jeopardizing the very meaning of democratic coexistence: *rather than societies of "people living together," our cities risk becoming societies of people who are rejected*, marginalized, uprooted, and oppressed. If we then look at the wider worldwide perspective, how can we fail to think that the very affirmation of the rights of individuals and peoples made in distinguished international assemblies is a merely futile exercise of rhetoric, if we fail to unmask the selfishness of the rich countries which exclude poorer countries from access to development or make such access dependent on arbitrary prohibitions against procreation, setting up an opposition between development and man himself? Should we not question the very economic models often adopted by States which, also as a result of international pressures and forms of conditioning, cause and aggravate situations of injustice and violence in which the life of whole peoples is degraded and trampled upon?

19. What are *the roots of this remarkable contradiction*? We can find them in an overall assessment of a cultural and moral nature, beginning with the mentality which *carries the concept of subjectivity to an extreme* and even distorts it, and recognizes as a subject of rights only the person who enjoys full or at least incipient autonomy and who emerges from a state of total dependence on others. But how can we reconcile this approach with *the exaltation of man as a being who is "not to be used"*? The theory of human rights is based precisely on the affirmation that the human person, unlike animals and things, cannot be subjected to domination by others. We must also mention the mentality which tends to *equate personal dignity with the capacity for verbal and explicit*, or at least perceptible, *communication*. It is clear that on the basis of these presuppositions there is no place in the world for anyone who, like the unborn or the dying, is a weak element in the social structure, or for anyone who appears completely at the mercy of others and radically dependent on them, and can only communicate through the silent language of a profound sharing of affection. In this case it is force which becomes the criterion for choice and action in interpersonal relations and in social life. But this is the exact opposite of what a state ruled by law, as a community in which the "reasons of force" are replaced by the "force of reason," historically intended to affirm.

At another level, the roots of the contradiction between the solemn affirmation of human rights and their tragic denial in practice lies in a *notion of freedom* which exalts the isolated individual in an absolute way, and gives no place to solidarity, to openness to others and service of them. While it is true that the taking of life not yet born or in its final stages is sometimes marked by a mistaken sense of altruism and human compassion, it cannot be denied that such a culture of death, taken as a whole, betrays a completely individualistic concept of freedom, which ends up by becoming the freedom of "the strong" against the weak who have no choice but to submit.

It is precisely in this sense that Cain's answer to the Lord's question: "Where is Abel your brother?" can be interpreted: "I do not know; *am I my brother's keeper?*" (Gen. 4:9). Yes, every man is his "brother's keeper," because God entrusts us to one another. And it is also in view of this entrusting that God gives everyone freedom, a freedom which possesses an *inherently relational dimension*. This is a great gift of the Creator, placed as it is at the service of the person and of his fulfillment through the gift of self and openness to others; but when freedom is made absolute in an individualistic way, it is emptied of its original content, and its very meaning and dignity are contradicted.

There is an even more profound aspect which needs to be emphasized: freedom negates and destroys itself, and becomes a factor leading to the destruction of others, when it no longer recognizes and respects its *essential link with the truth*. When freedom, out of a desire to emancipate itself from all forms of tradition and authority, shuts out even the most obvious evidence of an objective and universal truth, which is the foundation of personal and social life, then the person ends up by no longer taking as the sole and indisputable point of reference for his own choices the truth about good and evil, but only his subjective and changeable opinion or, indeed, his selfish interest and whim.

20. This view of freedom *leads to a serious distortion of life in society*. If the promotion of the self is understood in terms of absolute autonomy, people inevitably reach the point of rejecting one another. Everyone else is considered an enemy from whom one has to defend oneself. Thus society becomes a mass of individuals placed side by side, but without any mutual bonds. Each one wishes to assert himself independently of the other and in fact intends to make his own interests prevail. Still, in the face of other people's analogous interests, some kind of compromise must be found, if one wants a society in which the maximum possible freedom is guaranteed to each individual. In this way, any reference to common values and to a truth absolutely binding on everyone is lost, and social life ventures onto the shifting sands of complete relativism. At that point, *everything is negotiable, everything is open to bargaining*: even the first of the fundamental rights, the right to life.

This is what is happening also at the level of politics and government: the original and inalienable right to life is questioned or denied on the basis of a parliamentary vote or the will of one part of the people—even if it is the majority. This is the sinister result of a relativism which reigns unopposed: the "right" ceases to be such, because it is no longer firmly founded on the inviolable dignity of the person, but is made subject to the will of the stronger part. In this way democracy, contradicting its own principles, effectively moves towards a form of totalitarianism. The state is no longer the "common home" where all can live together on the basis of principles of fundamental equality, but is transformed into a *tyrant state*, which arrogates to itself the right to dispose of the life of the weakest and most defenseless members, from the unborn child to the elderly, in the name of a public interest which is really nothing but the interest of one part. The appearance of the strictest respect for legality is maintained, at least when the laws permitting abortion and euthanasia are the result of a ballot in accordance with what are generally seen as the rules of democracy. Really, what we have here is only the tragic caricature of legality; the democratic ideal, which is only truly such when it acknowledges and safeguards the dignity of every human person, *is betrayed in its very foundations*: "How is it still possible to speak of the dignity of every human person when the killing of the weakest and most innocent is permitted? In the name of what justice is the most unjust of discriminations practiced: some individuals are held to be deserving of defense and others are denied that dignity?"[16] When this happens, the process leading to the breakdown of a genuinely human co-existence and the disintegration of the State itself has already begun.

To claim the right to abortion, infanticide, and euthanasia, and to recognize that right in law, means to attribute to human freedom a *perverse* and *evil significance*: that of an *absolute power over others and against others*. This is the death of true freedom: "Truly, truly, I say to you, every one who commits sin is a slave to sin" (John 8:34).

"And from your face I shall be hidden" (Gen. 4:14):
The Eclipse of the Sense of God and of Man

21. In seeking the deepest roots of the struggle between the "culture of life" and the "culture of death," we cannot restrict ourselves to the perverse idea of freedom mentioned above. We have to go to the heart of the tragedy being experienced by modern man: *the eclipse of the sense of God and of man*, typical of a social and cultural climate dominated by secularism, which, with its ubiquitous tentacles, succeeds at times in putting Christian communities themselves to the test. Those who allow themselves to be influenced by this climate easily fall into a sad, vicious circle: *when the sense of God is lost, there is also a tendency to lose the sense of man*, of his dignity and his life; in turn, the systematic violation of the moral law, especially in the serious matter of respect for human life and its dignity, produces a kind of progressive darkening of the capacity to discern God's living and saving presence.

Once again we can gain insight from the story of Abel's murder by his brother. After the curse imposed on him by God, Cain thus addresses the Lord: "My punishment is greater than

I can bear. Behold, you have driven me this day away from the ground; and *from your face I shall be hidden*, and I shall be a fugitive and wanderer on the earth, and whoever finds me will slay me" (Gen. 4:13–14). Cain is convinced that his sin will not obtain pardon from the Lord and that his inescapable destiny will be to have to "hide his face" from Him. If Cain is capable of confessing that his fault is "greater than he can bear," it is because he is conscious of being in the presence of God and before God's just judgment. It is really only before the Lord that man can admit his sin and recognize its full seriousness. Such was the experience of David who, after "having committed evil in the sight of the Lord," and being rebuked by the Prophet Nathan, exclaimed: "My offenses truly I know them; my sin is always before me. Against you, you alone, have I sinned; what is evil in your sight I have done" (Ps. 51:5–6).

22. Consequently, when the sense of God is lost, the sense of man is also threatened and poisoned, as the Second Vatican Council concisely states: "Without the Creator the creature would disappear. ... But when God is forgotten the creature itself grows unintelligible." [17] Man is no longer able to see himself as "mysteriously different" from other earthly creatures; he regards himself merely as one more living being, as an organism which, at most, has reached a very high stage of perfection. Enclosed in the narrow horizon of his physical nature, he is somehow reduced to being "a thing," and no longer grasps the "transcendent" character of his "existence as man." He no longer considers life as a splendid gift of God, something "sacred" entrusted to his responsibility and thus also to his loving care and "veneration." Life itself becomes a mere "thing," which man claims as his exclusive property, completely subject to his control and manipulation.

Thus, in relation to life at birth or at death, man is no longer capable of posing the question of the truest meaning of his own existence, nor can he assimilate with genuine freedom these crucial moments of his own history. He is concerned only with "doing," and, using all kinds of technology, he busies himself with programming, controlling, and dominating birth and death. Birth and death, instead of being primary experiences demanding to be "lived," become things to be merely "possessed" or "rejected."

Moreover, once all reference to God has been removed, it is not surprising that the meaning of everything else becomes profoundly distorted. Nature itself, from being "*mater*" (mother), is now reduced to being "matter," and is subjected to every kind of manipulation. This is the direction in which a certain technical and scientific way of thinking, prevalent in present-day culture, appears to be leading when it rejects the very idea that there is a truth of creation which must be acknowledged or a plan of God for life which must be respected. Something similar happens when concern about the consequences of such a "freedom without law" leads some people to the opposite position of a "law without freedom,"

as for example in ideologies which consider it unlawful to interfere in any way with nature, practically "divinizing" it. Again, this is a misunderstanding of nature's dependence on the plan of the Creator. Thus it is clear that the loss of contact with God's wise design is the deepest root of modern man's confusion, both when this loss leads to a freedom without rules and when it leaves man in "fear" of his freedom.

By living "as if God did not exist," man not only loses sight of the mystery of God, but also of the mystery of the world and the mystery of his own being.

23. The eclipse of the sense of God and of man inevitably leads to a *practical materialism*, which breeds individualism, utilitarianism, and hedonism. Here too we see the permanent validity of the words of the Apostle: "And since they did not see fit to acknowledge God, God gave them up to a base mind and to improper conduct" (Rom. 1:28). The values of *being* are replaced by those of *having*. The only goal which counts is the pursuit of one's own material well-being. The so-called "quality of life" is interpreted primarily or exclusively as economic efficiency, inordinate consumerism, physical beauty, and pleasure, to the neglect of the more profound dimensions—interpersonal, spiritual, and religious—of existence.

In such a context, *suffering*, an inescapable burden of human existence but also a factor of possible personal growth, is "censored," rejected as useless, indeed opposed as an evil, always and in every way to be avoided. When it cannot be avoided and the prospect of even some future well-being vanishes, then life appears to have lost all meaning and the temptation grows in man to claim the right to suppress it.

Within this same cultural climate, the *body* is no longer perceived as a properly personal reality, a sign and place of relations with others, with God, and with the world. It is reduced to pure materiality: it is simply a complex of organs, functions, and energies to be used according to the sole criteria of pleasure and efficiency. Consequently, *sexuality* too is depersonalized and exploited: from being the sign, place, and language of love, that is, of the gift of self and acceptance of another, in all the other's richness as a person, it increasingly becomes the occasion and instrument for self-assertion and the selfish satisfaction of personal desires and instincts. Thus the original import of human sexuality is distorted and falsified, and the two meanings, unitive and procreative, inherent in the very nature of the conjugal act, are artificially separated: in this way the marriage union is betrayed and its fruitfulness is subjected to the caprice of the couple. *Procreation* then becomes the "enemy" to be avoided in sexual activity: if it is welcomed, this is only because it expresses a desire, or indeed the intention, to have a child "at all costs," and not because it signifies the complete acceptance of the other and therefore an openness to the richness of life which the child represents.

In the materialistic perspective described so far, *interpersonal relations are seriously impoverished.* The first to be harmed are women, children, the sick or suffering, and the elderly. The criterion of personal dignity—which demands respect, generosity, and service—is replaced by the criterion of efficiency, functionality, and usefulness: others are considered not for what they "are," but for what they "have, do, and produce." This is the supremacy of the strong over the weak.

24. *It is at the heart of the moral conscience* that the eclipse of the sense of God and of man, with all its various and deadly consequences for life, is taking place. It is a question, above all, of the *individual* conscience, as it stands before God in its singleness and uniqueness.[18] But it is also a question, in a certain sense, of the "moral conscience" *of society*: in a way it too is responsible, not only because it tolerates or fosters behavior contrary to life, but also because it encourages the "culture of death," creating and consolidating actual "structures of sin" which go against life. The moral conscience, both individual and social, is today subjected, also as a result of the penetrating influence of the media, to *an extremely serious and mortal danger*: that of *confusion between good and evil*, precisely in relation to the fundamental right to life. A large part of contemporary society looks sadly like that humanity which Paul describes in his Letter to the Romans. It is composed "of men who by their wickedness suppress the truth" (1:18): having denied God and believing that they can build the earthly city without Him, "they became futile in their thinking" so that "their senseless minds were darkened" (1:21); "claiming to be wise, they became fools" (1:22), carrying out works deserving of death, and "they not only do them but approve those who practice them" (1:32). When conscience, this bright lamp of the soul (cf. Matt. 6:22–23), calls "evil good and good evil" (Isa. 5:20), it is already on the path to the most alarming corruption and the darkest moral blindness.

And yet all the conditioning and efforts to enforce silence fail to stifle the voice of the Lord echoing in the conscience of every individual: it is always from this intimate sanctuary of the conscience that a new journey of love, openness, and service to human life can begin.

"You have come to the sprinkled blood"
(cf. Heb 12: 22, 24):
Signs of Hope and Invitation to Commitment

25. ... The blood of Christ, while it reveals the grandeur of the Father's love, *shows how precious man is in God's eyes and how priceless the value of his life*. The Apostle Peter reminds us of this: "You know that you were ransomed from the futile ways inherited from your fathers, not with perishable things such as silver or gold, but with the precious blood of Christ, like that of a lamb without blemish or spot" (1 Peter 1:18–19). Precisely by contemplating the precious blood of Christ, the sign of his self-giving love (cf. John 13:1), the believer learns to recognize and appreciate the almost divine dignity of every human being and can exclaim with ever renewed and grateful wonder: "How precious must man be in the eyes of the Creator, if he 'gained so great a Redeemer' (*Exsultet* of the Easter Vigil), and if God 'gave his only Son' in order that man 'should not perish but have eternal life!'" (cf. John 3:16).[20]

Furthermore, Christ's blood reveals to man that his greatness, and therefore his vocation, consists in *the sincere gift of self*. Precisely because it is poured out as the gift of life, the blood of Christ is no longer a sign of death, of definitive separation from the brethren, but the instrument of a communion which is richness of life for all. Whoever in the Sacrament of the Eucharist drinks this blood and abides in Jesus (cf. John 6:56) is drawn into the dynamism of his love and gift of life, in order to bring to its fullness the original vocation to love which belongs to everyone (cf. Gen. 1:27; 2:18–24).

It is from the blood of Christ that all draw *the strength to commit themselves to promoting life*. It is precisely this blood that is *the most powerful source of hope, indeed it is the foundation of the absolute certitude that in God's plan life will be victorious*. "And death shall be no more," exclaims the powerful voice which comes from the throne of God in the Heavenly Jerusalem (Rev. 21:4). And Saint Paul assures us that the present victory over sin is a sign and anticipation of the definitive victory over death, when there "shall come to pass the saying that is written: 'Death is swallowed up in victory.' 'O death, where is your victory? O death, where is your sting?'" (1 Cor. 15:54–55)

26. In effect, signs which point to this victory are not lacking in our societies and cultures, strongly marked though they are by the "culture of death." It would therefore be to give a one-sided picture, which could lead to sterile discouragement, if the condemnation of the threats to life were not accompanied by the presentation of the *positive signs* at work in humanity's present situation.

Unfortunately it is often hard to see and recognize these positive signs, perhaps also because they do not receive sufficient attention in the communications media. Yet, how many initiatives of help and support for people who are weak and defenseless have sprung up and continue to spring up in the Christian community and in civil society, at the local, national, and international levels, through the efforts of individuals, groups, movements, and organizations of various kinds!

There are still many *married couples* who, with a generous sense of responsibility, are ready to accept children as "the supreme gift of marriage."[21] Nor is there a lack of *families* which, over and above their everyday service to life, are willing to accept abandoned children, boys and girls and teenagers in difficulty, handicapped persons, elderly men and women who have been left alone. Many *centers in support of life*, or similar institutions, are sponsored by individuals and groups which, with admirable dedication and sacrifice, offer moral and material support to mothers who are in difficulty and are tempted to have recourse to abortion. Increasingly, there are appearing in many places *groups of volunteers* prepared to offer hospitality to persons without a family, who find themselves in conditions of particular distress or who need a supportive environment to help them to overcome destructive habits and discover anew the meaning of life.

Medical science, thanks to the committed efforts of researchers and practitioners, continues in its efforts to discover ever more effective remedies: treatments which were once inconceivable but which now offer much promise for the future are today being developed for the unborn, the suffering, and those in an acute or terminal stage of sickness. Various agencies and organizations are mobilizing their efforts to bring the benefits of the most advanced medicine to countries most afflicted by poverty and endemic diseases. In a similar way national and international associations of physicians are being organized to bring quick relief to peoples affected by natural disasters, epidemics, or wars. Even if a just international distribution of medical resources is still far from being a reality, how can we not recognize in the steps taken so far the sign of a growing solidarity among peoples, a praiseworthy human and moral sensitivity and a greater respect for life?

27. In view of laws which permit abortion and in view of efforts, which here and there have been successful, to legalize euthanasia, *movements and initiatives to raise social awareness in defense of life* have sprung up in many parts of the world. When, in accordance with their principles, such movements act resolutely, but without resorting to violence, they promote a wider and more profound consciousness of the value of life, and evoke and bring about a more determined commitment to its defense.

Furthermore, how can we fail to mention *all those daily gestures of openness, sacrifice, and unselfish care* which countless people lovingly make in families, hospitals, orphanages, homes for the elderly, and other centers or communities which defend life? Allowing herself to be guided by the example of Jesus the "Good Samaritan" (cf. Luke 10:29–37) and upheld by his strength, the Church has always been in the front line in providing charitable help: so many of her sons and daughters, especially men and women religious, in traditional and ever new forms, have consecrated and continue to consecrate their lives to God, freely giving of themselves out of love for their neighbor, especially for the weak and needy. These deeds strengthen the bases of the "civilization of love and life," without which the life of individuals and of society itself loses its most genuinely human quality. Even if they go unnoticed and remain hidden to most people, faith assures us that the Father "who sees in secret" (Matt. 6:6) not only will reward these actions but already here and now makes them produce lasting fruit for the good of all.

… Another welcome sign is the growing attention being paid to the *quality of life* and to *ecology*, especially in more developed societies, where people's expectations are no longer

concentrated so much on problems of survival as on the search for an overall improvement of living conditions. Especially significant is the reawakening of an ethical reflection on issues affecting life. The emergence and ever more widespread development of bioethics is promoting more reflection and dialogue—between believers and non-believers, as well as between followers of different religions—on ethical problems, including fundamental issues pertaining to human life.

28. This situation, with its lights and shadows, ought to make us all fully aware that we are facing an enormous and dramatic clash between good and evil, death and life, the "culture of death" and the "culture of life." We find ourselves not only "faced with" but necessarily "in the midst of" this conflict: we are all involved, and we all share in it, with the inescapable responsibility of *choosing to be unconditionally pro-life*.

… The unconditional choice for life reaches its full religious and moral meaning when it flows from, is formed by and nourished by *faith in Christ*. Nothing helps us so much to face positively the conflict between death and life in which we are engaged as faith in the Son of God who became man and dwelt among men so "that they may have life, and have it abundantly" (John 10:10). It is a matter of *faith in the Risen Lord, who has conquered death*; faith in the blood of Christ "that speaks more graciously than the blood of Abel" (Heb. 12:24).

With the light and strength of this faith, therefore, in facing the challenges of the present situation, the Church is becoming more aware of the grace and responsibility which come to her from her Lord of proclaiming, celebrating, and serving *the Gospel of life*.

Chapter II
I Came That They May Have Life:
The Christian Message Concerning Life

"The life was made manifest, and we saw it" (1 John 1:2): With Our Gaze Fixed on Christ, "The Word of Life"

29. Faced with the countless grave threats to life present in the modern world, one could feel overwhelmed by sheer powerlessness: good can never be powerful enough to triumph over evil!

At such times the People of God, and this includes every believer, is called to profess with humility and courage its faith in Jesus Christ, "the Word of life" (1 John 1:1). The *Gospel of life* is not simply a reflection, however new and profound, on human life. Nor is it merely a commandment aimed at raising awareness and bringing about significant changes in society. Still less is it an illusory promise of a better future. The *Gospel of life* is something concrete and personal, for it consists in the proclamation of *the very person of Jesus*. Jesus made himself known to the Apostle Thomas, and in him to every person, with the words: "I am the way, and the truth, and the life" (John 14:6). This is also how he spoke of himself to

Martha, the sister of Lazarus: "I am the resurrection and the life; he who believes in me, though he die, yet shall he live, and whoever lives and believes in me shall never die" (John 11:25–26). Jesus is the Son who from all eternity receives life from the Father (cf. John 5:26), and who has come among men to make them sharers in this gift: "I came that they may have life, and have it abundantly" (John 10:10).

Through the words, the actions, and the very person of Jesus, man is given the possibility of "knowing" *the complete truth* concerning the value of human life. From this "source" he receives, in particular, the capacity to "accomplish" this truth perfectly (cf. John 3:21), that is, to accept and fulfill completely the responsibility of loving and serving, of defending and promoting human life. In Christ, *the Gospel of life* is definitively proclaimed and fully given …

30. … In Jesus, the "Word of life," God's eternal life is thus proclaimed and given. Thanks to this proclamation and gift, our physical and spiritual life, also in its earthly phase, acquires its full value and meaning, for God's eternal life is in fact the end to which our living in this world is directed and called. In this way the *Gospel of life* includes everything that human experience and reason tell us about the value of human life, accepting it, purifying it, exalting it, and bringing it to fulfillment. …

"The name of Jesus … has made this man strong" (Acts 3:16): In the Uncertainties of Human Life, Jesus Brings Life's Meaning to Fulfilment

32. … The words and deeds of Jesus and those of his Church are not meant only for those who are sick or suffering or in some way neglected by society. On a deeper level, they affect *the very meaning of every person's life in its moral and spiritual dimensions.* Only those who recognize that their life is marked by the evil of sin can discover in an encounter with Jesus the Savior the truth and the authenticity of their own existence. Jesus himself says as much: "Those who are well have no need of a physician, but those who are sick; I have not come to call the righteous, but sinners to repentance" (Luke 5:31–32). …

33. … Life's contradictions and risks were fully accepted by Jesus: "though he was rich, yet for your sake he became poor, so that by his poverty you might become rich" (2 Cor. 8:9). The poverty of which Paul speaks is not only a stripping of divine privileges, but also a sharing in the lowliest and most vulnerable conditions of human life (cf. Phil. 2:6–7). Jesus lived this poverty throughout his life, until the culminating moment of the Cross: "he humbled himself and became obedient unto death, even death on a cross. Therefore God has highly exalted him and bestowed on him the name which is above every name" (Phil. 2:8–9). It is precisely *by his death that Jesus reveals all the splendor and value of life*, inasmuch as his self-oblation on the cross becomes the source of new life for all people (cf. John 12:32). In his journeying amid contradictions and in the very loss of his life, Jesus is guided by the certainty that his life is in the hands of the Father. Consequently, on the Cross, he can say to Him: "Father, into your hands I commend my spirit!" (Luke 23:46), that is, my life. Truly great must be the value of human life if the Son of God has taken it up and made it the instrument of the salvation of all humanity!

"Called … to be conformed to the image of his Son" (Rom. 8:28–29): God's Glory Shines on the Face of Man

34. Life is always a good. This is an instinctive perception and a fact of experience, and man is called to grasp the profound reason why this is so.

Why is life a good? This question is found everywhere in the Bible, and from the very first pages it receives a powerful and amazing answer. The life which God gives man is quite different from the life of all other living creatures, inasmuch as man, although formed from the dust of the earth (cf. Gen. 2:7, 3:19; Job 34:15; Pss. 103:14; 104:29), *is a manifestation of God in the world, a sign of his presence, a trace of his glory* (cf. Gen. 1:26–27; Ps. 8:6). This is what Saint Irenaeus of Lyons wanted to emphasize in his celebrated definition: "Man, living man, is the glory of God."[23] Man has been given a *sublime dignity*, based on the intimate bond which unites him to his Creator: in man there shines forth a reflection of God Himself. …

36. … The plan of life given to the first Adam finds at last its fulfillment in Christ. Whereas the disobedience of Adam had ruined and marred God's plan for human life and introduced death into the world, the redemptive obedience of Christ is the source of grace poured out upon the human race, opening wide to everyone the gates of the kingdom of life (cf. Rom. 5:12–21). As the Apostle Paul states: "The first man Adam became a living being; the last Adam became a life-giving spirit" (1 Cor. 15:45).

All who commit themselves to following Christ are given the fullness of life: the divine image is restored, renewed, and brought to perfection in them. God's plan for human beings is this, that they should "be conformed to the image of his Son" (Rom. 8:29). Only thus, in the splendor of this image, can man be freed from the slavery of idolatry, rebuild lost fellowship, and rediscover his true identity. …

38. Eternal life is therefore the life of God Himself and at the same time the *life of the children of God.* As they ponder this unexpected and inexpressible truth which comes to us from God in Christ, believers cannot fail to be filled with ever new wonder and unbounded gratitude. They can say in the words of the Apostle John: "See what love the Father has given us, that we should be called children of God; and so we are. … Beloved, we are God's children now; it does not yet appear what we shall be, but we know that when he appears we shall be like him, for we shall see him as he is" (1 John 3:1–2).

Here the Christian truth about life becomes most sublime. The dignity of this life is linked not only to its beginning, to the fact that it comes from God, but also to its final end, to its destiny of fellowship with God in knowledge and love of him. In the light of this truth Saint Irenaeus qualifies and completes his praise of man: "the glory of God" is indeed, "man, living man," but "the life of man consists in the vision of God."[27]

Immediate consequences arise from this for human life in its *earthly state*, in which, for that matter, eternal life already springs forth and begins to grow. Although man instinctively loves life because it is a good, this love will find further inspiration and strength, and new breadth and depth, in the divine dimensions of this good. Similarly, the love which every human being has for life cannot be reduced simply to a desire to have sufficient space for self-expression and for entering into relationships with others; rather, it develops in a joyous awareness that life can become the "place" where God manifests Himself, where we meet Him and enter into communion with Him. The life which Jesus gives in no way lessens the value of our existence in time; it takes it and directs it to its final destiny: "I am the resurrection and the life. . . . Whoever lives and believes in me shall never die" (John 11:25–26).

"From man in regard to his fellow man,
I will demand an accounting" (Gen. 9:5):
Reverence and Love for Every Human Life

39. Man's life comes from God; it is his gift, his image and imprint, a sharing in his breath of life. God therefore *is the sole Lord of this life*: man cannot do with it as he wills. God Himself makes this clear to Noah after the flood: "For your own lifeblood, too, I will demand an accounting . . . and from man in regard to his fellow man I will demand an accounting for human life" (Gen. 9:5). The biblical text is concerned to emphasize how the sacredness of life has its foundation in God and in his creative activity: "For God made man in his own image" (Gen. 9:6).

Human life and death are thus in the hands of God, in his power: "In his hand is the life of every living thing and the breath of all mankind," exclaims Job (12:10). "The Lord brings to death and brings to life; He brings down to Sheol and raises up" (1 Sam. 2:6). He alone can say: "It is I who bring both death and life" (Deut. 32:39).

But God does not exercise this power in an arbitrary and threatening way, but rather as part of his *care and loving concern for his creatures*. If it is true that human life is in the hands of God, it is no less true that these are loving hands, like those of a mother who accepts, nurtures, and takes care of her child: "I have calmed and quieted my soul, like a child quieted at its mother's breast; like a child that is quieted is my soul" (Ps. 131:2; cf. Isa. 49:15; 66:12–13; Hos. 11:4). Thus Israel does not see in the history of peoples and in the destiny of individuals the outcome of mere chance or of blind fate,

but rather the results of a loving plan by which God brings together all the possibilities of life and opposes the powers of death arising from sin: "God did not make death, and He does not delight in the death of the living. For He created all things that they might exist" (Wisd. 1:13–14).

40. The sacredness of life gives rise to its *inviolability, written from the beginning in man's heart*, in his conscience. The question: "What have you done?" (Gen. 4:10), which God addresses to Cain after he has killed his brother Abel, interprets the experience of every person: in the depths of his conscience, man is always reminded of the inviolability of life—his own life and that of others—as something which does not belong to him, because it is the property and gift of God the Creator and Father.

The commandment regarding the inviolability of human life reverberates *at the heart of the "ten words" in the covenant of Sinai* (cf. Exod. 34:28). In the first place that commandment prohibits murder: "You shall not kill" (Exod. 20:13); "do not slay the innocent and righteous" (Exod. 23:7). But, as is brought out in Israel's later legislation, it also prohibits all personal injury inflicted on another (cf. Exod. 21:12–27). Of course we must recognize that in the Old Testament this sense of the value of life, though already quite marked, does not yet reach the refinement found in the Sermon on the Mount. This is apparent in some aspects of the current penal legislation, which provided for severe forms of corporal punishment and even the death penalty. But the overall message, which the New Testament will bring to perfection, is a forceful appeal for respect for the inviolability of physical life and the integrity of the person. It culminates in the positive commandment which obliges us to be responsible for our neighbor as for ourselves: "You shall love your neighbor as yourself " (Lev. 19:18).

41. The commandment "You shall not kill," included and more fully expressed in the positive command of love for one's neighbor, is *reaffirmed in all its force by the Lord Jesus*. To the rich young man who asks him: "Teacher, what good deed must I do, to have eternal life?" Jesus replies: "If you would enter life, keep the commandments" (Matt. 19:16, 17). And he quotes, as the first of these: "You shall not kill" (Matt. 19:18). In the Sermon on the Mount, Jesus demands from his disciples a *righteousness which surpasses* that of the Scribes and Pharisees, also with regard to respect for life: "You have heard that it was said to the men of old, 'You shall not kill; and whoever kills shall be liable to judgment.' But I say to you that every one who is angry with his brother shall be liable to judgment" (Matt. 5:21–22).

By his words and actions, Jesus further unveils the positive requirements of the commandment regarding the inviolability of life. These requirements were already present in the Old Testament, where legislation dealt with protecting and defending life when it was weak and threatened: in the case of foreigners, widows, orphans, the sick, and the poor in general, including children in the womb (cf. Exod. 21:22; 22:20–26). With Jesus these positive requirements assume new force and urgency, and are revealed in all their breadth and depth: they range from caring for the life of one's *brother* (whether a blood brother, someone belonging to the same people, or a foreigner living in the land of Israel) to showing concern for the *stranger*, even to the point of loving one's *enemy*.

A stranger is no longer a stranger for the person who must *become a neighbor* to someone in need, to the point of accepting responsibility for his life, as the parable of the Good Samaritan shows so clearly (cf. Luke 10:25–37). Even an enemy ceases to be an enemy for the person who is obliged to love him (cf. Matt. 5:38–48; Luke 6:27–35), to "do good" to him (cf. Luke 6:27, 33, 35) and to respond to his immediate needs promptly and with no expectation of repayment (cf. Luke 6:34–35). The height of this love is to pray for one's enemy. By so doing we achieve harmony with the providential love of God: "But I say to you, love your enemies and pray for those who persecute you, so that you may be children of your Father who is in heaven; for He makes his sun rise on the evil and on the good and sends rain on the just and on the unjust" (Matt. 5:44–45; cf. Luke 6:28, 35).

Thus the deepest element of God's commandment to protect human life is the *requirement to show reverence and love* for every person and the life of every person. This is the teaching which the Apostle Paul, echoing the words of Jesus, addresses to the Christians in Rome: "The commandments, 'You shall not commit adultery, You shall not kill, You shall not steal, You shall not covet,' and any other commandment, are summed up in this sentence, '*You shall love your neighbor as yourself.*' Love does no wrong to a neighbor; therefore love is the fulfilling of the law" (Rom. 13:9–10).

"Be fruitful and multiply, and fill the earth and subdue it" (Gen 1:28): Man's Responsibility for Life

... 43. A certain sharing by man in God's lordship is also evident in the *specific responsibility* which he is given *for human life as such*. It is a responsibility which reaches its highest point in the giving of life *through procreation* by man and woman in marriage. As the Second Vatican Council teaches: "God Himself who said, 'It is not good for man to be alone' (Gen. 2:18) and 'who made man from the beginning male and female' (Matt. 19:4), wished to share with man a certain special participation in his own creative work. Thus he blessed male and female saying: 'Increase and multiply'" (Gen. 1:28). [30]

By speaking of "a certain special participation" of man and woman in the "creative work" of God, the council wishes to point out that having a child is an event which is deeply human and full of religious meaning, insofar as it involves both the spouses, who form "one flesh" (Gen. 2:24), and

God who makes Himself present. As I wrote in my *Letter to Families*: "When a new person is born of the conjugal union of the two, he brings with him into the world a particular image and likeness of God Himself: *the genealogy of the person is inscribed in the very biology of generation*. In affirming that the spouses, as parents, cooperate with God the Creator in conceiving and giving birth to a new human being, we are not speaking merely with reference to the laws of biology. Instead, we wish to emphasize that *God Himself is present in human fatherhood and motherhood* quite differently than He is present in all other instances of begetting 'on earth.' Indeed, God alone is the source of that 'image and likeness' which is proper to the human being, as it was received at Creation. Begetting is the continuation of Creation." [31]

This is what the Bible teaches in direct and eloquent language when it reports the joyful cry of the first woman, "the mother of all the living" (Gen. 3:20). Aware that God has intervened, Eve exclaims: "I have begotten a man with the help of the Lord" (Gen. 4:1). In procreation therefore, through the communication of life from parents to child, God's own image and likeness is transmitted, thanks to the creation of the immortal soul. [32] The beginning of the "book of the genealogy of Adam" expresses it in this way: "When God created man, He made him in the likeness of God. Male and female He created them, and He blessed them and called them man when they were created. When Adam had lived a hundred and thirty years, he became the father of a son in his own likeness, after his image, and named him Seth" (Gen. 5:1–3). It is precisely in their role as co-workers with God *who transmits his image to the new creature* that we see the greatness of couples who are ready "to cooperate with the love of the Creator and the Savior, who through them will enlarge and enrich his own family day by day." [33] This is why the bishop Amphilochius extolled "holy matrimony, chosen and elevated above all other earthly gifts" as "the begetter of humanity, the creator of images of God." [34]

Thus, a man and woman joined in matrimony become partners in a divine undertaking: through the act of procreation, God's gift is accepted and a new life opens to the future.

But over and above the specific mission of parents, *the task of accepting and serving life involves everyone; and this task must be fulfilled above all towards life when it is at its weakest*. It is Christ himself who reminds us of this when he asks to be loved and served in his brothers and sisters who are suffering in any way: the hungry, the thirsty, the foreigner, the naked, the sick, the imprisoned. ... Whatever is done to each of them is done to Christ himself (cf. Matt. 25:31–46).

"For you formed my inmost being" (Ps. 139:13): The Dignity of the Unborn Child

44. Human life finds itself most vulnerable when it enters the world and when it leaves the realm of time to embark upon eternity. The word of God frequently repeats the call to

show care and respect, above all where life is undermined by sickness and old age. Although there are no direct and explicit calls to protect human life at its very beginning, specifically life not yet born, and life nearing its end, this can easily be explained by the fact that the mere possibility of harming, attacking, or actually denying life in these circumstances is completely foreign to the religious and cultural way of thinking of the People of God.

In the Old Testament, sterility is dreaded as a curse, while numerous offspring are viewed as a blessing: "Sons are a heritage from the Lord, the fruit of the womb a reward" (Ps.127:3; cf. Ps. 128:3–4). This belief is also based on Israel's awareness of being the people of the Covenant, called to increase in accordance with the promise made to Abraham: "Look towards heaven, and number the stars, if you are able to number them, ... so shall your descendants be" (Gen. 15:5). But more than anything else, at work here is the certainty that the life which parents transmit has its origins in God. We see this attested in the many biblical passages which respectfully and lovingly speak of conception, of the forming of life in the mother's womb, of giving birth, and of the intimate connection between the initial moment of life and the action of God the Creator.

"Before I formed you in the womb I knew you, and before you were born I consecrated you" (Jer. 1:5): *the life of every individual, from its very beginning, is part of God's plan.* Job, from the depth of his pain, stops to contemplate the work of God who miraculously formed his body in his mother's womb. Here he finds reason for trust, and he expresses his belief that there is a divine plan for his life: "You have fashioned and made me; will you then turn and destroy me? Remember that you have made me of clay; and will you turn me to dust again? Did you not pour me out like milk and curdle me like cheese? You clothed me with skin and flesh, and knit me together with bones and sinews. You have granted me life and steadfast love; and your care has preserved my spirit" (Job 10:8–12). Expressions of awe and wonder at God's intervention in the life of a child in its mother's womb occur again and again in the Psalms.[35]

How can anyone think that even a single moment of this marvelous process of the unfolding of life could be separated from the wise and loving work of the Creator, and left prey to human caprice? Certainly the mother of the seven brothers did not think so; she professes her faith in God, both the source and guarantee of life from its very conception, and the foundation of the hope of new life beyond death: "I do not know how you came into being in my womb. It was not I who gave you life and breath, nor I who set in order the elements within each of you. Therefore the Creator of the world, who shaped the beginning of man and devised the origin of all things, will in his mercy give life and breath back to you again, since you now forget yourselves for the sake of his laws" (2 Macc. 7:22–23).

45. The New Testament revelation confirms the *indisputable recognition of the value of life from its very beginning.*

The exaltation of fruitfulness and the eager expectation of life resound in the words with which Elizabeth rejoices in her pregnancy: "The Lord has looked on me ... to take away my reproach among men" (Luke 1:25). And even more so, the value of the person from the moment of conception is celebrated in the meeting between the Virgin Mary and Elizabeth and between the two children whom they are carrying in the womb. It is precisely the children who reveal the advent of the Messianic age: in their meeting, the redemptive power of the presence of the Son of God among men first becomes operative. As Saint Ambrose writes: "The arrival of Mary and the blessings of the Lord's presence are also speedily declared. ... Elizabeth was the first to hear the voice; but John was the first to experience grace. She heard according to the order of nature; he leaped because of the mystery. She recognized the arrival of Mary; he the arrival of the Lord. The woman recognized the woman's arrival; the child, that of the child. The women speak of grace; the babies make it effective from within to the advantage of their mothers who, by a double miracle, prophesy under the inspiration of their children. The infant leaped, the mother was filled with the Spirit. The mother was not filled before the son, but after the son was filled with the Holy Spirit, he filled his mother too."[36]

"I kept my faith even when I said, 'I am greatly afflicted'" (Ps. 116:10): Life in Old Age and at Times of Suffering

46. With regard to the last moments of life too, it would be anachronistic to expect biblical revelation to make express reference to present-day issues concerning respect for elderly and sick persons, or to condemn explicitly attempts to hasten their end by force. The cultural and religious context of the Bible is in no way touched by such temptations; indeed, in that context the wisdom and experience of the elderly are recognized as a unique source of enrichment for the family and for society.

Old age is characterized by dignity and surrounded with reverence (cf. 2 Macc. 6:23). The just man does not seek to be delivered from old age and its burden; on the contrary his prayer is this: "You, O Lord, are my hope, my trust, O Lord, from my youth ... so even to old age and grey hairs, O God, do not forsake me, till I proclaim your might to all the generations to come" (Ps. 71:5, 18). The ideal of the Messianic age is presented as a time when "no more shall there be ... an old man who does not fill out his days" (Isa. 65:20).

In old age, how should one face the inevitable decline of life? *How should one act in the face of death? The believer knows that his life is in the hands of God:* "You, O Lord, hold my lot" (cf. Ps. 16:5), and he accepts from God the need to die: "This is the decree from the Lord for all flesh, and how can you reject the good pleasure of the Most High?" (Sir. 41:3–4). Man is not the master of life, nor is he the master of death. In life and in death, he has to entrust himself completely to the "good pleasure of the Most High," to his loving plan.

In moments of *sickness* too, man is called to have the same trust in the Lord and to renew his fundamental faith in the One who "heals all your diseases" (cf. Ps. 103:3). When every hope of good health seems to fade before a person's eyes—so as to make him cry out: "My days are like an evening shadow; I wither away like grass" (Ps. 102:11)—even then the believer is sustained by an unshakable faith in God's life-giving power. Illness does not drive such a person to despair and to seek death, but makes him cry out in hope: "I kept my faith, even when I said, 'I am greatly afflicted'" (Ps. 116:10); "O Lord my God, I cried to you for help, and you have healed me. O Lord, you have brought up my soul from Sheol, restored me to life from among those gone down to the pit" (Ps. 30:2–3).

47. The mission of Jesus, with the many healings he performed, shows *God's great concern even for man's bodily life*. Jesus, as "the physician of the body and of the spirit," [37] was sent by the Father to proclaim the good news to the poor and to heal the brokenhearted (cf. Luke 4:18; Isa. 61:1). Later, when he sends his disciples into the world, he gives them a mission, a mission in which healing the sick goes hand in hand with the proclamation of the Gospel: "And preach as you go, saying, 'The kingdom of heaven is at hand.' Heal the sick, raise the dead, cleanse lepers, cast out demons" (Matt. 10:7–8; cf. Mark 6:13; 16:18).

Certainly *the life of the body in its earthly state is not an absolute good* for the believer, especially as he may be asked to give up his life for a greater good. As Jesus says: "Whoever would save his life will lose it; and whoever loses his life for my sake and the gospel's will save it" (Mark 8:35). The New Testament gives many different examples of this. Jesus does not hesitate to sacrifice himself, and he freely makes of his life an offering to the Father (cf. John 10:17) and to those who belong to him (cf. John 10:15). The death of John the Baptist, precursor of the Savior, also testifies that earthly existence is not an absolute good; what is more important is remaining faithful to the word of the Lord even at the risk of one's life (cf. Mark 6:17–29). Stephen, losing his earthly life because of his faithful witness to the Lord's Resurrection, follows in the Master's footsteps and meets those who are stoning him with words of forgiveness (cf. Acts 7:59–60), thus becoming the first of a countless host of martyrs whom the Church has venerated since the very beginning.

No one, however, can arbitrarily choose whether to live or die; the absolute master of such a decision is the Creator alone, in whom "we live and move and have our being" (Acts 17:28).

"All who hold her fast will live" (Bar. 4:1):
From the Law of Sinai to the Gift of the Spirit

48. Life is indelibly marked by a truth of its own. By accepting God's gift, man is obliged to maintain life in this truth which is essential to it. To detach oneself from this truth is to condemn oneself to meaninglessness and unhappiness, and possibly to become a threat to the existence of others, since the barriers guaranteeing respect for life and the defense of life, in every circumstance, have been broken down.

The truth of life is revealed by God's commandment. The word of the Lord shows concretely the course which life must follow if it is to respect its own truth and to preserve its own dignity. The protection of life is not only ensured by the specific commandment "You shall not kill" (Exod. 20:13; Deut. 5:17); *the entire Law of the Lord* serves to protect life, because it reveals that truth in which life finds its full meaning.

It is not surprising, therefore, that God's Covenant with his people is so closely linked to the perspective of life, also in its body dimension. In that Covenant, God's *commandment* is offered as *the path of life*: "I have set before you this day life and good, death and evil. If you obey the commandments of the Lord your God which I command you this day, by loving the Lord your God, by walking in his ways, and by keeping his commandments and his statutes and his ordinances, then you shall live and multiply, and the Lord your God will bless you in the land which you are entering to take possession of" (Deut. 30:15–16). What is at stake is not only the land of Canaan and the existence of the people of Israel, but also the world of today and of the future, and the existence of all humanity. In fact, it is altogether impossible for life to remain authentic and complete once it is detached from the good; and the good, in its turn, is essentially bound to the commandments of the Lord, that is, to the "law of life" (Sir. 17:11). The good to be done is not added to life as a burden which weighs on it, since the very purpose of life is that good and only by doing it can life be built up.

It is thus *the Law as a whole* which fully protects human life. This explains why it is so hard to remain faithful to the commandment "You shall not kill" when the other "words of life" (cf. Acts 7:38) with which this commandment is bound up are not observed. Detached from this wider framework, the commandment is destined to become nothing more than an obligation imposed from without, and very soon we begin to look for its limits and try to find mitigating factors and exceptions. Only when people are open to the fullness of the truth about God, man, and history will the words "You shall not kill" shine forth once more as a good for man in himself and in his relations with others. In such a perspective we can grasp the full truth of the passage of the Book of Deuteronomy which Jesus repeats in reply to the first temptation: "Man does not live by bread alone, but . . . by everything that proceeds out of the mouth of the Lord" (Deut. 8:3; cf. Matt. 4:4).

It is by listening to the word of the Lord that we are able to live in dignity and justice. It is by observing the Law of God that we are able to bring forth fruits of life and happiness: "All who hold her fast will live, and those who forsake her will die" (Bar. 4:1).

…*"They shall look on him whom they have pierced" (John 19:37): The Gospel of Life Is Brought to Fulfillment on the Tree of the Cross*

50. At the end of this chapter, in which we have reflected on the Christian message about life, I would like to pause with each one of you to *contemplate the One who was pierced* and who draws all people to himself (cf. John 19:37; 12:32). Looking at "the spectacle" of the Cross (cf. Luke 23:48) we shall discover in this glorious tree the fulfillment and the complete revelation of the whole *Gospel of life*.

In the early afternoon of Good Friday, "there was darkness over the whole land … while the sun's light failed; and the curtain of the temple was torn in two" (Luke 23:44, 45). This is the symbol of a great cosmic disturbance and a massive conflict between the forces of good and the forces of evil, between life and death. Today, we too find ourselves in the midst of a dramatic conflict between the "culture of death" and the "culture of life." But the glory of the Cross is not overcome by this darkness; rather, it shines forth ever more radiantly and brightly, and is revealed as the center, meaning, and goal of all history and of every human life.

Jesus is nailed to the Cross and is lifted up from the earth. He experiences the moment of his greatest "powerlessness," and his life seems completely delivered to the derision of his adversaries and into the hands of his executioners: he is mocked, jeered at, insulted (cf. Mark 15:24–36). And yet, precisely amid all this, having seen him breathe his last, the Roman centurion exclaims: "Truly this man was the Son of God!" (Mark 15:39). It is thus, at the moment of his greatest weakness, that the Son of God is revealed for who he is: *on the Cross, his glory is made manifest.*

By his death, Jesus sheds light on the meaning of the life and death of every human being. Before he dies, Jesus prays to the Father, asking forgiveness for his persecutors (cf. Luke 23:34), and to the criminal who asks him to remember him in his kingdom he replies: "Truly, I say to you, today you will be with me in Paradise" (Luke 23:43). After his death "the tombs also were opened, and many bodies of the saints who had fallen asleep were raised" (Matt. 27:52). The salvation wrought by Jesus is the bestowal of life and resurrection. Throughout his earthly life, Jesus had indeed bestowed salvation by healing and doing good to all (cf. Acts 10:38). But his miracles, healings and even his raising of the dead were signs of another salvation, a salvation which consists in the forgiveness of sins, that is, in setting man free from his greatest sickness and in raising him to the very life of God.

On the Cross, the miracle of the serpent lifted up by Moses in the desert (John 3:14–15; cf. Num. 21:8–9) is renewed and brought to full and definitive perfection. Today too, by looking upon the one who was pierced, every person whose life is threatened encounters the sure hope of finding freedom and redemption. …

Chapter III
You Shall Not Kill: God's Holy Law

"If you would enter life, keep the commandments" (Matt. 19:17): Gospel and Commandment

52. "And behold, one came up to him, saying, 'Teacher, what good deed must I do, to have eternal life?'" (Matt. 19:6). Jesus replied, "If you would enter life, keep the commandments" (Matt. 19:17). The Teacher is speaking about eternal life, that is, a sharing in the life of God Himself. This life is attained through the observance of the Lord's commandments, including the commandment "You shall not kill." This is the first precept from the Decalogue which Jesus quotes to the young man who asks him what commandments he should observe: "Jesus said, 'You shall not kill, you shall not commit adultery, you shall not steal …'" (Matt. 19:18).

God's commandment is never detached from his love: it is always a gift meant for man's growth and joy. As such, it represents an essential and indispensable aspect of the Gospel, actually becoming "gospel" itself: joyful good news. The *Gospel of life* is both a great gift of God and an exacting task for humanity. It gives rise to amazement and gratitude in the person graced with freedom, and it asks to be welcomed, preserved, and esteemed, with a deep sense of responsibility. In giving life to man, God demands that he love, respect, and promote life. *The gift thus becomes a commandment, and the commandment is itself a gift.*

Man, as the living image of God, is willed by his Creator to be ruler and lord. Saint Gregory of Nyssa writes that "God made man capable of carrying out his role as king of the earth. … Man was created in the image of the One who governs the universe. Everything demonstrates that from the beginning man's nature was marked by royalty. … Man is a king. Created to exercise dominion over the world, he was given a likeness to the king of the universe; he is the living image who participates by his dignity in the perfection of the divine archetype."[38] Called to be fruitful and multiply, to subdue the earth, and to exercise dominion over other lesser creatures (cf. Gen. 1:28), man is ruler and lord not only over things but especially over himself,[39] and in a certain sense, over the life which he has received and which he is able to transmit through procreation, carried out with love and respect for God's plan. Man's *lordship* however is not absolute, but *ministerial*: it is a real reflection of the unique and infinite lordship of God. Hence man must exercise it with *wisdom and love*, sharing in the boundless wisdom and love of God. And this comes about through obedience to God's holy Law: a free and joyful obedience (cf. Ps. 119), born of and fostered by an awareness that the precepts of the Lord are a gift of grace entrusted to man always and solely for his good, for the preservation of his personal dignity, and the pursuit of his happiness.

With regard to things, but even more with regard to life, man is not the absolute master and final judge, but rather—and this is where his incomparable greatness lies—he is the "minister of God's plan."[40]

Life is entrusted to man as a treasure which must not be squandered, as a talent which must be used well. Man must render an account of it to his Master (cf. Matt. 25:14–30; Luke 19:12–27).

"From man in regard to his fellow man I will demand an accounting for human life" (Gen. 9:5): Human Life Is Sacred and Inviolable

53. "Human life is sacred because from its beginning it involves 'the creative action of God,' and it remains forever in a special relationship with the Creator, who is its sole end. God alone is the Lord of life from its beginning until its end: no one can, in any circumstance, claim for himself the right to destroy directly an innocent human being."[41] With these words the instruction *Donum vitae* sets forth the central content of God's revelation on the sacredness and inviolability of human life.

Sacred Scripture in fact presents the precept "You shall not kill" as a divine commandment (Exod. 20:13; Deut. 5:17). As I have already emphasized, this commandment is found in the Decalogue, at the heart of the Covenant which the Lord makes with his chosen people; but it was already contained in the original covenant between God and humanity after the purifying punishment of the Flood, caused by the spread of sin and violence (cf. Gen. 9:5–6).

God proclaims that He is absolute Lord of the life of man, who is formed in his image and likeness (cf. Gen. 1:26–28). Human life is thus given a sacred and inviolable character, which reflects the inviolability of the Creator Himself. Precisely for this reason God will severely judge every violation of the commandment "You shall not kill," the commandment which is at the basis of all life together in society. He is the "*goel*," the defender of the innocent (cf. Gen. 4:9–15; Isa. 41:14; Jer. 50:34; Ps. 19:14). God thus shows that he does not delight in the death of the living (cf. Wisd. 1:13). Only Satan can delight therein: for through his envy death entered the world (cf. Wisd. 2:24). He who is "a murderer from the beginning," is also "a liar and the father of lies" (John 8:44). By deceiving man, he leads him to projects of sin and death, making them appear as goals and fruits of life. ...

57. If such great care must be taken to respect every life, even that of criminals and unjust aggressors, the commandment "You shall not kill" has absolute value when it refers to the *innocent person*. And all the more so in the case of weak and defenseless human beings, who find their ultimate defense against the arrogance and caprice of others only in the absolute binding force of God's commandment.

In effect, the absolute inviolability of innocent human life is a moral truth clearly taught by Sacred Scripture, constantly upheld in the Church's Tradition and consistently proposed by her Magisterium. This consistent teaching is the evident result of that "supernatural sense of the faith" which, inspired and sustained by the Holy Spirit, safeguards the People of God from error when "it shows universal agreement in matters of faith and morals."[49]

Faced with the progressive weakening in individual consciences and in society of the sense of the absolute and grave moral illicitness of the direct taking of all innocent human life, especially at its beginning and at its end, *the Church's Magisterium* has spoken out with increasing frequency in defense of the sacredness and inviolability of human life. The papal magisterium, particularly insistent in this regard, has always been seconded by that of the bishops, with numerous and comprehensive doctrinal and pastoral documents issued either by episcopal conferences or by individual bishops. The Second Vatican Council also addressed the matter forcefully, in a brief but incisive passage.[50]

Therefore, by the authority which Christ conferred upon Peter and his successors, and in communion with the bishops of the Catholic Church, *I confirm that the direct and voluntary killing of an innocent human being is always gravely immoral.* This doctrine, based upon that unwritten law which man, in the light of reason, finds in his own heart (cf. Rom. 2:14–15), is reaffirmed by Sacred Scripture, transmitted by the Tradition of the Church and taught by the ordinary and universal magisterium.[51]

The deliberate decision to deprive an innocent human being of his life is always morally evil and can never be licit either as an end in itself or as a means to a good end. It is in fact a grave act of disobedience to the moral law, and indeed to God himself, the author and guarantor of that law; it contradicts the fundamental virtues of justice and charity. "Nothing and no one can in any way permit the killing of an innocent human being, whether a fetus or an embryo, an infant or an adult, an old person, or one suffering from an incurable disease, or a person who is dying. Furthermore, no one is permitted to ask for this act of killing, either for himself or herself or for another person entrusted to his or her care, nor can he or she consent to it, either explicitly or implicitly. Nor can any authority legitimately recommend or permit such an action."[52]

As far as the right to life is concerned, every innocent human being is absolutely equal to all others. This equality is the basis of all authentic social relationships which, to be truly such, can only be founded on truth and justice, recognizing and protecting every man and woman as a person and not as an object to be used. Before the moral norm which prohibits the direct taking of the life of an innocent human being "there are no privileges or exceptions for anyone. It makes no difference whether one is the master of the world or the 'poorest of the poor' on the face of the earth. Before the demands of morality we are all absolutely equal."[53]

"Your eyes beheld my unformed substance" (Ps. 139:16):
The Unspeakable Crime of Abortion

58. Among all the crimes which can be committed against life, procured abortion has characteristics making it particularly serious and deplorable. The Second Vatican Council defines abortion, together with infanticide, as an "unspeakable crime." [54]

But today, in many people's consciences, the perception of its gravity has become progressively obscured. The acceptance of abortion in the popular mind, in behavior and even in law itself, is a telling sign of an extremely dangerous crisis of the moral sense, which is becoming more and more incapable of distinguishing between good and evil, even when the fundamental right to life is at stake. Given such a grave situation, we need now more than ever to have the courage to look the truth in the eye and to *call things by their proper name*, without yielding to convenient compromises or to the temptation of self-deception. In this regard the reproach of the Prophet is extremely straightforward: "Woe to those who call evil good and good evil, who put darkness for light and light for darkness" (Isa. 5:20). Especially in the case of abortion there is a widespread use of ambiguous terminology, such as "interruption of pregnancy," which tends to hide abortion's true nature and to attenuate its seriousness in public opinion. Perhaps this linguistic phenomenon is itself a symptom of an uneasiness of conscience. But no word has the power to change the reality of things: procured abortion is *the deliberate and direct killing, by whatever means it is carried out, of a human being in the initial phase of his or her existence, extending from conception to birth.*

The moral gravity of procured abortion is apparent in all its truth if we recognize that we are dealing with murder and, in particular, when we consider the specific elements involved. The one eliminated is a human being at the very beginning of life. No one more absolutely *innocent* could be imagined. In no way could this human being ever be considered an aggressor, much less an unjust aggressor! He or she is *weak*, defenseless, even to the point of lacking that minimal form of defense consisting in the poignant power of a newborn baby's cries and tears. The unborn child is *totally entrusted* to the protection and care of the woman carrying him or her in the womb. And yet sometimes it is precisely the mother herself who makes the decision and asks for the child to be eliminated, and who then goes about having it done.

It is true that the decision to have an abortion is often tragic and painful for the mother, insofar as the decision to rid herself of the fruit of conception is not made for purely selfish reasons or out of convenience, but out of a desire to protect certain important values such as her own health or a decent standard of living for the other members of the family. Sometimes it is feared that the child to be born would live in such conditions that it would be better if the birth did not

take place. Nevertheless, these reasons and others like them, however serious and tragic, *can never justify the deliberate killing of an innocent human being.*

59. As well as the mother, there are often other people too who decide upon the death of the child in the womb. In the first place, the father of the child may be to blame, not only when he directly pressures the woman to have an abortion, but also when he indirectly encourages such a decision on her part by leaving her alone to face the problems of pregnancy: [55] in this way the family is thus mortally wounded and profaned in its nature as a community of love and in its vocation to be the "sanctuary of life." Nor can one overlook the pressures which sometimes come from the wider family circle and from friends. Sometimes the woman is subjected to such strong pressure that she feels psychologically forced to have an abortion: certainly in this case moral responsibility lies particularly with those who have directly or indirectly obliged her to have an abortion. Doctors and nurses are also responsible, when they place at the service of death skills which were acquired for promoting life.

But responsibility likewise falls on the legislators who have promoted and approved abortion laws, and, to the extent that they have a say in the matter, on the administrators of the health-care centers where abortions are performed. A general and no less serious responsibility lies with those who have encouraged the spread of an attitude of sexual permissiveness and a lack of esteem for motherhood, and with those who should have ensured—but did not—effective family and social policies in support of families, especially larger families and those with particular financial and educational needs. Finally, one cannot overlook the network of complicity which reaches out to include international institutions, foundations, and associations which systematically campaign for the legalization and spread of abortion in the world. In this sense abortion goes beyond the responsibility of individuals and beyond the harm done to them, and takes on a distinctly social dimension. It is a most serious *wound* inflicted on society and its culture by the very people who ought to be society's promoters and defenders. As I wrote in my *Letter to Families*, "we are facing an immense threat to life: not only to the life of individuals but also to that of civilization itself." [56] We are facing what can be called a *"structure of sin"* which opposes *human life not yet born.*

60. Some people try to justify abortion by claiming that the result of conception, at least up to a certain number of days, cannot yet be considered a personal human life. But in fact, "from the time that the ovum is fertilized, a life is begun which is neither that of the father nor the mother; it is rather the life of a new human being with his own growth. It would never be made human if it were not human already. This has always been clear, and ... modern genetic science offers clear confirmation. It has demonstrated that from the first instant there is established the program of what this liv-

ing being will be: a person, this individual person with his characteristic aspects already well determined. Right from fertilization the adventure of a human life begins, and each of its capacities requires time—a rather lengthy time—to find its place and to be in a position to act."[57] Even if the presence of a spiritual soul cannot be ascertained by empirical data, the results themselves of scientific research on the human embryo provide "a valuable indication for discerning, by the use of reason, a personal presence at the moment of the first appearance of a human life: how could a human individual not be a human person?"[58]

Furthermore, what is at stake is so important that, from the standpoint of moral obligation, the mere probability that a human person is involved would suffice to justify an absolutely clear prohibition of any intervention aimed at killing a human embryo. Precisely for this reason, over and above all scientific debates and those philosophical affirmations to which the magisterium has not expressly committed itself, the Church has always taught and continues to teach that the result of human procreation, from the first moment of its existence, must be guaranteed that unconditional respect which is morally due to the human being in his or her totality and unity as body and spirit: *"The human being is to be respected and treated as a person from the moment of conception*; and therefore from that same moment his rights as a person must be recognized, among which in the first place is the inviolable right of every innocent human being to life."[59]

61. The texts of *Sacred Scripture* never address the question of deliberate abortion and so do not directly and specifically condemn it. But they show such great respect for the human being in the mother's womb that they require as a logical consequence that God's commandment "You shall not kill" be extended to the unborn child as well.

Human life is sacred and inviolable at every moment of existence, including the initial phase which precedes birth. All human beings, from their mothers' womb, belong to God who searches them and knows them, who forms them and knits them together with his own hands, who gazes on them when they are tiny shapeless embryos and already sees in them the adults of tomorrow whose days are numbered and whose vocation is even now written in the "book of life" (cf. Ps. 139:1, 13–16). There too, when they are still in their mothers' womb—as many passages of the Bible bear witness[60]—they are the personal objects of God's loving and fatherly providence.

Christian Tradition—as the *Declaration* issued by the Congregation for the Doctrine of the Faith points out so well[61]— is clear and unanimous, from the beginning up to our own day, in describing abortion as a particularly grave moral disorder. From its first contacts with the Greco-Roman world, where abortion and infanticide were widely practiced, the first Christian community, by its teaching and practice,

radically opposed the customs rampant in that society, as is clearly shown by the Didache mentioned earlier.[62] Among the Greek ecclesiastical writers, Athenagoras records that Christians consider as murderesses women who have recourse to abortifacient medicines, because children, even if they are still in their mother's womb, "are already under the protection of Divine Providence."[63] Among the Latin authors, Tertullian affirms: "It is anticipated murder to prevent someone from being born; it makes little difference whether one kills a soul already born or puts it to death at birth. He who will one day be a man is a man already."[64]

Throughout Christianity's two-thousand-year history, this same doctrine has been constantly taught by the Fathers of the Church and by her pastors and Doctors. Even scientific and philosophical discussions about the precise moment of the infusion of the spiritual soul have never given rise to any hesitation about the moral condemnation of abortion.

62. The more recent *Papal Magisterium* has vigorously reaffirmed this common doctrine. Pius XI in particular, in his encyclical *Casti connubii*, rejected the specious justifications of abortion.[65] Pius XII excluded all direct abortion, i.e., every act tending directly to destroy human life in the womb "whether such destruction is intended as an end or only as a means to an end."[66] John XXIII reaffirmed that human life is sacred because "from its very beginning it directly involves God's creative activity."[67] The Second Vatican Council, as mentioned earlier, sternly condemned abortion: "From the moment of its conception, life must be guarded with the greatest care, while abortion and infanticide are unspeakable crimes."[68]

The Church's *canonical discipline*, from the earliest centuries, has inflicted penal sanctions on those guilty of abortion. This practice, with more or less severe penalties, has been confirmed in various periods of history. The 1917 *Code of Canon Law* punished abortion with excommunication.[69] The revised canonical legislation continues this tradition when it decrees that "a person who actually procures an abortion incurs automatic (*latae sententiae*) excommunication."[70] The excommunication affects all those who commit this crime with knowledge of the penalty attached, and thus includes those accomplices without whose help the crime would not have been committed.[71] By this reiterated sanction, the Church makes clear that abortion is a most serious and dangerous crime, thereby encouraging those who commit it to seek without delay the path of conversion. In the Church, the purpose of the penalty of excommunication is to make an individual fully aware of the gravity of a certain sin and then to foster genuine conversion and repentance.

Given such unanimity in the doctrinal and disciplinary tradition of the Church, Paul VI was able to declare that this tradition is unchanged and unchangeable.[72] Therefore, by the authority which Christ conferred upon Peter and his successors, in communion with the bishops—who on various occasions have condemned abortion and who in the aforementioned consultation, albeit dispersed throughout the world, have shown unanimous agreement concerning this doctrine *declare that direct abortion, that is, abortion willed as an end or as a means, always constitutes a grave moral disorder*, since it is the deliberate killing of an innocent human being. This doctrine is based upon the natural law and upon the written Word of God, is transmitted by the Church's Tradition, and is taught by the ordinary and universal magisterium.[73]

No circumstance, no purpose, no law whatsoever can ever make licit an act which is intrinsically illicit, since it is contrary to the Law of God which is written in every human heart, knowable by reason itself, and proclaimed by the Church.

63. This evaluation of the morality of abortion is to be applied also to the recent forms of *intervention on human embryos* which, although carried out for purposes legitimate in themselves, inevitably involve the killing of those embryos. This is the case with *experimentation on embryos*, which is becoming increasingly widespread in the field of biomedical research and is legally permitted in some countries. Although "one must uphold as licit procedures carried out on the human embryo which respect the life and integrity of the embryo and do not involve disproportionate risks for it, but rather are directed to its healing, the improvement of its condition of health, or its individual survival,"[74] it must nonetheless be stated that the use of human embryos or fetuses as an object of experimentation constitutes a crime against their dignity as human beings who have a right to the same respect owed to a child once born, just as to every person.[75]

This moral condemnation also regards procedures that exploit living human embryos and fetuses—sometimes specifically "produced" for this purpose by *in vitro* fertilization—either to be used as "biological material" or as *providers of organs or tissue for transplants* in the treatment of certain diseases. The killing of innocent human creatures, even if carried out to help others, constitutes an absolutely unacceptable act.

Special attention must be given to evaluating the morality of *prenatal diagnostic techniques* which enable the early detection of possible anomalies in the unborn child. In view of the complexity of these techniques, an accurate and systematic moral judgment is necessary. When they do not involve disproportionate risks for the child and the mother, and are meant to make possible early therapy or even to favor a serene and informed acceptance of the child not yet born, these techniques are morally licit. But since the possibilities of prenatal therapy are today still limited, it not infrequently happens that these techniques are used with a eugenic intention which accepts selective abortion in order to prevent the birth of children affected by various types of anomalies. Such an attitude is shameful and utterly reprehensible, since it presumes to measure the value of a human life only within the parameters of "normality" and physical well-being, thus opening the way to legitimizing infanticide and euthanasia as well.

And yet the courage and the serenity with which so many of our brothers and sisters suffering from serious disabilities lead their lives when they are shown acceptance and love bears eloquent witness to what gives authentic value to life and makes it, even in difficult conditions, something precious for them and for others. The Church is close to those married couples who, with great anguish and suffering, willingly accept gravely handicapped children. She is also grateful to all those families which, through adoption, welcome children abandoned by their parents because of disabilities or illnesses.

"It is I who bring both death and life" (Deut. 32:39): The Tragedy of Euthanasia

64. At the other end of life's spectrum, men and women find themselves facing the mystery of death. Today, as a result of advances in medicine and in a cultural context frequently closed to the transcendent, the experience of dying is marked by new features. When the prevailing tendency is to value life only to the extent that it brings pleasure and well-being, suffering seems like an unbearable setback, something from which one must be freed at all costs. Death is considered "senseless" if it suddenly interrupts a life still open to a future of new and interesting experiences. But it becomes a "rightful liberation" once life is held to be no longer meaningful because it is filled with pain and inexorably doomed to even greater suffering.

Furthermore, when he denies or neglects his fundamental relationship to God, man thinks he is his own rule and measure, with the right to demand that society should guarantee him the ways and means of deciding what to do with his life in full and complete autonomy. It is especially people in the developed countries who act in this way: they feel encouraged to do so also by the constant progress of medicine and its ever more advanced techniques. By using highly sophisticated systems and equipment, science and medical practice today are able not only to attend to cases formerly considered untreatable and to reduce or eliminate pain, but also to sustain and prolong life even in situations of extreme frailty, to resuscitate artificially patients whose basic biological functions have undergone sudden collapse, and to use special procedures to make organs available for transplanting.

In this context the temptation grows to have recourse to euthanasia, that is, *to take control of death and bring it about before its time, "gently"* ending one's own life or the life of others. In reality, what might seem logical and humane, when looked at more closely, is seen to be *senseless and inhumane*. Here we are faced with one of the more alarming symptoms of the "culture of death," which is advancing above all in prosperous societies, marked by an attitude of excessive preoccupation with efficiency and which sees the growing number of elderly and disabled people as intolerable and too burdensome. These people are very often isolated by their families and by society, which are organized almost exclusively on the basis of criteria of productive efficiency, according to which a hopelessly impaired life no longer has any value.

65. For a correct moral judgment on euthanasia, in the first place a clear definition is required. *Euthanasia in the strict sense* is understood to be an action or omission which of itself and by intention causes death, with the purpose of eliminating all suffering. "Euthanasia's terms of reference, therefore, are to be found in the intention of the will and in the methods used."[76]

Euthanasia must be distinguished from the decision to forgo so-called "aggressive medical treatment," in other words, medical procedures which no longer correspond to the real situation of the patient, either because they are by now disproportionate to any expected results or because they impose an excessive burden on the patient and his family. In such situations, when death is clearly imminent and inevitable, one can in conscience "refuse forms of treatment that would only secure a precarious and burdensome prolongation of life, so long as the normal care due to the sick person in similar cases is not interrupted."[77] Certainly there is a moral obligation to care for oneself and to allow oneself to be cared for, but this duty must take account of concrete circumstances. It needs to be determined whether the means of treatment available are objectively proportionate to the prospects for improvement. To forgo extraordinary or disproportionate means is not the equivalent of suicide or euthanasia; it rather expresses acceptance of the human condition in the face of death.[78]

In modern medicine, increased attention is being given to what are called "methods of palliative care," which seek to make suffering more bearable in the final stages of illness and to ensure that the patient is supported and accompanied in his or her ordeal. Among the questions which arise in this context is that of the licitness of using various types of painkillers and sedatives for relieving the patient's pain when this involves the risk of shortening life. While praise may be due to the person who voluntarily accepts suffering by forgoing treatment with painkillers in order to remain fully lucid and, if a believer, to share consciously in the Lord's Passion, such "heroic" behavior cannot be considered the duty of everyone. Pius XII affirmed that it is licit to relieve pain by narcotics, even when the result is decreased consciousness and a shortening of life, "if no other means exist, and if, in the given circumstances, this does not prevent the carrying out of other religious and moral duties."[79] In such a case, death is not willed or sought, even though for reasonable motives one runs the risk of it: there is simply a desire to ease pain effectively by using the analgesics which medicine provides. All the same, "it is not right to deprive the dying person of consciousness without a serious reason"[80]: as they approach death people ought to be able to satisfy their moral and family duties, and above all they ought to be able to prepare in a fully conscious way for their definitive meeting with God.

Taking into account these distinctions, in harmony with the magisterium of my predecessors[81] and in communion with the bishops of the Catholic Church, *I confirm that euthanasia is a grave violation of the law of God*, since it is the deliberate and morally unacceptable killing of a human person. This doctrine is based upon the natural law and upon the written word of God, is transmitted by the Church's Tradition and taught by the ordinary and universal magisterium.[82]

Depending on the circumstances, this practice involves the malice proper to suicide or murder.

66. Suicide is always as morally objectionable as murder. The Church's tradition has always rejected it as a gravely evil choice.[83] Even though a certain psychological, cultural, and social conditioning may induce a person to carry out an action which so radically contradicts the innate inclination to life, thus lessening or removing subjective responsibility, *suicide*, when viewed objectively, is a gravely immoral act. In fact, it involves the rejection of love of self and the renunciation of the obligation of justice and charity towards one's neighbor, towards the communities to which one belongs, and towards society as a whole.[84] In its deepest reality, suicide represents a rejection of God's absolute sovereignty over life and death, as proclaimed in the prayer of the ancient sage of Israel: "You have power over life and death; you lead men down to the gates of Hades and back again" (Wisd. 16:13; cf. Tob. 13:2).

To concur with the intention of another person to commit suicide and to help in carrying it out through so-called "assisted suicide" means to cooperate in, and at times to be the actual perpetrator of, an injustice which can never be excused, even if it is requested. In a remarkably relevant passage Saint Augustine writes that "it is never licit to kill another: even if he should wish it, indeed if he request it because, hanging between life and death, he begs for help in freeing the soul struggling against the bonds of the body and longing to be released; nor is it licit even when a sick person is no longer able to live."[85] Even when not motivated by a selfish refusal to be burdened with the life of someone who is suffering, euthanasia must be called a false mercy, and indeed a disturbing "perversion" of mercy. True compassion leads to sharing another's pain; it does not kill the person whose suffering we cannot bear. Moreover, the act of euthanasia appears all the more perverse if it is carried out by those, like relatives, who are supposed to treat a family member with patience and love, or by those, such as doctors, who by virtue of their specific profession are supposed to care for the sick person even in the most painful terminal stages.

The choice of euthanasia becomes more serious when it takes the form of a *murder* committed by others on a person who has in no way requested it and who has never consented to it. The height of arbitrariness and injustice is reached when certain people, such as physicians or legislators, arrogate to themselves the power to decide who ought to live and who ought to die. Once again we find ourselves before the temptation of Eden: to become like God who "knows good and evil" (cf. Gen. 3:5). God alone has the power over life and death: "It is I who bring both death and life" (Deut. 32:39; cf. 2 Kings 5:7; 1 Sam. 2:6). But he only exercises this power in accordance with a plan of wisdom and love. When man usurps this power, being enslaved by a foolish and selfish way of thinking, he inevitably uses it for injustice and death. Thus the life of the person who is weak is put into the hands of the one who is strong; in society the sense of justice is lost, and mutual trust, the basis of every authentic interpersonal relationship, is undermined at its root.

67. Quite different from this is the *way of love and true mercy*, which our common humanity calls for, and upon which faith in Christ the Redeemer, who died and rose again, sheds ever new light. The request which arises from the human heart in the supreme confrontation with suffering and death, especially when faced with the temptation to give up in utter desperation, is above all a request for companionship, sympathy, and support in the time of trial. It is a plea for help to keep on hoping when all human hopes fail. As the Second Vatican Council reminds us: "It is in the face of death that the riddle of human existence becomes most acute" and yet "man rightly follows the intuition of his heart when he abhors and repudiates the absolute ruin and total disappearance of his own person. Man rebels against death because he bears in himself an eternal seed which cannot be reduced to mere matter."[86]

This natural aversion to death and this incipient hope of immortality are illumined and brought to fulfillment by Christian faith, which both promises and offers a share in the victory of the Risen Christ: it is the victory of the One who, by his redemptive death, has set man free from death, "the wages of sin" (Rom. 6:23), and has given him the Spirit, the pledge of resurrection and of life (cf. Rom. 8:11). The certainty of future immortality and *hope in the promised resurrection* cast new light on the mystery of suffering and death, and fill the believer with an extraordinary capacity to trust fully in the plan of God.

The Apostle Paul expressed this newness in terms of belonging completely to the Lord who embraces every human condition: "None of us lives to himself, and none of us dies to himself. If we live, we live to the Lord, and if we die, we die to the Lord; so then, whether we live or whether we die, we are the Lord's" (Rom. 14:7–8). *Dying to the Lord* means experiencing one's death as the supreme act of obedience to the Father (cf. Phil. 2:8), being ready to meet death at the "hour" willed and chosen by Him (cf. John 13:1), which can only mean when one's earthly pilgrimage is completed. *Living to the Lord* also means recognizing that suffering, while still an evil and a trial in itself, can always become a source of good. It becomes such if it is experienced for love and with love through sharing, by God's gracious gift and one's own personal and free choice, in the

suffering of Christ crucified. In this way, the person who lives his suffering in the Lord grows more fully conformed to him (cf. Phil. 3:10; 1 Pet. 2:21) and more closely associated with his redemptive work on behalf of the Church and humanity.[87] This was the experience of Saint Paul, which every person who suffers is called to relive: "I rejoice in my sufferings for your sake; and in my flesh I complete what is lacking in Christ's afflictions for the sake of his Body, that is, the Church" (Col.1:24).

"We must obey God rather than men" (Acts 5:29): Civil Law and the Moral Law

68. One of the specific characteristics of present-day attacks on human life—as has already been said several times—consists in the trend to demand a *legal justification* for them, as if they were rights which the state, at least under certain conditions, must acknowledge as belonging to citizens. Consequently, there is a tendency to claim that it should be possible to exercise these rights with the safe and free assistance of doctors and medical personnel.

It is often claimed that the life of an unborn child or a seriously disabled person is only a relative good: according to a proportionalist approach, or one of sheer calculation, this good should be compared with and balanced against other goods. It is even maintained that only someone present and personally involved in a concrete situation can correctly judge the goods at stake: consequently, only that person would be able to decide on the morality of his choice. The state therefore, in the interest of civil coexistence and social harmony, should respect this choice, even to the point of permitting abortion and euthanasia.

At other times, it is claimed that civil law cannot demand that all citizens should live according to moral standards higher than what all citizens themselves acknowledge and share. Hence the law should always express the opinion and will of the majority of citizens and recognize that they have, at least in certain extreme cases, the right even to abortion and euthanasia. Moreover the prohibition and the punishment of abortion and euthanasia in these cases would inevitably lead—so it is said—to an increase of illegal practices: and these would not be subject to necessary control by society and would be carried out in a medically unsafe way. The question is also raised whether supporting a law which in practice cannot be enforced would not ultimately undermine the authority of all laws.

Finally, the more radical views go so far as to maintain that in a modern and pluralistic society people should be allowed complete freedom to dispose of their own lives as well as of the lives of the unborn: it is asserted that it is not the task of the law to choose between different moral opinions, and still less can the law claim to impose one particular opinion to the detriment of others.

69. In any case, in the democratic culture of our time it is commonly held that the legal system of any society should

limit itself to taking account of and accepting the convictions of the majority. It should therefore be based solely upon what the majority itself considers moral and actually practices. Furthermore, if it is believed that an objective truth shared by all is *de facto* unattainable, then respect for the freedom of the citizens—who in a democratic system are considered the true rulers—would require that on the legislative level the autonomy of individual consciences be acknowledged. Consequently, when establishing those norms which are absolutely necessary for social coexistence, the only determining factor should be the will of the majority, whatever this may be. Hence every politician, in his or her activity, should clearly separate the realm of private conscience from that of public conduct.

As a result we have what appear to be two diametrically opposed tendencies. On the one hand, individuals claim for themselves in the moral sphere the most complete freedom of choice and demand that the State should not adopt or impose any ethical position but limit itself to guaranteeing maximum space for the freedom of each individual, with the sole limitation of not infringing on the freedom and rights of any other citizen. On the other hand, it is held that, in the exercise of public and professional duties, respect for other people's freedom of choice requires that each one should set aside his or her own convictions in order to satisfy every demand of the citizens which is recognized and guaranteed by law; in carrying out one's duties the only moral criterion should be what is laid down by the law itself. Individual responsibility is thus turned over to the civil law, with a renouncing of personal conscience, at least in the public sphere.

70. At the basis of all these tendencies lies the ethical *relativism* which characterizes much of present-day culture. There are those who consider such relativism an essential condition of democracy, inasmuch as it alone is held to guarantee tolerance, mutual respect between people, and acceptance of the decisions of the majority, whereas moral norms considered to be objective and binding are held to lead to authoritarianism and intolerance.

But it is precisely the issue of respect for life which shows what misunderstandings and contradictions, accompanied by terrible practical consequences, are concealed in this position.

It is true that history has known cases where crimes have been committed in the name of "truth." But equally grave crimes and radical denials of freedom have also been committed and are still being committed in the name of "ethical relativism." When a parliamentary or social majority decrees that it is legal, at least under certain conditions, to kill unborn human life, is it not really making a "tyrannical" decision with regard to the weakest and most defenseless of human beings? Everyone's conscience rightly rejects those crimes against humanity of which our century has had such sad experience. But would these crimes cease to be crimes if, instead of being committed by unscrupulous tyrants, they were legitimated by popular consensus?

Democracy cannot be idolized to the point of making it a substitute for morality or a panacea for immorality. Fundamentally, democracy is a "system" and as such is a means and not an end. Its "moral" value is not automatic, but depends on conformity to the moral law to which it, like every other form of human behavior, must be subject: in other words, its morality depends on the morality of the ends which it pursues and of the means which it employs. If today we see an almost universal consensus with regard to the value of democracy, this is to be considered a positive "sign of the times," as the Church's magisterium has frequently noted.[88] But the value of democracy stands or falls with the values which it embodies and promotes. Of course, values such as the dignity of every human person, respect for inviolable and inalienable human rights, and the adoption of the "common good" as the end and criterion regulating political life are certainly fundamental and not to be ignored.

The basis of these values cannot be provisional and changeable "majority" opinions, but only the acknowledgment of an objective moral law which, as the "natural law" written in the human heart, is the obligatory point of reference for civil law itself. If, as a result of a tragic obscuring of the collective conscience, an attitude of skepticism were to succeed in bringing into question even the fundamental principles of the moral law, the democratic system itself would be shaken in its foundations, and would be reduced to a mere mechanism for regulating different and opposing interests on a purely empirical basis.[89]

Some might think that even this function, in the absence of anything better, should be valued for the sake of peace in society. While one acknowledges some element of truth in this point of view, it is easy to see that without an objective moral grounding not even democracy is capable of ensuring a stable peace, especially since peace which is not built upon the values of the dignity of every individual and of solidarity between all people frequently proves to be illusory. Even in participatory systems of government, the regulation of interests often occurs to the advantage of the most powerful, since they are the ones most capable of maneuvering not only the levers of power but also of shaping the formation of consensus. In such a situation, democracy easily becomes an empty word.

71. It is therefore urgently necessary, for the future of society and the development of a sound democracy, to rediscover those essential and innate human and moral values which flow from the very truth of the human being and express and safeguard the dignity of the person: values which no individual, no majority and no state can ever create, modify, or destroy, but must only acknowledge, respect, and promote.

Consequently there is a need to recover the *basic elements of a vision of the relationship between civil law and moral law,* which are put forward by the Church, but which are also part of the patrimony of the great juridical traditions of humanity.

Certainly the *purpose of civil law* is different and more limited in scope than that of the moral law. But "in no sphere of life can the civil law take the place of conscience or dictate norms concerning things which are outside its competence,"[90] which is that of ensuring the common good of people through the recognition and defense of their fundamental rights, and the promotion of peace and of public morality.[91] The real purpose of civil law is to guarantee an ordered social coexistence in true justice, so that all may "lead a quiet and peaceable life, godly and respectful in every way" (1 Tim. 2:2). Precisely for this reason, civil law must ensure that all members of society enjoy respect for certain fundamental rights which innately belong to the person, rights which every positive law must recognize and guarantee. First and fundamental among these is the inviolable right to life of every innocent human being. While public authority can sometimes choose not to put a stop to something which—were it prohibited—would cause more serious harm,[92] it can never presume to legitimize as a right of individuals—even if they are the majority of the members of society—an offense against other persons caused by the disregard of so fundamental a right as the right to life. The legal toleration of abortion or of euthanasia can in no way claim to be based on respect for the conscience of others, precisely because society has the right and the duty to protect itself against the abuses which can occur in the name of conscience and under the pretext of freedom.[93]

In the encyclical *Pacem in Terris*, John XXIII pointed out that "it is generally accepted today that the common good is best safeguarded when personal rights and duties are guaranteed. The chief concern of civil authorities must therefore be to ensure that these rights are recognized, respected, coordinated, defended, and promoted, and that each individual is enabled to perform his duties more easily. For 'to safeguard the inviolable rights of the human person, and to facilitate the performance of his duties, is the principal duty of every public authority.' Thus any government which refused to recognize human rights or acted in violation of them would not only fail in its duty; its decrees would be wholly lacking in binding force."[94]

72. The doctrine on the necessary conformity of civil law with the moral law is in continuity with the whole tradition of the Church. This is clear once more from John XXIII's encyclical: "Authority is a postulate of the moral order and derives from God. Consequently, laws and decrees enacted in contravention of the moral order, and hence of the divine will, can have no binding force in conscience . . . ; indeed, the passing of such laws undermines the very nature of authority and results in shameful abuse."[95] This is the clear teaching of Saint Thomas Aquinas, who writes that "human law is law inasmuch as it is in conformity with right reason and thus derives from the eternal law. But when a law is contrary to reason, it is called

an unjust law; but in this case it ceases to be a law and becomes instead an act of violence."[96] And again: "Every law made by man can be called a law insofar as it derives from the natural law. But if it is somehow opposed to the natural law, then it is not really a law but rather a corruption of the law."[97]

Now the first and most immediate application of this teaching concerns a human law which disregards the fundamental right and source of all other rights which is the right to life, a right belonging to every individual. Consequently, laws which legitimize the direct killing of innocent human beings through abortion or euthanasia are in complete opposition to the inviolable right to life proper to every individual; they thus deny the equality of everyone before the law. It might be objected that such is not the case in euthanasia, when it is requested with full awareness by the person involved. But any State which made such a request legitimate and authorized it to be carried out would be legalizing a case of suicide-murder, contrary to the fundamental principles of absolute respect for life and of the protection of every innocent life. In this way the State contributes to lessening respect for life and opens the door to ways of acting which are destructive of trust in relations between people. Laws which authorize and promote abortion and euthanasia are therefore radically opposed not only to the good of the individual but also to the common good; as such they are completely lacking in authentic juridical validity. Disregard for the right to life, precisely because it leads to the killing of the person whom society exists to serve, is what most directly conflicts with the possibility of achieving the common good. Consequently, a civil law authorizing abortion or euthanasia ceases by that very fact to be a true, morally binding civil law.

73. Abortion and euthanasia are thus crimes which no human law can claim to legitimize. There is no obligation in conscience to obey such laws; instead there is a *grave and clear obligation to oppose them by conscientious objection.* From the very beginnings of the Church, the apostolic preaching reminded Christians of their duty to obey legitimately constituted public authorities (cf. Rom. 13:7; 1 Pet. 2:13–14), but at the same time it firmly warned that "we must obey God rather than men" (Acts 5:29). In the Old Testament, precisely in regard to threats against life, we find a significant example of resistance to the unjust command of those in authority. After Pharaoh ordered the killing of all newborn males, the Hebrew midwives refused, "They did not do as the king of Egypt commanded them, but let the male children live" (Exod. 1:17). But the ultimate reason for their action should be noted: "*the midwives feared God*" (ibid.). It is precisely from obedience to God—to whom alone is due that fear which is acknowledgment of his absolute sovereignty—that the strength and the courage to resist unjust human laws are born. It is the strength and the courage of those prepared even to be imprisoned or put to the sword, in the certainty that this is what makes for "the endurance and faith of the saints" (Rev. 13:10).

In the case of an intrinsically unjust law, such as a law permitting abortion or euthanasia, it is therefore never licit to obey it, or to "take part in a propaganda campaign in favor of such a law, or vote for it."[98]

A particular problem of conscience can arise in cases where a legislative vote would be decisive for the passage of a more restrictive law, aimed at limiting the number of authorized abortions, in place of a more permissive law already passed or ready to be voted on. Such cases are not infrequent. It is a fact that while in some parts of the world there continue to be campaigns to introduce laws favoring abortion, often supported by powerful international organizations, in other nations—particularly those which have already experienced the bitter fruits of such permissive legislation—there are growing signs of a rethinking in this matter. In a case like the one just mentioned, when it is not possible to overturn or completely abrogate a pro-abortion law, an elected official, whose absolute personal opposition to procured abortion was well known, could licitly support proposals aimed at *limiting the harm* done by such a law and at lessening its negative consequences at the level of general opinion and public morality. This does not in fact represent an illicit cooperation with an unjust law, but rather a legitimate and proper attempt to limit its evil aspects.

74. The passing of unjust laws often raises difficult problems of conscience for morally upright people with regard to the issue of cooperation, since they have a right to demand not to be forced to take part in morally evil actions. Sometimes the choices which have to be made are difficult; they may require the sacrifice of prestigious professional positions or the relinquishing of reasonable hopes of career advancement. In other cases, it can happen that carrying out certain actions, which are provided for by legislation that overall is unjust, but which in themselves are indifferent, or even positive, can serve to protect human lives under threat. There may be reason to fear, however, that willingness to carry out such actions will not only cause scandal and weaken the necessary opposition to attacks on life, but will gradually lead to further capitulation to a mentality of permissiveness.

In order to shed light on this difficult question, it is necessary to recall the general principles concerning *cooperation in evil actions*. Christians, like all people of good will, are called upon under grave obligation of conscience not to cooperate formally in practices which, even if permitted by civil legislation, are contrary to God's law. Indeed, from the moral standpoint, it is never licit to cooperate formally in evil. Such cooperation occurs when an action, either by its very nature or by the form it takes in a concrete situation, can be defined as a direct participation in an act against innocent human life or a sharing in the immoral intention of the person committing it. This cooperation can never be justified either by invoking respect for the freedom of others or by appealing to the fact that civil law permits it or requires it. Each individual in fact has moral responsibility for the acts which he personally performs; no one can be exempted from this responsibility, and on the basis of it everyone will be judged by God himself (cf. Rom. 2:6; 14:12).

To refuse to take part in committing an injustice is not only a moral duty; it is also a basic human right. Were this not so, the human person would be forced to perform an action intrinsically incompatible with human dignity, and in this way human freedom itself, the authentic meaning and purpose of which are found in its orientation to the true and the good, would be radically compromised. What is at stake therefore is an essential right which, precisely as such, should be acknowledged and protected by civil law. In this sense, the opportunity to refuse to take part in the phases of consultation, preparation, and execution of these acts against life should be guaranteed to physicians, health-care personnel, and directors of hospitals, clinics, and convalescent facilities. Those who have recourse to conscientious objection must be protected not only from legal penalties but also from any negative effects on the legal, disciplinary, financial, and professional plane.

"You shall love your neighbor as yourself" (Luke 10:27): *"Promote"* Life

75. God's commandments teach us the way of life. The *negative moral precepts*, which declare that the choice of certain actions is morally unacceptable, have an absolute value for human freedom: they are valid always and everywhere, without exception. They make it clear that the choice of certain ways of acting is radically incompatible with the love of God and with the dignity of the person created in his image. Such choices cannot be redeemed by the goodness of any intention or of any consequence; they are irrevocably opposed to the bond between persons; they contradict the fundamental decision to direct one's life to God.[99]

In this sense, the negative moral precepts have an extremely important positive function. The "no" which they unconditionally require makes clear the absolute limit beneath which free individuals cannot lower themselves. At the same time they indicate the minimum which they must respect and from which they must start out in order to say "yes" over and over again, a "yes" which will gradually embrace the *entire horizon of the good* (cf. Matt. 5:48). The commandments, in particular the negative moral precepts, are the beginning and the first necessary stage of the journey towards freedom. As Saint Augustine writes, "the beginning of freedom is to be free from crimes . . . like murder, adultery, fornication, theft, fraud, sacrilege, and so forth. Only when one stops committing these crimes (and no Christian should commit them), one begins to lift up one's head towards freedom. But this is only the beginning of freedom, not perfect freedom."[100]

76. The commandment "You shall not kill" thus establishes the point of departure for the start of true freedom. It leads us to promote life actively, and to develop particular ways of thinking and acting which serve life. In this way we exercise our responsibility towards the persons entrusted to us and we show, in deeds and in truth, our gratitude to God for the great gift of life (cf. Ps. 139:13–14). The Creator has entrusted man's life to his responsible concern, not to make arbitrary use of it, but to preserve it with wisdom and to care for it with loving fidelity. The God of the Covenant has entrusted the life of every individual to his or her fellow human beings, brothers and sisters, according to the law of reciprocity in giving and receiving, of self-giving and of the acceptance of others. In the fullness of time, by taking flesh and giving his life for us, the Son of God showed what heights and depths this law of reciprocity can reach. With the gift of his Spirit, Christ gives new content and meaning to the law of reciprocity, to our being entrusted to one another. The Spirit who builds up communion in love creates between us a new fraternity and solidarity, a true reflection of the mystery of mutual self-giving and receiving proper to the Most Holy Trinity. The Spirit becomes the new law which gives strength to believers and awakens in them a responsibility for sharing the gift of self and for accepting others, as a sharing in the boundless love of Jesus Christ himself.

77. This new law also gives spirit and shape to the commandment "You shall not kill." For the Christian it involves an absolute imperative to respect, love, and promote the life of every brother and sister, in accordance with the requirements of God's bountiful love in Jesus Christ. "He laid down his life for us; and we ought to lay down our lives for the brethren" (1 John 3:16).

The commandment "You shall not kill," even in its more positive aspects of respecting, loving, and promoting human life, is binding on every individual human being. It resounds in the moral conscience of everyone as an irrepressible echo of the original covenant of God the Creator with mankind. It can be recognized by everyone through the light of reason; and it can be observed thanks to the mysterious working of the Spirit who, blowing where he wills (cf. John 3:8), comes to and involves every person living in this world.

It is therefore a service of love which we are all committed to ensure to our neighbor, that his or her life may be always defended and promoted, especially when it is weak or threatened. It is not only a personal but a social concern which we must all foster: a concern to make unconditional respect for human life the foundation of a renewed society.

We are asked to love and honor the life of every man and woman and to work with perseverance and courage so that our time, marked by all too many signs of death, may at last witness the establishment of a new culture of life, the fruit of the culture of truth and of love.

Chapter IV
You Did It to Me:
For a New Culture of Human Life

… *"That which we have seen and heard we proclaim also to you" (1 Jn 1:3): Proclaiming the Gospel of Life*

80. … Enlightened by this *Gospel of life*, we feel a need to proclaim it and to bear witness to it in all its *marvelous newness*. Since it is one with Jesus himself, who makes all things new [103] and conquers the "oldness" which comes from sin and leads to death,[104] this Gospel exceeds every human expectation and reveals the sublime heights to which the dignity of the human person is raised through grace. This is how Saint Gregory of Nyssa understands it: "Man, as a being, is of no account; he is dust, grass, vanity. But once he is adopted by the God of the universe as a son, he becomes part of the family of that Being, whose excellence and greatness no one can see, hear, or understand. What words, thoughts, or flight of the spirit can praise the superabundance of this grace? Man surpasses his nature: mortal, he becomes immortal; perishable, he becomes imperishable; fleeting, he becomes eternal; human, he becomes divine." [105]

Gratitude and joy at the incomparable dignity of man impel us to share this message with everyone: "that which we have seen and heard we proclaim also to you, so that you may have fellowship with us" (1 John 1:3). We need to bring the *Gospel of life* to the heart of every man and woman and to make it penetrate every part of society.

81. This involves above all proclaiming *the core* of this Gospel. It is the proclamation of a living God who is close to us, who calls us to profound communion with Himself and awakens in us the certain hope of eternal life. It is the affirmation of the inseparable connection between the person, his life, and his bodiliness. It is the presentation of human life as a life of relationship, a gift of God, the fruit and sign of his love. It is the proclamation that Jesus has a unique relationship with every person, which enables us to see in every human face the face of Christ. It is the call for a "sincere gift of self" as the fullest way to realize our personal freedom.

It also involves making clear all *the consequences* of this Gospel. These can be summed up as follows: human life, as a gift of God, is sacred and inviolable. For this reason procured abortion and euthanasia are absolutely unacceptable. Not only must human life not be taken, but it must be protected with loving concern. The meaning of life is found in giving and receiving love, and in this light human sexuality and procreation reach their true and full significance. Love also gives meaning to suffering and death; despite the mystery which surrounds them, they can become saving events. Respect for life requires that science and technology should always be at the service of man and his integral development. Society as a whole must respect, defend, and promote the dignity of every human person, at every moment and in every condition of that person's life.

82. To be truly a people at the service of life we must propose these truths constantly and courageously. ...

"I give you thanks that I am fearfully,
wonderfully made" (Ps. 139:14):
Celebrating the Gospel of Life

83. Because we have been sent into the world as a "people for life," our proclamation must also become *a genuine celebration of the Gospel of life*. This celebration, with the evocative power of its gestures, symbols, and rites, should become a precious and significant setting in which the beauty and grandeur of this Gospel is handed on.

For this to happen, we need first of all to *foster*, in ourselves and in others, *a contemplative outlook*.[107] Such an outlook arises from faith in the God of life, who has created every individual as a "wonder" (cf. Ps. 139:14). It is the outlook of those who see life in its deeper meaning, who grasp its utter gratuitousness, its beauty, and its invitation to freedom and responsibility. It is the outlook of those who do not presume to take possession of reality but instead accept it as a gift, discovering in all things the reflection of the Creator and seeing in every person his living image (cf. Gen. 1:27; Ps. 8:5). This outlook does not give in to discouragement when confronted by those who are sick, suffering, outcast, or at death's door. Instead, in all these situations it feels challenged to find meaning, and precisely in these circumstances it is open to perceiving in the face of every person a call to encounter, dialogue, and solidarity.

It is time for all of us to adopt this outlook, and with deep religious awe to rediscover the ability to *revere and honor every person*, as Paul VI invited us to do in one of his first Christmas messages.[108] Inspired by this contemplative outlook, the new people of the redeemed cannot but respond with songs of joy, praise, and thanksgiving for the priceless gift of life, for the mystery of every individual's call to share through Christ in the life of grace and in an existence of unending communion with God our Creator and Father.

84. *To celebrate the Gospel of life means to celebrate the God of life, the God who gives life*: "We must celebrate Eternal Life, from which every other life proceeds. From this, in proportion to its capacities, every being which in any way participates in life, receives life. This Divine Life, which is above every other life, gives and preserves life. Every life and every living movement proceed from this Life which transcends all life and every principle of life. It is to this that souls owe their incorruptibility and because of this all animals and plants live, which receive only the faintest glimmer of life. To men, beings made of spirit and matter, Life grants life. Even if we should abandon Life, because of its overflowing love for

man, it converts us and calls us back to itself. Not only this: it promises to bring us, soul and body, to perfect life, to immortality. It is too little to say that this Life is alive: it is the Principle of life, the Cause and sole Wellspring of life. Every living thing must contemplate it and give it praise: it is Life which overflows with life." [109]

Like the Psalmist, we too, in our *daily prayer* as individuals and as a community, praise and bless God our Father, who knitted us together in our mother's womb, and saw and loved us while we were still without form (cf. Ps. 139:13, 15–16). We exclaim with overwhelming joy: "I give you thanks that I am fearfully, wonderfully made; wonderful are your works. You know me through and through" (Ps. 139:14). Indeed, "despite its hardships, its hidden mysteries, its suffering, and its inevitable frailty, this mortal life is a most beautiful thing, a marvel ever new and moving, an event worthy of being exalted in joy and glory." [110] Moreover, man and his life appear to us not only as one of the greatest marvels of creation: for God has granted to man a dignity which is near to divine (Ps. 8:5–6). In every child which is born and in every person who lives or dies we see the image of God's glory. We celebrate this glory in every human being, a sign of the living God, an icon of Jesus Christ.

We are called to express wonder and gratitude for the gift of life and to welcome, savor, and share the *Gospel of life* not only in our personal and community prayer, but above all in the *celebrations of the liturgical year*. Particularly important in this regard are the *Sacraments*, the efficacious signs of the presence and saving action of the Lord Jesus in Christian life. The Sacraments make us sharers in divine life, and provide the spiritual strength necessary to experience life, suffering, and death in their fullest meaning. Thanks to a genuine rediscovery and a better appreciation of the significance of these rites, our liturgical celebrations, especially celebrations of the Sacraments, will be ever more capable of expressing the full truth about birth, life, suffering, and death, and will help us to live these moments as a participation in the Paschal Mystery of the Crucified and Risen Christ.

85. In celebrating the *Gospel of life* we also need to *appreciate and make good use of the wealth of gestures and symbols present in the traditions and customs of different cultures and peoples*. There are special times and ways in which the peoples of different nations and cultures express joy for a newborn life, respect for and protection of individual human lives, care for the suffering or needy, closeness to the elderly and the dying, participation in the sorrow of those who mourn, and hope and desire for immortality.

In view of this and following the suggestion made by the cardinals in the consistory of 1991, I propose that a *Day for Life* be celebrated each year in every country, as already established by some episcopal conferences. The celebration of this day should be planned and carried out with the active participation of all sectors of the local Church. Its primary purpose should be to foster in individual consciences, in families, in the Church, and in civil society a recognition of the meaning and value of human life at every stage and in every condition. Particular attention should be drawn to the seriousness of abortion and euthanasia, without neglecting other aspects of life which from time to time deserve to be given careful consideration, as occasion and circumstances demand.

86. As part of the spiritual worship acceptable to God (cf. Rom. 12:1), *the Gospel of life* is to be celebrated above all in *daily living*, which should be filled with self-giving love for others. In this way, our lives will become a genuine and responsible acceptance of the gift of life and a heartfelt song of praise and gratitude to God who has given us this gift. This is already happening in the many different acts of selfless generosity, often humble and hidden, carried out by men and women, children and adults, the young and the old, the healthy and the sick.

It is in this context, so humanly rich and filled with love, that *heroic actions* too are born. These are *the most solemn celebration of the Gospel of life*, for they proclaim it *by the total gift of self.* They are the radiant manifestation of the highest degree of love, which is to give one's life for the person loved (cf. John 15:13). They are a sharing in the mystery of the Cross, in which Jesus reveals the value of every person, and how life attains its fullness in the sincere gift of self. Over and above such outstanding moments, there is an everyday heroism, made up of gestures of sharing, big or small, which build up an authentic culture of life. A particularly praiseworthy example of such gestures is the donation of organs, performed in an ethically acceptable manner, with a view to offering a chance of health and even of life itself to the sick who sometimes have no other hope. ...

*"What does it profit, my brethren, if a man says
he has faith but has not works?" (James 2:14):
Serving the Gospel of Life*

87. By virtue of our sharing in Christ's royal mission, our support and promotion of human life must be accomplished through the *service of charity*, which finds expression in personal witness, various forms of volunteer work, social activity, and political commitment. This is a *particularly pressing need at the present time*, when the "culture of death" so forcefully opposes the "culture of life," and often seems to have the upper hand. But even before that it is a need which springs from "faith working through love" (Gal. 5:6). As the Letter of James admonishes us: "What does it profit, my brethren, if a man says he has faith but has not works? Can his faith save him? If a brother or sister is ill-clad and in lack of daily food, and one of you says to them, 'Go in peace, be warmed and filled,' without giving them the things needed for the body, what does it profit? So faith by itself, if it has no works, is dead" (2:14–17).

In our service of charity, *we must be inspired and distinguished by a specific attitude*: we must care for the other as a person for whom God has made us responsible. As disciples of Jesus, we are called to become neighbors to everyone (cf. Luke 10:29–37), and to show special favor to those who are poorest, most alone, and most in need. In helping the hungry, the thirsty, the foreigner, the naked, the sick, the imprisoned—as well as the child in the womb and the old person who is suffering or near death—we have the opportunity to serve Jesus. He himself said: "As you did it to one of the least of these my brethren, you did it to me" (Matt. 25:40). Hence we cannot but feel called to account and judged by the ever relevant words of Saint John Chrysostom: "Do you wish to honor the body of Christ? Do not neglect it when you find it naked. Do not do it homage here in the church with silk fabrics only to neglect it outside where it suffers cold and nakedness."[113]

Where life is involved, the service of charity must be profoundly consistent. It cannot tolerate bias and discrimination, for human life is sacred and inviolable at every stage and in every situation; it is an indivisible good. We need then to "show care" *for all life and for the life of everyone.* Indeed, at an even deeper level, we need to go to the very roots of life and love.

It is this deep love for every man and woman which has given rise down the centuries to an *outstanding history of charity*, a history which has brought into being in the Church and society many forms of service to life which evoke admiration from all unbiased observers. Every Christian community, with a renewed sense of responsibility, must continue to write this history through various kinds of pastoral and social activity. To this end, appropriate and effective programs of *support for new life* must be implemented, with special closeness to mothers who, even without the help of the father, are not afraid to bring their child into the world and to raise it. Similar care must be shown for the life of the marginalized or suffering, especially in its final phases.

88. All of this involves a patient and fearless *work of education* aimed at encouraging one and all to bear each other's burdens (cf. Gal. 6:2). It requires a continuous promotion of *vocations to service*, particularly among the young. It involves the implementation of long-term practical *projects and initiatives* inspired by the Gospel.

Many are the *means* towards this end which *need to be developed* with skill and serious commitment. At the first stage of life, *centers for natural methods of regulating fertility* should be promoted as a valuable help to responsible parenthood, in which all individuals, and in the first place the child, are recognized and respected in their own right, and where every decision is guided by the ideal of the sincere gift of self. *Marriage and family counseling agencies* by their specific work of guidance and prevention, carried out in accordance with an anthropology consistent with the Christian vision of the person, of the couple, and of sexuality, also offer valuable help in rediscovering the meaning of love and life, and in supporting and accompanying every family in its mission as the "sanctuary of life." Newborn life is also served by *centers of assistance and homes or centers where new life receives a welcome.* Thanks to the work of such centers, many unmarried mothers and couples in difficulty discover new hope and find assistance and support in overcoming hardship and the fear of accepting a newly conceived life or life which has just come into the world.

When life is challenged by conditions of hardship, maladjustment, sickness, or rejection, other programs—such as *communities for treating drug addiction, residential communities for minors or the mentally ill, care and relief centers for AIDS patients, associations for solidarity especially towards the disabled*—are eloquent expressions of what charity is able to devise in order to give everyone new reasons for hope and practical possibilities for life.

And when earthly existence draws to a close, it is again charity which finds the most appropriate means for enabling the *elderly*, especially those who can no longer look after themselves, and the *terminally ill* to enjoy genuinely humane assistance and to receive an adequate response to their needs, in particular their anxiety and their loneliness. In these cases the role of families is indispensable; yet families can receive much help from social welfare agencies and, if necessary, from recourse to *palliative care*, taking advantage of suitable medical and social services available in public institutions or in the home.

In particular, the role of *hospitals, clinics, and convalescent homes* needs to be reconsidered. These should not merely be institutions where care is provided for the sick or the dying. Above all they should be places where suffering, pain, and death are acknowledged and understood in their human and specifically Christian meaning. This must be especially evident and effective in *institutes staffed by religious or in any way connected with the Church.*

89. Agencies and centers of service to life, and all other initiatives of support and solidarity which circumstances may from time to time suggest, need to be directed by *people who are generous in their involvement and fully aware* of the importance of the *Gospel of life* for the good of individuals and society.

A unique responsibility belongs to health-care personnel: doctors, pharmacists, nurses, chaplains, men and women religious, administrators, and volunteers. Their profession calls for them to be guardians and servants of human life. In today's cultural and social context, in which science and the practice of medicine risk losing sight of their inherent ethical dimension, health-care professionals can be strongly tempted at times to become manipulators of life, or even agents of death. In the face of this temptation their responsibility today is greatly increased. Its deepest inspiration and strongest support lie in the intrinsic and undeniable ethical dimension of the health-care profession, something already recognized by the ancient and still relevant *Hippocratic Oath*, which requires every doctor to commit himself to absolute respect for human life and its sacredness.

Absolute respect for every innocent human life also requires the *exercise of conscientious objection* in relation to procured abortion and euthanasia. "Causing death" can never be considered a form of medical treatment, even when the intention is solely to comply with the patient's request. Rather, it runs completely counter to the health-care profession, which is meant to be an impassioned and unflinching affirmation of life. Biomedical research too, a field which promises great benefits for humanity, must always reject experimentation, research, or applications which disregard the inviolable dignity of the human being, and thus cease to be at the service of people and become instead means which, under the guise of helping people, actually harm them.

90. *Volunteer workers* have a specific role to play: they make a valuable contribution to the service of life when they combine professional ability and generous, selfless love. The *Gospel of life* inspires them to lift their feelings of good will towards others to the heights of Christ's charity; to renew every day, amid hard work and weariness, their awareness of the dignity of every person; to search out people's needs and, when necessary, to set out on new paths where needs are greater but care and support weaker.

If charity is to be realistic and effective, it demands that the *Gospel of life* be implemented also by means of certain *forms of social activity and commitment in the political field,* as a way of defending and promoting the value of life in our ever more complex and pluralistic societies. *Individuals, families, groups, and associations*, albeit for different reasons and in different ways, all have a responsibility for shaping society and developing cultural, economic, political, and legislative projects which, with respect for all and in keeping with democratic principles, will contribute to the building of a society in which the dignity of each person is recognized and protected and the lives of all are defended and enhanced.

This task is the particular responsibility of *civil leaders.* Called to serve the people and the common good, they have a duty to make courageous choices in support of life, especially through *legislative measures*. In a democratic system, where laws and decisions are made on the basis of the consensus of many, the sense of personal responsibility in the consciences of individuals invested with authority may be weakened. But no one can ever renounce this responsibility, especially when he or she has a legislative or decision-making mandate, which calls that person to answer to God, to his or her own conscience, and to the whole of society for choices which may be contrary to the common good. Although laws are not the only means of protecting human life, nevertheless they do play a very important and sometimes decisive role in influencing patterns of thought and behavior. I repeat once more that a law which violates an innocent person's natural right to life is unjust and, as such, is not valid as a law. For this reason I urgently appeal once more to all political leaders not to pass laws which, by disregarding the dignity of the person, undermine the very fabric of society.

The Church well knows that it is difficult to mount an effective legal defense of life in pluralistic democracies, because of the presence of strong cultural currents with differing outlooks. At the same time, certain that moral truth cannot fail to make its presence deeply felt in every conscience, the Church encourages political leaders, starting with those who are Christians, not to give in, but to make those choices which, taking into account what is realistically attainable, will lead to the re-establishment of a just order in the defense and promotion of the value of life. Here it must be noted that it is not enough to remove unjust laws. The underlying causes of attacks on life have to be eliminated, especially by ensuring proper support for families and motherhood. *A family policy must be the basis and driving force of all social policies.* For this reason there need to be set in place social and political initiatives capable of guaranteeing conditions of true freedom of choice in matters of parenthood. It is also necessary to rethink labor, urban, residential, and social service policies so as to harmonize working schedules with time available for the family, so that it becomes effectively possible to take care of children and the elderly.

91. Today an important part of policies which favor life is the *issue of population growth.* Certainly public authorities have a responsibility to "intervene to orient the demography of the population."[114] But such interventions must always take into account and respect the primary and inalienable responsibility of married couples and families, and cannot employ methods which fail to respect the person and fundamental human rights, beginning with the right to life of every innocent human being. It is therefore morally unacceptable to encourage, let alone impose, the use of methods such as contraception, sterilization, and abortion in order to regulate births. The ways of solving the population problem are quite different. Governments and the various international agencies must above all strive to create economic, social, public health, and cultural conditions which will enable married couples to make their choices about procreation in full freedom and with genuine responsibility. They must then make efforts to ensure "greater opportunities and a fairer distribution of wealth so that everyone can share equitably in the goods of creation. Solutions must be sought on the global level by establishing a *true economy of communion and sharing of goods,* in both the national and international order."[115] This is the only way to respect the dignity of persons and families, as well as the authentic cultural patrimony of peoples.

Service of the *Gospel of life* is thus an immense and complex task. This service increasingly appears as a valuable and fruitful area for positive cooperation with our brothers and sisters of other churches and ecclesial communities, in accordance with the *practical ecumenism* which the Second Vatican Council authoritatively encouraged.[116] It also appears as a providential area for dialogue and joint efforts with the followers of other religions and with all people of good will. *No single person or group has a monopoly on the defense and promotion of life. These are everyone's task and responsibility.* On the eve of the Third Millennium, the challenge facing us is an arduous one: only the concerted efforts of all those who believe in the value of life can prevent a setback of unforeseeable consequences for civilization.

....."Walk as children of light" (Eph. 5:8): Bringing About a Transformation of Culture

95. "Walk as children of light ... and try to learn what is pleasing to the Lord. Take no part in the unfruitful works of darkness" (Eph. 5:8, 10–11). In our present social context, marked by a dramatic struggle between the "culture of life" and the "culture of death," there is need to *develop a deep critical sense,* capable of discerning true values and authentic needs.

What is urgently called for is a *general mobilization of consciences and a united ethical effort to activate a great campaign in support of life. All together, we must build a new culture of life*: new, because it will be able to confront and solve today's unprecedented problems affecting human life; new, because it will be adopted with deeper and more dynamic conviction by all Christians; new, because it will be capable of bringing about a serious and courageous cultural dialogue among all parties. While the urgent need for such a cultural transformation is linked to the present historical situation, it is also rooted in the Church's mission of evangelization. The purpose of the Gospel, in fact, is "to transform humanity from within and to make it new."[123] Like the yeast which leavens the whole measure of dough (cf. Matt. 13:33), the Gospel is meant to permeate all cultures and give them life from within,[124] so that they may express the full truth about the human person and about human life.

We need to begin with *the renewal of a culture of life within Christian communities themselves.* Too often it happens that believers, even those who take an active part in the life of the Church, end up by separating their Christian faith from its ethical requirements concerning life, and thus fall into moral subjectivism and certain objectionable ways of acting. With great openness and courage, we need to question how widespread is the culture of life today among individual Christians, families, groups, and communities in our dioceses. With equal clarity and determination, we must identify the steps we are called to take in order to serve life in all its truth. At the same time, we need to promote a serious and in-depth exchange about basic issues of human life with everyone, including non-believers, in intellectual circles, in the various professional spheres, and at the level of people's everyday life.

96. The first and fundamental step towards this cultural transformation consists in *forming consciences* with regard to the incomparable and inviolable worth of every human life. It is of the greatest importance to *re-establish the essential connection between life and freedom*. These are inseparable goods: where one is violated, the other also ends up being violated. There is no true freedom where life is not welcomed and loved; and there is no fullness of life except in freedom. Both realities have something inherent and specific which links them inextricably: the vocation to love. Love, as a sincere gift of self,[125] is what gives the life and freedom of the person their truest meaning.

No less critical in the formation of conscience is *the recovery of the necessary link between freedom and truth*. As I have frequently stated, when freedom is detached from objective truth it becomes impossible to establish personal rights on a firm rational basis; and the ground is laid for society to be at the mercy of the unrestrained will of individuals or the oppressive totalitarianism of public authority.[126]

It is therefore essential that man should acknowledge his inherent condition as a creature to whom God has granted being and life as a gift and a duty. Only by admitting his innate dependence can man live and use his freedom to the full, and at the same time respect the life and freedom of every other person. Here especially one sees that "at the heart of every culture lies the attitude man takes to the greatest mystery: the mystery of God."[127] Where God is denied and people live as though he did not exist, or his commandments are not taken into account, the dignity of the human person and the inviolability of human life also end up being rejected or compromised. ...

98. In a word, we can say that the cultural change which we are calling for demands from everyone the courage to *adopt a new life-style*, consisting in making practical choices—at the personal, family, social, and international levels—on the basis of a correct scale of values: *the primacy of being over having*,[130] *of the person over things*.[131] This renewed life-style involves a passing from *indifference to concern for others, from rejection to acceptance of them*. Other people are not rivals from whom we must defend ourselves, but brothers and sisters to be supported. They are to be loved for their own sakes, and they enrich us by their very presence. ...

...*"We are writing this that our joy may be complete" (1 John 1:4):*
The Gospel of Life Is for the Whole of Human Society

101. "We are writing you this that our joy may be complete" (1 John 1:4). The revelation of the *Gospel of life* is given to us as a good to be shared with all people: so that all men and women may have fellowship with us and with the Trinity (cf. 1 John 1:3). Our own joy would not be complete if we failed to share this Gospel with others but kept it only for ourselves.

The Gospel of life is not for believers alone: *it is for everyone*. The issue of life and its defense and promotion is not a concern of Christians alone. Although faith provides special light and strength, this question arises in every human conscience which seeks the truth and which cares about the future of humanity. Life certainly has a sacred and religious value, but in no way is that value a concern only of believers. The value at stake is one which every human being can grasp by the light of reason; thus it necessarily concerns everyone.

Consequently, all that we do as the "people of life and for life" should be interpreted correctly and welcomed with favor. When the Church declares that unconditional respect for the right to life of every innocent person—from conception to natural death—is one of the pillars on which every civil society stands, she "wants simply to *promote a human state*. A state which recognizes the defense of the fundamental rights of the human person, especially of the weakest, as its primary duty."[136]

The Gospel of life is for the whole of human society. To be actively pro-life is to contribute to the *renewal of society* through the promotion of the common good. It is impossible to further the common good without acknowledging and defending the right to life, upon which all the other inalienable rights of individuals are founded and from which they develop. A society lacks solid foundations when, on the one hand, it asserts values such as the dignity of the person, justice, and peace, but then, on the other hand, radically acts to the contrary by allowing or tolerating a variety of ways in which human life is devalued and violated, especially where it is weak or marginalized. Only respect for life can be the foundation and guarantee of the most precious and essential goods of society, such as democracy and peace.

There can be no *true democracy* without a recognition of every person's dignity and without respect for his or her rights.

Nor can there be *true peace* unless *life is defended and promoted*. As Paul VI pointed out: "Every crime against life is an attack on peace, especially if it strikes at the moral conduct of people. ... But where human rights are truly professed and publicly recognized and defended, peace becomes the joyful and operative climate of life in society."[137]

The "people of life" rejoices in being able to share its commitment with so many others. Thus may the "people for life" constantly grow in number and may a new culture of love and solidarity develop for the true good of the whole of human society.

Conclusion

... 105 ... And as we, the pilgrim people, the people of life and for life, make our way in confidence towards "a new heaven and a new earth" (Rev. 21:1), we look to her who is for us "a sign of sure hope and solace."[142]

O Mary,
bright dawn of the new world,
Mother of the living,
to you do we entrust the *cause of life*:
Look down, O Mother,
upon the vast numbers
of babies not allowed to be born,
of the poor whose lives are made difficult,
of men and women
who are victims of brutal violence,
of the elderly and the sick killed
by indifference or out of misguided mercy.
Grant that all who believe in your Son
may *proclaim the Gospel of life*
with honesty and love
to the people of our time.
Obtain for them the grace
to *accept that Gospel*
as a gift ever new,
the joy *of celebrating* it with gratitude
throughout their lives
and the courage to *bear witness to it*
resolutely, in order to build,
together with all people of good will,
the civilization of truth and love,
to the praise and glory of God,
the Creator and lover of life.

Given at Rome, at Saint Peter's, on March 25, the Solemnity of the Annunciation of the Lord, in the year 1995, the seventeenth of my pontificate.

Notes

[1] The expression "Gospel of life" is not found as such in Sacred Scripture. But it does correspond to an essential dimension of the biblical message.

[2] Second Vatican Ecumenical Council, Pastoral Constitution on the Church in the Modern World *Gaudium et spes*, n. 22.

[3] Cf. John Paul II, encyclical letter *Redemptor hominis* (March 4, 1979), n. 10, AAS 71 (1979): 275.

[4] Cf. *ibid.*, n. 14.

[5] Second Vatican Ecumenical Council, Pastoral Constitution on the Church in the Modern World *Gaudium et spes*, n. 27.

... [14] Cf. Congregation for the Doctrine of the Faith, Instruction on Respect for Human Life in its Origin and on the Dignity of Procreation *Donum vitae, AAS* 80 (1988): 70–102.

[15] Address during the Prayer Vigil for the Eighth World Youth Day, Denver (August 14, 1993), 11, 3, *AAS* 86 (1994): 419.

[16] John Paul II, address to the participants at the study conference on "The Right to Life and Europe," December 18, 1987, *Insegnamenti*, X, 3 (1987): 1446–1447.

[17] Second Vatican Ecumenical Council, *Gaudium et spes*, n. 36.

[18] Cf. ibid., 16.

... [20] John Paul II, *Redemptor hominis*, n. 10, AAS 71 (1979): 274.

[21] Second Vatican Ecumenical Council, *Gaudium et spes*, n. 50.

... [23] "Gloria Dei vivens homo": *Adversus Haereses*, IV, 20, 7, SCh 100/2, 648–649.

... [27] "Vita autem hominis visio Dei": *Adversus Haereses*, IV, 20, 7, *SCh* 100/12, 648–649.

... [30] Second Vatican Ecumenical Council, *Gaudium et spes*, n. 50.

[31] *Gratissimam sane*, n. 9, *AAS* 86 (1994): 878; cf. Pius XII, encyclical letter *Humani generis* (August 12, 1950), *AAS* 42 (1950): 574.

[32] "Animas enim a Deo immediate creari catholica fides nos retinere iubet": Pius XII, *Humani generis, AAS* 42 (1950): 575.

[33] Second Vatican Ecumenical Council, *Gaudium et spes*, n. 50; cf. John Paul II, post-synodal apostolic exhortation *Familiaris consortio* (November 22, 1981), n. 28, *AAS* 74 (1982): 114.

[34] *Homilies*, 11, 1; CCSG 3, 39.

[35] See, for example, Pss. 22:10–11; 71:6; 139:13–14.

[36] *Expositio Evangelii secundum Lucam*, II, 22–23, CCL, 14, 40–41.

[37] Saint Ignatius of Antioch, *Letter to the Ephesians*, 7, 2, in *Patres Apostolici*, ed. F. X. Funk, vol. II, 82.

[38] *De Hominis Opificio*, 4, PG 44, 136.

[39] Cf. Saint John Damascene, *De fide orthodoxa*, 2, 12, PG 94, 920–922, quoted in Saint Thomas Aquinas, *Summa theologiae*, I-II, prologue.

[40] Paul VI, encyclical letter *Humanae vitae* (July 25, 1968), n. 13, *AAS* 60 (1968): 489.

[41] Congregation for the Doctrine of the Faith, *Donum vitae*, intro., n. 5, *AAS* 80 (1988): 76–77; cf. *Catechism of the Catholic Church*, n. 2258.

... [49] Second Vatican Ecumenical Council, Dogmatic Constitution on the Church *Lumen gentium*, n. 12.

[50] Cf. Second Vatican Ecumenical Council, *Gaudium et spes*, n. 27.

[51] Cf. Second Vatican Ecumenical Council, *Lumen gentium*, n. 25.

[52] Congregation for the Doctrine of the Faith, Declaration on Euthanasia *Iura et bona* (May 5, 1980), II, *AAS* 72 (1980): 546.

[53] John Paul II, encyclical letter *Veritatis splendor* (August 6, 1993), n. 96, *AAS* 85 (1993): 1209.

[54] Second Vatican Ecumenical Council, *Gaudium et spes*, n. 51: "Abortus necnon infanticidium nefanda sunt crimina."

[55] Cf. John Paul II, apostolic letter *Mulieris dignitatem* (August 15, 1988), n. 14, *AAS* 80 (1988): 1686.

[56] N. 21, *AAS* 86 (1994): 920.

[57] Congregation for the Doctrine of the Faith, *Declaration on Procured Abortion* (November 18, 1974), nn. 12–13, *AAS* 66 (1974): 738.

[58] Congregation for the Doctrine of the Faith, *Donum vitae*, I, n. 1, AAS 80 (1988): 78–79.

[59] Ibid., 79.

[60] Hence the Prophet Jeremiah: "The word of the Lord came to me saying: 'Before I formed you in the womb I knew you, and before you were born I consecrated you; I appointed you a prophet to the nations'" (1:4–5). The Psalmist, for his part, addresses the Lord in these words: "Upon you I have leaned from my birth; you are he who took me from my mother's womb" (Ps. 71:6; cf. Isa. 46:3; Job 10:8–12; Ps. 22:10–11). So too the Evangelist Luke in the magnificent episode of the meeting of the two mothers, Elizabeth and Mary, and their two sons, John the Baptist and Jesus, still hidden in their mothers' wombs (cf. 1:39–45) emphasizes how even before their birth the two little ones are able to communicate: the child recognizes the coming of the Child and leaps for joy.

[61] Cf. Congregation for the Doctrine of the Faith, *Declaration on Procured Abortion*, n. 7, AAS 66 (1974): 740–747.

[62] "You shall not kill a child by abortion nor shall you kill it once it is born": V, 2, *Patres Apostolici*, ed. F. X. Funk, I, 17.

[63] Apologia on behalf of the Christians, 35, PG 6, 969.

[64] *Apologeticum*, IX, 8, CSEL 69, 24.

[65] Cf. encyclical letter *Casti connubii* (December 31, 1930), II, AAS 22 (1930): 562–592.

[66] Address to the Biomedical Association "San Luca" (November 12, 1944), *Discorsi e Radiomessaggi* VI (1944–1945): 191; cf. address to the Italian Catholic Union of Midwives (October 29, 1951), n. 2, *AAS* 43 (1951): 838.

[67] Encyclical letter *Mater et magistra* (May 15, 1961), 3, *AAS* 53 (1961): 447.

[68] Second Vatican Ecumenical Council, *Gaudium et spes*, n. 51.

[69] Can. 2350 §1.

[70] 1983 Code of Canon Law, can. 1398; cf. Code of Canons of the Eastern Churches, canon 1450 § 2.

[71] Cf. 1983 Code of Canon Law, can. 1329; also Code of Canons of the Eastern Churches, can. 1417.

[72] Cf. address to the National Congress of Italian jurists (December 9, 1972), *AAS* 64 (1972): 777; idem, encyclical letter *Humanae vitae*, n. 14, AAS 60 (1968): 490.

[73] Cf. Second Vatican Ecumenical Council, *Lumen gentium*, n. 25.

[74] Congregation for the Doctrine of the Faith, *Donum vitae*, I, 3, *AAS* 80 (1988): 80.

[75] Charter of the Rights of the Family (October 22, 1983) (Vatican Polyglot Press, 1983), art. 4b.

[76] Congregation for the Doctrine of the Faith, *Iura et bona*, II, *AAS* 72 (1980): 546.

[77] Ibid., IV.

[78] Cf. ibid.

[79] Pius XII, address to an international group of physicians (February 24, 1957), III, *AAS* 49 (1957): 147; cf. Congregation for the Doctrine of the Faith, *Iura et bona*, III, *AAS* 72 (1980): 547–548.

[80] Pius XII, address to an international group of physicians, III, *AAS* 49 (1957): 145.

[81] Cf. Pius XII, address to an international group of physicians, *loc. cit.*, 129–147; Congregation of the Holy Office, *Decretum de directa insontium occisione* (December 2, 1940), AAS 32 (1940): 553–554; Paul VI, message to French television: "Every life is sacred" (January 27, 1971), *Insegnamenti* IX (1971): 57–58; idem, address to the International College of Surgeons (June 1, 1972), *AAS* 64 (1972): 432–436; Second Vatican Ecumenical Council, *Gaudium et spes*, n. 27.

[82] Cf. Second Vatican Ecumenical Council, *Lumen gentium*, n. 25.

[83] Cf. Saint Augustine, *De civitate Dei* I, 20, CCL 47, 22; Aquinas, *Summa theologiae*, II-II, q. 6.5.

[84] Congregation for the Doctrine of the Faith, *Iura et bona*, I, AAS 72 (1980): 545; *Catechism of the Catholic Church*, nn. 2281–2283.

[85] *Ep.* 204, 5, *CSEL* 57, 320.

[86] Second Vatican Ecumenical Council, *Gaudium et spes*, n. 18.

[87] Cf. John Paul II, apostolic letter *Salvifici doloris* (February 11, 1984), nn. 14–24, *AAS* 76 (1984): 214–234.

[88] Cf. John Paul II, *Centesimus annus*, 46, AAS 83 (1991): 850; Pius XII, Christmas Radio Message (December 24, 1944), *AAS* 37 (1945): 10–20.

[89] Cf. John Paul II, *Veritatis splendor*, nn. 97 and 99, *AAS* 85 (1993): 1209–1211.

[90] Congregation for the Doctrine of the Faith, *Donum vitae*, III, AAS 80 (1988): 98.

[91] Cf. Second Vatican Ecumenical Council, Declaration on Religious Freedom *Dignitatis humanae*, n. 7.

[92] Cf. Aquinas, *Summa theologiae* I-II, q. 96.2.

[93] Cf. Second Vatican Ecumenical Council, *Dignitatis humanae*, n. 7.

[94] Encyclical letter *Pacem in terris* (April 11, 1963), II, *AAS* 55 (1963): 273–274. The internal quote is from Pius XII, radio message of Pentecost 1941 (June 1, 1941), *AAS* 33 (1941): 200. On this topic, the encyclical cites: Pius XI, encyclical letter *Mit brennender Sorge* (March 14, 1937), *AAS* 29 (1937): 159; encyclical letter *Divini redemptoris* (March 19, 1937), III, AAS 29 (1937): 79; Pius XII, Christmas radio message (December 24, 1942), *AAS* 35 (1943): 9–24.

[95] Encyclical letter *Pacem in terris* (April 11, 1963), II, *AAS* 55 (1963): 271.

[96] *Summa theologiae*, I-II, q. 93.3, ad 2.

[97] Ibid., I-II, q. 95.2. Aquinas quotes Saint Augustine: "Non videtur esse lex, quae iusta non fuerit," De libero arbitrio, I, 5, 11, PL 32, 1227.

[98] Congregation for the Doctrine of the Faith, *Declaration on Procured Abortion*, n. 22, AAS 66 (1974):744.

[99] Cf. *Catechism of the Catholic Church*, nn. 1753–1755; John Paul II, *Veritatis splendor*, nn. 81–82, AAS 85 (1993): 1198–1199.

[100] In Iohannis *Evangelium Tractatus*, 41, 10, CCL 36, 3 63; cf. John Paul II, *Veritatis splendor*, n. 13, AAS 85 (1993): 1144.

… [103] Cf. Saint Irenaeus: "Omnem novitatem attulit, semetipsum afferens, qui fuerat annuntiatus," *Adversus haereses*, IV, 34, 1, SCh 100/12, 846–847.

[104] Cf. Saint Thomas Aquinas, "Peccator inveterascit, recedens a novitate Christi," *In Psalmos Davidis lectura*, 6, 5.

[105] *De Beatitudinibus*, Oratio VII, PG 44, 1280.

… [107] Cf. John Paul II, *Centesimus annus*, n. 37, *AAS* 83 (1991): 840.

[108] Cf. message for Christmas 1967, *AAS* 60 (1968): 40.

[109] Pseudo-Dionysius the Areopagite, *On the Divine Names*, 6, 1–3, PG 3, 856–857.

[110] Paul VI, *Pensiero alla morte* (Brescia: Instituto Paolo VI, 1988), 24.

… [113] *In Matthaeum*, Hom. L, 3, PG 58, 508.

[114] *Catechism of the Catholic Church*, n. 2372.

[115] John Paul II, address to the Fourth General Conference of Latin American Bishops in Santo Domingo (October 12, 1992), n. 15, *AAS* 85 (1993): 819.

[116] Cf. Decree on Ecumenism *Unitatis redintegratio*, n. 12; Pastoral Constitution on the Church in the Modern World *Gaudium et spes*, n. 90.

… [123] Paul VI, apostolic exhortation *Evangelii nuntiandi* (December 8, 1975), n. 18, *AAS* 68 (1976): 17.

[124] Cf. ibid., n. 20.

[125] Cf. Second Vatican Ecumenical Council, *Gaudium et spes*, n. 24.

[126] Cf. John Paul II, *Centesimus annus*, n. 17, AAS 83 (1991): 814; idem, *Veritatis splendor*, nn. 95–101, AAS 85 (1993): 1208–1213.

[127] John Paul II, *Centesimus annus*, n. 24, AAS 83 (1991): 822.

… [130] Cf. Second Vatican Ecumenical Council, *Gaudium et spes*, n. 35; Paul VI, encyclical letter *Populorum progressio* (March 26, 1967), n. 15, *AAS* 59 (1967): 265.

[131] Cf. John Paul II, *Gratissimam sane*, n. 13, *AAS* 86 (1994): 892.

… [136] John Paul II, address to participants in the Study Conference on "The Right to Life in Europe" (December 18, 1987), *Insegnamenti* X, 3 (1987): 1446.

[137] Message for the 1977 World Day of Peace, *AAS* 68 (1976): 711–712.

… [142] Second Vatican Ecumenical Council, *Lumen gentium*, n. 68.

APPENDIX X

Committee on Doctrine
National Conference of Catholic Bishops (U.S.)

Moral Principles concerning Infants with Anencephaly

September 19, 1996

Anencephaly is a congenital anomaly characterized by failure of development of the cerebral hemispheres and overlying skull and scalp, exposing the brain stem. This condition exists in varying degrees of severity. Most infants who have anencephaly do not survive for more than a few days after birth. Modern medical techniques usually can determine this condition with a high degree of certainty before birth. When anencephaly is detected some physicians recommend that the pregnancy be terminated in order to free the mother from the psychological anxiety and possible physical complications throughout the remainder of the pregnancy.

According to the well-established teaching of the Catholic Church, the rights of a mother and her unborn child deserve equal protection because they are based on the dignity of the human person whatever the condition of that person. Consequently, it can never be morally justified directly to cause the death of an innocent person no matter the age or condition of that person.

Some have attempted to argue that anencephalic children may be prematurely delivered, even when this would be inappropriate for other children. This argument is based on the opinion that because of their apparent lack of cognitive function, and in view of the probable brevity of their lives, these infants are not the subject of human rights, or at least have lives of less meaning or purpose than others. Doubts about the human dignity of the anencephalic infant, however, have no solid ground, and the benefit of any doubt must be in the child's favour. As a general rule, conditions of the human body, regardless of severity, in no way compromise human dignity or human rights.

The *Ethical and Religious Directives for Catholic Health Care Services (ERD)* Directive 45, states:

Abortion (that is, the directly intended termination of pregnancy before viability or the directly intended

destruction of a viable fetus) is never permitted. Every procedure whose sole immediate effect is the termination of pregnancy before viability is an abortion, which, in its moral context, includes the interval between conception and implantation of the embryo.

The phrase "sole immediate effect" is further explained by Directive 47 which states:

Operations, treatments, and medications that have as their direct purpose the cure of a proportionately serious pathological condition of a pregnant woman are permitted when they cannot be safely postponed until the unborn child is viable, even if they will result in the death of the unborn child.

In other words, it is permitted to treat directly a pathology of the mother even when this has the unintended side-effect of causing the death of her child, if this pathology left untreated would have life-threatening effects on both mother and child, but it is not permitted to terminate or gravely risk the child's life as a *means* of treating or protecting the mother.

Hence, it is clear that before "viability" it is never permitted to terminate the gestation of an anencephalic child as the *means* of avoiding psychological or physical risks to the mother. Nor is such termination permitted after "viability" if early delivery endangers the child's life due to complications of prematurity. In such cases, it cannot reasonably be maintained that such a termination is simply a side-effect of the treatment of a pathology of the mother (as described in Directive 47). Anencephaly is not a pathology of the mother, but of the child, and terminating her pregnancy cannot be a treatment of a pathology she does not have. Only if the complications of the pregnancy result in a life-threatening pathology of the mother, may the treatment of this pathology be permitted even at a risk to the child, and then only if the child's death is not a means to treating the mother.

The fact that the life of a child suffering from anencephaly will probably be brief cannot excuse directly causing death before "viability" or gravely endangering the child's life after "viability" as a result of the complications of prematurity.

The anencephalic child during his or her probably brief life after birth should be given the comfort and palliative care appropriate to all the dying. This failing life need not be further troubled by using extraordinary means to prolong it (see *ERD*, Directives 57 & 58). It is most commendable for parents to wish to donate the organs of an anencephalic child for transplants that may assist other children, but this may never be permitted before the donor child is certainly dead.

The profound and personal suffering of the parents of an anencephalic child gives us cause for concern and calls for compassionate pastoral and medical care as the parents prepare for the pain and emptiness that the certain death of their newborn child will bring. The mother who carries to term a child who will soon die deserves our every possible support. The baptism of the child assures the parents of the child's eternal happiness, and the provision of Christian burial of the deceased infant gives witness to the Church's unconditional respect for human life and the recognition that in the face of every human being is an encounter with God.

Pontifical Academy for Life

Declaration on the Production and the Scientific and Therapeutic Use of Human Embryonic Stem Cells

August 25, 2000

This document seeks to contribute to the debate on the production and use of *embryonic stem cells* which is now taking place in scientific and ethical literature and in public opinion. Given the growing relevance of the debate on the limits and liceity of the production and use of such cells, there is a pressing need to reflect on the ethical implications which are present.

The first section will very briefly set out the most recent scientific data on stem cells and the biotechnological data on their production and use. The second section will draw attention to the more relevant ethical problems raised by these new discoveries and their applications.

Scientific Aspects

Although some aspects need to be studied more thoroughly, a commonly accepted *definition* of "stem cell" describes it as a cell with two characteristics: 1) the *property of an unlimited self-maintenance*—that is, the ability to reproduce itself over a long period of time without becoming differentiated; and 2) the *capability to produce non-permanent progenitor cells*, with limited capacity for proliferation, from which derive *a variety of lineages of highly differentiated cells* (neural cells, muscle cells, blood cells, etc.). For about thirty years stem cells have provided a vast field of research in adult tissue,[1] in embryonic tissue and in *in vitro* cultures of embryonic stem cells of experimental animals.[2] But public attention has recently increased with a new milestone that has been reached: the production of human embryonic stem cells.

Human embryonic stem cells

Today, the *preparation of human embryonic stem cells* (human ES cells) implies the following[3]: 1) the *production of human embryos* and/or the *use* of the surplus embryos resulting from *in vitro* fertilization or of frozen embryos; 2) the *development* of these embryos to the stage of initial blastocysts; 3) the *isolation* of the embryoblast or inner cell mass (ICM)—which implies the *destruction of the embryo*; 4) *culturing* these cells on a feeder layer of irradiated mouse embryonic fibroblasts in a suitable medium, where they can multiply and coalesce to form colonies; 5) repeated *subculturing* of these colonies, which lead to the formation of *cell lines* capable of multiplying

indefinitely while preserving the characteristics of ES cells for months and years.

These ES cells, however, are only the point of departure for the preparation of *differentiated cell lines*, that is, of cells with the characteristics proper of the various tissues (muscle, neural, epithelial, haematic, germinal, etc.). Methods for obtaining them are still being studied;[4] but the injection of human ES cells into experimental animals (mice) or their culture *in vitro* in controlled environments to their confluence have shown that they are able to produce differentiated cells which, in a normal development, would derive from the three different embryonic tissue layers: endoderm (intestinal epithelium), mesoderm (cartilage, bone, smooth and striated muscle) and ectoderm (neural epithelium, squamous epithelium).[5]

The results of these experiments had a great impact on the world of both science and biotechnology—especially medicine and pharmacology—no less than the world of business and the mass media. There were high hopes that the application of this knowledge would lead to new and safer ways of treating serious diseases, something which had been sought for years.[6] But the impact was greatest in the political world.[7] In the United States in particular, in response to the long-standing opposition of Congress to the use of federal funds for research in which human embryos were destroyed, there came strong pressure from the National Institutes of Health (NIH), among others, to obtain funds for at least using stem cells produced by private groups; there came also recommendations from the National Bioethics Advisory Committee (NBAC), established by the Federal Government to study the problem, that public money should be given not only for research on embryonic stem cells but also for producing them. Indeed, persistent efforts are being made to rescind definitively the present legal ban on the use of federal funds for research on human embryos.

Similar pressures are being brought to bear also in England, Japan and Australia.

Therapeutic cloning

It had become clear that the therapeutic use of ES cells, as such, entailed significant risks, since—as had been observed in experiments on mice—tumours resulted. It would have been necessary therefore to prepare specialized lines of *differentiated cells* as they were needed; and it did not appear that this could be done in a short period of time. But, even if successful, it would have been very difficult to be certain that the inoculation or therapeutic implant was free of stem cells, which would entail the corresponding risks. Moreover there would have been a need for further treatment to overcome immunological incompatibility. For these reasons, three methods of *therapeutic cloning*[8] were proposed, suitable for preparing pluripotent human embryonic stem cells with well defined genetic information from which desired differentiation would then follow.

1. *The replacement of the nucleus of an oocyte with the nucleus of an adult cell of a given subject,* followed by embryonic development to the stage of blastocyst and the use of the inner cell mass (ICM) in order to obtain ES cells and, from these, the desired differentiated cells.

2. *The transfer of a nucleus of a cell of a given subject into an oocite of another animal.* An eventual success in this procedure should lead—it is presumed—to the development of a human embryo, to be used as in the preceding case.

3. *The reprogramming of the nucleus of a cell of a given subject by fusing the ES cytoplast with a somatic cell karyoplast, thus obtaining a "cybrid".* This is a possibility which is still under study. In any event, this method too would seem to demand a prior preparation of ES cells from human embryos.

Current scientific research is looking to the first of these possibilities as the preferred method, but it is obvious that—from a moral point of view, as we shall see—all three proposed solutions are unacceptable.

Adult stem cells

From studies on adult stem cells (ASC) in the last thirty years it had been clearly shown that many adult tissues contain stem cells, but stem cells capable of producing only cells proper to a given tissue. That is, it was not thought that these cells could be reprogrammed. In more recent years,[9] however, *pluripotent stem cells* were also discovered in various human tissues—in bone marrow (HSCs), in the brain (NSCs), in the mesenchyme (MSCs) of various organs, and in umbilical cord blood (P/CB, placental/cord blood); these are cells capable of producing different types of cells, mostly blood cells, muscle cells and neural cells. It was learnt how to recognize them, select them, maintain them in development, and induce them to form different types of mature cells by means of growth factors and other regulating proteins. Indeed noteworthy progress has already been made in the experimental field, applying the most advanced methods of genetic engineering and molecular biology in analyzing the genetic programme at work in stem cells,[10] and in importing the desired genes into stem cells or progenitor cells which, when implanted, are able

to restore specific functions to damaged tissue.[11] It is sufficient to mention, on the basis of the reported references, that in human beings the stem cells of bone marrow, from which the different lines of blood cells are formed, have as their marker the molecule CD34; and that, when purified, these cells are able to restore entirely the normal blood count in patients who receive ablative doses of radiation and chemotherapy, and this with a speed which is in proportion to the quantity of cells used. Furthermore, there are already indications on how to guide the development of neural stem cells (NSCs) through the use of various proteins—among them neuroregulin and bone morphogenetic protein 2 (BMP2)—which can direct NSCs to become neurons or glia (myelin-producing neural support cells) or even smooth muscle tissue.

The note of satisfaction, albeit cautious, with which many of the cited works conclude is an indication of the great promise that "adult stem cells" offer for effective treatment of many pathologies. Thus the affirmation made by D. J. Watt and G. E. Jones: "The muscle stem cell, whether it be of the embryonic myoblast lineage, or of the adult satellite status, may well turn out to be a cell with far greater importance to tissues other than its tissue of origin and may well hold the key to future therapies for diseases other than those of a myogenic nature" (p. 93). As J. A. Nolta and D. B. Kohn emphasize: "Progress in the use of gene transfer into haemotopoietic cells has led to initial clinical trials. Information developed by these early efforts will be used to guide future developments. Ultimately, gene therapy may allow a number of genetic and acquired diseases to be treated, without the current complications from bone marrow transplantation with allogeneic cells." (p. 460); and the confirmation offered by D. L. Clarke and J. Frisén: "These studies suggest that stem cells in different adult tissues may be more similar than previously thought and perhaps in some cases have a developmental repertoire close to that of ES cells" (p. 1663) and "demonstrates that an adult neural stem cell has a very broad developmental capacity and may potentially be used to generate a variety of cell types for transplantation in different diseases" (p. 1660).

The progress and results obtained in the field of adult stem cells (ASC) show not only their great plasticity but also their many possible uses, in all likelihood no different from those of embryonic stem cells, since plasticity depends in large part upon genetic information, which can be reprogrammed.

Obviously, it is not yet possible to compare the therapeutic results obtained and obtainable using embryonic stem cells and adult stem cells. For the latter, various pharmaceutical firms are already conducting clinical experiments[12] which are showing success and raising genuine hopes for the not too distant future. With embryonic stem cells, even if various experimental approaches prove positive,[13] their application in the clinical field—owing precisely to the serious ethical and legal problems which arise—needs to be seriously reconsidered and requires a great sense of responsibility before the dignity of every human being.

Ethical Problems

Given the nature of this article, the key ethical problems implied by these new technologies are presented briefly, with an indication of the responses which emerge from a careful consideration of the human subject from the moment of conception. It is this consideration which underlies the position affirmed and put forth by the Magisterium of the Church.

The *first ethical problem*, which is fundamental, can be formulated thus: *Is it morally licit to produce and/or use living human embryos for the preparation of ES cells?*

The answer is negative, for the following reasons:

1. On the basis of a complete biological analysis, the living human embryo is—from the moment of the union of the gametes—a *human subject* with a well defined identity, which from that point begins its own *coordinated, continuous and gradual development*, such that at no later stage can it be considered as a simple mass of cells.[14]

2. From this it follows that as a *"human individual"* it has the *right* to its own life; and therefore every intervention which is not in favour of the embryo is an act which violates that right. Moral theology has always taught that in the case of *"jus certum tertii"* the system of probabilism does not apply.[15]

3. Therefore, the ablation of the inner cell mass (ICM) of the blastocyst, which critically and irremediably damages the human embryo, curtailing its development, is a *gravely immoral* act and consequently is *gravely illicit.*

4. *No end believed to be good*, such as the use of stem cells for the preparation of other differentiated cells to be used in what look to be promising therapeutic procedures, *can justify an intervention of this kind.* A good end does not make right an action which in itself is wrong.

5. For Catholics, this position is explicitly confirmed by the Magisterium of the Church which, in the Encyclical *Evangelium Vitae,* with reference to the Instruction *Donum Vitae* of the Congregation for the Doctrine of the Faith, affirms: "The Church has always taught and continues to teach that the result of human procreation, from the first moment of its existence, must be guaranteed that unconditional respect which is morally due to the human being in his or her totality and unity in body and spirit: >The human being is to be respected and treated as a person from the moment of conception; and therefore from that same moment his rights as a person must be recognized, among which in the first place is the inviolable right of every innocent human being to life'"(No. 60).[16]

The *second ethical problem* can be formulated thus: *Is it morally licit to engage in so-called "therapeutic cloning" by producing cloned human embryos and then destroying them in order to produce ES cells?*

The answer is negative, for the following reason: Every type of therapeutic cloning, which implies producing human embryos and then destroying them in order to obtain stem cells, is illicit; for there is present the ethical problem examined above, which can only be answered in the negative.[17]

The *third ethical problem* can be formulated thus: *Is it morally licit to use ES cells, and the differentiated cells obtained from them, which are supplied by other researchers or are commercially obtainable?*

The answer is negative, since: prescinding from the participation—formal or otherwise—in the morally illicit intention of the principal agent, the case in question entails a proximate material cooperation in the production and manipulation of human embryos on the part of those producing or supplying them.

In conclusion, it is not hard to see the seriousness and gravity of the ethical problem posed by the desire to extend to the field of human research the production and/or use of human embryos, even from an humanitarian perspective.

The possibility, now confirmed, of using *adult stem cells* to attain the same goals as would be sought with embryonic stem cells—even if many further steps in both areas are necessary before clear and conclusive results are obtained—indicates that adult stem cells represent a more reasonable and human method for making correct and sound progress in this new field of research and in the therapeutic applications which it promises. These applications are undoubtedly a source of great hope for a significant number of suffering people.

The President
Prof. Juan de Dios Vial Correa
The Vice President
S.E. Mons. Elio Sgreccia

Notes

[1]Cf. M. LOEFFLER, C. S. POTTEN, *Stem Cells and Cellular Pedigrees—a Conceptual Introduction*, in C. S. POTTEN (ed.), *Stem Cells*, Academic Press, London (1997), pp.1-27; D. Van der KOOY, S. WEISS, *Why Stem Cells?*, Science 2000, 287, 1439-1441.

[2]Cf. T: NAKANO, H. KODAMA, T. HONJO, *Generation of Lymphohematopoietic Cells from Embryonic Stem Cells in Culture*, Science 1994, 265, 1098-1101; G. KELLER, *In Vitro Differentiation of Embryonic Stem Cells*, Current Opinion in Cell Biology 1995, 7, 862-869; S. ROBERTSON, M. KENNEDY, G. KELLER, *Hematopoietic Commitment During Embryogenesis*, Annals of the New York Academy of Sciences 1999, 872, 9-16.

[3]Cf. J.A .Thomson, J. Itskovitz-Eldor, S.S. Shapiro et al., *Embryonic Stem Cell Lines Derived from Human Blastocysts*, Science 1998, 282, 1145-1147; G. VOGEL, *Harnessing the Power of Stem Cells*, Science 1999, 283, 1432-1434.

[4]Cf. F. M. WATT, B. L. M. HOGAN, *Out of Eden: Stem Cells and Their Niches*, Science 2000, 287, 1427-1430.

[5]Cf. J. A. THOMSON, J. ITSKOVITZ-ELDOR, S. S. SHAPIRO et al., *op. cit.*

[6]Cf. U.S. CONGRESS, OFFICE OF TECHNOLOGY ASSESSMENT, *Neural Grafting: Repairing the Brain and Spinal Cord*, OTA-BA-462, Washington, DC, U.S. Government Printing Office, 1990; A. McLAREN, *Stem Cells: Golden Opportunities with Ethical Baggage*, Science 2000, 288, 1778.

[7]Cf. E. MARSHALL, *A Versatile Cell Line Raises Scientific Hopes, Legal Questions*, Science 1998, 282, 1014-1015; J. GEARHART, *New Potential for Human Embryonic Stem Cells*, ibid., 1061-1062; E. MARSHALL, *Britain Urged to Expand Embryo Studies*, ibid., 2167-2168; 73 SCIENTISTS, *Science Over Politics*, Science 1999, 283, 1849-1850; E. MARSHALL, *Ethicists Back Stem Cell Research, White House Treads Cautiously*, Science 1999, 285, 502; H. T. SHAPIRO, *Ethical Dilemmas and Stem Cell Research*, ibid., 2065; G. VOGEL, *NIH Sets Rules for Funding Embryonic Stem Cell Research*, Science 1999, 286, 2050; G. KELLER, H. R. SNODGRASS, *Human Embryonic Stem Cells: the Future Is Now*, Nature Medicine 1999, 5, 151-152; G.J. ANNAS, A. CAPLAN, S. ELIAS, *Stem Cell Politics, Ethics and Medical Progress*, ibid., 1339-1341; G. VOGEL, *Company Gets Rights to Cloned Human Embryos*, Science 2000, 287, 559; D. NORMILE, *Report Would Open Up Research in Japan*, ibid., 949; M. S. FRANKEL, *In Search of Stem Cell Policy*, ibid., 1397; D. PERRY, *Patients Voices: the Powerful Sound in the Stem Cell Debate*, ibid., 1423; N. LENOIR, *Europe Confronts the Embryonic Stem Cell Research Challenge*, ibid., 1425-1427; F. E. YOUNG, *A Time for Restraint*, ibid., 1424; EDITORIAL, *Stem Cells*, Nature Medicine 2000, 6, 231.

[8]D. DAVOR, J. GEARHART, *Putting Stem Cells to Work*, Science 1999, 283, 1468-1470.

[9]Cf. C. S. POTTEN (ed.), *Stem Cells*, Academic Press, London 1997, p. 474; D. ORLIC, T. A. BOCK, L. KANZ, *Hemopoietic Stem Cells: Biology and Transplantation*, Ann. N. Y. Acad. Sciences, vol. 872, New York 1999, p. 405; M. F. PITTENGER, A. M. MACKAY, S.C. BECK et al., *Multilineage Potential of Adult Human Mesenchymal Stem Cells*, Science 1999, 284, 143-147; C. R. R. BJORNSON, R.L. RIETZE, B. A. REYNOLDS et al., *Turning Brain into Blood: a Hematopoietic Fate Adopted by Adult Neural Stem Cells* in vivo, Science 1999, 283, 534-536; V. OUREDNIK, J. OUREDNIK, K. I. PARK, E. Y. SNYDER, *Neural Stem Cells—a Versatile Tool for Cell Replacement and Gene Therapy in the Central Nervous System*, Clinical Genetics 1999, 56, 267-278; I. LEMISCHKA, *Searching for Stem Cell Regulatory Molecules: Some General Thoughts and Possible Approaches*, Ann. N.Y. Acad. Sci. 1999, 872, 274-288; H. H. GAGE, *Mammalian Neural Stem Cells*, Science 2000, 287, 1433-1438; D. L. CLARKE, C. B. JOHANSSON, J. FRISEN et al., *Generalized Potential of Adult Neural Stem Cells*, Science 2000, 288, 1660-1663; G. VOGEL, *Brain Cells Reveal Surprising Versatility*, ibid., 1559-1561.

[10]Cf. R. L. PHILLIPS, R. E. ERNST, I. R. LEMISCHKA, et al., *The Genetic Program of Hematopoietic Stem Cells*, Science 2000, 288, 1635-1640.

[11]Cf. D. J. WATT, G. E. JONES, *Skeletal Muscle Stem Cells: Function and Potential Role in Therapy*, in C. S. POTTEN, *Stem Cells, op. cit.*, 75-98; J. A. NOLTA, D. B. KOHN, *Haematopoietic Stem Cells for Gene Therapy*, ibid., 447-460; Y. REISNER, E. BACHAR-LUSTIG, H-W. LI et al., *The Role of Megadose CD34+ Progenitor Cells in the Treatment of Leukemia Patients Without a Matched Donor and in Tolerance Induction for Organ Transplantation*, Ann. N.Y. Acad. Sci. 1999, 872, 336-350; D. W. EMERY, G. STAMATOYANNOPOULOS, *Stem Cell Gene Therapy for the ß-Chain Hemoglobinopathies*, ibid., 94-108; M. GRIFFITH, R. OSBORNE, R. MUNGER, *Functional Human Corneal Equivalents Constructed from Cell Lines*, Science 1999, 286, 2169-2172; N. S. ROY, S. WANG, L. JIANG et al., In vitro *Neurogenesis by Progenitor Cells Isolated from the Adult Hippocampus*, Nature Medicine 2000, 6, 271-277; M. NOBLE, *Can Neural Stem Cells Be Used as Therapeutic Vehicles in the Treatment of Brain Tumors?*, ibid., 369-370; I. L. WEISSMAN, *Translating Stem and Progenitor Cell Biology to the Clinic: Barriers and Opportunities*, Science 2000, 287, 1442-1446; P. SERUP, *Panning for Pancreatic Stem Cells*, Nature Genetics 2000, 25, 134-135.

[12]E. MARSHALL, *The Business of Stem Cells*, Science 2000, 287, 1419-1421.

[13]Cf. O. BRUSTLE, K. N. JONES, R. D. LEARISH et al., *Embryonic Stem Cell-Derived Glial Precursors: a Source of Myelinating Transplants*, Science 1999, 285, 754-756; J. W. McDONALD, X-Z LIU, Y. QU et al., *Transplanted Embryonic Stem Cells Survive, Differentiate and Promote Recovery in Injured Rat Spinal Cord*, Nature Medicine 1999, 5, 1410-1412.

[14]Cf. A. SERRA , R. COLOMBO, *Identità e Statuto dell'Embrione Umano: il Contributo della Biologia*, in PONTIFICIA ACADEMIA PRO VITA, *Identità e Statuto dell'Embrione Umano*, Libreria Editrice Vaticana, Città del Vaticano 1998, pp.106-158.

[15]Cf. I. CARRASCO de PAULA, *Il Rispetto Dovuto all'Embrione Umano: Prospettiva Storico-Dottrinale*, in ibid., pp. 9-33; R. LUCAS LUCAS, *Statuto Antropologico dell'Embrione Umano*, in ibid., pp.159-185; M. COZZOLI, *L'Embrione Umano: Aspetti Etico-Normativi*, in ibid., pp.237-273; L. EUSEBI, *La Tutela dell'Embrione Umano: Profili Giuridici*, in ibid., pp. 274-286.

[16]JOHN PAUL II, *Encyclical Letter "Evangelium Vitae"* (25 March 1995), Acta Apostolicae Sedis 1995, 87, 401-522; cf. also CONGREGATION FOR THE DOCTRINE OF THE FAITH, *Instruction on Respect for Human Life in Its Origins and on the Dignity of Procreation "Donum Vitae"* (22 February 1987), Acta Apostolicae Sedis 1988, 80, 70-102.

[17]CONGREGATION FOR THE DOCTRINE OF THE FAITH, *op. cit.*, I, no. 6; C.B.COHEN (ed.), *Special Issue: Ethics and the Cloning of Human Embryos*, Kennedy Institute of Ethics Journal 1994, n.4, 187-282; H. T. SHAPIRO, *Ethical and Policy Issues of Human Cloning*, Science 1997, 277, 195-196; M.L. DI PIETRO, *Dalla Clonazione Animale alla Clonazione dell'Uomo?*, Medicina e Morale 1997, no. 6, 1099-2005; A. SERRA, *Verso la Clonazione dell'Uomo? Una Nuova Frontiera della Scienza*, La Civiltà Cattolica 1998 I, 224-234; ibid., *La Clonazione Umana in Prospettiva "Sapienziale"*, ibid., 329-339.

APPENDIX XII

Pope John Paul II

Address to the Eighteenth International Congress of the Transplantation Society

August 29, 2000

Distinguished Ladies and Gentlemen,

1. I am happy to greet all of you at this International Congress, which has brought you together for a reflection on the complex and delicate theme of transplants. I thank Professor Raffaello Cortesini and Professor Oscar Salvatierra for their kind words, and I extend a special greeting to the Italian Authorities present.

To all of you I express my gratitude for your kind invitation to take part in this meeting and I very much appreciate the serious consideration you are giving to the moral teaching of the Church. With respect for science and being attentive above all to the law of God, the Church has no other aim but the integral good of the human person.

Transplants are a great step forward in science's service of man, and not a few people today owe their lives to an organ transplant. Increasingly, the technique of transplants has proven to be a valid means of attaining the primary goal of all medicine - the service of human life. That is why in the Encyclical Letter *Evangelium vitae* I suggested that one way of nurturing a genuine culture of life "is the donation of organs, performed in an ethically acceptable manner, with a view to offering a chance of health and even of life itself to the sick who sometimes have no other hope" (No. 86).

2. As with all human advancement, this particular field of medical science, for all the hope of health and life it offers to many, also presents *certain critical issues* that need to be examined in the light of a discerning anthropological and ethical reflection.

In this area of medical science too the fundamental criterion must be *the defence and promotion of the integral good of the human person*, in keeping with that unique dignity which is ours by virtue of our humanity. Consequently, it is evident that every medical procedure performed on the human person is subject to limits: not just the limits of what it is technically possible, but also limits determined by respect for human nature itself, understood in its fullness: "what is technically possible is not for that reason alone morally admissible" (Congregation for the Doctrine of the Faith, *Donum vitae,* 4).

3. It must first be emphasized, as I observed on another occasion, that every organ transplant has its source in a decision of great ethical value: "the decision to offer without reward a part of one's own body for the health and well-being of another person" (*Address to the Participants in a Congres on Organ Transplants,* 20 June 1991, No. 3). Here precisely lies the nobility of the gesture, a gesture which is a genuine act of love. It is not just a matter of giving away something that belongs to us but of giving something of ourselves, for "by virtue of its substantial union with a spiritual soul, the human body cannot be considered as a mere complex of tissues, organs and functions . . . rather it is a constitutive part of the person who manifests and expresses himself through it" (Congregation for the Doctrine of the Faith, *Donum vitae,* 3).

Accordingly, any procedure which tends to commercialize human organs or to consider them as items of exchange or trade must be considered morally unacceptable, because to use the body as an "object" is to violate the dignity of the human person.

This first point has an immediate consequence of great ethical import: *the need for informed consent.* The human "authenticity" of such a decisive gesture requires that individuals be properly informed about the processes involved, in order to be in a position to consent or decline in a free and conscientious manner. The consent of relatives has its own ethical validity in the absence of a decision on the part of the donor. Naturally, an analogous consent should be given by the recipients of donated organs.

4. Acknowledgement of the unique dignity of the human person has a further underlying consequence: *vital organs which occur singly in the body can be removed only after death*, that is from the body of someone who is certainly dead. This requirement is self-evident, since to act otherwise would mean intentionally to cause the death of the donor in disposing of his organs. This gives rise to one of the most debated issues in contemporary bioethics, as well as to serious concerns in the minds of ordinary people. I refer to the problem of *ascertaining the fact of death*. When can a person be considered dead with complete certainty?

In this regard, it is helpful to recall that *the death of the person* is a single event, consisting in the total disintegration of that unitary and integrated whole that is the personal self. It results from the separation of the life-principle (or soul) from the corporal reality of the person. The death of the person, understood in this primary sense, is an event which *no scientific technique or empirical method can identify directly.*

Yet human experience shows that once death occurs *certain biological signs inevitably follow*, which medicine has learnt to recognize with increasing precision. In this sense, the "criteria" for ascertaining death used by medicine today should not be understood as the technical-scientific determination of the *exact moment* of a person's death, but as a scientifically secure means of identifying *the biological signs that a person has indeed died.*

5. It is a well-known fact that for some time certain scientific approaches to ascertaining death have shifted the emphasis from the traditional cardio-respiratory signs to the so-called *"neurological" criterion.* Specifically, this consists in establishing, according to clearly determined parameters commonly held by the international scientific community, the complete and irreversible cessation of all brain activity (in the cerebrum, cerebellum and brain stem). This is then considered the sign that the individual organism has lost its integrative capacity.

With regard to the parameters used today for ascertaining death—whether the "encephalic" signs or the more traditional cardio-respiratory signs—the Church does not make technical decisions. She limits herself to the Gospel duty of comparing the data offered by medical science with the Christian understanding of the unity of the person, bringing out the similarities and the possible conflicts capable of endangering respect for human dignity.

Here it can be said that the criterion adopted in more recent times for ascertaining the fact of death, namely the *complete* and *irreversible* cessation of all brain activity, if rigorously applied, does not seem to conflict with the essential elements of a sound anthropology. Therefore a health-worker professionally responsible for ascertaining death can use these criteria in each individual case as the basis for arriving at that degree of assurance in ethical judgement which moral teaching describes as "moral certainty". This moral certainty is considered the necessary and sufficient basis for an ethically correct course of action Only where such certainty exists, and where informed consent has already been given by the donor or the donor's legitimate representatives, is it morally right to initiate the technical procedures required for the removal of organs for transplant.

6. Another question of great ethical significance is that of *the allocation of donated organs* through waiting-lists and the assignment of priorities. Despite efforts to promote the practice of organ-donation, the resources available in many countries are currently insufficient to meet medical needs. Hence there is a need to compile waiting-lists for transplants on the basis of clear and properly reasoned criteria.

From the moral standpoint, an obvious principle of justice requires that the criteria for assigning donated organs should in no way be "discriminatory" (i.e. based on age, sex, race, religion, social standing, etc.) or "utilitarian" (i.e. based on work capacity, social usefulness, etc.). Instead, in determining who should have precedence in receiving an organ, *judgements should be made on the basis of immunological and clinical factors.*Any other criterion would prove wholly arbitrary and subjective, and would fail to recognize the intrinsic value of each human person as such, a value that is independent of any external circumstances.

7. A final issue concerns a possible alternative solution to the problem of finding human organs for transplantion, something still very much in the experimental stage, namely *xenotransplants*, that is, organ transplants from other animal species.

It is not my intention to explore in detail the problems connected with this form of intervention. I would merely recall that already in 1956 Pope Pius XII raised the question of their legitimacy. He did so when commenting on the scientific possibility, then being presaged, of transplanting animal corneas to humans. His response is still enlightening for us today: in principle, he stated, for a *xenotransplant* to be licit, the transplanted organ must not impair the integrity of the psychological or genetic identity of the person receiving it; and there must also be a proven biological possibility that the transplant will be successful and will not expose the recipient to inordinate risk (cf. *Address to the Italian Association of Cornea Donors and to Clinical Oculists and Legal Medical Practitioners*, 14 May 1956).

8. In concluding, I express the hope that, thanks to the work of so many generous and highly-trained people, scientific and technological research in the field of transplants will continue to progress, and extend to *experimentation with new therapies which can replace organ transplants*, as some recent developments in prosthetics seem to promise. In any event, methods that fail to respect the dignity and value of the person must always be avoided. I am thinking in particular of attempts at human cloning with a view to obtaining organs for transplants: these techniques, insofar as they involve the manipulation and destruction of human embryos, are not morally acceptable, even when their proposed goal is good in itself. Science itself points to other forms of *therapeutic intervention* which would not involve cloning or the use of embryonic cells, but rather would make use of stem cells taken from adults. This is the direction that research must follow if it wishes to respect the dignity of each and every human being, even at the embryonic stage.

In addressing these varied issues, *the contribution of philosophers and theologians* is important. Their careful and competent reflection on the ethical problems associated with transplant therapy can help to clarify the criteria for assessing what kinds of transplants are morally acceptable and under what conditions, especially with regard to the protection of each individual's personal identity.

I am confident that social, political and educational leaders will renew their commitment to fostering a genuine culture of generosity and solidarity. There is a need to instil in people's hearts, especially in the hearts of the young, a genuine and deep appreciation of the need for brotherly love, a love that can find expression in the decision to become an organ donor.

May the Lord sustain each one of you in your work, and guide you in the service of authentic human progress. I accompany this wish with my Blessing.

APPENDIX XIII

United States Conference of Catholic Bishops

Ethical and Religious Directives for Catholic Health Care Services

Fourth Edition, 2001

This fourth edition of the *Ethical and Religious Directives for Catholic Health Care Services* was developed by the Committee on Doctrine of the National Conference of Catholic Bishops and approved as the national code by the full body of bishops at their June 2001 general meeting. This edition of the *Directives*, which replaces all previous editions, is recommended for implementation by the diocesan bishop and is authorized for publication by the undersigned.

Monsignor William P. Fay
General Secretary
NCCB/USCC

Preamble

Health care in the United States is marked by extraordinary change. Not only is there continuing change in clinical practice due to technological advances, but the health-care system in the United States is being challenged by both institutional and social factors as well. At the same time, there are a number of developments within the Catholic Church affecting the ecclesial mission of health care. Among these are significant changes in religious orders and congregations, the increased involvement of lay men and women, a heightened awareness of the Church's social role in the world, and developments in moral theology since the Second Vatican Council. A contemporary understanding of the Catholic health-care ministry must take into account the new challenges presented by transitions both in the Church and in American society.

Throughout the centuries, with the aid of other sciences, a body of moral principles has emerged that expresses the Church's teaching on medical and moral matters and has proven to be pertinent and applicable to the ever-changing circumstances of health care and its delivery. In response to today's challenges, these same moral principles of Catholic teaching provide the rationale and direction for this revision of the *Ethical and Religious Directives for Catholic Health Care Services.*

These directives presuppose our statement *Health and Health Care* published in 1981.[1] There we presented the theological principles that guide the Church's vision of health care, called for all Catholics to share in the healing mission of the Church, expressed our full commitment to the health care ministry, and offered encouragement to all those who are involved in it. Now, with American health care facing even more dramatic changes, we reaffirm the Church's commitment to health-care ministry and the distinctive Catholic identity of the Church's institutional health-care services.[2] The purpose of these *Ethical and Religious Directives* then is twofold: first, to reaffirm the ethical standards of behavior in health care that flow from the Church's teaching about the dignity of the human person; second, to provide authoritative guidance on certain moral issues that face Catholic health care today.

The *Ethical and Religious Directives* are concerned primarily with institutionally based Catholic health care services. They address the sponsors, trustees, administrators, chaplains, physicians, health-care personnel, and patients or residents of these institutions and services. Since they express the Church's moral teaching, these directives also will be helpful to Catholic professionals engaged in health care services in other settings. The moral teachings that we profess here flow principally from the natural law, understood in the light of the revelation Christ has entrusted to his Church. From this source the Church has derived its understanding of the nature of the human person, of human acts, and of the goals that shape human activity.

The directives have been refined through an extensive process of consultation with bishops, theologians, sponsors, administrators, physicians, and other health-care providers. While providing standards and guidance, the directives do not cover in detail all of the complex issues that confront Catholic health care today. Moreover, the directives will be reviewed periodically by the National Conference of Catholic Bishops, in the light of authoritative Church teaching, in order to address new insights from theological and medical research or new requirements of public policy.

The directives begin with a general introduction that presents a theological basis for the Catholic health-care ministry. Each of the six parts that follow is divided into two sections. The first section is in expository form; it serves as an introduction and provides the context in which concrete issues can be discussed from the perspective of the Catholic faith. The second section is in prescriptive form; the directives promote and protect the truths of the Catholic faith as those truths are brought to bear on concrete issues in health care.

General Introduction

The Church has always sought to embody our Savior's concern for the sick. The gospel accounts of Jesus' ministry draw special attention to his acts of healing: he cleansed a man with leprosy (Mt 8:1–4; Mk 1:40–42); he gave sight to two people who were blind (Mt 20:29–34; Mk 10:46–52); he enabled one who was mute to speak (Lk 11:14); he cured a woman who was hemorrhaging (Mt 9:20–22; Mk 5:25–34); and he brought a young girl back to life (Mt 9:18, 23–25; Mk 5:35–42). Indeed, the Gospels are replete with examples of how the Lord cured every kind of ailment and disease (Mt 9:35). In the account of Matthew, Jesus' mission fulfilled the prophecy of Isaiah: "He took away our infirmities and bore our diseases" (Mt 8:17; cf. Is 53:4).

Jesus' healing mission went further than caring only for physical affliction. He touched people at the deepest level of their existence; he sought their physical, mental, and spiritual healing (Jn 6:35, 11:25–27). He "came so that they might have life and have it more abundantly" (Jn 10:10).

The mystery of Christ casts light on every facet of Catholic health care: to see Christian love as the animating principle of health care; to see healing and compassion as a continuation of Christ's mission; to see suffering as a participation in the redemptive power of Christ's passion, death, and resurrection; and to see death, transformed by the Resurrection, as an opportunity for a final act of communion with Christ.

For the Christian, our encounter with suffering and death can take on a positive and distinctive meaning through the redemptive power of Jesus' suffering and death. As St. Paul says, we are "always carrying about in the body the dying of Jesus, so that the life of Jesus may also be manifested in our body" (2 Cor 4:10). This truth does not lessen the pain and fear, but gives confidence and grace for bearing suffering rather than being overwhelmed by it. Catholic health-care ministry bears witness to the truth that, for those who are in Christ, suffering and death are the birth pangs of the new creation. "God Himself will always be with them [as their God]. He will wipe every tear from their eyes, and there shall be no more death or mourning, wailing or pain, [for] the old order has passed away" (Rev 21:3–4).

In faithful imitation of Jesus Christ, the Church has served the sick, suffering, and dying in various ways throughout history. The zealous service of individuals and communities has provided shelter for the traveler; infirmaries for the sick; and homes for children, adults, and the elderly.[3] In the United States, the many religious communities as well as dioceses that sponsor and staff this country's Catholic health-care institutions and services have established an effective Catholic presence in health care. Modeling their efforts on the gospel parable of the Good Samaritan, these communities of women and men have exemplified authentic neighborliness to those in need (Lk 10:25–37). The Church seeks to ensure that the service offered in the past will be continued into the future.

While many religious communities continue their commitment to the health-care ministry, lay Catholics increasingly have stepped forward to collaborate in this ministry. Inspired by the example of Christ and mandated by the Second Vatican Council, lay faithful are invited to a broader and more intense field of ministries than in the past.[4] By virtue of their Baptism, lay faithful are called to participate actively in the Church's life and mission.[5] Their participation and leadership in the health care ministry, through new forms of sponsorship and governance of institutional Catholic health care, are essential for the Church to continue her ministry of healing and compassion. They are joined in the Church's health-care mission by many men and women who are not Catholic.

Catholic health care expresses the healing ministry of Christ in a specific way within the local church. Here the diocesan bishop exercises responsibilities that are rooted in his office as pastor, teacher, and priest. As the center of unity in the diocese and coordinator of ministries in the local church, the diocesan bishop fosters the mission of Catholic health care in a way that promotes collaboration among health care leaders, providers, medical professionals, theologians, and other specialists. As pastor, the diocesan bishop is in a unique position to encourage the faithful to greater responsibility in the healing ministry of the Church. As teacher, the diocesan bishop ensures the moral and religious identity of the health care ministry in whatever setting it is carried out in the diocese. As priest, the diocesan bishop oversees the sacramental care of the sick. These responsibilities will require that Catholic health-care providers and the diocesan bishop engage in ongoing communication on ethical and pastoral matters that require his attention.

In a time of new medical discoveries, rapid technological developments, and social change, what is new can either be an opportunity for genuine advancement in human culture, or it can lead to policies and actions that are contrary to the true dignity and vocation of the human person. In consultation with medical professionals, church leaders review these developments, judge them according to the principles of right reason and the ultimate standard of revealed truth, and offer authoritative teaching and guidance about the moral and pastoral responsibilities entailed by the Christian faith.[6] While the Church cannot furnish a ready answer to every moral dilemma, there are many questions about which she provides normative guidance and direction. In the absence of a determination by the magisterium, but never contrary to Church teaching, the guidance of approved authors can offer appropriate guidance for ethical decision making.

Created in God's image and likeness, the human family shares in the dominion that Christ manifested in his healing ministry. This sharing involves a stewardship over all material creation (Gn 1:26) that should neither abuse nor squander nature's resources. Through science the human race comes to understand God's wonderful work; and through technology it must conserve, protect, and perfect nature in harmony with God's purposes. Health-care professionals pursue a special vocation to share in carrying forth God's life-giving and healing work.

The dialogue between medical science and Christian faith has for its primary purpose the common good of all human persons. It presupposes that science and faith do not contradict each other. Both are grounded in respect for truth and freedom. As new knowledge and new technologies expand, each person must form a correct conscience based on the moral norms for proper health care.

PART ONE
The Social Responsibility of
Catholic Health-Care Services

Their embrace of Christ's healing mission has led institutionally based Catholic health-care services in the United States to become an integral part of the nation's health-care system. Today, this complex health-care system confronts a range of economic, technological, social, and moral challenges. The response of Catholic health-care institutions and services to these challenges is guided by normative principles that inform the Church's healing ministry.

First, Catholic health-care ministry is rooted in a commitment to promote and defend human dignity; this is the foundation of its concern to respect the sacredness of every human life from the moment of conception until death. The first right of the human person, the right to life, entails a right to the means for the proper development of life, such as adequate health care.[7]

Second, the biblical mandate to care for the poor requires us to express this in concrete action at all levels of Catholic health care. This mandate prompts us to work to ensure that our country's health-care delivery system provides adequate health care for the poor. In Catholic institutions, particular attention should be given to the health care needs of the poor, the uninsured, and the underinsured.[8]

Third, Catholic health-care ministry seeks to contribute to the common good. The common good is realized when economic, political, and social conditions ensure protection for the fundamental rights of all individuals and enable all to fulfill their common purpose and reach their common goals.[9]

Fourth, Catholic health-care ministry exercises responsible stewardship of available health-care resources. A just health-care system will be concerned both with promoting equity of care—to assure that the right of each person to basic health care is respected—and with promoting the good health of all in the community. The responsible stewardship of health-care resources can be accomplished best in dialogue with people from all levels of society, in accordance with the principle of subsidiarity and with respect for the moral principles that guide institutions and persons.

Fifth, within a pluralistic society, Catholic health care services will encounter requests for medical procedures contrary to the moral teachings of the Church. Catholic health care does not offend the rights of individual conscience by refusing to provide or permit medical procedures that are judged morally wrong by the teaching authority of the Church.

Directives

1. A Catholic institutional health-care service is a community that provides health care to those in need of it. This service must be animated by the Gospel of Jesus Christ and guided by the moral tradition of the Church.

2. Catholic health care should be marked by a spirit of mutual respect among care-givers that disposes them to deal with those it serves and their families with the compassion of Christ, sensitive to their vulnerability at a time of special need.

3. In accord with its mission, Catholic health care should distinguish itself by service to and advocacy for those

people whose social condition puts them at the margins of our society and makes them particularly vulnerable to discrimination: the poor; the uninsured and the underinsured; children and the unborn; single parents; the elderly; those with incurable diseases and chemical dependencies; racial minorities; immigrants and refugees. In particular, the person with mental or physical disabilities, regardless of the cause or severity, must be treated as a unique person of incomparable worth, with the same right to life and to adequate health care as all other persons.

4. A Catholic health-care institution, especially a teaching hospital, will promote medical research consistent with its mission of providing health care and with concern for the responsible stewardship of health-care resources. Such medical research must adhere to Catholic moral principles.

5. Catholic health care services must adopt these directives as policy, require adherence to them within the institution as a condition for medical privileges and employment, and provide appropriate instruction regarding the directives for administration, medical and nursing staff, and other personnel.

6. A Catholic health-care organization should be a responsible steward of the health-care resources available to it. Collaboration with other health care providers, in ways that do not compromise Catholic social and moral teaching, can be an effective means of such stewardship.[10]

7. A Catholic health-care institution must treat its employees respectfully and justly. This responsibility includes: equal employment opportunities for anyone qualified for the task, irrespective of a person's race, sex, age, national origin, or disability; a workplace that promotes employee participation; a work environment that ensures employee safety and well-being; just compensation and benefits; and recognition of the rights of employees to organize and bargain collectively without prejudice to the common good.

8. Catholic health-care institutions have a unique relationship to both the Church and the wider community they serve. Because of the ecclesial nature of this relationship, the relevant requirements of canon law will be observed with regard to the foundation of a new Catholic health-care institution; the substantial revision of the mission of an institution; and the sale, sponsorship transfer, or closure of an existing institution.

9. Employees of a Catholic health-care institution must respect and uphold the religious mission of the institution and adhere to these directives. They should maintain professional standards and promote the institution's commitment to human dignity and the common good.

PART TWO
The Pastoral and Spiritual Responsibility of Catholic Health Care

The dignity of human life flows from creation in the image of God (Gn 1:26), from redemption by Jesus Christ (Eph 1:10; 1 Tm 2:4–6), and from our common destiny to share a life with God beyond all corruption (1 Cor 15:42–57). Catholic health care has the responsibility to treat those in need in a way that respects the human dignity and eternal destiny of all. The words of Christ have provided inspiration for Catholic health care: "I was ill and you cared for me" (Mt 25:36). The care provided assists those in need to experience their own dignity and value, especially when these are obscured by the burdens of illness or the anxiety of imminent death.

Since a Catholic health-care institution is a community of healing and compassion, the care offered is not limited to the treatment of a disease or bodily ailment but embraces the physical, psychological, social, and spiritual dimensions of the human person. The medical expertise offered through Catholic health care is combined with other forms of care to promote health and relieve human suffering. For this reason, Catholic health care extends to the spiritual nature of the person. "Without health of the spirit, high technology focused strictly on the body offers limited hope for healing the whole person."[11] Directed to spiritual needs that are often appreciated more deeply during times of illness, pastoral care is an integral part of Catholic health care. Pastoral care encompasses the full range of spiritual services, including a listening presence; help in dealing with powerlessness, pain, and alienation; and assistance in recognizing and responding to God's will with greater joy and peace. It should be acknowledged, of course, that technological advances in medicine have reduced the length of hospital stays dramatically. It follows, therefore, that the pastoral care of patients, especially administration of the sacraments, will be provided more often than not at the parish level, both before and after one's hospitalization. For this reason, it is essential that there be very cordial and cooperative relationships between the personnel of pastoral care departments and the local clergy and ministers of care.

Priests, deacons, religious, and laity exercise diverse but complementary roles in this pastoral care. Since many areas of pastoral care call upon the creative response of these pastoral care-givers to the particular needs of patients or residents, the following directives address only a limited number of specific pastoral activities.

Directives

10. A Catholic health-care organization should provide pastoral care to minister to the religious and spiritual needs of all those it serves. Pastoral care personnel— clergy, religious, and lay alike—should have appropriate

professional preparation, including an understanding of these directives.

11. Pastoral care personnel should work in close collaboration with local parishes and community clergy. Appropriate pastoral services and/or referrals should be available to all in keeping with their religious beliefs or affiliation.

12. For Catholic patients or residents, provision for the sacraments is an especially important part of Catholic health-care ministry. Every effort should be made to have priests assigned to hospitals and health care institutions to celebrate the Eucharist and provide the sacraments to patients and staff.

13. Particular care should be taken to provide and to publicize opportunities for patients or residents to receive the sacrament of Penance.

14. Properly prepared lay Catholics can be appointed to serve as extraordinary ministers of Holy Communion, in accordance with canon law and the policies of the local diocese. They should assist pastoral care personnel— clergy, religious, and laity—by providing supportive visits, advising patients regarding the availability of priests for the sacrament of Penance, and distributing Holy Communion to the faithful who request it.

15. Responsive to a patient's desires and condition, all involved in pastoral care should facilitate the avail- ability of priests to provide the sacrament of Anointing of the Sick, recognizing that through this sacrament Christ provides grace and support to those who are seriously ill or weakened by advanced age. Normally, the sacrament is celebrated when the sick person is fully conscious. It may be conferred upon the sick who have lost consciousness or the use of reason, if there is reason to believe that they would have asked for the sacrament while in control of their faculties.

16. All Catholics who are capable of receiving Communion should receive Viaticum when they are in danger of death, while still in full possession of their faculties.[12]

17. Except in cases of emergency (i.e., danger of death), any request for Baptism made by adults or for infants should be referred to the chaplain of the institution. Newly born infants in danger of death, including those miscarried, should be baptized if this is possible.[13] In case of emergency, if a priest or a deacon is not available, anyone can validly baptize.14 In the case of emergency Baptism, the chaplain or the director of pastoral care is to be notified.

18. When a Catholic who has been baptized but not yet confirmed is in danger of death, any priest may confirm the person.[15]

19. A record of the conferral of Baptism or Confirmation should be sent to the parish in which the institution is located and posted in its Baptism/Confirmation registers.

20. Catholic discipline generally reserves the reception of the sacraments to Catholics. In accord with canon 844, § 3, Catholic ministers may administer the sacraments of Eucharist, Penance, and Anointing of the Sick to members of the oriental churches that do not have full communion with the Catholic Church, or of other churches that in the judgment of the Holy See are in the same condition as the oriental churches, if such persons ask for the sacraments on their own and are properly disposed.

With regard to other Christians not in full communion with the Catholic Church, when the danger of death or other grave necessity is present, the four conditions of canon 844, § 4, also must be present, namely, they cannot approach a minister of their own community; they ask for the sacraments on their own; they manifest Catholic faith in these sacraments; and they are properly disposed. The diocesan bishop has the responsibility to oversee this pastoral practice.

21. The appointment of priests and deacons to the pastoral care staff of a Catholic institution must have the explicit approval or confirmation of the local bishop in collaboration with the administration of the institution. The appointment of the director of the pastoral care staff should be made in consultation with the diocesan bishop.

22. For the sake of appropriate ecumenical and interfaith relations, a diocesan policy should be developed with regard to the appointment of non-Catholic members to the pastoral care staff of a Catholic health care institution. The director of pastoral care at a Catholic institution should be a Catholic; any exception to this norm should be approved by the diocesan bishop.

PART THREE
The Professional-Patient Relationship

A person in need of health care and the professional health-care provider who accepts that person as a patient enter into a relationship that requires, among other things, mutual respect, trust, honesty, and appropriate confidentiality. The resulting free exchange of information must avoid manipu- lation, intimidation, or condescension. Such a relationship enables the patient to disclose personal information needed for effective care and permits the health-care provider to use his or her professional competence most effectively to maintain or restore the patient's health. Neither the health care profes- sional nor the patient acts independently of the other; both participate in the healing process.

Today, a patient often receives health care from a team of providers, especially in the setting of the modern acute-care hospital. But the resulting multiplication of relationships does not alter the personal character of the interaction between health-care providers and the patient. The relationship of the person seeking health care and the professionals providing that care is an important part of the foundation on which diagnosis and care are provided. Diagnosis and care, therefore, entail a series of decisions with ethical as well as medical dimensions. The health-care professional has the knowledge and experience to pursue the goals of healing, the maintenance of health, and the compassionate care of the dying, taking into account the patient's convictions and spiritual needs, and the moral responsibilities of all concerned. The person in need of health care depends on the skill of the health-care provider to assist in preserving life and promoting health of body, mind, and spirit. The patient, in turn, has a responsibility to use these physical and mental resources in the service of moral and spiritual goals to the best of his or her ability.

When the health-care professional and the patient use institutional Catholic health care, they also accept its public commitment to the Church's understanding of and witness to the dignity of the human person. The Church's moral teaching on health care nurtures a truly interpersonal professional-patient relationship. This professional-patient relationship is never separated, then, from the Catholic identity of the health-care institution. The faith that inspires Catholic health care guides medical decisions in ways that fully respect the dignity of the person and the relationship with the health-care professional.

Directives

23. The inherent dignity of the human person must be respected and protected regardless of the nature of the person's health problem or social status. The respect for human dignity extends to all persons who are served by Catholic health care.

24. In compliance with federal law, a Catholic health care institution will make available to patients information about their rights, under the laws of their state, to make an advance directive for their medical treatment. The institution, however, will not honor an advance directive that is contrary to Catholic teaching. If the advance directive conflicts with Catholic teaching, an explanation should be provided as to why the directive cannot be honored.

25. Each person may identify in advance a representative to make health-care decisions as his or her surrogate in the event that the person loses the capacity to make health-care decisions. Decisions by the designated surrogate should be faithful to Catholic moral principles and to the person's intentions and values or, if the person's intentions are unknown, to the person's best interests. In the event that an advance directive is not executed, those who are in a position to know best the patient's wishes—usually family members and loved ones—should participate in the treatment decisions for the person who has lost the capacity to make health-care decisions.

26. The free and informed consent of the person or the person's surrogate is required for medical treatments and procedures, except in an emergency situation when consent cannot be obtained and there is no indication that the patient would refuse consent to the treatment.

27. Free and informed consent requires that the person or the person's surrogate receive all reasonable information about the essential nature of the proposed treatment and its benefits; its risks, side-effects, consequences, and cost; and any reasonable and morally legitimate alternatives, including no treatment at all.

28. Each person or the person's surrogate should have access to medical and moral information and counseling so as to be able to form his or her conscience. The free and informed health-care decision of the person or the person's surrogate is to be followed so long as it does not contradict Catholic principles.

29. All persons served by Catholic health care have the right and duty to protect and preserve their bodily and functional integrity.[16] The functional integrity of the person may be sacrificed to maintain the health or life of the person when no other morally permissible means is available.[17]

30. The transplantation of organs from living donors is morally permissible when such a donation will not sacrifice or seriously impair any essential bodily function and the anticipated benefit to the recipient is proportionate to the harm done to the donor. Furthermore, the freedom of the prospective donor must be respected, and economic advantages should not accrue to the donor.

31. No one should be the subject of medical or genetic experimentation, even if it is therapeutic, unless the person or surrogate first has given free and informed consent. In instances of nontherapeutic experimentation, the surrogate can give this consent only if the experiment entails no significant risk to the person's well-being. Moreover, the greater the person's incompetency and vulnerability, the greater the reasons must be to perform any medical experimentation, especially nontherapeutic.

32. While every person is obliged to use ordinary means to preserve his or her health, no person should be obliged to submit to a health-care procedure that the person has judged, with a free and informed conscience, not to provide a reasonable hope of benefit without imposing excessive risks and burdens on the patient or excessive expense to family or community.[18]

33. The well-being of the whole person must be taken into account in deciding about any therapeutic intervention or use of technology. Therapeutic procedures that are likely to cause harm or undesirable side-effects can be justified only by a proportionate benefit to the patient.

34. Health-care providers are to respect each person's privacy and confidentiality regarding information related to the person's diagnosis, treatment, and care.

35. Health-care professionals should be educated to recognize the symptoms of abuse and violence and are obliged to report cases of abuse to the proper authorities in accordance with local statutes.

36. Compassionate and understanding care should be given to a person who is the victim of sexual assault. Health care providers should cooperate with law-enforcement officials and offer the person psychological and spiritual support as well as accurate medical information. A female who has been raped should be able to defend herself against a potential conception from the sexual assault. If, after appropriate testing, there is no evidence that conception has occurred already, she may be treated with medications that would prevent ovulation, sperm capacitation, or fertilization. It is not permissible, however, to initiate or to recommend treatments that have as their purpose or direct effect the removal, destruction, or interference with the implantation of a fertilized ovum.[19]

37. An ethics committee or some alternate form of ethical consultation should be available to assist by advising on particular ethical situations, by offering educational opportunities, and by reviewing and recommending policies. To these ends, there should be appropriate standards for medical ethical consultation within a particular diocese that will respect the diocesan bishop's pastoral responsibility as well as assist members of ethics committees to be familiar with Catholic medical ethics and, in particular, these directives.

PART FOUR
Issues in Care for the Beginning of Life

The Church's commitment to human dignity inspires an abiding concern for the sanctity of human life from its very beginning, and with the dignity of marriage and of the marriage act by which human life is transmitted. The Church cannot approve medical practices that undermine the biological, psychological, and moral bonds on which the strength of marriage and the family depends.

Catholic health-care ministry witnesses to the sanctity of life "from the moment of conception until death."[20] The Church's defense of life encompasses the unborn and the care of women and their children during and after pregnancy. The Church's commitment to life is seen in its willingness to collaborate with others to alleviate the causes of the high infant mortality rate and to provide adequate health care to mothers and their children before and after birth.

The Church has the deepest respect for the family, for the marriage covenant, and for the love that binds a married couple together. This includes respect for the marriage act by which husband and wife express their love and cooperate with God in the creation of a new human being. The Second Vatican Council affirms:

This love is an eminently human one. ... It involves the good of the whole person. ... The actions within marriage by which the couple are united intimately and chastely are noble and worthy ones. Expressed in a manner which is truly human, these actions signify and promote that mutual self-giving by which spouses enrich each other with a joyful and a thankful will.[21]

Marriage and conjugal love are by their nature ordained toward the begetting and educating of children. Children are really the supreme gift of marriage and contribute very substantially to the welfare of their parents. ... Parents should regard as their proper mission the task of transmitting human life and educating those to whom it has been transmitted ... They are thereby cooperators with the love of God the Creator and are, so to speak, the interpreters of that love.[22]

For legitimate reasons of responsible parenthood, married couples may limit the number of their children by natural means. The Church cannot approve contraceptive interventions that "either in anticipation of the marital act, or in its accomplishment or in the development of its natural consequences, have the purpose, whether as an end or a means, to render procreation impossible."[23] Such interventions violate "the inseparable connection, willed by God ... between the two meanings of the conjugal act: the unitive and procreative meanings."[24]

With the advance of the biological and medical sciences, society has at its disposal new technologies for responding to the problem of infertility. While we rejoice in the potential for good inherent in many of these technologies, we cannot assume that what is technically possible is always morally right. Reproductive technologies that substitute for the marriage act are not consistent with human dignity. Just as the marriage act is joined naturally to procreation, so procreation is joined naturally to the marriage act. As Pope John XXIII observed:

The transmission of human life is entrusted by nature to a personal and conscious act and as such is subject to all the holy laws of God: the immutable and inviolable laws which must be recognized and observed. For this reason, one cannot use means and follow methods which could be licit in the transmission of the life of plants and animals.[25]

Because the moral law is rooted in the whole of human nature, human persons, through intelligent reflection on their own spiritual destiny, can discover and cooperate in the plan of the Creator.[26]

Directives

38. When the marital act of sexual intercourse is not able to attain its procreative purpose, assistance that does not separate the unitive and procreative ends of the act, and does not substitute for the marital act itself, may be used to help married couples conceive.[27]

39. Those techniques of assisted conception that respect the unitive and procreative meanings of sexual intercourse and do not involve the destruction of human embryos, or their deliberate generation in such numbers that it is clearly envisaged that all cannot implant and some are simply being used to maximize the chances of others implanting, may be used as therapies for infertility.

40. Heterologous fertilization (that is, any technique used to achieve conception by the use of gametes coming from at least one donor other than the spouses) is prohibited because it is contrary to the covenant of marriage, the unity of the spouses, and the dignity proper to parents and the child.[28]

41. Homologous artificial fertilization (that is, any technique used to achieve conception using the gametes of the two spouses joined in marriage) is prohibited when it separates procreation from the marital act in its unitive significance (e.g., any technique used to achieve extra-corporeal conception).[29]

42. Because of the dignity of the child and of marriage, and because of the uniqueness of the mother-child relationship, participation in contracts or arrangements for surrogate motherhood is not permitted. Moreover, the commercialization of such surrogacy denigrates the dignity of women, especially the poor.[30]

43. A Catholic health-care institution that provides treatment for infertility should offer not only technical assistance to infertile couples but also should help couples pursue other solutions (e.g., counseling, adoption).

44. A Catholic health-care institution should provide prenatal, obstetric, and postnatal services for mothers and their children in a manner consonant with its mission.

45. Abortion (that is, the directly intended termination of pregnancy before viability or the directly intended destruction of a viable fetus) is never permitted. Every procedure whose sole immediate effect is the termination of pregnancy before viability is an abortion, which, in its moral context, includes the interval between conception and implantation of the embryo. Catholic health care institutions are not to provide abortion services, even based upon the principle of material cooperation. In this context, Catholic health care institutions need to be concerned about the danger of scandal in any association with abortion providers.

46. Catholic health care providers should be ready to offer compassionate physical, psychological, moral, and spiritual care to those persons who have suffered from the trauma of abortion.

47. Operations, treatments, and medications that have as their direct purpose the cure of a proportionately serious pathological condition of a pregnant woman are permitted when they cannot be safely postponed until the unborn child is viable, even if they will result in the death of the unborn child.

48. In case of extrauterine pregnancy, no intervention is morally licit which constitutes a direct abortion.[31]

49. For a proportionate reason, labor may be induced after the fetus is viable.

50. Prenatal diagnosis is permitted when the procedure does not threaten the life or physical integrity of the unborn child or the mother and does not subject them to disproportionate risks; when the diagnosis can provide information to guide preventative care for the mother or pre- or postnatal care for the child; and when the parents, or at least the mother, give free and informed consent. Prenatal diagnosis is not permitted when undertaken with the intention of aborting an unborn child with a serious defect.[32]

51. Nontherapeutic experiments on a living embryo or fetus are not permitted, even with the consent of the parents. Therapeutic experiments are permitted for a proportionate reason with the free and informed consent of the parents or, if the father cannot be contacted, at least of the mother. Medical research that will not harm the life or physical integrity of an unborn child is permitted with parental consent.[33]

52. Catholic health institutions may not promote or condone contraceptive practices but should provide, for married couples and the medical staff who counsel them, instruction both about the Church's teaching on responsible parenthood and in methods of natural family planning.

53. Direct sterilization of either men or women, whether permanent or temporary, is not permitted in a Catholic health-care institution. Procedures that induce sterility are permitted when their direct effect is the cure or alleviation of a present and serious pathology and a simpler treatment is not available.[34]

54. Genetic counseling may be provided in order to promote responsible parenthood and to prepare for the proper treatment and care of children with genetic defects, in accordance with Catholic moral teaching and the intrinsic rights and obligations of married couples regarding the transmission of life.

PART FIVE
Issues in Care for the Dying

Christ's redemption and saving grace embrace the whole person, especially in his or her illness, suffering, and death.[35] The Catholic health-care ministry faces the reality of death with the confidence of faith. In the face of death—for many, a time when hope seems lost—the Church witnesses to her belief that God has created each person for eternal life.[36]

Above all, as a witness to its faith, a Catholic health care institution will be a community of respect, love, and support to patients or residents and their families as they face the reality of death. What is hardest to face is the process of dying itself, especially the dependency, the helplessness, and the pain that so often accompany terminal illness. One of the primary purposes of medicine in caring for the dying is the relief of pain and the suffering caused by it. Effective management of pain in all its forms is critical in the appropriate care of the dying.

The truth that life is a precious gift from God has profound implications for the question of stewardship over human life. We are not the owners of our lives and, hence, do not have absolute power over life. We have a duty to preserve our life and to use it for the glory of God, but the duty to preserve life is not absolute, for we may reject life-prolonging procedures that are insufficiently beneficial or excessively burdensome. Suicide and euthanasia are never morally acceptable options.

The task of medicine is to care even when it cannot cure. Physicians and their patients must evaluate the use of the technology at their disposal. Reflection on the innate dignity of human life in all its dimensions and on the purpose of medical care is indispensable for formulating a true moral judgment about the use of technology to maintain life. The use of life-sustaining technology is judged in light of the Christian meaning of life, suffering, and death. Only in this way are two extremes avoided: on the one hand, an insistence on useless or burdensome technology even when a patient may legitimately wish to forgo it and, on the other hand, the withdrawal of technology with the intention of causing death.[37]

Some state Catholic conferences, individual bishops, and the NCCB Committee on Pro-Life Activities have addressed the moral issues concerning medically assisted hydration and nutrition. The bishops are guided by the Church's teaching forbidding euthanasia, which is "an action or an omission which of itself or by intention causes death, in order that all suffering may in this way be eliminated."[38] These statements agree that hydration and nutrition are not morally obligatory either when they bring no comfort to a person who is imminently dying or when they cannot be assimilated by a person's body. The NCCB Committee on Pro-Life Activities's report, in addition, points out the necessary distinctions between questions already resolved by the magisterium and those requiring further reflection, as, for example, the morality of withdrawing medically assisted hydration and nutrition from a person who is in the condition that is recognized by physicians as the "persistent vegetative state" (PVS).[39]

Directives

55. Catholic health-care institutions offering care to persons in danger of death from illness, accident, advanced age, or similar condition should provide them with appropriate opportunities to prepare for death. Persons in danger of death should be provided with whatever information is necessary to help them understand their condition and have the opportunity to discuss their condition with their family members and care providers. They should also be offered the appropriate medical information that would make it possible to address the morally legitimate choices available to them. They should be provided the spiritual support as well as the opportunity to receive the sacraments in order to prepare well for death.

56. A person has a moral obligation to use ordinary or proportionate means of preserving his or her life. Proportionate means are those that in the judgment of the patient offer a reasonable hope of benefit and do not entail an excessive burden or impose excessive expense on the family or the community.[40]

57. A person may forgo extraordinary or disproportionate means of preserving life. Disproportionate means are those that in the patient's judgment do not offer a reasonable hope of benefit, or entail an excessive burden, or impose excessive expense on the family or the community.[41]

58. There should be a presumption in favor of providing nutrition and hydration to all patients, including patients who require medically assisted nutrition and hydration, as long as this is of sufficient benefit to outweigh the burdens involved to the patient.

59. The free and informed judgment made by a competent adult patient concerning the use or withdrawal of life-sustaining procedures should always be respected and normally complied with, unless it is contrary to Catholic moral teaching.

60. Euthanasia is an action or omission that of itself or by intention causes death in order to alleviate suffering. Catholic health-care institutions may never condone or participate in euthanasia or assisted suicide in any way. Dying patients who request euthanasia should receive loving care, psychological and spiritual support, and appropriate remedies for pain and other symptoms so that they can live with dignity until the time of natural death.[42]

61. Patients should be kept as free of pain as possible so that they may die comfortably and with dignity, and in the place where they wish to die. Since a person has the right to prepare for his or her death while fully conscious, he or she should not be deprived of consciousness without a compelling reason. Medicines capable of alleviating or suppressing pain may be given to a dying person, even if this therapy may indirectly shorten the person's life so long as the intent is not to hasten death. Patients experiencing suffering that cannot be alleviated should be helped to appreciate the Christian understanding of redemptive suffering.

62. The determination of death should be made by the physician or competent medical authority in accordance

with responsible and commonly accepted scientific criteria.

63. Catholic health-care institutions should encourage and provide the means whereby those who wish to do so may arrange for the donation of their organs and bodily tissue, for ethically legitimate purposes, so that they may be used for donation and research after death.

64. Such organs should not be removed until it has been medically determined that the patient has died. In order to prevent any conflict of interest, the physician who determines death should not be a member of the transplant team.

65. The use of tissue or organs from an infant may be permitted after death has been determined and with the informed consent of the parents or guardians.

66. Catholic health-care institutions should not make use of human tissue obtained by direct abortions even for research and therapeutic purposes.[43]

PART SIX
Forming New Partnerships with Health Care Organizations and Providers

Until recently, most health-care providers enjoyed a degree of independence from one another. In ever-increasing ways, Catholic health-care providers have become involved with other health-care organizations and providers. For instance, many Catholic health-care systems and institutions share in the joint purchase of technology and services with other local facilities or physicians' groups. Another phenomenon is the growing number of Catholic health-care systems and institutions joining or co-sponsoring integrated delivery networks or managed care organizations in order to contract with insurers and other health-care payers. In some instances, Catholic health-care systems sponsor a health-care plan or health maintenance organization. In many dioceses, new partnerships will result in a decrease in the number of health-care providers, at times leaving the Catholic institution as the sole provider of health-care services. At whatever level, new partnerships forge a variety of interwoven relationships: between the various institutional partners, between health-care providers and the community, between physicians and health-care services, and between health care services and payers.

On the one hand, new partnerships can be viewed as opportunities for Catholic health-care institutions and services to witness to their religious and ethical commitments and so influence the healing profession. For example, new partnerships can help to implement the Church's social teaching. New partnerships can be opportunities to realign the local delivery system in order to provide a continuum of health care to the community; they can witness to a responsible stewardship of limited health care resources; and they can be opportunities to provide to poor and vulnerable persons a more equitable access to basic care.

On the other hand, new partnerships can pose serious challenges to the viability of the identity of Catholic health care institutions and services, and their ability to implement these directives in a consistent way, especially when partnerships are formed with those who do not share Catholic moral principles. The risk of scandal cannot be underestimated when partnerships are not built upon common values and moral principles. Partnership opportunities for some Catholic health care providers may even threaten the continued existence of other Catholic institutions and services, particularly when partnerships are driven by financial considerations alone. Because of the potential dangers involved in the new partnerships that are emerging, an increased collaboration among Catholic-sponsored health-care institutions is essential and should be sought before other forms of partnerships.

The significant challenges that new partnerships may pose, however, do not necessarily preclude their possibility on moral grounds. The potential dangers require that new partnerships undergo systematic and objective moral analysis, which takes into account the various factors that often pressure institutions and services into new partnerships that can diminish the autonomy and ministry of the Catholic partner. The following directives are offered to assist institutionally based, Catholic health-care services in this process of analysis. To this end, the National Conference of Catholic Bishops has established the Ad Hoc Committee on Health Care Issues and the Church as a resource for bishops and health-care leaders.

This new edition of the *Ethical and Religious Directives* omits the appendix concerning cooperation, which was contained in the 1995 edition. Experience has shown that the brief articulation of the principles of cooperation that was presented there did not sufficiently forestall certain possible misinterpretations and in practice gave rise to problems in concrete applications of the principles. Reliable theological experts should be consulted in interpreting and applying the principles governing cooperation, with the proviso that, as a rule, Catholic partners should avoid entering into partnerships that would involve them in cooperation with the wrongdoing of other providers.

Directives

67. Decisions that may lead to serious consequences for the identity or reputation of Catholic health care services, or entail the high risk of scandal, should be made in consultation with the diocesan bishop or his health care liaison.

68. Any partnership that will affect the mission or religious and ethical identity of Catholic health-care institutional services must respect Church teaching and discipline. Diocesan bishops and other Church authorities should be involved as such partnerships are developed, and the diocesan bishop should give the appropriate authorization before they are completed. The diocesan bishop's

approval is required for partnerships sponsored by institutions subject to his governing authority; for partnerships sponsored by religious institutes of pontifical right, his *nihil obstat* should be obtained.

69. If a Catholic health care organization is considering entering into an arrangement with another organization that may be involved in activities judged morally wrong by the Church, participation in such activities must be limited to what is in accord with the moral principles governing cooperation.

70. Catholic health care organizations are not permitted to engage in immediate material cooperation in actions that are intrinsically immoral, such as abortion, euthanasia, assisted suicide, and direct sterilization.[44]

71. The possibility of scandal must be considered when applying the principles governing cooperation.[45] Cooperation, which in all other respects is morally licit, may need to be refused because of the scandal that might be caused. Scandal can sometimes be avoided by an appropriate explanation of what is in fact being done at the health care facility under Catholic auspices. The diocesan bishop has final responsibility for assessing and addressing issues of scandal, considering not only the circumstances in his local diocese but also the regional and national implications of his decision.[46]

72. The Catholic partner in an arrangement has the responsibility periodically to assess whether the binding agreement is being observed and implemented in a way that is consistent with Catholic teaching.

Conclusion

Sickness speaks to us of our limitations and human frailty. It can take the form of infirmity resulting from the simple passing of years or injury from the exuberance of youthful energy. It can be temporary or chronic, debilitating, and even terminal. Yet the follower of Jesus faces illness and the consequences of the human condition aware that our Lord always shows compassion toward the infirm.

Jesus not only taught his disciples to be compassionate, but he also told them who should be the special object of their compassion. The parable of the feast with its humble guests was preceded by the instruction: "When you hold a banquet, invite the poor, the crippled, the lame, the blind" (Lk 14:13). These were people whom Jesus healed and loved.

Catholic health care is a response to the challenge of Jesus to go and do likewise. Catholic health-care services rejoice in the challenge to be Christ's healing compassion in the world and see their ministry not only as an effort to restore and preserve health but also as a spiritual service and a sign of that final healing that will one day bring about the new creation that is the ultimate fruit of Jesus' ministry and God's love for us.

Notes

[1] National Conference of Catholic Bishops (NCCB), *Health and Health Care: A Pastoral Letter of the American Catholic Bishops* (Washington, D.C.: United States Catholic Conference, 1981).

[2] Health-care services under Catholic auspices are carried out in a variety of institutional settings (e.g., hospitals, clinics, out-patient facilities, urgent care centers, hospices, nursing homes, and parishes). Depending on the context, these directives will employ the terms "institution" and/or "services" in order to encompass the variety of settings in which Catholic health care is provided.

[3] NCCB, *Health and Health Care*, 5.

[4] Second Vatican Ecumenical Council, *Decree on the Apostolate of the Laity (Apostolicam Actuositatem)* (1965), n. 1.

[5] Pope John Paul II, post-synodal apostolic exhortation, *On the Vocation and the Mission of the Lay Faithful in the Church and in the World (Christifideles Laici)* (Washington, D.C.: United States Catholic Conference, 1988), n. 29.

[6] As examples, see Congregation for the Doctrine of the Faith (CDF), *Declaration on Procured Abortion* (1974); idem, *Declaration on Euthanasia* (1980); idem, *Instruction on Respect for Human Life in its Origin and on the Dignity of Procreation: Replies to Certain Questions of the Day (Donum vitae)* (Washington, D.C.: United States Catholic Conference, 1987).

[7] Pope John XXIII, encyclical letter, *Peace on Earth (Pacem in Terris)* (Washington, D.C.: United States Catholic Conference, 1963), n. 11; NCCB, *Health and Health Care*, 5, 17–18; *Catechism of the Catholic Church*, 2nd ed. (Washington, D.C.: United States Catholic Conference, 2000), n. 2211.

[8] Pope John Paul II, *On Social Concern: Encyclical Letter on the Occasion of the Twentieth Anniversary of "Populorum Progressio," (Sollicitudo Rei Socialis)* (Washington, D.C.: United States Catholic Conference, 1988), n. 43.

[9] National Conference of Catholic Bishops, *Economic Justice for All: Pastoral Letter on Catholic Social Teaching and the U.S. Economy* (Washington, D.C.: United States Catholic Conference, 1986), n. 80.

[10] The duty of responsible stewardship demands responsible collaboration. But in collaborative efforts, Catholic institutionally based health-care services must be attentive to occasions when the policies and practices of other institutions are not compatible with the Church's authoritative moral teaching. At such times, Catholic health-care institutions should determine whether or to what degree collaboration would be morally permissible. To make that judgment, the governing boards of Catholic institutions should adhere to the moral principles on cooperation. See pt. 6.

[11] NCCB, *Health and Health Care*, 12.

[12] Cf. *Code of Canon Law*, cc. 921–923.

[13] Cf. ibid., c. 867, § 2; and c. 871.

[14] To confer Baptism in an emergency, one must have the proper intention (to do what the Church intends by Baptism) and pour water on the head of the person to be baptized, meanwhile pronouncing the words: "I baptize you in the name of the Father,

and of the Son, and of the Holy Spirit."

[15] Cf. *Code of Canon Law*, c. 883, 3E.

[16] For example, while the donation of a kidney represents loss of biological integrity, such a donation does not compromise functional integrity since human beings are capable of functioning with only one kidney.

[17] Cf. dir. 53.

[18] CDF, *Declaration on Euthanasia*, IV; cf. also dirs. 56–57.

[19] It is recommended that a sexually assaulted woman be advised of the ethical restrictions that prevent Catholic hospitals from using abortifacient procedures; cf. Pennsylvania Catholic Conference, "Guidelines for Catholic Hospitals Treating Victims of Sexual Assault," *Origins* 22 (1993): 810.

[20] Pope John Paul II, Address of October 29, 1983, to the 35th General Assembly of the World Medical Association, *Acta Apostolicae Sedis* 76 (1984): 390.

[21] Second Vatican Ecumenical Council, Pastoral Constitution on the Church in the Modern World *(Gaudium et Spes)* (1965), n. 49.

[22] Ibid., n. 50.

[23] Pope Paul VI, encyclical letter, *On the Regulation of Birth (Humanae vitae)* (Washington, D.C.: United States Catholic Conference, 1968), n. 14.

[24] Ibid., n. 12.

[25] Pope John XXIII, encyclical letter, *Mater et Magistra* (1961), n. 193, quoted in Congregation for the Doctrine of the Faith, *Donum vitae*, n. 4.

[26] Pope John Paul II, encyclical letter, *The Splendor of Truth (Veritatis Splendor)* (Washington, D.C.: United States Catholic Conference, 1993), n. 50.

[27] "Homologous artificial insemination within marriage cannot be admitted except for those cases in which the technical means is not a substitute for the conjugal act but serves to facilitate and to help so that the act attains its natural purpose." *Donum vitae*, II, B, n. 6; cf. also I, nn. 1, 6.

[28] Ibid., II, A, n. 2.

[29] "Artificial insemination as a substitute for the conjugal act is prohibited by reason of the voluntarily achieved dissociation of the two meanings of the conjugal act. Masturbation, through which the sperm is normally obtained, is another sign of this dissociation: even when it is done for the purpose of procreation, the act remains deprived of its unitive meaning: 'It lacks the sexual relationship called for by the moral order, namely, the relationship which realizes "the full sense of mutual self-giving and human procreation in the context of true love."' Ibid., II, B, n. 6.

[30] Ibid., II, A, n. 3.

[31] Cf. dir. 45.

[32] CDF, *Donum vitae*, I, n. 2.

[33] Cf. ibid., n. 4.

[34] Cf. Congregation for the Doctrine of the Faith, "Responses on Uterine Isolation and Related Matters" (July 31, 1993), *Origins* 24 (1994): 211–212.

[35] Pope John Paul II, apostolic letter, *On the Christian Meaning of Human Suffering (Salvifici Doloris)* (Washington, D.C.: United States Catholic Conference, 1984), nn. 25–27.

[36] National Conference of Catholic Bishops, *Order of Christian Funerals* (Collegeville, MN.: The Liturgical Press, 1989), n. 1.

[37] CDF, *Declaration on Euthanasia*.

[38] Ibid., II, p. 4.

[39] Committee for Pro-Life Activities, National Conference of Catholic Bishops, *Nutrition and Hydration: Moral and Pastoral Reflections* (Washington, D.C.: United States Catholic Conference, 1992). On the importance of consulting authoritative teaching in the formation of conscience and in taking moral decisions, see John Paul II, *Veritatis splendor*, nn. 63–64.

[40] CDF, *Declaration on Euthanasia*, IV.

[41] Ibid.

[42] Cf. ibid.

[43] CDF, *Donum vitae*, I, n. 4.

[44] While there are many acts of varying moral gravity that can be identified as intrinsically evil, in the context of contemporary health care the most pressing concerns are currently abortion, euthanasia, assisted suicide, and direct sterilization. See Pope John Paul II's *Ad Limina* Address to the bishops of Texas, Oklahoma, and Arkansas (Region X), in *Origins* 28 (1998): 283. See also "Reply of the Sacred Congregation for the Doctrine of the Faith on Sterilization in Catholic Hospitals" *(Quaecumque Sterilizatio)*, March 13, 1975, *Origins* 10 (1976): 33–35: "Any cooperation institutionally approved or tolerated in actions which are in themselves, that is, by their nature and condition, directed to a contraceptive end ... is absolutely forbidden. For the official approbation of direct sterilization and, *a fortiori*, its management and execution in accord with hospital regulations, is a matter which, in the objective order, is by its very nature (or intrinsically) evil." This directive supersedes the "Commentary on the Reply of the Sacred Congregation for the Doctrine of the Faith on Sterilization in Catholic Hospitals" published by the National Conference of Catholic Bishops on September 15, 1977, in *Origins* 11 (1977): 399–400.

[45] See *Catechism of the Catholic Church*: "Scandal is an attitude or behavior which leads another to do evil" (n. 2284); "Anyone who uses the power at his disposal in such a way that it leads others to do wrong becomes guilty of scandal and responsible for the evil that he has directly or indirectly encouraged" (n. 2287).

[46] See "The Pastoral Role of the Diocesan Bishop in Catholic Health Care Ministry," *Origins* 26 (1997): 703.

APPENDIX XIV

Pope John Paul II

Address to the Participants in the International Congress on Life-Sustaining Treatments and Vegetative State: Scientific Advances and Ethical Dilemmas

March 20, 2004

1. I cordially greet all of you who took part in the International Congress: *"Life-Sustaining Treatments and Vegetative State: Scientific Advances and Ethical Dilemmas."* I wish to extend a special greeting to Bishop Elio Sgreccia, Vice-President of the Pontifical Academy for Life, and to Prof. Gian Luigi Gigli, President of the International Federation of Catholic Medical Associations and selfless champion of the fundamental value of life, who has kindly expressed your shared feelings.

This important Congress, organized jointly by the Pontifical Academy for Life and the International Federation of Catholic Medical Associations, is dealing with a very significant issue: *the clinical condition called the "vegetative state".* The complex scientific, ethical, social and pastoral implications of such a condition require in-depth reflections and a fruitful interdisciplinary dialogue, as evidenced by the intense and carefully structured programme of your work sessions.

2. With deep esteem and sincere hope, the Church encourages the efforts of men and women of science who, sometimes at great sacrifice, daily dedicate their task of study and research to the improvement of the diagnostic, therapeutic, prognostic and rehabilitative possibilities confronting those patients who rely completely on those who care for and assist them. The person in a vegetative state, in fact, shows no evident sign of self-awareness or of awareness of the environment, and seems unable to interact with others or to react to specific stimuli.

Scientists and researchers realize that one must, first of all, arrive at a correct diagnosis, which usually requires prolonged and careful observation in specialized centres, given also the high number of diagnostic errors reported in the literature. Moreover, not a few of these persons, with appropriate treatment and with specific rehabilitation programmes, have been able to emerge from a vegetative state. On the contrary, many others unfortunately remain prisoners of their condition even for long stretches of time and without needing technological support.

In particular, the term *permanent vegetative state* has been coined to indicate the condition of those patients whose "vegetative state" continues for over a year. Actually, there is no different diagnosis that corresponds to such a definition, but only a conventional prognostic judgment, relative to the fact that the recovery of patients, statistically speaking, is ever more difficult as the condition of vegetative state is prolonged in time.

However, we must neither forget nor underestimate that there are well-documented cases of at least partial recovery even after many years; we can thus state that medical science, up until now, is still unable to predict with certainty who among patients in this condition will recover and who will not.

3. Faced with patients in similar clinical conditions, there are some who cast doubt on the persistence of the "human quality" itself, almost as if the adjective "vegetative" (whose use is now solidly established), which symbolically describes a clinical state, could or should be instead applied to the sick as such, actually demeaning their value and personal dignity. In this sense, it must be noted that this term, even when confined to the clinical context, is certainly not the most felicitous when applied to human beings.

In opposition to such trends of thought, I feel the duty to reaffirm strongly that the intrinsic value and personal dignity of every human being do not change, no matter what the concrete circumstances of his or her life. *A man, even if seriously ill or disabled in the exercise of his highest functions, is and always will be a man*, and he will never become a "vegetable" or an "animal".

Even our brothers and sisters who find themselves in the clinical condition of a "vegetative state" retain their human dignity in all its fullness. The loving gaze of God the Father continues to fall upon them, acknowledging them as his sons and daughters, especially in need of help.

4. Medical doctors and health-care personnel, society and the Church have moral duties toward these persons from which they cannot exempt themselves without lessening the demands both of professional ethics and human and Christian solidarity.

The sick person in a vegetative state, awaiting recovery or a natural end, still has the right to basic health care (nutrition, hydration, cleanliness, warmth, etc.), and to the prevention of complications related to his confinement to bed. He also has the right to appropriate rehabilitative care and to be monitored for clinical signs of eventual recovery.

I should like particularly to underline how the administration of water and food, even when provided by artificial means, always represents a *natural means* of preserving life, not a *medical act*. Its use, furthermore, should be considered, in principle, *ordinary* and *proportionate*, and as such morally obligatory, insofar as and until it is seen to have attained its proper finality, which in the present case consists in providing nourishment to the patient and alleviation of his suffering.

The obligation to provide the "normal care due to the sick in such cases" (Congregation for the Doctrine of the Faith, *Iura et Bona*, p. IV) includes, in fact, the use of nutrition and hydration (cf. Pontifical Council "Cor Unum", *Dans le Cadre*, 2, 4, 4; Pontifical Council for Pastoral Assistance to Health Care Workers, *Charter of Health Care Workers*, n. 120). The evaluation of probabilities, founded on waning hopes for recovery when the vegetative state is prolonged beyond a year, cannot ethically justify the cessation or interruption of *minimal care* for the patient, including nutrition and hydration. Death by starvation or dehydration is, in fact, the only possible outcome as a result of their withdrawal. In this sense it ends up becoming, if done knowingly and willingly, true and proper euthanasia by omission.

In this regard, I recall what I wrote in the Encyclical *Evangelium vitae*, making it clear that "by *euthanasia in the true and proper sense* must be understood an action or omission which by its very nature and intention brings about death, with the purpose of eliminating all pain"; such an act is always "a *serious violation of the law of God*, since it is the deliberate and morally unacceptable killing of a human person" (n. 65).

Besides, the moral principle is well known, according to which even the simple doubt of being in the presence of a living person already imposes the obligation of full respect and of abstaining from any act that aims at anticipating the person's death.

5. Considerations about the "quality of life", often actually dictated by psychological social and economic pressures, cannot take precedence over general principles.

First of all, no evaluation of costs can outweigh the value of the fundamental good which we are trying to protect, that of human life. Moreover, to admit that decisions regarding man's life can be based on the external acknowledgment of its quality, is the same as acknowledging that increasing and decreasing levels of quality of life, and therefore of human dignity, can be attributed from an external perspective to any subject, thus introducing into social relations a discriminatory and eugenic principle.

Moreover, it is not possible to rule out *a priori* that the withdrawal of nutrition and hydration, as reported by authoritative studies, is the source of considerable suffering for the sick person, even if we can see only the reactions at the level of the autonomic nervous system or of gestures. Modern clinical neurophysiology and neuro-imaging techniques, in fact, seem to point to the lasting quality in these patients of elementary forms of communication and analysis of stimuli.

6. However, it is not enough to reaffirm the general principle according to which the value of a man's life cannot be made subordinate to any judgment of its quality expressed by other men; it is necessary to promote the *taking of positive actions* as a stand against pressures to withdraw hydration and nutrition as a way to put an end to the lives of these patients.

It is necessary, above all, *to support those families* who have had one of their loved ones struck down by this terrible clinical condition. They cannot be left alone with their heavy human, psychological and financial burden. Although the care for these patients is not, in general, particularly costly, society must allot sufficient resources for the care of this sort of frailty, by way of bringing about appropriate, concrete initiatives such as, for example, the creation of a network of awakening centres with specialized treatment and rehabilitation programmes; financial support and home assistance for families when patients are moved back home at the end of intensive rehabilitation programmes; the establishment of facilities which can accommodate those cases in which there is no family able to deal with the problem or to provide "breaks" for those families who are at risk of psychological and moral burn-out.

Proper care for these patients and their families should, moreover, include the presence and the witness of a medical doctor and an entire team, who are asked to help the family understand that they are there as allies who are in this struggle with them. The participation of volunteers represents a basic support to enable the family to break out of its isolation and to help it to realize that it is a precious and not a forsaken part of the social fabric.

In these situations, then, spiritual counselling and pastoral aid are particularly important as help for recovering the deepest meaning of an apparently desperate condition.

7. Distinguished Ladies and Gentlemen, in conclusion I exhort you, as men and women of science responsible for the dignity of the medical profession, to guard jealously the principle according to which the true task of medicine is "to cure if possible, always to care".

As a pledge and support of this, your authentic humanitarian mission to give comfort and support to your suffering brothers and sisters, I remind you of the words of Jesus: "Amen, I say to you, whatever you did for one of these least brothers of mine, you did for me" (Mt 25: 40).

In this light, I invoke upon you the assistance of him, whom a meaningful saying of the Church Fathers describes as *Christus medicus*, and in entrusting your work to the protection of Mary, Consoler of the sick and Comforter of the dying, I lovingly bestow on all of you a special Apostolic Blessing.

APPENDIX XV

Pontifical Academy for Life

Moral Reflections on Vaccines Prepared from Cells Derived from Aborted Human Fetuses

June 5, 2005

The matter in question regards the lawfulness of production, distribution, and use of certain vaccines whose production is connected with acts of procured abortion. It concerns vaccines containing live viruses which have been prepared from human cell lines of fetal origin, using tissues from aborted human fetuses as a source of such cells. The best known, and perhaps the most important due to its vast distribution and its use on an almost universal level, is the vaccine against rubella (German measles).

Rubella and Its Vaccine

Rubella (German measles)[1] is a viral illness caused by a togavirus of the genus *Rubivirus* and is characterized by a maculopapular rash. It consists of an infection which is common in infancy and has no clinical manifestations in one case out of two, is self-limiting and usually benign. Nonetheless, the German measles virus is one of the most pathological infective agents for the embryo and fetus. When a woman catches the infection during pregnancy, especially during the first trimester, the risk of fetal infection is very high (approximately 95 percent). The virus replicates itself in the placenta and infects the fetus, causing the constellation of abnormalities denoted by the name of *congenital rubella syndrome*. For example, the severe epidemic of German measles which affected a huge part of the United States in 1964 caused 20,000 cases of congenital rubella,[2] resulting in 11,250 abortions (spontaneous or surgical), 2,100 neonatal deaths, 11,600 cases of deafness, 3,580 cases of blindness, and 1,800 cases of mental retardation. It was this epidemic that pushed for the development and introduction on the market of an effective vaccine against rubella, thus permitting an effective prophylaxis against this infection.

The severity of congenital rubella and the handicaps which it causes justify systematic vaccination against such a sickness. It is very difficult, perhaps even impossible, to avoid the infection of a pregnant woman, even if the rubella infection of a person in contact with this woman is diagnosed from the first day of the eruption of the rash. Therefore, one tries to prevent transmission by suppressing the reservoir of infection among children who have not been vaccinated, by means of early immunization of all children (universal vaccination). Universal vaccination has resulted in a considerable fall in the incidence of congenital rubella, with a general incidence reduced to less than 5 cases per 100,000 live births. Nevertheless, this progress remains fragile. In the United States, for example, after an overwhelming reduction in the number of cases of congenital rubella to only a few cases annually, i.e., less than 0.1 per 100,000 live births, a new epidemic wave came on in 1991, with an incidence that rose to 0.8 per 100,000. Such waves of resurgence of German measles were also seen in 1997 and in the year 2000. These periodic episodes of resurgence make it evident that there is a persistent circulation of the virus among young adults, which is the consequence of insufficient vaccination coverage. The latter situation allows a significant proportion of vulnerable subjects to persist, who are a source of periodic epidemics which put women in the fertile age group who have not been immunized at risk. Therefore, the reduction to the point of eliminating congenital rubella is considered a priority in public health care.

Vaccines Currently Produced Using Human Cell Lines That Come from Aborted Fetuses

To date, there are two human diploid cell lines which were originally prepared from tissues of aborted fetuses (in 1964 and 1970) and are used for the preparation of vaccines based on live attenuated virus: the first one is the WI-38 line (Wistar Institute 38), with human diploid lung fibroblasts coming from a female fetus that was aborted because the family felt they had too many children.[3] It was prepared and developed by Leonard Hayflick in 1964[4] and bears the ATCC [American Type Culture Collection] number CCL-75. WI-38 has been used for the preparation of the historical vaccine RA 27/3 against rubella.[5] The second human cell line is MRC-5 (Medical Research Council 5; human, lung, embryonic; ATCC number CCL-171), with human lung fibroblasts coming from a fourteen-week male fetus aborted for "psychiatric reasons" from a twenty-seven-year-old woman in the United Kingdom. MRC-5 was prepared and developed by J.P. Jacobs in 1966.[6] Other human cell lines have been developed for pharmaceutical needs, but are not involved in the vaccines actually available.[7]

The vaccines that are incriminated today as using human cell lines from aborted fetuses, WI-38 and MRC-5, are the following[8]:

A. Live vaccines against rubella:[9]

- The monovalent vaccines against rubella Meruvax II (Merck, U.S.), Rudivax (Sanofi Pasteur, France), and Ervevax ([using]RA 27/3, GlaxoSmithKline, Belgium)

- The combined vaccine MR against rubella and measles, commercialized with the name of M-R-VAX (Merck), and Rudi-Rouvax (Aventis Pasteur, France)

- The combined vaccine against rubella and mumps marketed under the name of Biavax II (Merck)

- The combined vaccine MMR (measles, mumps, rubella) against rubella, mumps, and measles, marketed under the name of M-M-R II (Merck), R.O.R., Trimovax (Sanofi Pasteur, France), and Priorix (GlaxoSmithKline, U.K.)

B. Other vaccines, also prepared using human cell lines from aborted fetuses:

- Two vaccines against hepatitis A, one produced by Merck (Vaqta), the other one produced by GlaxoSmithKline (Havrix), both of them being prepared using MRC-5

- One vaccine against chicken pox, Varivax, produced by Merck using WI-38 and MRC-5

- One vaccine against poliomyelitis, the inactivated polio virus vaccine Poliovax (Aventis Pasteur) using MRC-5

- One vaccine against rabies, Imovax, produced by Aventis Pasteur, harvested from infected human diploid cells, MRC-5 strain

- One vaccine against smallpox, AC AM 1000, prepared by Acambis using MRC-5, still on trial

The Position of the Ethical Problem Related to These Vaccines

From the point of view of prevention of viral diseases such as German measles, mumps, measles, chicken pox, and hepatitis A, it is clear that the making of effective vaccines against diseases such as these, as well as their use in the fight against these infections, up to the point of eradication, by means of an obligatory vaccination of all the population at risk, undoubtedly represents a milestone in the secular fight of man against infective and contagious diseases.

However, as the same vaccines are prepared from viruses taken from the tissues of fetuses that had been infected and voluntarily aborted, and the viruses were subsequently attenuated and cultivated from human cell lines which come likewise from procured abortions, they do not cease to pose ethical problems. The need to articulate a moral reflection on the matter in question arises mainly from the connection which exists between the vaccines mentioned above and the procured abortions from which biological material necessary for their preparation was obtained.

If someone rejects every form of voluntary abortion of human fetuses, would such a person not contradict himself or herself by allowing the use of these vaccines of live attenuated viruses on their children? Would it not be a matter of true (and illicit) cooperation in evil, even though this evil was carried out forty years ago?

Before proceeding to consider this specific case, we need to recall briefly the principles assumed in classical moral doctrine with regard to the problem of *cooperation in evil*,[10] a problem which arises every time that a moral agent perceives the existence of a link between his own acts and a morally evil action carried out by others.

The Principle of Licit Cooperation in Evil

The first fundamental distinction to be made is that between *formal* and *material cooperation. Formal cooperation* is carried out when the moral agent cooperates with the immoral action of another person, sharing in the latter's evil intention. On the other hand, when a moral agent cooperates with the immoral action of another person without sharing his or her evil intention, it is a case of *material cooperation.*

Material cooperation can be further divided into categories of *immediate* (direct) and *mediate* (indirect), depending on whether the cooperation is in the execution of the sinful action per se, or whether the agent acts by fulfilling the conditions—either by providing instruments or products—which make it possible to commit the immoral act. Furthermore, forms of *proximate cooperation* and *remote cooperation* can be distinguished, in relation to the "distance" (be it in terms of *temporal* space or *material* connection) between the act of cooperation and the sinful act committed by someone else. *Immediate material cooperation* is always *proximate*, while *mediate material cooperation* can be *either proximate* or *remote*.

Formal cooperation is always morally illicit because it represents a form of direct and intentional participation in the sinful action of another person.[11] *Material cooperation* can sometimes be illicit (depending on the conditions of the "double effect" or "indirect voluntary" action), but when *immediate material cooperation* concerns grave attacks on human life, it is always to be considered illicit, given the precious nature of the value in question.[12]

A further distinction made in classical morality is that between *active* (or positive) cooperation in evil and *passive* (or negative) cooperation in evil, the former referring to the performance of an act of cooperation in a sinful action that is carried out by another person, while the latter refers to the omission of an act of denunciation or impediment of a sinful action carried out by another person, insomuch as there was a moral duty to do that which was omitted.[13] Passive cooperation can also be formal or material, immediate or mediate, proximate or remote. Obviously, every type of formal passive cooperation is to be considered illicit, but even passive material cooperation should generally be avoided, although it is admitted (by many authors) that there is not a rigorous obligation to avoid it in a case in which it would be greatly difficult to do so.

Application to the Use of Vaccines Prepared from Cells Coming from Embryos or Fetuses Aborted Voluntarily

In the specific case under examination, there are three categories of people who are involved in the cooperation in evil, evil which is obviously represented by the action of a voluntary abortion performed by others: (a) those who prepare the vaccines using human cell lines coming from voluntary abortions; (b) who participate in the mass marketing of such vaccines; (c) those who need to use them for health reasons.

Firstly, one must consider morally illicit every form of *formal* cooperation (sharing the evil intention) in the action of those who have performed a voluntary abortion, which in turn has allowed the retrieval of fetal tissues, required for the preparation of vaccines. Therefore, whoever—regardless of the category to which he belongs—cooperates in some way, sharing its intention, in the performance of a voluntary abortion with the aim of producing the above-mentioned vaccines, participates, in actuality, in the same moral evil as the person who has performed that abortion. Such participation would also take place in the case where someone sharing the intention of the abortion refrains from denouncing or criticizing this illicit action, although having the moral duty to do so (*passive formal cooperation*).

In a case where there is no such formal sharing of the immoral intention of the person who has performed the abortion, any form of cooperation would be *material*, with the following specifications.

As regards the preparation, distribution, and marketing of vaccines produced as a result of the use of biological material whose origin is connected with cells coming from fetuses voluntarily aborted, such a process is stated, as a matter of principle, morally illicit, because it could contribute in encouraging the performance of other voluntary abortions, with the purpose of the production of such vaccines. Nevertheless, it should be recognized that, within the chain of production-distribution-marketing, the various cooperating agents can have different moral responsibilities.

However, there is another aspect to be considered, and that is the form of *passive material cooperation* which would be carried out by the producers of these vaccines, if they do not denounce and reject publicly the original immoral act (the voluntary abortion), and if they do not dedicate themselves together to research and promote alternative ways, exempt from moral evil, for the production of vaccines for the same

infections. Such *passive material cooperation*, if it should occur, is equally illicit.

As regards those who need to use such vaccines for reasons of health, it must be emphasized that, apart from every form *of formal cooperation*, in general, doctors or parents who resort to the use of these vaccines for their children, in spite of knowing their origin (voluntary abortion), carry out a form of *very remote mediate material cooperation*, and thus very mild, in the performance of the original act of abortion, and a *mediate material cooperation*, with regard to the marketing of cells coming from abortions, and *immediate*, with regard to the marketing of vaccines produced with such cells. The cooperation is therefore more intense on the part of the authorities and national health systems that accept the use of the vaccines.

However, in this situation, the aspect *of passive cooperation* is that which stands out most. It is up to the faithful and citizens of upright conscience (fathers of families, doctors) to oppose, even by making an objection of conscience, the ever more widespread attacks against life and the "culture of death" which underlies them. From this point of view, the use of vaccines whose production is connected with procured abortion constitutes at least a mediate remote passive material cooperation to the abortion, and an immediate passive material cooperation with regard to their marketing. Furthermore, on a cultural level, the use of such vaccines contributes in the creation of a generalized social consensus to the operation of the pharmaceutical industries which produce them in an immoral way.

Therefore, doctors and fathers of families have a duty to take recourse to alternative vaccines[14] (if they exist), putting pressure on the political authorities and health systems so that other vaccines without moral problems become available. They should take recourse, if necessary, to the use of conscientious objection[15] with regard to the use of vaccines produced by means of cell lines of aborted human fetal origin. Equally, they should oppose by all means (in writing, through the various associations, mass media) the vaccines which do not yet have morally acceptable alternatives, creating pressure so that alternative vaccines are prepared, which are not connected with the abortion of a human fetus, and requesting rigorous legal control of the pharmaceutical industry producers.

As regards the diseases against which there are no alternative vaccines which are available and ethically acceptable, it is right to abstain from using these vaccines if it can be done without causing children, and indirectly the population as a whole, to undergo significant risks to their health. However, if the latter are exposed to considerable dangers to their health, vaccines with moral problems pertaining to them may also be used on a temporary basis. The moral reason is that the duty to avoid *passive material cooperation* is not obligatory if there is grave inconvenience. Moreover, we find, in such a case, *a proportional reason,* in order to accept the use of these vaccines in the presence of the danger of favoring the spread of the pathological agent, due to the lack of vaccination of children. This is particularly true in the case of vaccination against German measles.[16]

In any case, there remains a moral duty to continue to fight and to employ every lawful means in order to make life difficult for the pharmaceutical industries which act unscrupulously and unethically. However, the burden of this important battle cannot and must not fall on innocent children and on the health situation of the population—especially with regard to pregnant women.

To summarize, it must be confirmed that:

- There is a grave responsibility to use alternative vaccines and to make a conscientious objection with regard to those which have moral problems.

- As regards the vaccines without an alternative, the need to contest so that others may be prepared must be reaffirmed, as should be the lawfulness of using the former in the meantime insomuch as is necessary in order to avoid a serious risk not only for one's own children but also, and perhaps more specifically, for the health conditions of the population as a whole—especially for pregnant women.

- The lawfulness of the use of these vaccines should not be misinterpreted as a declaration of the lawfulness of their production, marketing, and use, but is to be understood as being a passive material cooperation and, in its mildest and remotest sense, also active, morally justified as an *extrema ratio* due to the necessity to provide for the good of one's children and of the people who come in contact with the children (pregnant women).

- Such cooperation occurs in a context of moral coercion of the conscience of parents, who are forced to choose to act against their conscience or otherwise, to put the health of their children and of the population as a whole at risk. This is an unjust alternative choice, which must be eliminated as soon as possible.

Notes

[1] J. E. Banatvala and D. W. G. Brown, "Rubella," *Lancet* 363.9415 (April 3, 2004): 1127–1137.

[2] "Rubella," *Morbidity and Mortality Weekly Report* 13 (1964): 93; S. A. Plotkin, "Virologic Assistance in the Management of German Measles in Pregnancy," *Journal of the American Medical Association* 190 (October 26, 1964): 265–268.

[3] G. Sven, S. Plotkin, and K. McCarthy, "Gamma Globulin Prophylaxis; Inactivated Rubella Virus; Production and Biological Control of Live Attenuated Rubella Virus Vaccines," *American Journal of Diseases of Children* 118.2 (August 1969): 372–381.

[4] L. Hayflick, "The Limited In Vitro Lifetime of Human Diploid Cell Strains," *Experimental Cell Research* 37.3 (March 1965): 614–636; G. Sven, "Gamma Globulin Prophylaxis."

[5] S. A. Plotkin, D. Cornfeld, and T. H. Ingalls, "Studies of Immunization with Living Rubella Virus, Trials in Children with a Strain Coming from an Aborted Fetus," *American Journal of Diseases in Children* 110.4 (October 1965): 381–389.

[6] J. P. Jacobs, C. M. Jones, and J. P. Bailie, "Characteristics of a Human Diploid Cell Designated MRC-5," *Nature* 277.5254 (July 11, 1970): 168–170.

[7] Two other human cell lines that are permanent, HEK 293 aborted fetal cell line, from primary human embryonic kidney cells transformed by sheared adenovirus type 5 (the fetal kidney material was obtained from an aborted fetus, in 1972 probably), and PER.C6, a fetal cell line created using retinal tissue from an aborted baby of eighteen-weeks' gestation, have been developed for the pharmaceutical manufacturing of adenovirus vectors (for gene therapy). They have not been involved in the making of any of the attenuated live viruses vaccines presently in use, because of their capacity to develop tumorigenic cells in the recipient. However, some vaccines, still at the developmental stage, against ebola virus (Crucell N.V. and the Vaccine Research Center of the National Institutes of Health's Allergy and Infectious Diseases, NIAID), HIV (Merck), influenza (MedImmune and Sanofi Pasteur), Japanese encephalitis (Crucell N.V. and Rhein Biotech N.V.) are prepared using PER.C6 cell line (Crucell N.V., Leiden, the Netherlands).

[8] Against these various infectious diseases, there are some alternative vaccines that are prepared using animals' cells or tissues, and are therefore ethically acceptable. Their availability depends on the country in question. Concerning the particular case of the United States, there are no options for the time being in that country for the vaccination against rubella, chickenpox, and hepatitis A, other than the vaccines proposed by Merck, prepared using the human cell lines WI-38 and MRC-5. There is a vaccine against smallpox prepared with the Vero cell line (derived from the kidney of an African green monkey), ACAM 2000 (Acambis-Baxter; a second-generation smallpox vaccine, stockpiled, not approved in the United States), which offers, therefore, an alternative to the Acambis 1000. There are alternative vaccines against mumps (Mumpsvax, Merck), measles (Attenuvax, Merck), and rabies (RabAvert, Chiron Therapeutics), prepared from chicken embryos (however, serious allergies have occurred with such vaccines), poliomyelitis (IPOL, Aventis-Pasteur, prepared with monkey kidney cells), and smallpox (a third-generation smallpox vaccine MVA [modified vaccinia ankara], Acambis-Baxter). In Europe and in Japan, there are other vaccines available against rubella and hepatitis A, produced using nonhuman cell lines. The Kitasato Institute produce four vaccines against rubella, called Takahashi, [TCRB19], TO-336, and Matuba, prepared with cells from rabbit kidney, and one (Matuura) prepared with cells from a quail embryo. … Kaketsuken produces another vaccine against hepatitis A, called Ainmugen, prepared with cells from monkey kidney. The only remaining problem is with the vaccine Varivax against chicken pox, for which there is no alternative.

[9] The vaccine against rubella using the strain Wistar RA 27/3 of live attenuated rubella virus, adapted and propagated in WI-38 human diploid lung fibroblasts, is at the center of the present con-

troversy regarding the morality of the use of vaccines prepared with the help of human cell lines coming from aborted fetuses.

[10] D. M. Prummer O. P., "De cooperatione ad malum," in *Manuale Theologiae Moralis secundum Principia S. Thomae Aquinatis*, tomus I (Friburgi Brisgoviae: Herder & Co., 1923), pars I, trat. IX, caput. III, no. 2, 429–434. K. H. Peschke, "Cooperation in the Sins of Others," in *Christian Ethics: Moral Theology in the Light of Vatican II*, vol. 1 of *General Moral Theology*, rev. ed. (Alcester, U.K.: C. Goodliffe Neale, 1986): 320–324.

[11] A. Fisher, "Cooperation in Evil," *Catholic Medical Quarterly* (1994): 15–22; D. Tettamanzi, "Cooperazione," in *Dizionario di Bioetica*, eds. S. Leone and S. Privitera (Acireale, Italy: Istituto Siciliano di Bioetica, 1994): 194–198; L. Melina, "La cooperazione con azioni moralmente cattive contra la vita umana," in *Commentario Interdisciplinare alia "Evangelium Vitae,"* eds. E. Sgreccia and Ramon Luca Lucas (Vatican City: Libreria Editrice Vaticana, 1997): 467–490; E. Sgreccia, *Manuale di Bioetica*, 3rd ed., vol. I, (Milan: Vita e Pensiero, 1999): 362–363.

[12] See John Paul II, *Evangelium vitae*, n. 74.

[13] *Catechism of the Catholic Church*, n. 1868.

[14] The alternative vaccines in question are those that are prepared by means of cell lines which are not of human origin, for example, the Vero cell line (from monkeys) (D. Vinnedge, "The Smallpox Vaccine," *National Catholic Bioethics Quarterly* 2.1 [Spring 2000]: 2), the kidney cells of rabbits or monkeys, or the cells of chicken embryos. However, it should be noted that grave forms of allergy have occurred with some of the vaccines prepared in this way. The use of recombinant DNA technology could lead to the development of new vaccines in the near future which will no longer require the use of cultures of human diploid cells for the attenuation of the virus and its growth, for such vaccines will not be prepared from a basis of attenuated virus, but from the genome of the virus and from the antigens thus developed. G. C. Woodrow, "An Overview of Biotechnology as Applied to Vaccine Development," in *New Generation Vaccines*, eds. W. M. McDonnell and M. M. Levine (New York: Marcel Dekker, 1990), 32–37; F. K. Askarim "Immunization," *JAMA* 278.22 (December 10, 1997): 2005–2006. Some experimental studies have already been done using vaccines developed from DNA that has been derived from the genome of the German measles virus. Moreover, some Asiatic researchers are trying to use the varicella virus as a vector for the insertion of genes which codify the viral antigens of rubella. These studies are still at a preliminary phase and the refinement of vaccine preparations which can be used in clinical practice will require a lengthy period of time and will be at high costs.

[15] Such a duty may lead, as a consequence, to taking recourse to "objection of conscience" when the action recognized as illicit is an act permitted or even encouraged by the laws of the country and poses a threat to human life. The encyclical letter *Evangelium vitae* underlined this "obligation to oppose" the laws which permit abortion or euthanasia "by conscientious objection" (n. 73).

[16] This is particularly true in the case of vaccination against German measles, because of the danger of congenital rubella syndrome. This could occur, causing grave congenital malformations in the fetus, when a pregnant woman enters into contact, even if it is brief, with children who have not been immunized and are carriers of the virus. In this case, the parents who did not accept the vaccination of their own children become responsible for the malformations in question, and for the subsequent abortion of fetuses, when they have been discovered to be malformed.

APPENDIX XVI

Congregation for the Doctrine of the Faith

Responses to Certain Questions of the United States Conference of Catholic Bishops concerning Artificial Nutrition and Hydration, with Commentary

August 1, 2007

First question: *Is the administration of food and water (whether by natural or artificial means) to a patient in a "vegetative state" morally obligatory except when they cannot be assimilated by the patient's body or cannot be administered to the patient without causing significant physical discomfort?*

Response: Yes. The administration of food and water even by artificial means is, in principle, an ordinary and proportionate means of preserving life. It is therefore obligatory to the extent to which, and for as long as, it is shown to accomplish its proper finality, which is the hydration and nourishment of the patient. In this way suffering and death by starvation and dehydration are prevented.

Second question: *When nutrition and hydration are being supplied by artificial means to a patient in a "permanent vegetative state", may they be discontinued when competent physicians judge with moral certainty that the patient will never recover consciousness?*

Response: No. A patient in a "permanent vegetative state" is a person with fundamental human dignity and must, therefore, receive ordinary and proportionate care which includes, in principle, the administration of water and food even by artificial means.

The Supreme Pontiff Benedict XVI, at the Audience granted to the undersigned Cardinal Prefect of the Congregation for the Doctrine of the Faith, approved these Responses, adopted in the Ordinary Session of the Congregation, and ordered their publication.

Rome, from the Offices of the
Congregation for the Doctrine of the Faith,
August 1, 2007

William Cardinal Levada
Prefect

Angelo Amato, S.D.B.
Titular Archbishop of Sila
Secretary

Commentary

The Congregation for the Doctrine of the Faith has formulated responses to questions presented by His Excellency the Most Reverend William S. Skylstad, President of the United States Conference of Catholic Bishops, in a letter of July 11, 2005, regarding the nutrition and hydration of patients in the condition commonly called a "vegetative state." The object of the questions was whether the nutrition and hydration of such patients, especially if provided by artificial means, would constitute an excessively heavy burden for the patients, for their relatives, or for the health-care system, to the point where it could be considered, also in the light of the moral teaching of the Church, a means that is extraordinary or disproportionate and therefore not morally obligatory.

The Address of Pope Pius XII to a Congress on Anesthesiology, given on November 24, 1957, is often invoked in favor of the possibility of abandoning the nutrition and hydration of such patients. In this address, the Pope restated two general ethical principles. On the one hand, natural reason and Christian morality teach that, in the case of a grave illness, the patient and those caring for him or her have the right and the duty to provide the care necessary to preserve health and life. On the other hand, this duty in general includes only the use of those means which, considering all the circumstances, are ordinary, that is to say, which do not impose an extraordinary burden on the patient or on others. A more severe obligation would be too burdensome for the majority of persons and would make it too difficult to attain more important goods. Life, health and all temporal activities are subordinate to spiritual ends. Naturally, one is not forbidden to do more than is strictly obligatory to preserve life and health, on condition that one does not neglect more important duties.

One should note, first of all, that the answers given by Pius XII referred to the use and interruption of techniques of resuscitation. However, the case in question has nothing to do with such techniques. Patients in a "vegetative state" breathe spontaneously, digest food naturally, carry on other metabolic functions, and are in a stable situation. But they are not able to feed themselves. If they are not provided artificially with food and liquids, they will die, and the cause of their death will be neither an illness nor the "vegetative state" itself, but solely starvation and dehydration. At the same time, the artificial administration of water and food generally does not impose a heavy burden either on the patient or on his or her relatives. It does not involve excessive expense; it is within the capacity of an average health-care system, does not of itself require hospitalization, and is proportionate to accomplishing its purpose, which is to keep the patient from dying of starvation and dehydration. It is not, nor is it meant to be, a treatment that cures the patient, but is rather ordinary care aimed at the preservation of life.

What may become a notable burden is when the "vegetative state" of a family member is prolonged over time. It is a burden like that of caring for a quadriplegic, someone with serious mental illness, with advanced Alzheimer's disease, and so on. Such persons need continuous assistance for months or even for years. But the principle formulated by Pius XII cannot, for obvious reasons, be interpreted as meaning that in such cases those patients, whose ordinary care imposes a real burden on their families, may licitly be left to take care of themselves and thus abandoned to die. This is not the sense in which Pius XII spoke of extraordinary means.

Everything leads to the conclusion that the first part of the principle enunciated by Pius XII should be applied to patients in a "vegetative state": in the case of a serious illness, there is the right and the duty to provide the care necessary for preserving health and life. The development of the teaching of the Church's Magisterium, which has closely followed the progress of medicine and the questions which this has raised, fully confirms this conclusion.

The *Declaration on Euthanasia*, published by the Congregation for the Doctrine of the Faith on May 5, 1980, explained the distinction between proportionate and disproportionate means, and between therapeutic treatments and the normal care due to the sick person: "When inevitable death is imminent in spite of the means used, it is permitted in conscience to take the decision to refuse forms of treatment that would only secure a precarious and burdensome prolongation of life, so long as the normal care due to the sick person in similar cases is not interrupted" (Part IV). Still less can one interrupt the ordinary means of care for patients who are not facing an imminent death, as is generally the case of those in a "vegetative state"; for these people, it would be precisely the interruption of the ordinary means of care which would be the cause of their death.

On June 27, 1981, the Pontifical Council *Cor Unum* published a document entitled *Some Ethical Questions Relating to the Gravely Ill and the Dying*, in which, among other things, it is stated that "There remains the strict obligation to administer at all costs those means which are called 'minimal': that is, those that normally and in usual conditions are aimed at maintaining life (nourishment, blood transfusions, injections, etc.). The discontinuation of these minimal measures would mean in effect willing the end of the patient's life" (no. 2.4.4.).

In an Address to participants in an international course on forms of human preleukemia on November 15, 1985, Pope John Paul II, recalling the *Declaration on Euthanasia,* stated clearly that, in virtue of the principle of proportionate care, one may not relinquish "the commitment to valid treatment for sustaining life nor assistance with the normal means of preserving life", which certainly includes the administration of food and liquids. The Pope also noted that those omissions are not licit which are aimed "at shortening life in order to spare the patient or his family from suffering".

In 1995 the Pontifical Council for Pastoral Assistance to Health Care Workers published the *Charter for Health Care Workers*, paragraph 120 of which explicitly affirms: "The administration of food and liquids, even artificially, is part of the normal treatment always due to the patient when this is not burdensome for him or her; their undue interruption can have the meaning of real and true euthanasia".

The Address of John Paul II to a group of Bishops from the United States of America on a visit *ad limina*, on October 2, 1998, is quite explicit: nutrition and hydration are to be considered as normal care and ordinary means for the preservation of life. It is not acceptable to interrupt them or to withhold them, if from that decision the death of the patient will follow. This would be euthanasia by omission (cf. no. 4).

In his Address of March 20, 2004, to the participants of an International Congress on "Life-sustaining Treatments and the Vegetative State: scientific progress and ethical dilemmas", John Paul II confirmed in very clear terms what had been said in the documents cited above, clarifying also their correct interpretation. The Pope stressed the following points:

1) "The term *permanent vegetative state* has been coined to indicate the condition of those patients whose 'vegetative state' continues for over a year. Actually, there is no different diagnosis that corresponds to such a definition, but only a conventional prognostic judgment, relative to the fact that the recovery of patients, statistically speaking, is ever more difficult as the condition of vegetative state is prolonged in time" (no. 2).[1]

2) In response to those who doubt the "human quality" of patients in a "permanent vegetative state", it is necessary to reaffirm that "the intrinsic value and personal dignity of every human being do not change, no matter what the concrete circumstances of his or her life. *A man, even if seriously ill or disabled in the exercise of his highest functions, is and always will be a man*, and he will never become a 'vegetable' or an 'animal'" (no. 3).

3) "The sick person in a vegetative state, awaiting recovery or a natural end, still has the right to basic health care (nutrition, hydration, cleanliness, warmth, etc.), and to the prevention of

complications related to his confinement to bed. He also has the right to appropriate rehabilitative care and to be monitored for clinical signs of possible recovery. I should like particularly to underline how the administration of water and food, even when provided by artificial means, always represents a *natural means* of preserving life, not a *medical act*. Its use, furthermore, should be considered, in principle, *ordinary* and *proportionate*, and as such morally obligatory, to the extent to which, and for as long as, it is shown to accomplish its proper finality, which in the present case consists in providing nourishment to the patient and alleviation of his suffering" (no. 4).

4) The preceding documents were taken up and interpreted in this way: "The obligation to provide the 'normal care due to the sick in such cases' (Congregation for the Doctrine of the Faith, *Declaration on Euthanasia*, p. IV) includes, in fact, the use of nutrition and hydration (cf. Pontifical Council *Cor Unum, Some Ethical Questions Relating to the Gravely Ill and the Dying*, no. 2, 4, 4; Pontifical Council for Pastoral Assistance to Health Care Workers, *Charter for Health Care Workers*, no. 120). The evaluation of probabilities, founded on waning hopes for recovery when the vegetative state is prolonged beyond a year, cannot ethically justify the cessation or interruption of *minimal care* for the patient, including nutrition and hydration. Death by starvation or dehydration is, in fact, the only possible outcome as a result of their withdrawal. In this sense it ends up becoming, if done knowingly and willingly, true and proper euthanasia by omission" (n. 4).

Therefore, the Responses now given by the Congregation for the Doctrine of the Faith continue the direction of the documents of the Holy See cited above, and in particular the Address of John Paul II of March 20, 2004. The basic points are two. It is stated, first of all, that the provision of water and food, even by artificial means, is in principle an ordinary and proportionate means of preserving life for patients in a "vegetative state": "It is therefore obligatory, to the extent to which,

and for as long as, it is shown to accomplish its proper finality, which is the hydration and nourishment of the patient". It is made clear, secondly, that this ordinary means of sustaining life is to be provided also to those in a "permanent vegetative state", since these are persons with their fundamental human dignity.

When stating that the administration of food and water is morally obligatory *in principle*, the Congregation for the Doctrine of the Faith does not exclude the possibility that, in very remote places or in situations of extreme poverty, the artificial provision of food and water may be physically impossible, and then *ad impossibilia nemo tenetur*. However, the obligation to offer the minimal treatments that are available remains in place, as well as that of obtaining, if possible, the means necessary for an adequate support of life. Nor is the possibility excluded that, due to emerging complications, a patient may be unable to assimilate food and liquids, so that their provision becomes altogether useless. Finally, the possibility is not absolutely excluded that, in some rare cases, artificial nourishment and hydration may be excessively burdensome for the patient or may cause significant physical discomfort, for example resulting from complications in the use of the means employed.

These exceptional cases, however, take nothing away from the general ethical criterion, according to which the provision of water and food, even by artificial means, always represents a *natural means* for preserving life, and is not a *therapeutic treatment*. Its use should therefore be considered *ordinary and proportionate*, even when the "vegetative state" is prolonged.

Note

[1] Terminology concerning the different phases and forms of the "vegetative state" continues to be discussed, but this is not important for the moral judgment involved.

APPENDIX XVII

Congregation for the Doctrine of the Faith

Instruction Dignitas personae *on Certain Bioethical Questions*

June 20, 2008

Introduction

1. The dignity of a person must be recognized in every human being from conception to natural death. This fundamental principle expresses *a great "yes" to human life* and must be at the center of ethical reflection on biomedical research, which has an ever greater importance in today's world. The Church's Magisterium has frequently intervened to clarify and resolve moral questions in this area. The Instruction *Donum vitae* was particularly significant.[1] And now, twenty years after its publication, it is appropriate to bring it up to date.

The teaching of *Donum vitae* remains completely valid, both with regard to the principles on which it is based and the moral evaluations which it expresses. However, new biomedical technologies which have been introduced in the critical area of human life and the family have given rise to further questions, in particular in the field of research on human embryos, the use of stem cells for therapeutic purposes, as well as in other areas of experimental medicine. These new questions require answers. The pace of scientific developments in this area and the publicity they have received have raised expectations and concerns in large sectors of public opinion. Legislative assemblies have been asked to make decisions on these questions in order to regulate them by law; at times, wider popular consultation has also taken place.

These developments have led the Congregation for the Doctrine of the Faith to prepare a *new doctrinal Instruction* which addresses some recent questions in the light of the criteria expressed in the Instruction *Donum vitae* and which also examines some issues that were treated earlier, but are in need of additional clarification.

2. In undertaking this study, the Congregation for the Doctrine of the Faith has benefited from the analysis of the Pontifical Academy for Life and has consulted numerous experts with regard to the scientific aspects of these questions, in order to address them with the principles of Christian anthropology. The Encyclicals *Veritatis splendor*[2] and *Evangelium vitae*[3] of John Paul II, as well as other interventions of the Magisterium, offer clear indications with regard to both the method and the content of the examination of the problems under consideration.

In the current multifaceted philosophical and scientific context, a considerable number of scientists and philosophers, in the spirit of the *Hippocratic Oath*, see in medical science a service to human fragility aimed at the cure of disease, the relief of suffering and the equitable extension of necessary care to all people. At the same time, however, there are also persons in the world of philosophy and science who view advances in biomedical technology from an essentially eugenic perspective.

3. In presenting principles and moral evaluations regarding biomedical research on human life, the Catholic Church draws upon *the light both of reason and of faith* and seeks to set forth an integral vision of man and his vocation, capable of incorporating everything that is good in human activity, as well as in various cultural and religious traditions which not infrequently demonstrate a great reverence for life.

The Magisterium also seeks to offer a word of support and encouragement for the perspective on culture which considers *science an invaluable service to the integral good of the life and dignity of every human being*. The Church therefore views scientific research with hope and desires that many Christians will dedicate themselves to the progress of biomedicine and will bear witness to their faith in this field. She hopes moreover that the results of such research may also be made available in areas of the world that are poor and afflicted by disease, so that those who are most in need will receive humanitarian assistance. Finally, the Church seeks to draw near to every human being who is suffering, whether in body or in spirit, in order to bring not only comfort, but also light and hope. These give meaning to moments of sickness and to the experience of death, which indeed are part of human life and are present in the story of every person, opening that story to the mystery of the Resurrection. Truly, the gaze of the Church is full of trust because "Life will triumph: this is a sure hope for us. Yes, life will triumph because truth, goodness, joy and true progress are on the side of life. God, who loves life and gives it generously, is on the side of life."[4]

The present Instruction is addressed to the Catholic faithful and to all who seek the truth.[5] It has three parts: the first recalls some anthropological, theological and ethical elements of fundamental importance; the second addresses new problems regarding procreation; the third examines new procedures involving the manipulation of embryos and the human genetic patrimony.

First Part:
Anthropological, Theological and Ethical Aspects of Human Life and Procreation

4. In recent decades, medical science has made significant strides in understanding human life in its initial stages. Human biological structures and the process of human generation are better known. These developments are certainly positive and worthy of support when they serve to overcome or correct pathologies and succeed in re-establishing the normal functioning of human procreation. On the other hand, they are negative and cannot be utilized when they involve the destruction of human beings or when they employ means which contradict the dignity of the person or when they are used for purposes contrary to the integral good of man.

The body of a human being, from the very first stages of its existence, can never be reduced merely to a group of cells. The embryonic human body develops progressively according to a well-defined program with its proper finality, as is apparent in the birth of every baby.

It is appropriate to recall the *fundamental ethical criterion* expressed in the Instruction *Donum vitae* in order to evaluate all moral questions which relate to procedures involving the human embryo: "Thus the fruit of human generation, from the first moment of its existence, that is to say, from the moment the zygote has formed, demands the unconditional respect that is morally due to the human being in his bodily and spiritual totality. The human being is to be respected and treated as a person from the moment of conception; and therefore from that same moment his rights as a person must be recognized, among which in the first place is the inviolable right of every innocent human being to life."[6]

5. This ethical principle, which reason is capable of recognizing as true and in conformity with the natural moral law, should be the basis for all legislation in this area.[7] In fact, *it presupposes a truth of an ontological character*, as *Donum vitae* demonstrated from solid scientific evidence, regarding the continuity in development of a human being.

If *Donum vitae*, in order to avoid a statement of an explicitly philosophical nature, did not define the embryo as a person, it nonetheless did indicate that there is an intrinsic connection between the ontological dimension and the specific value of every human life. Although the presence of the spiritual soul cannot be observed experimentally, the conclusions of science regarding the human embryo give "a valuable indication for discerning by the use of reason a personal presence at the moment of the first appearance of a human life: how could a human individual not be a human person?"[8] Indeed, the reality of the human being for the entire span of life, both before and after birth, does not allow us to posit either a change in nature or a gradation in moral value, since it possesses full anthropological and ethical status. The human embryo has, therefore, from the very beginning, the dignity proper to a person.

6. Respect for that dignity is owed to every human being because each one carries in an indelible way his own dignity and value. *The origin of human life has its authentic context in marriage and in the family,* where it is generated through an act which expresses the reciprocal love between a man and a woman. Procreation which is truly responsible vis-à-vis the child to be born "must be the fruit of marriage."[9]

Marriage, present in all times and in all cultures, "is in reality something wisely and providently instituted by God the Creator with a view to carrying out his loving plan in human beings. Thus, husband and wife, through the reciprocal gift of themselves to the other—something which is proper and exclusive to them—bring about that communion of persons by which they perfect each other, so as to cooperate with God in the procreation and raising of new lives."[10] In the fruitfulness of married love, man and woman "make it clear that at the origin of their spousal life there is a genuine 'yes', which is pronounced and truly lived in reciprocity, remaining ever open to life ... Natural law, which is at the root of the recognition of true equality between persons and peoples, deserves to be recognized as the source that inspires the relationship between the spouses in their responsibility for begetting new children. The transmission of life is inscribed in nature and its laws stand as an unwritten norm to which all must refer."[11]

7. It is the Church's conviction that what is human is not only received and respected by *faith*, but is also purified, elevated and perfected. God, after having created man in his image and likeness (cf. Gen 1:26), described his creature as "very good" (Gen 1:31), so as to be assumed later in the Son (cf. Jn 1:14). In the mystery of the Incarnation, the Son of God confirmed the dignity of the body and soul which constitute the human being. Christ did not disdain human bodiliness, but instead fully disclosed its meaning and value: "In reality, it is only in the mystery of the incarnate Word that the mystery of man truly becomes clear."[12]

By becoming one of us, the Son makes it possible for us to become "sons of God" (Jn 1:12), "sharers in the divine nature" (2 Pet 1:4). This new dimension does not conflict with the dignity of the creature which everyone can recognize by the use of reason, but elevates it into a wider horizon of life which is proper to God, giving us the ability to reflect more profoundly on human life and on the acts by which it is brought into existence.[13]

The respect for the individual human being, which reason requires, is further enhanced and strengthened in the light of these truths of faith: thus, we see that there is no contradiction between the affirmation of the dignity and the affirmation of the sacredness of human life. "The different ways in which God, acting in history, cares for the world and for mankind are not mutually exclusive; on the contrary, they support each other and intersect. They have their origin and goal in the eternal, wise and loving counsel whereby God predestines men and women 'to be conformed to the image of his Son' (Rom 8:29)."[14]

8. By taking the interrelationship of these two dimensions, *the human and the divine*, as the starting point, one understands better why it is that man has unassailable value: *he possesses an eternal vocation* and *is called to share in the trinitarian love of the living God.*

This value belongs to all without distinction. By virtue of the simple fact of existing, every human being must be fully respected. The introduction of discrimination with regard to human dignity based on biological, psychological, or educational development, or based on health-related criteria, must be excluded. At every stage of his existence, man, created in the image and likeness of God, reflects "the face of his Only begotten Son ... This boundless and almost incomprehensible love of God for the human being reveals the degree to which the human person deserves to be loved in himself, independently of any other consideration—intelligence, beauty, health, youth, integrity, and so forth. In short, human life is always a good, for *it 'is a manifestation of God in the world, a sign of his presence, a trace of his glory'* (*Evangelium vitae*, 34)."[15]

9. These two dimensions of life, the natural and the supernatural, allow us to understand better the sense in which *the acts that permit a new human being to come into existence*, in which a man and a woman give themselves to each other, *are a reflection of trinitarian love.* "God, who is love and life, has inscribed in man and woman the vocation to share in a special way in his mystery of personal communion and in his work as Creator and Father."[16]

Christian marriage is rooted "in the natural complementarity that exists between man and woman, and is nurtured through the personal willingness of the spouses to share their entire life-project, what they have and what they are: for this reason such communion is the fruit and the sign of a profoundly human need. But in Christ the Lord, God takes up this human need, confirms it, purifies it and elevates it, leading it to perfection through the sacrament of matrimony: the Holy Spirit who is poured out in the sacramental celebration offers Christian couples the gift of a new communion of love that is the living and real image of that unique unity which makes of the Church the indivisible Mystical Body of the Lord Jesus."[17]

10. The Church, by expressing an ethical judgment on some developments of recent medical research concerning man and his beginnings, does not intervene in the area proper to medical science itself, but rather calls everyone to ethical and social responsibility for their actions. She reminds them that the ethical value of biomedical science is gauged in reference to both *the unconditional respect owed to every human being*

at every moment of his or her existence, and the *defense of the specific character of the personal act which transmits life.* The intervention of the Magisterium falls within its mission of *contributing to the formation of conscience*, by authentically teaching the truth which is Christ and at the same time by declaring and confirming authoritatively the principles of the moral order which spring from human nature itself.[18]

Second Part:
New Problems Concerning Procreation

11. In light of the principles recalled above, certain questions regarding procreation which have emerged and have become more clear in the years since the publication of *Donum vitae* can now be examined.

Techniques for assisting fertility

12. With regard to the *treatment of infertility*, new medical techniques must respect three fundamental goods: (a) the right to life and to physical integrity of every human being from conception to natural death; (b) the unity of marriage, which means reciprocal respect for the right within marriage to become a father or mother only together with the other spouse;[19] (c) the specifically human values of sexuality which require "that the procreation of a human person be brought about as the fruit of the conjugal act specific to the love between spouses."[20] Techniques which assist procreation "are not to be rejected on the grounds that they are artificial. As such, they bear witness to the possibilities of the art of medicine. But they must be given a moral evaluation in reference to the dignity of the human person, who is called to realize his vocation from God to the gift of love and the gift of life."[21]

In light of this principle, all techniques of heterologous artificial fertilization,[22] as well as those techniques of homologous artificial fertilization[23] which substitute for the conjugal act, are to be excluded. On the other hand, techniques which act *as an aid to the conjugal act and its fertility* are permitted. The Instruction *Donum vitae* states: "The doctor is at the service of persons and of human procreation. He does not have the authority to dispose of them or to decide their fate. A medical intervention respects the dignity of persons when it seeks to assist the conjugal act either in order to facilitate its performance or in order to enable it to achieve its objective once it has been normally performed."[24] And, with regard to homologous artificial insemination, it states: "Homologous artificial insemination within marriage cannot be admitted except for those cases in which the technical means is not a substitute for the conjugal act, but serves to facilitate and to help so that the act attains its natural purpose."[25]

13. Certainly, techniques aimed at removing obstacles to natural fertilization, as for example, hormonal treatments for infertility, surgery for endometriosis, unblocking of fallopian tubes or their surgical repair, are licit. All these techniques may

be considered *authentic treatments* because, once the problem causing the infertility has been resolved, the married couple is able to engage in conjugal acts resulting in procreation, without the physician's action directly interfering in that act itself. None of these treatments replaces the conjugal act, which alone is worthy of truly responsible procreation.

In order to come to the aid of the many infertile couples who want to have children, adoption should be encouraged, promoted and facilitated by appropriate legislation so that the many children who lack parents may receive a home that will contribute to their human development. In addition, research and investment directed at the *prevention of sterility* deserve encouragement.

In vitro fertilization and the deliberate destruction of embryos

14. The fact that the process of in vitro fertilization very frequently involves the deliberate destruction of embryos was already noted in the Instruction *Donum vitae*.[26] There were some who maintained that this was due to techniques which were still somewhat imperfect. Subsequent experience has shown, however, that all techniques of in vitro fertilization proceed as if the human embryo were simply a mass of cells to be used, selected and discarded.

It is true that approximately a third of women who have recourse to artificial procreation succeed in having a baby. It should be recognized, however, that given the proportion between the total number of embryos produced and those eventually born, *the number of embryos sacrificed is extremely high*.[27] These losses are accepted by the practitioners of in vitro fertilization as the price to be paid for positive results. In reality, it is deeply disturbing that research in this area aims principally at obtaining better results in terms of the percentage of babies born to women who begin the process, but does not manifest a concrete interest in the right to life of each individual embryo.

15. It is often objected that the loss of embryos is, in the majority of cases, unintentional or that it happens truly against the will of the parents and physicians. They say that it is a question of risks which are not all that different from those in natural procreation; to seek to generate new life without running any risks would in practice mean doing nothing to transmit it. It is true that not all the losses of embryos in the process of in vitro fertilization have the same relationship to the will of those involved in the procedure. But it is also true that in many cases the abandonment, destruction and loss of embryos are foreseen and willed.

Embryos produced in vitro which have defects are directly discarded. Cases are becoming ever more prevalent in which couples who have no fertility problems are using artificial means of procreation in order to engage in genetic selection of their offspring. In many countries, it is now common to stimulate ovulation so as to obtain a large number of oocytes which are then fertilized. Of these, some are transferred into the woman's uterus, while the others are frozen for future use. The reason for multiple transfer is to increase the probability that at least one embryo will implant in the uterus. In this technique, therefore, the number of embryos transferred is greater than the single child desired, in the expectation that some embryos will be lost and multiple pregnancy may not occur. In this way, the practice of multiple embryo transfer implies *a purely utilitarian treatment of embryos*. One is struck by the fact that, in any other area of medicine, ordinary professional ethics and the health-care authorities themselves would never allow a medical procedure which involved such a high number of failures and fatalities. In fact, techniques of in vitro fertilization are accepted based on the presupposition that the individual embryo is not deserving of full respect in the presence of the competing desire for offspring which must be satisfied.

This sad reality, which often goes unmentioned, is truly deplorable: the "various techniques of artificial reproduction, which would seem to be at the service of life and which are frequently used with this intention, actually open the door to new threats against life."[28]

16. The Church moreover holds that it is ethically unacceptable to *dissociate procreation from the integrally personal context of the conjugal act*[29]: human procreation is a personal act of a husband and wife, which is not capable of substitution. The blithe acceptance of the enormous number of abortions involved in the process of in vitro fertilization vividly illustrates how the replacement of the conjugal act by a technical procedure—in addition to being in contradiction with the respect that is due to procreation as something that cannot be reduced to mere reproduction—leads to a weakening of the respect owed to every human being. Recognition of such respect is, on the other hand, promoted by the intimacy of husband and wife nourished by married love.

The Church recognizes the legitimacy of the desire for a child and understands the suffering of couples struggling with problems of fertility. Such a desire, however, should not override the dignity of every human life to the point of absolute supremacy. The desire for a child cannot justify the "production" of offspring, just as the desire not to have a child cannot justify the abandonment or destruction of a child once he or she has been conceived.

In reality, it seems that some researchers, lacking any ethical point of reference and aware of the possibilities inherent in technological progress, surrender to the logic of purely subjective desires[30] and to economic pressures which are so strong in this area. In the face of this manipulation of the human being in his or her embryonic state, it needs to be repeated that "God's love does not differentiate between the newly conceived infant still in his or her mother's womb and the child or young person, or the adult and the elderly person. God does not distinguish between them because he sees an impression of his own image and likeness (Gen 1:26) in each one ... Therefore, the Magisterium of the Church has constantly proclaimed the sacred and inviolable character of every human life from its conception until its natural end."[31]

Intracytoplasmic sperm injection (ICSI)

17. Among the recent techniques of artificial fertilization which have gradually assumed a particular importance is *intracytoplasmic sperm injection*.[32] This technique is used with increasing frequency given its effectiveness in overcoming various forms of male infertility.[33]

Just as in general with in vitro fertilization, of which it is a variety, ICSI is intrinsically illicit: it causes *a complete separation between procreation and the conjugal act*. Indeed ICSI takes place "outside the bodies of the couple through actions of third parties whose competence and technical activity determine the success of the procedure. Such fertilization entrusts the life and identity of the embryo into the power of doctors and biologists and establishes the domination of technology over the origin and destiny of the human person. Such a relationship of domination is in itself contrary to the dignity and equality that must be common to parents and children. Conception in vitro is the result of the technical action which presides over fertilization. Such fertilization is neither in fact achieved nor positively willed as the expression and fruit of a specific act of the conjugal union."[34]

Freezing embryos

18. One of the methods for improving the chances of success in techniques of in vitro fertilization is the multiplication of attempts. In order to avoid repeatedly taking oocytes from the woman's body, the process involves a single intervention in which multiple oocytes are taken, followed by cryopreservation of a considerable number of the embryos conceived in vitro.[35] In this way, should the initial attempt at achieving pregnancy not succeed, the procedure can be repeated or additional pregnancies attempted at a later date. In some cases, even the embryos used in the first transfer are frozen because the hormonal ovarian stimulation used to obtain the oocytes has certain effects which lead physicians to wait until the woman's physiological conditions have returned to normal before attempting to transfer an embryo into her womb.

Cryopreservation is *incompatible with the respect owed to human embryos*; it presupposes their production in vitro; it exposes them to the serious risk of death or physical harm, since a high percentage does not survive the process of freezing and thawing; it deprives them at least temporarily of maternal reception and gestation; it places them in a situation in which they are susceptible to further offense and manipulation.[36]

The majority of embryos that are not used remain "orphans". Their parents do not ask for them and at times all trace of the parents is lost. This is why there are thousands upon thousands of frozen embryos in almost all countries where in vitro fertilization takes place.

19. With regard to the large number of *frozen embryos already in existence* the question becomes: what to do with them? Some of those who pose this question do not grasp its ethical nature, motivated as they are by laws in some countries that require cryopreservation centers to empty their storage tanks periodically. Others, however, are aware that a grave injustice has been perpetrated and wonder how best to respond to the duty of resolving it.

Proposals to *use these embryos for research or for the treatment of disease* are obviously unacceptable because they treat the embryos as mere "biological material" and result in their destruction. The proposal to thaw such embryos without reactivating them and use them for research, as if they were normal cadavers, is also unacceptable.[37]

The proposal that these embryos could be put at the disposal of infertile couples as a *treatment for infertility* is not ethically acceptable for the same reasons which make artificial heterologous procreation illicit as well as any form of surrogate motherhood;[38] this practice would also lead to other problems of a medical, psychological and legal nature.

It has also been proposed, solely in order to allow human beings to be born who are otherwise condemned to destruction, that there could be a form of "*prenatal adoption*". This proposal, praiseworthy with regard to the intention of respecting and defending human life, presents however various problems not dissimilar to those mentioned above.

All things considered, it needs to be recognized that the thousands of abandoned embryos represent *a situation of injustice which in fact cannot be resolved*. Therefore John Paul II made an "appeal to the conscience of the world's scientific authorities and in particular to doctors, that the production of human embryos be halted, taking into account that there seems to be no morally licit solution regarding the human destiny of the thousands and thousands of 'frozen' embryos which are and remain the subjects of essential rights and should therefore be protected by law as human persons."[39]

The freezing of oocytes

20. In order avoid the serious ethical problems posed by the freezing of embryos, the freezing of oocytes has also been advanced in the area of techniques of in vitro fertilization.[40] Once a sufficient number of oocytes has been obtained for a series of attempts at artificial procreation, only those which are to be transferred into the mother's body are fertilized while the others are frozen for future fertilization and transfer should the initial attempts not succeed.

In this regard it needs to be stated that *cryopreservation of oocytes for the purpose of being used in artificial procreation is to be considered morally unacceptable*.

The reduction of embryos

21. Some techniques used in artificial procreation, above all the transfer of multiple embryos into the mother's womb, have caused a significant increase in the frequency of multiple pregnancy. This situation gives rise in turn to the practice of so-called embryo reduction, a procedure in which embryos or fetuses in the womb are directly exterminated. The decision to eliminate human lives, given that it was a human life that was desired in the first place, represents a contradiction that can often lead to suffering and feelings of guilt lasting for years.

From the ethical point of view, *embryo reduction is an intentional selective abortion.* It is in fact the deliberate and direct elimination of one or more innocent human beings in the initial phase of their existence and as such it always constitutes a grave moral disorder.[41]

The ethical justifications proposed for embryo reduction are often based on analogies with natural disasters or emergency situations in which, despite the best intentions of all involved, it is not possible to save everyone. Such analogies cannot in any way be the basis for an action which is directly abortive. At other times, moral principles are invoked, such as those of the lesser evil or double effect, which are likewise inapplicable in this case. It is never permitted to do something which is intrinsically illicit, not even in view of a good result: *the end does not justify the means.*

Preimplantation diagnosis

22. Preimplantation diagnosis is a form of prenatal diagnosis connected with techniques of artificial fertilization in which embryos formed in vitro undergo genetic diagnosis before being transferred into a woman's womb. Such diagnosis is done *in order to ensure that only embryos free from defects or having the desired sex or other particular qualities are transferred.*

Unlike other forms of prenatal diagnosis, in which the diagnostic phase is clearly separated from any possible later elimination and which provide therefore a period in which a couple would be free to accept a child with medical problems, in this case, the diagnosis before implantation is immediately followed by the elimination of an embryo suspected of having genetic or chromosomal defects, or not having the sex desired, or having other qualities that are not wanted. Preimplantation diagnosis – connected as it is with artificial fertilization, which is itself always intrinsically illicit – is directed toward the *qualitative selection and consequent destruction of embryos,* which constitutes an act of abortion. Preimplantation diagnosis is therefore the expression of a *eugenic mentality* that "accepts selective abortion in order to prevent the birth of children affected by various types of anomalies. Such an attitude is shameful and utterly reprehensible, since it presumes to measure the value of a human life only within the parameters of 'normality' and physical well-being, thus opening the way to legitimizing infanticide and euthanasia as well."[42]

By treating the human embryo as mere "laboratory material", *the concept itself of human dignity is also subjected to alteration and discrimination.* Dignity belongs equally to every single human being, irrespective of his parents' desires, his social condition, educational formation or level of physical development. If at other times in history, while the concept and requirements of human dignity were accepted in general, discrimination was practiced on the basis of race, religion or social condition, today there is a no less serious and unjust form of discrimination which leads to the non-recognition of the ethical and legal status of human beings suffering from serious diseases or disabilities. It is forgotten that sick and disabled people are not some separate category of humanity; in fact, sickness and disability are part of the human condition and affect every individual, even when there is no direct experience of it. Such discrimination is immoral and must therefore be considered legally unacceptable, just as there is a duty to eliminate cultural, economic and social barriers which undermine the full recognition and protection of disabled or ill people.

New forms of interception and contragestation

23. Alongside methods of preventing pregnancy which are, properly speaking, contraceptive, that is, which prevent conception following from a sexual act, there are other technical means which act after fertilization, when the embryo is already constituted, either before or after implantation in the uterine wall. Such methods are *interceptive* if they interfere with the embryo before implantation and *contragestative* if they cause the elimination of the embryo once implanted.

In order to promote wider use of interceptive methods,[43] it is sometimes stated that the way in which they function is not sufficiently understood. It is true that there is not always complete knowledge of the way that different pharmaceuticals operate, but scientific studies indicate that *the effect of inhibiting implantation is certainly present,* even if this does not mean that such interceptives cause an abortion every time they are used, also because conception does not occur after every act of sexual intercourse. It must be noted, however, that anyone who seeks to prevent the implantation of an embryo which may possibly have been conceived and who therefore either requests or prescribes such a pharmaceutical, generally intends abortion.

When there is a delay in menstruation, a contragestative is used,[44] usually one or two weeks after the non-occurrence of the monthly period. The stated aim is to re-establish menstruation, but what takes place in reality is the *abortion of an embryo which has just implanted.*

As is known, abortion is "the deliberate and direct killing, by whatever means it is carried out, of a human being in the initial phase of his or her existence, extending from conception to birth."[45] Therefore, the use of means of interception and contragestation fall within the *sin of abortion* and are gravely immoral. Furthermore, when there is certainty that an abortion has resulted, there are serious penalties in canon law.[46]

Third Part:
New Treatments Which Involve
the Manipulation of the Embryo
or the Human Genetic Patrimony

24. Knowledge acquired in recent years has opened new perspectives for both regenerative medicine and for the treatment of genetically based diseases. In particular, *research on embryonic stem cells* and its possible future uses have prompted great interest, even though up to now such research has not produced effective results, as distinct from *research on adult stem cells*. Because some maintain that the possible medical advances which might result from research on embryonic stem cells could justify various forms of manipulation and destruction of human embryos, a whole range of questions has emerged in the area of gene therapy, from cloning to the use of stem cells, which call for attentive moral discernment.

Gene therapy

25. Gene therapy commonly refers to techniques of genetic engineering applied to human beings for therapeutic purposes, that is to say, with the aim of curing genetically based diseases, although recently gene therapy has been attempted for diseases which are not inherited, for cancer in particular.

In theory, it is possible to use gene therapy on two levels: somatic cell gene therapy and germ line cell therapy. *Somatic cell gene therapy* seeks to eliminate or reduce genetic defects on the level of somatic cells, that is, cells other than the reproductive cells, but which make up the tissue and organs of the body. It involves procedures aimed at certain individual cells with effects that are limited to a single person. *Germ line cell therapy* aims instead at correcting genetic defects present in germ line cells with the purpose of transmitting the therapeutic effects to the offspring of the individual. Such methods of gene therapy, whether somatic or germ line cell therapy, can be undertaken on a fetus *before his or her birth* as gene therapy in the uterus or *after birth* on a child or adult.

26. For a moral evaluation the following distinctions need to be kept in mind. *Procedures used on somatic cells for strictly therapeutic purposes are in principle morally licit.* Such actions seek to restore the normal genetic configuration of the patient or to counter damage caused by genetic anomalies or those related to other pathologies. Given that gene therapy can involve significant risks for the patient, the ethical principle must be observed according to which, in order to proceed to a therapeutic intervention, it is necessary to establish beforehand that the person being treated will not be exposed to risks to his health or physical integrity which are excessive or disproportionate to the gravity of the pathology for which a cure is sought. The informed consent of the patient or his legitimate representative is also required.

The moral evaluation of *germ line cell therapy* is different. Whatever genetic modifications are effected on the germ cells of a person will be transmitted to any potential offspring. Because the risks connected to any genetic manipulation are considerable and as yet not fully controllable, *in the present state of research, it is not morally permissible to act in a way that may cause possible harm to the resulting progeny*. In the hypothesis of gene therapy on the embryo, it needs to be added that this only takes place in the context of in vitro fertilization and thus runs up against all the ethical objections to such procedures. For these reasons, therefore, it must be stated that, in its current state, germ line cell therapy in all its forms is morally illicit.

27. *The question of using genetic engineering for purposes other than medical treatment also calls for consideration.* Some have imagined the possibility of using techniques of genetic engineering to introduce alterations with the presumed aim of improving and strengthening the gene pool. Some of these proposals exhibit a certain dissatisfaction or even rejection of the value of the human being as a finite creature and person. Apart from technical difficulties and the real and potential risks involved, such manipulation would promote a eugenic mentality and would lead to indirect social stigma with regard to people who lack certain qualities, while privileging qualities that happen to be appreciated by a certain culture or society; such qualities do not constitute what is specifically human. This would be in contrast with the fundamental truth of the equality of all human beings which is expressed in the principle of justice, the violation of which, in the long run, would harm peaceful coexistence among individuals. Furthermore, one wonders who would be able to establish which modifications were to be held as positive and which not, or what limits should be placed on individual requests for improvement since it would be materially impossible to fulfil the wishes of every single person. Any conceivable response to these questions would, however, derive from arbitrary and questionable criteria. All of this leads to the conclusion that the prospect of such an intervention would end sooner or later by harming the common good, by favouring the will of some over the freedom of others. Finally it must also be noted that in the attempt to create *a new type of human being* one can recognize an ideological element in which man tries to take the place of his Creator.

In stating the ethical negativity of these kinds of interventions which imply *an unjust domination of man over man*, the Church also recalls the need to return to an attitude of care for people and of education in accepting human life in its concrete historical finite nature.

Human cloning

28. Human cloning refers to the asexual or agametic reproduction of the entire human organism in order to produce

one or more "copies" which, from a genetic perspective, are substantially identical to the single original.[47]

Cloning is proposed for two basic purposes: reproduction, that is, in order to obtain the birth of a baby, and *medical therapy* or research. In theory, reproductive cloning would be able to satisfy certain specific desires, for example, control over human evolution, selection of human beings with superior qualities, pre-selection of the sex of a child to be born, production of a child who is the "copy" of another, or production of a child for a couple whose infertility cannot be treated in another way. Therapeutic cloning, on the other hand, has been proposed as a way of producing embryonic stem cells with a predetermined genetic patrimony in order to overcome the problem of immune system rejection; this is therefore linked to the issue of the use of stem cells.

Attempts at cloning have given rise to genuine concern throughout the entire world. Various national and international organizations have expressed negative judgments on human cloning and it has been prohibited in the great majority of nations.

Human cloning is intrinsically illicit in that, by taking the ethical negativity of techniques of artificial fertilization to their extreme, it seeks to *give rise to a new human being without a connection to the act of reciprocal self-giving between the spouses* and, more radically, *without any link to sexuality*. This leads to manipulation and abuses gravely injurious to human dignity.[48]

29. If cloning were to be done for *reproduction*, this would impose on the resulting individual a predetermined genetic identity, subjecting him—as has been stated—to a form of *biological slavery*, from which it would be difficult to free himself. The fact that someone would arrogate to himself the right to determine arbitrarily the genetic characteristics of another person represents *a grave offense to the dignity of that person as well as to the fundamental equality of all people*.

The originality of every person is a consequence of the particular relationship that exists between God and a human being from the first moment of his existence and carries with it the obligation to respect the singularity and integrity of each person, even on the biological and genetic levels. In the encounter with another person, we meet a human being who owes his existence and his proper characteristics to the love of God, and only the love of husband and wife constitutes a mediation of that love in conformity with the plan of the Creator and heavenly Father.

30. From the ethical point of view, so-called therapeutic cloning is even more serious. To create embryos with the intention of destroying them, even with the intention of helping the sick, is completely incompatible with human dignity, because it makes the existence of a human being at the embryonic stage nothing more than a means to be used and destroyed. It is *gravely immoral to sacrifice a human life for therapeutic ends*.

The ethical objections raised in many quarters to therapeutic cloning and to the use of human embryos formed in vitro have led some researchers to propose new techniques which are presented as capable of producing stem cells of an embryonic type without implying the destruction of true human embryos.[49] These proposals have been met with questions of both a scientific and an ethical nature regarding above all the ontological status of the "product" obtained in this way. Until these doubts have been clarified, the statement of the Encyclical *Evangelium vitae* needs to be kept in mind: "what is at stake is so important that, from the standpoint of moral obligation, the mere probability that a human person is involved would suffice to justify an absolutely clear prohibition of any intervention aimed at killing a human embryo."[50]

The therapeutic use of stem cells

31. Stem cells are undifferentiated cells with two basic characteristics: (a) the prolonged capability of multiplying themselves while maintaining the undifferentiated state; (b) the capability of producing transitory progenitor cells from which fully differentiated cells descend, for example, nerve cells, muscle cells and blood cells.

Once it was experimentally verified that when stem cells are transplanted into damaged tissue they tend to promote cell growth and the regeneration of the tissue, new prospects opened for regenerative medicine, which have been the subject of great interest among researchers throughout the world.

Among the sources for human stem cells which have been identified thus far are: the embryo in the first stages of its existence, the fetus, blood from the umbilical cord and various tissues from adult humans (bone marrow, umbilical cord, brain, mesenchyme from various organs, etc.) and amniotic fluid. At the outset, studies focused on *embryonic stem cells*, because it was believed that only these had significant capabilities of multiplication and differentiation. Numerous studies, however, show that *adult stem cells* also have a certain versatility. Even if these cells do not seem to have the same capacity for renewal or the same plasticity as stem cells taken from embryos, advanced scientific studies and experimentation indicate that these cells give more positive results than embryonic stem cells. Therapeutic protocols in force today provide for the use of adult stem cells and many lines of research have been launched, opening new and promising possibilities.

32. With regard to the ethical evaluation, it is necessary to consider the *methods of obtaining stem cells* as well as *the risks connected with their clinical and experimental use*.

In these methods, the origin of the stem cells must be taken into consideration. Methods which do not cause serious harm to the subject from whom the stem cells are taken are to be considered licit. This is generally the case when tissues are taken from: (a) an adult organism; (b) the blood of the umbilical cord at the time of birth; (c) fetuses who have died of natural causes. The obtaining of stem cells from a living human embryo, on the other hand, invariably causes the death of the embryo and is consequently gravely illicit: "research, in such cases, irrespective of efficacious therapeutic results, is not truly at the service of humanity. In fact, this research advances through the suppression of human lives that are equal in dignity to the lives of other human individuals and to the lives of the researchers themselves. History itself has condemned such a science in the past and will condemn it in the future, not only because it lacks the light of God but also because it lacks humanity."[51]

The use of embryonic stem cells or differentiated cells derived from them—even when these are provided by other researchers through the destruction of embryos or when such cells are commercially available—presents serious problems from the standpoint of cooperation in evil and scandal.[52]

There are no moral objections to the clinical use of stem cells that have been obtained licitly; however, the common criteria of medical ethics need to be respected. Such use should be characterized by scientific rigor and prudence, by reducing to the bare minimum any risks to the patient and by facilitating the interchange of information among clinicians and full disclosure to the public at large.

Research initiatives involving the use of adult stem cells, since they do not present ethical problems, should be encouraged and supported.[53]

Attempts at hybridization

33. Recently animal oocytes have been used for reprogramming the nuclei of human somatic cells—this is generally called *hybrid cloning*—in order to extract embryonic stem cells from the resulting embryos without having to use human oocytes.

From the ethical standpoint, such procedures represent an offense against the dignity of human beings on account of *the admixture of human and animal genetic elements capable of disrupting the specific identity of man*. The possible use of the stem cells, taken from these embryos, may also involve additional health risks, as yet unknown, due to the presence of animal genetic material in their cytoplasm. To consciously expose a human being to such risks is morally and ethically unacceptable.

The use of human "biological material" of illicit origin

34. For scientific research and for the production of vaccines or other products, cell lines are at times used which are the result of an illicit intervention against the life or physical integrity of a human being. The connection to the unjust act may be either mediate or immediate, since it is generally a question of cells which reproduce easily and abundantly. This "material" is sometimes made available commercially or distributed freely to research centers by governmental agencies having this function under the law. All of this gives rise to *various ethical problems with regard to cooperation in evil and with regard to scandal*. It is fitting therefore to formulate general principles on the basis of which people of good conscience can evaluate and resolve situations in which they may possibly be involved on account of their professional activity.

It needs to be remembered above all that the category of abortion "is to be applied also to the recent forms of *intervention on human embryos* which, although carried out for purposes legitimate in themselves, inevitably involve the killing of those embryos. This is the case with *experimentation on embryos*, which is becoming increasingly widespread in the field of biomedical research and is legally permitted in some countries … [T]he use of human embryos or fetuses as an object of experimentation constitutes a crime against their dignity as human beings who have a right to the same respect owed to a child once born, just as to every person."[54] These forms of experimentation always constitute a grave moral disorder.[55]

35. A different situation is created when researchers use "biological material" of illicit origin which has been produced apart from their research center or which has been obtained commercially. The Instruction *Donum vitae* formulated the general principle which must be observed in these cases: "The corpses of human embryos and fetuses, whether they have been deliberately aborted or not, must be respected just as the remains of other human beings. In particular, they cannot be subjected to mutilation or to autopsies if their death has not yet been verified and without the consent of the parents or of the mother. Furthermore, the moral requirements must be safeguarded that there be no complicity in deliberate abortion and that the risk of scandal be avoided."[56]

In this regard, *the criterion of independence as it has been formulated by some ethics committees is not sufficient*. According to this criterion, the use of "biological material" of illicit origin would be ethically permissible provided there is a clear separation between those who, on the one hand, produce, freeze and cause the death of embryos and, on the other, the researchers involved in scientific experimentation. The criterion of independence is not sufficient to avoid a contradiction in the attitude of the person who says that he does not approve of the injustice perpetrated by others, but at the same time accepts for his own work the "biological material" which the others have obtained by means of that injustice. When the illicit action is endorsed by the laws which regulate health care and scientific research, it is necessary to distance oneself from the evil aspects of that system in order not to give the impression of a certain toleration or tacit acceptance of actions which are gravely unjust.[57] Any appearance of acceptance would in fact contribute to the growing indifference to, if not the approval of, such actions in certain medical and political circles.

At times, the objection is raised that the above-mentioned considerations would mean that people of good conscience involved in research would have the duty to oppose actively all the illicit actions that take place in the field of medicine, thus excessively broadening their ethical responsibility. In reality, the duty to avoid cooperation in evil and scandal relates to their ordinary professional activities, which they must pursue in a just manner and by means of which they must give witness to the value of life by their opposition to gravely unjust laws. Therefore, it needs to be stated that there is a duty to refuse to use such "biological material" even when there is no close connection between the researcher and the actions of those who performed the artificial fertilization or the abortion, or when there was no prior agreement with the centers in which the artificial fertilization took place. This duty springs from the necessity to *remove oneself*, within the area of one's own research, *from a gravely unjust legal situation and to affirm with clarity the value of human life*. Therefore, the above-mentioned criterion of independence is necessary, but may be ethically insufficient.

Of course, within this general picture there exist *differing degrees of responsibility*. Grave reasons may be morally proportionate to justify the use of such "biological material". Thus, for example, danger to the health of children could permit parents to use a vaccine which was developed using cell lines of illicit origin, while keeping in mind that everyone has the duty to make known their disagreement and to ask that their health-care system make other types of vaccines available. Moreover, in organizations where cell lines of illicit origin are being utilized, the responsibility of those who make the decision to use them is not the same as that of those who have no voice in such a decision.

In the context of the urgent need to *mobilize consciences in favour of life*, people in the field of health care need to be reminded that "their responsibility today is greatly increased. Its deepest inspiration and strongest support lie in the intrinsic and undeniable ethical dimension of the health-care profession, something already recognized by the ancient and still relevant *Hippocratic Oath*, which requires every doctor to commit himself to absolute respect for human life and its sacredness."[58]

Conclusion

36. There are those who say that the moral teaching of the Church contains too many prohibitions. In reality, however, her teaching is based on the recognition and promotion of all the gifts which the Creator has bestowed on man: such as life, knowledge, freedom and love. Particular appreciation is due not only to man's intellectual activities, but also to those which are practical, like work and technological activities. By these, in fact, he participates in the creative power of God and is called to transform creation by ordering its many resources toward the dignity and wellbeing of all human beings and of the human person in his entirety. In this way, man acts as the steward of the value and intrinsic beauty of creation.

Human history shows, however, how man has abused and can continue to abuse the power and capabilities which God has entrusted to him, giving rise to *various forms of unjust discrimination and oppression* of the weakest and most defenseless: the daily attacks on human life; the existence of large regions of poverty where people are dying from hunger and disease, excluded from the intellectual and practical resources available in abundance in many countries; technological and industrial development which is creating the real risk of a collapse of the ecosystem; the use of scientific research in the areas of physics, chemistry and biology for purposes of waging war; the many conflicts which still divide peoples and cultures; these sadly are only some of the most obvious signs of how man can make bad use of his abilities and become his own worst enemy by losing the awareness of his lofty and specific vocation to collaborate in the creative work of God.

At the same time, human history has also shown real *progress in the understanding and recognition of the value and dignity of every person* as the foundation of the rights and ethical imperatives by which human society has been, and continues to be structured. Precisely in the name of promoting human dignity, therefore, practices and forms of behaviour harmful to that dignity have been prohibited. Thus, for example, there are legal and political—and not just ethical—prohibitions of racism, slavery, unjust discrimination and marginalization of women, children, and ill and disabled people. Such prohibitions bear witness to the inalienable value and intrinsic dignity of every human being and are a sign of genuine progress in human history. In other words, the legitimacy of every prohibition is based on the need to protect an authentic moral good.

37. If initially human and social progress was characterized primarily by industrial development and the production of consumer goods, today it is distinguished by developments in information technologies, research in genetics, medicine and biotechnologies for human benefit, which are areas of great importance for the future of humanity, but in which there are also evident and unacceptable abuses. "Just as a century ago it was the working classes which were oppressed in their fundamental rights, and the Church courageously came to their defense by proclaiming the sacrosanct rights of the worker as person, so now, when another category of persons is being oppressed in the fundamental right to life, the Church feels in duty bound to speak out with the same courage on behalf of those who have no voice. Hers is always the evangelical cry in defense of the world's poor, those who are threatened and despised and whose human rights are violated."[59]

In virtue of the Church's doctrinal and pastoral mission, the Congregation for the Doctrine of the Faith has felt obliged to reiterate both the dignity and the fundamental and inalienable rights of every human being, including those in the initial stages of their existence, and to state explicitly the need for protection and respect which this dignity requires of everyone.

The fulfillment of this duty implies courageous opposition to all those practices which result in grave and unjust discrimination against unborn human beings, who have the dignity of a person, created like others in the image of God. *Behind every "no" in the difficult task of discerning between good and evil, there shines a great "yes" to the recognition of the dignity and inalienable value of every single and unique human being called into existence.*

The Christian faithful will commit themselves to the energetic promotion of a new culture of life by receiving the contents of this Instruction with the religious assent of their spirit, knowing that God always gives the grace necessary to observe his commandments and that, in every human being, above all in the least among us, one meets Christ himself (cf. Mt 25:40). In addition, all persons of good will, in particular physicians and researchers open to dialogue and desirous of knowing what is true, will understand and agree with these principles and judgments, which seek to safeguard the vulnerable condition of human beings in the first stages of life and to promote a more human civilization.

The Sovereign Pontiff Benedict XVI, in the Audience granted to the undersigned Cardinal Prefect on 20 June 2008, approved the present Instruction, adopted in the Ordinary Session of this Congregation, and ordered its publication.

Rome, from the Offices of the Congregation for the Doctrine of the Faith,
8 September 2008,
Feast of the Nativity of the Blessed Virgin Mary.

William Card. Levada
Prefect
+ Luis F. Ladaria, S.I.
Titular Archbishop of Thibica
Secretary

Notes

[1] Congregation for the Doctrine of the Faith, Instruction *Donum vitae* on respect for human life at its origins and for the dignity of procreation (22 February 1987): AAS 80 (1988), 70-102.

[2] John Paul II, Encyclical Letter *Veritatis splendor* regarding certain fundamental questions of the Church's moral teaching (6 August 1993): AAS 85 (1993), 1133-1228.

[3] John Paul II, Encyclical Letter *Evangelium vitae* on the value and inviolability of human life (25 March 1995): AAS 87 (1995), 401-522.

[4] John Paul II, Address to the participants in the Seventh Assembly of the Pontifical Academy of Life (3 March 2001), 3: AAS 93 (2001), 446.

[5] Cf. John Paul II, Encyclical Letter *Fides et ratio* on the relationship between faith and reason (14 September 1998), 1: AAS 91 (1999), 5.

[6] Congregation for the Doctrine of the Faith, Instruction *Donum vitae*, I, 1: AAS 80 (1988), 79.

[7] Human rights, as Pope Benedict XVI has recalled, and in particular the right to life of every human being "are based on the natural law inscribed on human hearts and present in different cultures and civilizations. Removing human rights from this context would mean restricting their range and yielding to a relativistic conception, according to which the meaning and interpretation of rights could vary and their universality would be denied in the name of different cultural, political, social and even religious outlooks. This great variety of viewpoints must not be allowed to obscure the fact that not only rights are universal, but so too is the human person, the subject of those rights" (Address to the General Assembly of the United Nations [18 April 2008]: AAS 100 [2008], 334).

[8] Congregation for the Doctrine of the Faith, Instruction *Donum vitae*, I, 1: AAS 80 (1988), 78-79.

[9] Congregation for the Doctrine of the Faith, Instruction *Donum vitae*, II, A, 1: AAS 80 (1988), 87.

[10] Paul VI, Encyclical Letter *Humanae vitae* (25 July 1968), 8: AAS 60 (1968), 485-486.

[11] Benedict XVI, Address to the Participants in the International Congress organized by the Pontifical Lateran University on the 40th Anniversary of the Encyclical *Humanae vitae*, 10 May 2008: *L'Osservatore Romano*, 11 May 2008, p. 1; cf. John XXIII, Encyclical Letter *Mater et magistra* (15 May 1961), III: AAS 53 (1961), 447.

[12] Second Vatican Council, Pastoral Constitution *Gaudium et spes*, 22.

[13] Cf. John Paul II, Encyclical Letter *Evangelium vitae*, 37-38: AAS 87 (1995), 442-444.

[14] John Paul II, Encyclical Letter *Veritatis splendor*, 45: AAS 85 (1993), 1169.

[15] Benedict XVI, Address to the General Assembly of the Pontifical Academy for Life and International Congress on "The Human Embryo in the Pre-implantation Phase" (27 February 2006): AAS 98 (2006), 264.

[16] Congregation for the Doctrine of the Faith, Instruction *Donum vitae*, Introduction, 3: AAS 80 (1988), 75.

[17] John Paul II, Apostolic Exhortation *Familiaris consortio* on the role of the Christian family in the modern world (22 September 1981), 19: AAS 74 (1982), 101-102.

[18] Cf. Second Vatican Council, Declaration *Dignitatis humanae*, 14.

[19] Cf. Congregation for the Doctrine of the Faith, Instruction *Donum vitae*, II, A, 1: AAS 80 (1988), 87.

[20] Congregation for the Doctrine of the Faith, Instruction *Donum vitae*, II, B, 4: AAS 80 (1988), 92.

[21] Congregation for the Doctrine of the Faith, Instruction *Donum vitae*, Introduction, 3: AAS 80 (1988), 75.

[22] The term *heterologous artificial fertilization or procreation* refers to "techniques used to obtain a human conception

artificially by the use of gametes coming from at least one donor other than the spouses who are joined in marriage" (Instruction *Donum vitae*, II: AAS 80 [1988], 86).

²³The term *homologous artificial fertilization or procreation* refers to "the technique used to obtain a human conception using the gametes of the two spouses joined in marriage" (Instruction *Donum vitae*, II: AAS 80 [1988], 86).

²⁴Congregation for the Doctrine of the Faith, Instruction *Donum vitae*, II, B, 7: AAS 80 (1988), 96; cf. Pius XII, Address to those taking part in the Fourth International Congress of Catholic Doctors (29 September 1949): AAS 41 (1949), 560.

²⁵Congregation for the Doctrine of the Faith, Instruction *Donum vitae*, II, B, 6: AAS 80 (1988), 94.

²⁶Cf. Congregation for the Doctrine of the Faith, Instruction *Donum vitae*, II: AAS 80 (1988), 86.

²⁷Currently the number of embryos sacrificed, even in the most technically advanced centers of artificial fertilization, hovers above 80%.

²⁸John Paul II, Encyclical Letter *Evangelium vitae*, 14: AAS 87 (1995), 416.

²⁹Cf. Pius XII, Address to the Second World Congress in Naples on human reproduction and sterility (19 May 1956): AAS 48 (1956), 470; Paul VI, Encyclical Letter *Humanae vitae*, 12: AAS 60 (1968), 488-489; Congregation for the Doctrine of the Faith, Instruction *Donum vitae*, II, B, 4-5: AAS 80 (1988), 90-94.

³⁰An increasing number of persons, even those who are unmarried, are having recourse to techniques of artificial reproduction in order to have a child. These actions weaken the institution of marriage and cause babies to be born in environments which are not conducive to their full human development.

³¹Benedict XVI, Address to the General Assembly of the Pontifical Academy for Life and International Congress on "The Human Embryo in the Pre-implantation Phase" (27 February 2006): AAS 98 (2006), 264.

³²*Intracytoplasmic sperm injection* is similar in almost every respect to other forms of in vitro fertilization with the difference that in this procedure fertilization in the test tube does not take place on its own, but rather by means of the injection into the oocyte of a single sperm, selected earlier, or by the injection of immature germ cells taken from the man.

³³There is ongoing discussion among specialists regarding the health risks which this method may pose for children conceived in this way.

³⁴Congregation for the Doctrine of the Faith, Instruction *Donum vitae*, II, B, 5: AAS 80 (1988), 93.

³⁵Cryopreservation of embryos refers to freezing them at extremely low temperatures, allowing long term storage.

³⁶Cf. Congregation for the Doctrine of the Faith, Instruction *Donum vitae*, I, 6: AAS 80 (1988), 84-85.

³⁷Cf. numbers 34-35 below.

³⁸Cf. Congregation for the Doctrine of the Faith, Instruction *Donum vitae*, II, A, 1-3: AAS 80 (1988), 87-89.

³⁹John Paul II, Address to the participants in the Symposium on "*Evangelium vitae* and Law" and the Eleventh International Colloquium on Roman and Canon Law (24 May 1996), 6: AAS

88 (1996), 943-944.

⁴⁰Cryopreservation of oocytes is also indicated in other medical contexts which are not under consideration here. The term oocyte refers to the female germ cell (gametocyte) not penetrated by the spermatozoa.

⁴¹Cf. Second Vatican Council, Pastoral Constitution *Gaudium et spes*, n. 51; John Paul II, Encyclical Letter *Evangelium vitae*, 62: AAS 87 (1995), 472.

⁴²John Paul II, Encyclical Letter *Evangelium vitae*, 63: AAS 87 (1995), 473.

⁴³The interceptive methods which are best known are the IUD (intrauterine device) and the so-called "morning-after pills".

⁴⁴The principal means of contragestation are RU-486 (mifepristone), synthetic prostaglandins or methotrexate.

⁴⁵John Paul II, Encyclical Letter *Evangelium vitae*, 58: AAS 87 (1995), 467.

⁴⁶Cf. CIC, can. 1398 and CCEO, can. 1450 § 2; cf. also CIC, can. 1323-1324. The Pontifical Commission for the Authentic Interpretation of the Code of Canon Law declared that the canonical concept of abortion is "the killing of the fetus in whatever way or at whatever time from the moment of conception" (*Response* of 23 May 1988: AAS 80 [1988], 1818).

⁴⁷In the current state of knowledge, the techniques which have been proposed for accomplishing human cloning are two: artificial embryo twinning and cell nuclear transfer. *Artificial embryo twinning* consists in the artificial separation of individual cells or groups of cells from the embryo in the earliest stage of development. These are then transferred into the uterus in order to obtain identical embryos in an artificial manner. *Cell nuclear transfer*, or cloning properly speaking, consists in introducing a nucleus taken from an embryonic or somatic cell into an denucleated oocyte. This is followed by stimulation of the oocyte so that it begins to develop as an embryo.

⁴⁸Cf. Congregation for the Doctrine of the Faith, Instruction *Donum vitae*, I, 6: AAS 80 (1988), 84; John Paul II, Address to Members of the Diplomatic Corps accredited to the Holy See (10 January 2005), 5: AAS 97 (2005), 153.

⁴⁹The new techniques of this kind are, for example, the use of human parthenogenesis, altered nuclear transfer (ANT) and oocyte assisted reprogramming (OAR).

⁵⁰John Paul II, Encyclical Letter *Evangelium vitae*, 60: AAS 87 (1995), 469.

⁵¹Benedict XVI, Address to the participants in the Symposium on the topic: "Stem Cells: what is the future for therapy?" organized by the Pontifical Academy for Life (16 September 2006): AAS 98 (2006), 694.

⁵²Cf. numbers 34-35 below.

⁵³Cf. Benedict XVI, Address to the participants in the Symposium on the topic: "Stem Cells: what is the future for therapy?" organized by the Pontifical Academy for Life (16 September 2006): AAS 98 (2006), 693-695.

⁵⁴John Paul II, Encyclical Letter *Evangelium vitae*, 63: AAS 87 (1995), 472-473.

⁵⁵Cf. John Paul II, Encyclical Letter *Evangelium vitae*, 62:

AAS 87 (1995), 472.

[56] Congregation for the Doctrine of the Faith, Instruction *Donum vitae*, I, 4: AAS 80 (1988), 83.

[57] Cf. John Paul II, Encyclical Letter *Evangelium vitae*, 73: AAS 87 (1995), 486: "Abortion and euthanasia are thus crimes which no human law can claim to legitimize. There is no obligation in conscience to obey such laws; instead there is a *grave and clear obligation to oppose them by conscientious objection*". The right of conscientious objection, as an expression of the right to freedom of conscience, should be protected by law.

[58] John Paul II, Encyclical Letter *Evangelium vitae*, 63: AAS 89 (1995), 502.

[59] John Paul II, Letter to all the Bishops on "The Gospel of Life" (19 May 1991): AAS 84 (1992), 319.

BIBLIOGRAPHY

GENERAL REFERENCES

Aquinas, Thomas. *Summa theologiae*, translated by the Fathers of the English Dominican Province. Westminster, MD: Christian Classics, 1981.

Ashley, Benedict M., O.P., and Kevin D. O'Rourke, O.P. *Health Care Ethics: A Theological Analysis*, 4th ed. Washington, D.C.: Georgetown University Press, 1997.

Ashley, Benedict M., O.P., Jean DeBlois, and Kevin D. O'Rourke, O.P. *Health Care Ethics: A Catholic Theological Analysis*, 5th ed. Washington, D.C.: Georgetown University Press, 2006.

Cataldo, Peter J. "The Principle of the Double Effect." *Ethics & Medics* 20.3 (March 1995): 1–3.

Catechism of the Catholic Church, 2nd ed., translated by the United States Conference of Catholic Bishops. Vatican City: Libreria Editrice Vaticana, 1994, 1997.

Congregation for the Doctrine of the Faith. *Donum vitae*. February 22, 1987. Vatican edition.

Congregation for the Doctrine of the Faith. *Quaecumque sterilizatio* (Reply of the Sacred Congregation for the Doctrine of the Faith on Sterilization in Catholic Hospitals). March 13, 1975. Vatican edition.

Congregation for the Doctrine of the Faith. Responses to Certain Questions of the United States Conference of Catholic Bishops concerning Artificial Nutrition and Hydration. August 1, 2007. Reprinted in *Ethics & Medics* 32.11 (November 2007): 1–3.

Congregation for the Doctrine of the Faith. Responses to Questions Proposed Concerning "Uterine Isolation" and Related Matters." July 31, 1993. In *L'Osservatore Romano* (English), August 3, 1994, 2.

Griese, Orville N. *Catholic Identity in Health Care: Principles and Practice*. Braintree, MA: Pope John Center, 1987.

Hoffmann, Diane E. "Evaluating Ethics Committees: A View from the Outside."*Milbank Quarterly* 71.4 (1993): 677–701.

Hoffmann, Diane E. "Regulating Ethics Committees in Health Care Institutions—Is It Time?" *Maryland Law Review* 50.3 (1991): 746–749.

John Paul II. Address to the 18th International Congress of the Transplantation Society. August 29, 2000. Vatican edition.

John Paul II, Pope. *Evangelium vitae*. March 25, 1995. Vatican edition.

John Paul II, Pope. *Fides et ratio*. September 14, 1998. Vatican edition.

John Paul II, Pope. *Redemptor hominis*. March 4, 1979. Vatican edition.

John Paul II, Pope. *Veritatis splendor*. August 6, 1993. Vatican edition.

Joint Commission for Accreditation of Healthcare Organizations. *Comprehensive Accreditation Manual for Hospitals*. Oakbrook Terrace, IL: JCAHO, 1996. Annual editions with updates are published by the Joint Commission.

Kelly, Gerald, S.J. *Medico-Moral Problems*. St. Louis, MO: Catholic Hospital Association of the United States and Canada, 1958.

Kelly, Margaret John, and Donald McCarthy, eds. *Ethics Committees: A Challenge for Catholic Health Care*. St. Louis, MO: Pope John Center and Catholic Health Association of the United States, 1984.

Monks of Solesmes, eds. *The Human Body: Papal Teachings*. Boston: St. Paul Editions, 1960.

National Institutes of Health (NIH). *State-of-the-Science Conference on Improving End-of-Life Care*. Bethesda, MD: NIH, 2004.

O'Donnell, Thomas J., S.J. *Medicine and Christian Morality*, 3rd ed. New York: Alba House, 1996.

Pius XI, Pope. *Casti connubii*. December 31, 1930.

Pontifical Academy for Life. *Declaration on the Production and the Scientific and Therapeutic Use of Human Embryonic Stem Cells*. August 25, 2000. Vatican edition.

President's Commission for Ethics in Medicine and Behavioral and Biomedical Research. *Deciding to Forgo Life-Sustaining Treatment: Ethical, Medical, and Legal Issues in Treatment Decisions*. Washington, D.C.: U.S. Government Printing Office, 1983.

Takahashi, K., and S. Yamanaka. "Induction of Pluripotent Stem Cells from Mouse Embryonic and Adult Fibroblast Cultures by Defined Factors." *Cell* 126.4 (August 25, 2006): 1–14.

U.S. Conference of Catholic Bishops. *Ethical and Religious Directives for Catholic Health Care Services*, 4th ed. Washington, D.C.: U.S. Conference of Catholic Bishops, 2001.

Veatch, Robert M. *A Theory of Medical Ethics*. New York: Basic Books, 1981.

PART ONE Foundational Principles

American Hospital Association, Technical Panel on Biomedical Ethics. *Values in Conflict: Resolving Ethical Issues in Health Care*, 2nd ed. Chicago: American Hospital Association, 1994.

American Medical Association, Council on Ethical and Judicial Affairs. *Code of Medical Ethics: Current Opinions with Annotations, 2008–2009*. Chicago: American Medical Association Press, 2008.

Aristotle. *Nichomachean Ethics*, translated by Martin Ostwald. New York: Macmillan, 1987.

Ashley, Benedict M., O.P. "Elements of a Catholic Conscience." In *Catholic Conscience: Foundation and Formation*, edited by Russell E. Smith, 39–58. Braintree, MA: Pope John Center, 1991.

Ashley, Benedict M., O.P. *Living the Truth in Love: A Biblical Introduction to Moral Theology*. New York: Alba House, 1996.

Benedict XVI, Pope. *Spe salvi*. November 30, 2007. Vatican edition.

Benjamin, Martin, and Joy Curtis. "Virtue and the Practice of Nursing." In *Virtue and Medicine*, edited by Earl E. Shelp, 257–273. Dordrecht, Netherlands: D. Reidel, 1985.

Blum, Lawrence. "Compassion." In *Explaining Emotions*, edited by Amelie Rorty, 507–518. Berkeley: University of California Press, 1980. Reprinted in *The Virtues: Contemporary Essays on Moral Character*, edited by Robert B. Kruschwitz and Robert C. Roberts, 229–236. Belmont, CA: Wadsworth, 1987.

Bohr, David. *Catholic Moral Tradition: In Christ, A New Creation*. Huntington, IN: Our Sunday Visitor, 1990.

Bourke, Vernon J. *Ethics: A Textbook in Moral Philosophy*. New York: Macmillan Company, 1951.

Callahan, Daniel. "Autonomy: A Moral Good, Not a Moral Obsession." *Hastings Center Report* 14.5 (October 1984): 40–42.

Canadian Catholic Conference. *Statement on the Formation of Conscience*. December 1, 1973. Boston: Daughters of St. Paul, 1974.

Cessario, Romanus, O.P. *Introduction to Moral Theology.* Washington, D.C.: Catholic University of America Press, 2001.

Congregation for the Doctrine of the Faith. *Declaration on Euthanasia.* May 5, 1980. Vatican edition.

DeLugo, John. *De Justitia et Jure.* Lyons, 1642.

Diamond, Eugene F. *A Catholic Guide to Medical Ethics: Catholic Principles in Clinical Practice.* Palos Park, IL: Linacre Institute, 2001.

DiPietro, Melanie, S.C. *Congregational Sponsorship.* Madison, WI: Catholic Health Association of Wisconsin, 1985.

Edelstein, Ludwig. *The Hippocratic Oath: Text, Translation, and Interpretation.* Baltimore: Johns Hopkins Press, 1943.

Ford, John C., S.J., and Gerald Kelly, S.J. *Contemporary Moral Theology.* Vol. 1, *Questions in Fundamental Moral Theology.* Westminster, MD: Newman Press, 1958.

Gallagher, David M. "Object and Intention in Moral Actions." *Ethics & Medics* 24.1 (January 1999): 1–2.

Gallagher, John, C.S.B. "The Principles of Totality: Man's Stewardship of His Body." In *Moral Theology Today: Certitudes and Doubts*, edited by Donald G. McCarthy, 217–242. St. Louis: Pope John Center, 1984.

Galot, J., S.J. *Inspiriter of the Community.* New York: Alba House, 1971.

Gonsalves, Milton. *Fagothey's Right and Reason: Ethics in Theory and Practice*, 9th ed. St. Louis, MO: Merrill, 1989.

Haas, John. "The Totality and Integrity of the Body." *Ethics & Medics* 20.2 (February 1995): 1–3.

Henry, Charles W., O.S.B. "The Place of Prudence in Medical Decision Making." *Journal of Religion and Health* 3.1 (Spring 1993): 27–37.

Hibbs, Thomas. "Principles and Prudence: The Aristotelianism of Thomas' Account of Moral Knowledge." *New Scholasticism* 61 (1987): 271–284.

John Paul II, Pope. "Address to Pontifical Academy of Sciences." October 23, 1982. *Origins* 12.21 (November 4, 1982): 342.

John Paul II, Pope. "The Human Person—Beginning and End of Scientific Research." Address to the Pontifical Academy of Sciences, Rome. October 28, 1994. *The Pope Speaks* (March–April 1995): 80–84.

Kelly, David F. *Contemporary Health Care Ethics.* Washington, D.C.: Georgetown University Press, 2004.

Kelly, Gerald, S.J. "Pope Pius XII and the Principle of Totality." *Theological Studies* 16 (1955): 373–396.

Kucharek, Cass. *To Settle Your Conscience.* Huntington, IN: Our Sunday Visitor, 1974.

Lobo, George V., S.J. *Guide to Christian Living: A New Compendium of Moral Theology.* Westminster, MD: Christian Classics, 1989.

Lynch, J. J. "Totality, Principle of." In *New Catholic Encyclopedia*, vol. 14, 211–212. Washington, D.C.: Catholic University of America Press, 1967.

Mangan, Joseph T., S.J. "An Historical Analysis of the Principle of Double Effect." *Theological Studies* 10.1 (March 1949): 41–61.

May, William E. *Becoming Human: An Invitation to Christian Ethics.* Dayton, OH: Pflaum Publishing, 1975.

May, William E. *Catholic Bioethics and the Gift of Human Life*, 2nd edition. Huntingdon, IN: Our Sunday Visitor, 2008.

May, William E. "The Magisterium and Bioethics." *Ethics & Medics* 12.8 (August 1987): 1–3.

McCarthy, Edward J. Bayer, and John A. Leies, eds. *Handbook on Critical Life Issues*, rev. ed. Braintree, MA: Pope John Center, 1988.

McInerny Ralph M. *Aquinas on Human Action: A Theory of Practice.* Washington, D.C.: Catholic University of America Press, 1992.

Mullady, Brian, O.P. "The Moral Act: Object, Circumstances, Intention." *Ethics & Medics* 19.9 (September 1994): 1–2.

National Conference of Catholic Bishops. *Code of Medical Ethics for Catholic Hospitals.* Washington, D.C.: United States Catholic Conference, 1954.

National Conference of Catholic Bishops. *Ethical and Religious Directives for Catholic Health Care Facilities.* Washington, D.C.: NCCB, 1971 (rev. 1975).

O'Keefe, Martin D., S.J. *Known from the Things That Are: Fundamental Theory of the Moral Life.* Houston: Center for Thomistic Studies, 1987.

O'Rourke, Kevin D., O.P., T. Kopfensteiner, and R. Hamel, and Philip Boyle. *Medical Ethics: Sources of Catholic Teaching*, 2nd ed. Washington, D.C.: Georgetown University Press, 1993.

Pellegrino, Edmund D. "The Virtuous Physician, and the Ethics of Medicine." In *Virtue and Medicine*, edited by Earl E. Shelp, 237–255. Dordrecht: D. Reidel, 1985.

Pellegrino, Edmund D., and David C. Thomasma. *The Christian Virtues in Medical Practice.* Washington, D.C.: Georgetown University Press, 1996.

Pellegrino, Edmund D., and David C. Thomasma. *The Virtues in Medical Practice.* New York: Oxford University Press, 1993.

Percival, Thomas. "Of Professional Conduct." In *Ethics in Medicine: Historical Perspectives and Contemporary Concerns*, edited by Stanley J. Reiser, Arthur J. Dyck, and William J. Curran, 18–25. Cambridge: MIT Press, 1977.

Pinckaers, Servais, O.P.. *Morality: The Catholic View*, translated by Michael Sherwin, O.P. South Bend, IN: St. Augustine's Press, 2001.

Pinckaers, Servais, O.P. "Natural Law and Freedom." In *Morality: The Catholic View.* South Bend, IN: St. Augustine's Press, 2003.

Pius XII, Pope. "The Intangibility of the Human Person." Address to the First International Congress of Histopathology. September 13, 1952. In *The Human Body*, edited by the Monks of Solesmes, 194–208. Boston: St. Paul Editions, 1979.

Pius XII, Pope. "Removal of a Healthy Organ." Address to Delegates at the Twenty-Sixth Congress of Urology. October 8, 1953. In *The Human Body*, edited by the Monks of Solesmes, 277–281. Boston: St. Paul Editions, 1979.

Pontifical Council for Pastoral Assistance to Health Care Workers. *Charter for Health Care Workers.* Boston: Pauline Books & Media, 1994.

Ratzinger, Joseph Cardinal. "Conscience and Truth." In *Catholic Conscience: Foundation and Formation*, edited by Russell E. Smith, 7–28. Braintree, MA: Pope John Center, 1991.

Ratzinger, Joseph Cardinal. "La bioetica nella prospettiva cristiana." *La Civiltà Cattolica* (September 21, 1991): 465–474.

Ratzinger, Joseph Cardinal. *On Conscience.* Philadelphia: National Catholic Bioethics Center, 2007.

Regan, Robert. *Professional Secrecy.* Washington, D.C.: Augustinian Press, 1943.

Shelp, Earl E., ed. *Virtue and Medicine.* Dordrecht: D. Reidel, 1985.

Smith, Russell E., ed. *Catholic Conscience: Foundation and Formation.* Braintree, MA: Pope John Center, 1991.

Sullivan, Francis A., S.J. *Magisterium: Teaching Authority in the Catholic Church.* Dublin: Gill and Macmillan, 1983.

Sullivan, Scott M. "A History of Extraordinary Means." *Ethics & Medics* 31.11 (November 2006): 3–4.

Thomson, John C. ed. *The New York Code of Civil Procedure*, 37th ed. Albany, NY: Matthew Bender, 1912.

Vatican Council II. *Gaudium et spes*. December 7, 1965.

Veatch, Robert M. *Medical Ethics*. Boston: Jones and Bartlett Publishers, 1989.

Viafora, Corrado. "I principi della bioetica." In *Bioetica e Cultura*, edited by Salvatore Privitera, 9–37. Palermo, Italy: Instituto Siciliano di Bioetica 2, 1993.

World Medical Association, *Declaration of Helsinki: Ethical Principles for Medical Research Involving Human Subjects*. Helsinki, Finland: WMA, June 1964.

Wuerl, Donald. "The Bishop, Conscience, and Moral Teaching." In *Catholic Conscience: Foundation and Formation*, edited by Russell E. Smith, 123–140. Braintree, MA: Pope John Center, 1991.

PART TWO Ethics Committees

American Society for Bioethics and Humanities. *Core Competencies for Health Care Ethics Consultation*. Glenview, IL: ASBH, 1998.

Armstrong, P. W. "Legal and Judicial Issues of Ethics Committees." In *Ethics Committees: A Challenge for Catholic Health Care*, 44–54. St. Louis, MO: Pope John Center and Catholic Health Association of the United States, 1984.

Bernt, Francis, Peter Clark, Josita Starrs, and Patricia Talone, R.S.M. "Ethics Committees in Catholic Hospitals." *Health Progress* 87.2 (March–April 2006): 18–25.

Blake, David C. "Reinventing the Healthcare Ethics Committee." *HEC Forum* 12.1 (January 2000): 8–32.

Bosk, Charles L., and Joel Frader. "Institutional Ethics Committees: Sociological Oxymoron, Empirical Black Box." In *Bioethics and Society: Constructing the Ethical Enterprise*, edited by Raymond DeVries and Janardan Subedi, 94–116. Upper Saddle River, NJ: Prentice Hall, 1998.

Callahan, Sidney. "A Feminist Case Against Euthanasia." *Health Progress* 77.6 (November–December 1996): 21–29.

Catholic Hospital Association. *Ethical and Religious Directives for Catholic Hospitals*. St. Louis: Catholic Hospital Association, 1949.

Dubler, Nancy Neveloff, and Leonard J. Marcus. *Mediating Bioethical Disputes: A Practical Guide*. New York: United Hospital Fund of New York, 1994.

Ehleben, Carole M., Brian H. Childs, and Steven L. Saltzman. "HEC Self Assessment: What Is It Exactly that You Do? A Snapshot of an Ethicist at Work." *HEC Forum* 10.1 (March 1998): 71–74.

Fletcher, John C., and Diane E. Hoffmann. "Ethics Committees: Time to Experiment with Standards." *Annals of Internal Medicine* 120.4 (February 15, 1994): 335–338.

Foglia, Mary Beth, and Robert A. Pearlman. "Integrating Clinical and Organizational Ethics: A Systems Perspective Can Provide an Antidote to the 'Silo' Problem in Clinical Ethics Consultations." *Health Progress* 87.2 (March–April 2006): 31–35.

Fox, Ellen, Mary Beth Foglia, and Robert A. Pearlman, of the National Center for Ethics in Health Care (VHA), Washington, D.C. "Preventive Ethics: A Quality Improvement Approach to Health Care Ethics." Presentation at the 9th Annual Meeting of the American Society of Bioethics and Humanities (ASBH). October 18, 2007.

Friedman, Marilyn. "Beyond Caring: The De-Moralization of Gender." In *An Ethic of Care: Feminist and Interdisciplinary Perspective*, edited by Mary Jeanne Larrabee, 258–273. New York: Routledge, 1993.

Gilligan, Carol. *In A Different Voice: Psychological Theory and Women's Development*. Cambridge, MA: Harvard University Press, 1982.

Griener, Glenn G., and Janet L. Storch. "The Educational Needs of Ethics Committees." *Cambridge Quarterly of Healthcare Ethics* 3.3 (Summer 1994): 467–477.

Griener, Glenn G., and Janet L. Storch. "Hospital Ethics Committees: Problems in Evaluation." *HEC Forum* 4.1 (1992): 5–18.

Groopman, Jerome. *How Doctors Think*. New York: Houghton Mifflin, 2007.

Grubbs, Peggy A., and Barbara A. Blasband. *The Long-Term Care Nursing Assistant*, 2nd ed. Upper Saddle River, NJ: Prentice Hall Health, 2000.

Haddad, Amy, and George Annas. "Do Ethics Committees Work? Yes and No." *Hospitals and Health Networks* 68.9 (May 5, 1994): 6.

Hamel, Ron. "Ethics Committees: Pursuing Enhanced Effectiveness." *Health Progress* 87.2 (March–April 2006): 17.

Hayes, Gregory J. "Ethics Committees: Group Process Concerns and the Need for Research." *Cambridge Quarterly of Healthcare Ethics* 4.1 (Winter 1995): 83–91.

Ignatavicius, Donna D. *Introduction to Long Term Care Nursing: Principles and Practice*. Philadelphia: F. A. Davis Co., 1998.

Larrabee, Mary Jeanne, ed. *An Ethic of Care: Feminist and Interdisciplinary Perspectives*. New York: Routledge, 1993.

Lewthwaite, Barbara, and Sharon Erickson-Nesmith. "Needs Assessment for Healthcare Ethics Education." *HEC Forum* 10.1 (March 1998): 86–101.

Lowes, Robert. "Hospital Ethics Committees." *Medical World News* 35.1 (January 15, 1994): 24–25, 29–32, 37.

Lusky, Richard. "Educating Healthcare Ethics Committees (EHEC 1992–1996): The Evaluation Results." *HEC Forum* 8 (October 1996): 247–289.

Magill, Gerard, et al. *ASBH Task Force Report on Ethics Consultation Liability*. Glenview, IL: American Society for Bioethics and Humanities, 2004.

Merritt, Andrew L. "The Tort Liability of Hospital Ethics Committees." *Southern California Law Review* 60.5 (July 1987): 1239–1297.

Murphy, Kevin. "A 'Next Generation' Ethics Committee." *Health Progress* 87.2 (March–April 2006): 26–30.

Neff-Smith, M., S. Giles, E. M. Spencer, and J. C. Fletcher. "Ethics Program Evaluation: The Virginia Hospital Ethics Fellows Example." *HEC Forum* 9.4 (December 1997): 375–388.

O'Brien, Daniel, ed. *Ethics in Health Care: Ingredients for Effective Committees*. Ann Arbor, MI: Sisters of St. Joseph Health System, 1995.

O'Rourke, Kevin D., O.P., and D. Brodeur. *Medical Ethics: Common Ground for Understanding*. St. Louis: Catholic Health Association, 1987.

O'Rourke, Kevin D., O.P., T. Kopfensteiner, and R. Hamel. "A Brief History: A Summary of the Development of the Ethical and Religious Directives for Catholic Health Care Services." *Health Progress* 82.6 (November–December 2001): 18–21.

Povar, Gail J. "Evaluating Ethics Committees: What Do We Mean by Success?" *Maryland Law Review* 50.3 (1991): 904–919.

Ross, Judith Wilson. *Handbook for Hospital Ethics Committees*. Chicago: American Hospital Association, 1986.

Ross, Judith Wilson, John. W. Glaser, Dorothy Rasinski-Gregory, Joan McIver Gibson, Corrine Bayley and Giles R. Scofield. *Health Care Ethics Committees: The Next Generation*. Chicago: American Hospital Publishing, 1993.

Rueping, Janis, and Dan O. Dugan. "A Next Generation Ethics Program in Progress: Lessons from Experience." *HEC Forum,* 12.1 (January 2000): 49–56.

Scheirton, Linda S. "Determinants of Hospital Ethics Committee Success." *HEC Forum* 4.6 (1992): 342–359.

Scheirton, Linda S. "Measuring Hospital Ethics Committee Success." *Cambridge Quarterly of Healthcare Ethics* 2.4 (Fall 1993): 495–504.

Schick, Ida Critelli, and Sally Moore. "Ethics Committees Identify Four Key Factors for Success." *HEC Forum* 10.1 (March 1998): 75–85.

Silverman, Henry J. "Revitalizing a Hospital Ethics Committee." *HEC Forum* 6 (July 1994): 189–222.

Sontag, David N. "Are Clinical Ethics Consultants in Danger? An Analysis of the Potential Legal Liability of Individual Clinical Ethicists." *University of Pennsylvania Law Review* 151 (2002) 667.

Spicker, Stuart F. *The Healthcare Ethics Committee Experience: Selected Readings from HEC Forum.* Malabar, FL: Krieger, 1998.

Spielman, Bethany. "Has Faith in Health Care Ethics Consultants Gone Too Far? Risks of an Unregulated Practice and a Model Act to Contain Them." *Marquette Law Review* 85 (2001) 161.

Thomasma, David C. "Education of Ethics Committees." *Bioethics Forum* 10.4 (Fall 1994): 12–18.

Tronto, Joan C. "Beyond Gender Difference to a Theory of Care." In *An Ethic of Care: Feminist and Interdisciplinary Perspectives*, edited by Mary Jeanne Larrabee, 240–257. New York: Routledge, 1993.

Tropman, John E. *The Catholic Ethic in American Society: An Exploration of Values.* San Francisco: Jossey-Bass, 1995.

Tuohey, John. "Ethics Consultation in Portland." *Health Progress* 87.2 (March–April 2006): 36–41.

PART THREE Beginning-of-Life Issues

Alikani, M. "Micromanipulation of Human Gametes for Assisted Fertilization." *Current Opinion in Obstetrics and Gynecology* 5.5 (October 1993): 594–599.

Allegra A., A. Marino, F. Coffaro, P. Scaglione, F. Sammartano, G. Rizza, and A. Volpes. "GnRH Antagonist-Induced Inhibition of the Premature LH Surge Increases Pregnancy Rates in IUI-stimulated Cycles: A Prospective Randomized Trial." *Human Reproduction* 22.1 (January 2007): 101–108.

American Society for Reproductive Medicine. *Guidelines on Number of Embryos Transferred.* Birmingham, AL: ASRM, November 1999.

Andersen, A. N., V. Goossens, L. Gianaroli, R. Felberbaum, J. de Mouzon, and K. G. Nygren. "Assisted Reproductive Technology in Europe, 2003." *Human Reproduction* 22.6 (June 2007): 1513–1525.

Aquinas, Thomas. *Commentary on Aristotle's* Nicomachean Ethics, translated by C.I. Litzinger, O.P. Notre Dame, IN: Dumb Ox Books, 1993.

Aquinas, Thomas. *Summa contra gentiles*, translated by V. J. Bourke. Notre Dame, IN: University of Notre Dame Press, 1975.

Aristotle. *Nicomachean Ethics*, translated by W.D. Ross. In *The Basic Works of Aristotle*, edited by Richard McKeon, 935–1126. New York: Random House, 1941.

Arowojolu, A. O., I. A. Okewole, and A. O. Adekunle, "Comparative Evaluation of the Effectiveness and Safety of Two Regimens of Levonorgestrel for Emergency Contraception in Nigerians." *Contraception* 66.4 (October 2002): 269–273.

Ashley, Benedict M., O.P. and Albert S. Moraczewski, O.P. "Is the Biological Subject of Human Rights Present from Conception?" In *The Fetal Tissue Issue: Medical and Ethical Aspects*, edited by Peter J. Cataldo and Albert S. Moraczewski, O.P., 33–59. Braintree, MA: Pope John Center, 1994.

Ashley, Benedict M., O.P., and Kevin D. O'Rourke, O.P. *Health Care Ethics: A Theological Analysis*, 4th ed. Washington, D.C.: Georgetown University Press, 1997.

Austriaco, Nicanor Pier Giorgio, O.P. "Is Plan B an Abortifacient? A Critical Look at the Scientific Evidence." *National Catholic Bioethics Quarterly* 7.4 (Winter 2007): 703–707.

Barbieri, Robert L. "Gonadotropin Releasing Hormone Analogues for Contraception." In *Fertility Control*, 2nd ed., edited by Stephen L. Corson, Richard J. Derman, and Louise B. Tyrer, 247–253. Pearl River, NY: Parthenon, 1994.

Bayer, Edward J. "Isolating the Threatening Womb." *Ethics & Medics* 10.2 (February 1985): 3–4.

———. *Rape Within Marriage: A Moral Analysis Delayed*. Lanham, MD: University Press of America, 1985.

Beers, Mark H., ed. *The Merck Manual of Diagnosis and Therapy*, 18th ed. Whitehouse Station, NJ: Merck, 2006.

Benedict XVI, Pope. "Interview in Preparation for the Upcoming Journey to Bavaria." August 5, 2006. Vatican edition.

Berg, Thomas V., L.C., and Edward J. Furton. *Human Embryo Adoption: Biotechnology, Marriage, and the Right to Life*. Philadelphia, PA/Thornwood, NY: National Catholic Bioethics Center and Westchester Institute for Ethics & the Human Person, 2006.

Boyle, Joseph M., Jr. "Double Effect and a Certain Kind of Craniotomy." *Irish Theological Quarterly* 44 (1977): 303–318.

Brito, K.S., L. Bahamondes, J.A. Nascimento, L. de Santis, and M.J. Munuce. "The In Vitro Effect of Emergency Contraception Doses of Levonorgestrel on the Acrosome Reaction of Human Sperm." *Contraception* 72.3 (September 2005): 225–228.

Cannon, L., and H. Jesionowska. "Methotrexate Treatment of Tubal Pregnancy." *Fertility and Sterility* 55.6 (June 1991): 1033–1038.

Carlin, R., D. Davis, M. Weiss, B. Schultz, and D. Troyer. "Expression of Early Transcription Factors Oct-4, Sox-2 and Nanog by Porcine Umbilical Cord Matrix Cells." *Reproductive Biology and Endocrinology* 4.1 (February 6, 2006): 8.

Cataldo, Peter J. "GIFT as Assistance." *Ethics & Medics* 22.12 (December 1997): 3–4.

Cataldo, Peter J. "The Newest Reproductive Technologies: Applying Catholic Teaching." In *The Gospel of Life and the Vision of Health Care*, edited by Russell E. Smith, 61–94. Braintree, MA: Pope John Center, 1996.

Cataldo, Peter J. "Reproductive Technologies." *Ethics & Medics* 21.1 (January 1996): 1–3.

Cessario, Romanus, O.P. "Toward an Adequate Method for Catholic Bioethics," *National Catholic Bioethics Quarterly* 1.1 (Spring 2001): 51–62.

Cohlen, B.J., E.R. te Velde, R.J. van Kooij, C.W. Looman, and J.D. Habbema. "Controlled Ovarian Hyperstimulation and Intrauterine Insemination for Treating Male Subfertility: A Controlled Study." *Human Reproduction* 13.6 (June 1998): 1553–1558.

Congregation for the Doctrine of the Faith. *Declaration on Certain Questions Concerning Sexual Ethics* (Persona humana). December 29, 1975. Vatican edition.

Congregation for the Doctrine of the Faith. *Declaration on Procured Abortion*. November 18, 1974. Vatican edition.

Connecticut Bishops. "Statement on Plan B and Catholic Hospitals." September 27, 2007. Connecticut Catholic Conference, http://www.ctcatholic.org/Bishops-Statement-Plan-B.php.

Connell, Francis J., C.Ss.R. "Is Contraception Intrinsically Wrong?" *American Ecclesiastical Review* 150.6 (June 1964): 434–439.

Connell, Francis J., C.Ss.R. "The Sterilization of a Retarded Girl." *American Ecclesiastical Review* 152 (January–June 1966): 280–281.

Connery, John R., S.J. "Tubal Ligation: Good Medicine? Good Morality?" In *Readings in Moral Theology.* Vol. 8, *Dialogue about Catholic Sexual Teaching,* edited by Charles E. Curran and Richard McCormick, S.J., 217–219. New York: Paulist Press, 1993.

Cumming, D.C. "Pregnancy Rates following Intrauterine Insemination with Washed or Unwashed Sperm." *Fertility and Sterility* 49.4 (April 1988): 735–736.

Crockett S. A., J. DeCook, D. Harrison, C. Hersh. "Using Hormone Contraceptives Is a Decision Involving Science, Scripture, and Conscience." In *The Reproduction Revolution: A Christian Appraisal of Sexuality, Reproductive Technologies, and the Family,* edited by John F. Kilner, Paige C. Cunningham, and W. David Hager, 192–201. Grand Rapids, MI: Wm. B. Eerdmans, 2000.

Croxatto, H.B., V. Brache, M. Pavez, L. Cochon, M.L. Forcelledo, F. Alvarez, R. Massai, A. Faundes, A.M. Salvatierra. "Pituitary-Ovarian Function following the Standard Levonorgestrel Emergency Contraceptive Dose or a Single 0.75 mg Dose Given on the Days Preceding Ovulation." *Contraception* 70.6 (December 2004): 442–450.

DeMarco, Donald. *Biotechnology and the Assault on Parenthood.* San Francisco: Ignatius Press, 1991.

DeMarco, Donald. "GIFT as Replacement." *Ethics & Medics* 22.11 (November 1997): 3–4.

DeMarco, Donald. *In My Mother's Womb.* Manassas, VA: Trinity Communications, 1987.

Diamond, Eugene F. "Ovral in Rape Protocols." *Ethics & Medics* 21.10 (October 1996): 1–2.

Diamond, Eugene F. "Rape Protocol." *Linacre Quarterly* 60.3 (August 1993): 8–19.

Diamond, Eugene F. "Sterilization in Catholic Hospitals." *Linacre Quarterly* 55.1 (February 1988): 57–66.

Do Nascimento, J.A., M. Seppala, A. Perdigão, X. Espejo-Arce, M.J. Munuce, L. Hautala, R. Koistinen, L. Andrade, L. Bahamondes."In Vivo Assessment of the Human Sperm Acrosome Reaction and the Expression of Glycodelin-A in Human Endometrium after Levonorgestrel-Emergency Contraceptive Pill Administration." *Human Reproduction* 22.8 (August 2007): 2190–2195.

Doerfler, John F. "Technology and Human Reproduction." *Ethics & Medics* 24.8 (August 1999): 3–4.

Durand, M., M. Seppala, C. Cravioto Mdel, H. Koistinen, R. Koistinen, J. González-Macedo, F. Larrea. "Late Follicular Phase Administration of Levonorgestrel as an Emergency Contraceptive Changes the Secretory Pattern of Glycodelin in Serum and Endometrium during the Luteal Phase of the Menstrual Cycle." *Contraception* 71.6 (June 2005): 451–457.

Durand, M., M. del Carmen Cravioto, E. G. Raymond, O. Durán-Sánchez, M. De la Luz Cruz-Hinojosa, A. Castell-Rodríguez, R. Schiavon, F. Larrea. "On the Mechanisms of Action of Short-Term Levonorgestrel Administration in Emergency Contraception." *Contraception* 64.4 (October 2001): 227–234.

Ecochard, R., H. Boehringer, M. Rabilloud, H. Marret. "Chronological Aspects of Ultrasonic, Hormonal, and Other Indirect Indices of Ovulation." *BJOG* 108.8 (August 2001): 822–829.

Enserink, M. "Selling the Stem Cell Dream." *Science* 313.5784 (July 14, 2006): 160–163.

European Society of Human Reproduction and Embryology. The European IVF Monitoring Programme (EIM) for ESHRE. "Assisted Reproductive Technology and Intrauterine Inseminations in Europe, 2005: Results Generated from Eruopean Registers by ESHRE." *Human Reproduction* 24.6 (June 2009): 1267–1287.

Fackler, Martin. "Risk Taking Is in His Genes." *New York Times*, December 11, 2007.

Farmer, R. M., T. Kirschbaum, D. Potter, T. H. Strong, and A. L. Medearis. "Uterine Rupture during Trial of Labor after Previous Cesarean Section." *American Journal of Obstetrics and Gynecology* 165.4 (October 1991): 996–1001.

Flannery, Kevin L., S.J. "The Field of Moral Action According to Thomas Aquinas." *The Thomist* 69.1 (January 2005): 1–30.

Flannery, Kevin L., S.J. "What Is Included in a Means to an End?" *Gregorianum* 74.3 (1993): 499–513.

Fraser, Ian S. "Response to Letter to the Editor." *Contraception* 77.6 (June 2007): 464–465.

Freud, Sigmund. *A General Introduction to Psycho-Analysis,* translated by Joan Riviere. New York: Liverwright, 1935.

Gemzell-Danielsson, K., and L. Marions. "Mechanisms of Action of Mifepristone and Levonorgestrel When Used for Emergency Contraception." *Human Reproduction Update* 10.4 (July–August 2004): 341–348.

Gerrard, Thomas. "The Church and Eugenics." *The Catholic Encyclopedia.* Vol. 16. New York: Encyclopedia Press, 1914.

Goldzieher, Joseph W. *Hormonal Contraception: Pills, Injections & Implants.* Dallas: Essential Medical Information Systems, 1989.

Goodwin, T. M. "'Medicalizing' Moral Decisions in Reproductive Medicine." In *Faith and Challenges to the Family,* edited by Russell E. Smith, 79–99. Braintree, MA: Pope John Center, 1994.

Grisez, Germain. *Abortion: The Myths, the Realities, and the Arguments.* Cleveland, OH: Corpus Books, 1970.

Grisez, Germain. *The Way of the Lord Jesus.* Vol. 1, *Christian Moral Principles.* Chicago: Franciscan Herald Press, 1983.

Grisez, Germain. *The Way of the Lord Jesus.* Vol. 2, *Living a Christian Life.* Quincy, IL: Franciscan Press, 1993.

Grisez, Germain. "When Do People Begin?" *Proceedings of the American Catholic Philosophical Association* 63 (1989): 27–47.

Guan, K., K. Nayernia, L. S. Maier, S. Wagner, R. Dressel, J. H. Lee, J. Nolte, F. Wolf, M. Li, W. Engel, and G. Hasenfuss. "Pluripotency of Spermatogonial Stem Cells from Adult Mouse Testis." *Nature* 440.7088 (April 27, 2006): 1199–1203.

Guevin, Benedict, O.S.B. "A Theological Caution on NFP." *Ethics & Medics* 25.9 (September 2000): 2–4.

Haas, John. "GIFT? No!" *Ethics & Medics* 18.9 (September 1993): 2–3.

Hall, J. E., N. Bhatta, J. M. Adams, J. E. Rivier, W. W. Vale, W. F. Crowley Jr. "Variable Tolerance of the Developing Follicle and Corpus Luteum to Gonadotropin-Releasing Hormone Antagonist-Induced Gonadotropin Withdrawal in the Human." *Journal of Clinical Endocrinology and Metabolism* 72.5 (1991): 993–1000.

Hamoda, H., P. W. Ashok, C. Stalder, G. M. Flett, E. Kennedy, A. Templeton. "A Randomized Trial of Mifepristone (10 mg) and Levonorgestrel for Emergency Contraception." *Obstetrics & Gynecology* 104.6 (December 2004): 1307–1313.

Hapangama, D., A. F. Glasier, and D. T. Baird, "The Effects of Peri-Ovulatory Administration of Levonorgestrel on the Menstrual Cycle." *Contraception* 63.3 (March 2001): 123–129.

Highfield, Roger. "Dolly Creator Prof. Ian Wilmut Shuns Cloning." *London Telegraph.* November 16, 2007.

Hilgers, Thomas W. "Answers for Infertility." *Celebrate Life* (May–June 1995): 34.

Hilliard, Marie T. "Plan B's Abortifacient Effect." *National Catholic Bioethics Quarterly* 8.1 (Spring 2008): 9–13.

Ho, P. C., and M. S. Kwan. "A Prospective Randomized Comparison of Levonorgestrel with the Yuzpe Regimen in Post-Coital Contraception." *Human Reproduction* 8.3 (March 1993): 389–392.

Hoffman, D. I., G. L. Zellman, C. C. Fair, J. F. Mayer, J. G. Zeitz, W. E. Gibbons, and T. G. Turner Jr., for the Society for Assisted Reproduction (SART) and RAND. "Cryopreserved Embryos in the United States and Their Availability for Research." *Fertility and Sterility* 79.5 (May 2003): 1063–1069.

Holy See. *Charter of the Rights of the Family.* October 22, 1983. Vatican edition.

Holy See. Intervention at the Sixth Committee of the 58th General Assembly of the United Nations on the International Convention against the Cloning of Human Beings. Address of H.E. Msgr. Celestino Migliore. October 21, 2003. Vatican edition.

Holy See. Intervention at the Special Committee of the 57th General Assembly of the United Nations on Human Embryonic Cloning. September 23, 2002. Vatican edition.

Holy See. "The Views of the Holy See on Human Cloning." Statement of the Permanent Observer Mission of the Holy See to the United Nations. July 17, 2003. New York: Permanent Observer Mission of the Holy See to the United Nations, 2003.

Holy See. Message to Those Attending an International Congress Sponsored by the Pontifical Council for the Family, the Bioethics Institute of the Catholic University of the Sacred Heart, and the Pontifical Athenaeum Regina Apostolorum, for the Anniversary of the Encyclical *Evangelium vitae.* April 23, 1996.

Hwang, W. S., Y. J. Ryu, J. H. Park, E. S. Park, E. G. Lee, J. M. Koo, H. Y. Jeon, et al. "Evidence of a Pluripotent Human Embryonic Stem Cell Line Derived from a Cloned Blastocyst." *Science* 303.5664 (March 12, 2004): 1669–1674. Retracted in *Science.* 311.5759 (January 20, 2006): 335.

John Paul II, Pope. Message for the Celebration of the World Day of Peace. January 1, 2001. Vatican edition.

Kanatsu-Shinohara M., and T. Shinohara. "The Germ of Pluripotency." *Nature Biotechnology* 24.6 (June 2006): 663–664.

Kolata, Gina. "Man Who Helped Start Stem Cell War May End It." *New York Times.* November 22, 2007.

Lalitkumar, P. G. L., S. Lalitkumar, C. X. Meng, A. Stavreus-Evers, F. Hambiliki, U. Bentin-Ley, and Kristina Gemzell-Danielsson. "Mifepristone, But Not Levonorgestrel, Inhibits Human Blastocyst Attachment to an In Vitro Endometrial Three-Dimensional Cell Culture Model." *Human Reproduction* 22.11 (November 2007): 3031–3037.

Larimore, Walter L., and Randy Alcorn. "Using the Birth Control Pill Is Ethically Unacceptable." In *The Reproduction Revolution: A Christian Appraisal of Sexuality, Reproductive Technologies, and the Family*, edited by John F. Kilner, Paige C. Cunningham, and W. David Hager, 179–191. Grand Rapids, MI: Wm. B. Eerdmans, 2000.

Larimore, Walter L., and Joseph B. Stanford. "Postfertilization Effects of Oral Contraceptives and Their Relationship to Informed Consent." *Archives of Family Medicine* 9.2 (February 2000): 126–133.

Lee, Patrick. *Abortion and Unborn Human Life.* Washington, D.C.: Catholic University of America Press, 1996.

Leung, A. S., E. K. Leung, and R. H. Paul. "Uterine Rupture after Previous Cesarean Delivery: Maternal and Fetal Consequences." *American Journal of Obstetrics and Gynecology* 169.4 (October 1993): 945–950.

Ling, T., M. Kuo, C. Li, A. Yu, Y. Huang, T. Wu, Y. Lin, S. Chen, and J. Yu. "Identification of Pulmonary Oct-4+ Stem/Progenitor Cells and Demonstration of their Susceptibility to SARS Coronavirus (SARS-CoV) Infection In Vitro." *Proceedings of the National Academy of Sciences of the United States of America* 103.25 (June 20, 2006): 9530–9535.

Ling, W. Y., A. Robichaud, I. Zayid, W. Wrixon, S. C. MacLeod. "Mode of Action of dl-Norgestrel and Ethinylestradiol Combination in Postcoital Contraception." *Fertility and Sterility* 32.3 (September 1979): 297–302.

Lyons, Mary Louise. "The Management of Ectopic Pregnancies: A Moral Analysis." In *The Fetal Tissue Issue*, edited by Peter J. Cataldo and Albert S. Moraczewski, O.P., 121–148. Braintree, MA: Pope John Center, 1994.

Marions, L., S. Z. Cekan, M. Bygdeman, and K. Gemzell-Danielsson. "Effect of Emergency Contraception with Levonorgestrel or Mifepristone on Ovarian Function." *Contraception* 69.5 (May 2004): 373–377.

Marions L., K. Hultenby, I. Lindell, X. Sun, B. Ståbi, and K. Gemzell-Danielsson. "Emergency Contraception with Mifepristone and Levonorgestrel: Mechanism of Action." *Obstetrics & Gynecology* 100.1 (July 2002): 65–71.

Martinez, A. R., R. E. Bernardus, J. P. Vermeiden, and J. Schoemaker. "Basic Questions on Intrauterine Insemination." *Obstetrical and Gynecological Survey* 48.12 (December 1993): 811–828.

May, William E. "Catholic Teaching on the Laboratory Generation of Human Life." In *The Gift of Life*, edited by Thomas Hilgers and Marilyn Wallace, 77–92. Omaha, NB: Pope Paul VI Institute Press, 1990.

McCarthy, Donald G. "Catholic Moral Teaching and TOT/GIFT: Response." In *Reproductive Technologies, Marriage and the Church*, edited by Donald G. McCarthy, 140–145. Braintree, MA: Pope John Center, 1988.

McCarthy, Donald G. "GIFT? Yes!" *Ethics & Medics* 18.9 (September 1993): 3–4.

McCarthy, Donald G., ed. "Pastoral Concerns: Procreation and the Marital Act." In *Reproductive Technologies, Marriage and the Church*, 164–174. Braintree, MA: Pope John Center, 1988.

McCarthy, Donald G., and Albert S. Moraczewski, O.P., eds. *An Ethical Evaluation of Fetal Experimentation: An Interdisciplinary Study*. St. Louis: Pope John Center, 1976.

McCullough, Marie. "Stem Cells Without the Fuss? Possibly." *Detroit Free Press*. November 21, 2007.

McHugh, John A., O.P., and Charles J. Callan, O.P. *Moral Theology: A Complete Course*. Vol. 1, revised and enlarged by Edward P. Farrell, O.P. New York: Joseph F. Wagner, 1958.

McReavy, L. L. "The Dutch Hierarchy on Marriage Problems." *Clergy Review* 49 (February 1964): 113–115.

Meng, C. X., K. L. Andersson, U. Bentin-Ley, K. Gemzell-Danielsson, and P. G. Lalitkumar. "Effect of Levonorgestrel and Mifepristone on Endometrial Receptivity Markers in a Three-Dimensional Human Endometrial Cell Culture Model." *Fertility and Sterility* 91.1 (January 2009): 256–264.

Miech, Ralph. "A Proposed Novel Treatment for Rape Victims." *National Catholic Bioethics Quarterly* 5.4 (Winter 2005): 687–695.

Miech, Ralph. "Pathopharmacology of Excessive Hemorrhage in Mifepristone Abortions." *Annals of Pharmacotherapy* 41.12 (December 2007): 2002–2007.

Miech, Ralph. "Pathophysiology of Mifepristone-Induced Septic Shock due to *Clostridium sordellii*." *Annals of Pharmacotherapy* 39.9 (September 2005): 1483–1488.

Mikolajczyk, R. T., and J. B. Stanford. "Levonorgestrel Emergency Contraception: A Joint Analysis of Effectiveness and Mechanisms of Action." *Fertility and Sterility* 88.3 (September 2007): 565–571.

Mirkes, Renée, O.S.M. "Fictions, Fallacies, and Pro-Choice Rhetoric." *Ethics & Medics* 14.10 (October 1989): 1–2.

Mirkes, Renée, O.S.M. "PAS and the Second Victim of Abortion," Part 1. *Ethics & Medics* 14.11 (November 1989): 3–4.

Mirkes, Renée, O.S.M. "PAS and the Second Victim of Abortion," Part 2. *Ethics & Medics* 14.12 (December 1989): 3–4.

Moraczewski, Albert S., O.P. "Managing Tubal Pregnancies," Part 1. *Ethics & Medics* 21.6 (June 1996): 3–4.

Moraczewski, Albert S., O.P. "Managing Tubal Pregnancies," Part 2. *Ethics & Medics* 21.8 (August 1996): 3–4.

Müller A. L., C. M. Llados, and H. B. Croxatto. "Postcoital Treatment with Levonorgestrel Does Not Disrupt Post-Fertilization Events in the Rat." *Contraception* 67.5 (May 2003): 415–419.

Mulligan, James J. *Choose Life*. Braintree, MA: Pope John Center, 1991.

Mulligan, James J. *Commentary on the Reply of the Sacred Congregation for the Doctrine of the Faith to NCCB on Sterilization in Catholic Hospitals.* September 15, 1977. Washington D.C.: United States Catholic Conference, 1983.

Mulligan, James J. Statement on Tubal Ligation. Washington, D.C.: United States Catholic Conference, July 3, 1980.

National Research Council. *Scientific and Medical Aspects of Human Reproductive Cloning.* Washington, D.C.: National Academies Press, 2002.

Nickerson, Colin. "Breakthrough on Stem Cells: Reprogramming of Human Skin May Circumvent Ethics Controversy." *Boston Globe*, November 21, 2007.

Noonan, John T., Jr. *Contraception: A History of Its Treatment by the Catholic Theologians and Canonists.* New York: New American Library, 1965.

Novikova, N., E. Weisberg, F. Z. Stanczyk, H. B. Croxatto, and I. S. Fraser. "Effectiveness of Levonorgestrel Emergency Contraception Given Before or After Ovulation: A Pilot Study." *Contraception* 75.2 (February 2007): 112–118.

Ortiz, M. E., R. E. Ortiz, M. A. Fuentes, V. H. Parraguez, and H. B. Croxatto. "Postcoital Administration of Levonorgestrel Does Not Interfere with Post-Fertilization Events in the New-World Monkey *Cebus paella.*" *Human Reproduction* 19.6 (June 2004): 1352–1356.

Paddock, Catherine. "Reprogrammed Skin Cells Could Replace Embryonic Stem Cells." *Medical News Today*, November 26, 2007.

Pastor, John. "Healing Potential Discovered in Everyday Human Brain Cells." *Health Science Center News* (University of Florida), August 16, 2006.

Paul VI, Pope. *Humanae vitae.* July 25, 1968. In *Humanae Vitae: A Generation Later* by Janet E. Smith, 272–295. Washington, D.C.: Catholic University of America Press, 1991.

Pearlstone, Anthony C., and Eric S. Surrey. "The Temporal Relation Between the Urine LH Surge and Sonographic Evidence of Ovulation: Determinants and Clinical Significance." *Obstetrics & Gynecology* 83.2 (February 1994): 184–188.

Piccione, Joseph J. "A New Approach to Sexual Assault Treatment: Moral Considerations." In *Walk as Children of Light: The Challenge of Cooperation in a Pluralistic Society*, edited by Edward J. Furton, 187–203. Boston: National Catholic Bioethics Center, 2003.

Piccione, Joseph J. "Rape and the Peoria Protocol." *Ethics & Medics* 22.9 (September 1997): 1–2.

Pius XII, Pope. "Address to the Second World Congress on Fertility and Sterility." May 19, 1956. *AAS* 48 (1956): 471–473.

Piccione, Joseph J. "Christian Principles and the Medical Profession." Allocution to the Italian Medical-Biological Union of St. Luke, November 12, 1944. In *The Human Body*, edited by the Monks of Solesmes, 51–65. Boston: Saint Paul Editions, 1960.

Pontifical Academy for Life. "Moral Reflections on Vaccines Prepared from Cells Derived from Aborted Human Fetuses." June 5, 2005. Reprinted in *National Catholic Bioethics Quarterly* 6.3 (Autumn 2006): 541–549.

Pontifical Academy for Life. Reflections on Cloning. 1997. Vatican edition.

Pontifical Academy for Life. Statement on the So-Called Morning After Pill. October 31, 2000. Vatican edition.

Prentice, David. "Adult versus Embryonic Stem Cells." Testimony before the House Health and Government Operations Committee and House Appropriations Committee Maryland Legislature AGAINST House Bill 1183, "Maryland Stem Cell Research Act of 2005." March 2, 2005.

Pritts, E. A., and A. K. Atwood. "Luteal Phase Support in Infertility Treatment: A Meta-Analysis of the Randomized Trials." *Human Reproduction* 17.9 (September 2002): 2287–2299.

Rand Institute for Civil Justice and Rand Health. "How Many Frozen Embryos are Available for Research?" *Law & Health Research Brief* RB-9038 (2003).

Raymond, E., D. Taylor, J. Trussell, and M. J. Steiner. "Minimum Effectiveness of the Levonorgestrel Regimen of Emergency Contraception." *Contraception* 69.1 (January 2004): 79–81.

Rock, John A. "Ectopic Pregnancy." In *TeLinde's Operative Gynecology*, edited by John D. Thompson and John A. Rock, 422–423. Philadelphia: J. P. Lippincott Co., 1992.

Rohlfs, Steven P. "Pregnancy Prevention and Rape: Another View." *Ethics & Medics* 18.5 (May 1993): 1–2.

Seppälä, M., R. N. Taylor, H. Koistinen, R. Koistinen, and E. Milgrom. "Glycodelin: A Major Lipocalin Protein of the Reproductive Axis with Diverse Actions in Cell Recognition and Differentiation." *Endocrine Reviews* 23.4 (August 2002): 401–430.

Smith, William B. "Catholic Hospitals and Sterilization." *Linacre Quarterly* 44.2 (May 1977): 107–116.

Stanford, J. B., and R. T. Mikolajczyk. "Methodological Review of the Effectiveness of Emergency Contraception." *Current Women's Health Reviews* 1.2 (2005): 1–11.

Swahn, M. L., P. Westlund, E. Johannisson, and M. Bygdeman. "Effect of Post-Coital Contraceptive Methods on the Endometrium and the Menstrual Cycle." *Acta Obstetricia et Gynecologica Scandinavica* 75.8 (September 1996): 738–744.

Takahashi, K., K. Tanabe, M. Ohnuki, M. Narita, T. Ichisaka, K. Tomoda, and S. Yamanaka. "Induction of Pluripotent Stem Cells from Adult Human Fibroblasts by Defined Factors." *Cell* 131.5 (November 30, 2007): 861–872.

Task Force on Postovulatory Methods of Fertility Regulation. "Randomized Controlled Trial of Levonorgestrel versus the Yuzpe Regime of Combined Oral Contraceptives for Emergency Contraception." *Lancet* 352.9126 (August 8, 1998): 428–433.

te Velde, E. R., and B. J. Cohlen. "The Management of Infertility." *New England Journal of Medicine* 340.3 (January 21, 1999): 224–226.

Tirelli, A., A. Cagnacci, and A. Volpe. "Levonorgestrel Administration in Emergency Contraception: Bleeding Pattern and Pituitary-Ovarian Function." *Contraception* 77.5 (May 2008): 328–332.

Tonti-Filippini, Nicholas. "*Donum Vitae* and Gamete Intra-Fallopian Tube Transfer." *Linacre Quarterly* 57.2 (May 1990): 68–79.

Trussell, J., and E. G. Raymond. "Statistical Evidence about the Mechanism of Action of the Yuzpe Regimen of Emergency Contraception." *Obstetrics & Gynecology* 93.5 pt 2 (May 1999): 872–876.

Trussell, J., C. Ellertson, H. von Hertzen, A. Bigrigg, A. Webb, M. Evans, S. Ferden, and C. Leadbetter. "Estimating the Effectiveness of Emergency Contraceptive Pills." *Contraception* 67.4 (April 2003): 259–265.

United Nations General Assembly, Fifty-Ninth Session, Sixth Committee. "United Nations Declaration on Human Cloning" (A/RES/59/280). March 23, 2005.

United States Conference of Catholic Bishops. "Moral Principles Concerning Infants with Anencephaly." September 19, 1996. Washington, D.C.: USCCB, 1996.

U.S. Department of Health and Human Services. Centers for Disease Control and Prevention. *2004 Assisted Reproductive Technology Success Rates: National Summary and Fertility Clinic Reports*. Atlanta: U.S. Department of Health and Human Services, December 2006.

U.S. Food and Drug Administration. "FDA Approves Over-The-Counter Access for Plan B for Women 18 and Older, Prescription Remains Required for Women 17 and Under." *FDA News*, August 24, 2006.

Verpoest, W.M., D.J. Cahill, C.R. Harlow, and M.G. Hull. "Relationship between Midcycle Luteinizing Hormone Surge Quality and Oocyte Fertilization." *Fertility and Sterility* 73.1 (January 2000): 75–77.

von Hertzen H., G. Piaggio, J. Ding, J. Chen, S. Song, G. Bártfai, E. Ng, et al.; WHO Research Group on Post-ovulatory Methods of Fertility Regulation. "Low Dose Mifepristone and Two Regimens of Levonorgestrel for Emergency Contraception: A WHO Multicentre Randomised Trial." *Lancet* 360.9348 (December 7, 2002): 1803–1810.

Wade, Nicholas. "Some Scientists See Shift in Stem Cell Hopes." *New York Times*. August 14, 2006.

Welch, Lawrence J. "An Excessive Claim: Sterilization and Immediate Material Cooperation." *Linacre Quarterly* 66.4 (November 1999): 4–25.

Wilcox, A.J., D. Dunson, and D.D. Baird. "The Timing of the 'Fertile Window' in the Menstrual Cycle: Day Specific Estimates from a Prospective Study." *British Medical Journal* 321.7271 (November 18, 2000): 1259–1262.

Wilcox, A.J., C.R. Weinberg, and D.D. Baird. "Timing of Sexual Intercourse in Relation to Ovulation: Effects on the Probability of Conception, Survival of the Pregnancy, and Sex of the Baby." *New England Journal of Medicine* 333.23 (December 7, 1995): 1517–1521.

Yeung, Patrick, Jr., Erica Laethem, and Joseph Tham, L.C. "Is Plan B Abortifacient? Further Response" (letter). *National Catholic Bioethics Quarterly* 8.2 (Summer 2008): 217–221.

Yeung, Patrick, Jr., Erica Laethem, and Joseph Tham, L.C. "More on Plan B" (letter). *National Catholic Bioethics Quarterly* 8.3 (Autumn 2008): 418–424.

Yu, J., M.A. Vodyanik, K. Smuga-Otto, J. Antosiewicz-Bourget, J.L. Frane, S. Tian, J. Nie, et al. "Induced Pluripotent Stem Cell Lines Derived from Human Somatic Cells." *Science* 318.5858 (December 21, 2007): 1917–1920.

PART FOUR End-of-Life Issues

Aging with Dignity. "Five Wishes." Tallahassee, FL: Aging with Dignity, 2007.

Album, D., and S. Westin. "Do Diseases Have a Prestige Hierarchy? A Survey among Physicians and Medical Students." *Social Science and Medicine* 66.1 (January 2008): 182–188.

American Academy of Neurology. *Practice Parameters: Determining Brain Death in Adults*. St. Paul: American Academy of Neurology, 1994.

American Medical Association, Council on Ethical and Judicial Affairs. *Code of Medical Ethics: Current Opinions with Annotations, 2008–2009*. Chicago: American Medical Association Press, 2008.

Andrews, Keith, L. Murphy, R. Munday, and Clare Littlewood. "Misdiagnosis of the Vegetative State: Retrospective Study in a Rehabilitation Unit." *British Medical Journal* 313.7048 (July 6, 1996): 13–16.

Australian Catholic Bishops Conference. *Briefing Note on the Obligation to Provide Nutrition and Hydration*. September 3, 2004.

Battin, Margaret P. *The Least Worst Death: Essays in Bioethics on the End of Life*. New York: Oxford University Press, 1994.

Bauman, Z. *Mortality, Immortality, and Other Life Strategies*. Cambridge: Polity Press, 1992.

Beauchamp, Tom L., and James F. Childress. *Principles of Biomedical Ethics*, 4th ed. New York: Oxford University Press, 1994.

Becker, G. "Deadly Inequality in the Health Care 'Safety Net': Uninsured Ethnic Minorities Struggle to Live with Life-Threatening Illnesses." *Medical Anthropology Quarterly* 18.2 (June 2004): 258–275.

Berkman, John. "Medically Assisted Nutrition and Hydration in Medicine and Moral Theology: A Contextualization of Its Past and a Direction for Its Future." *The Thomist* 68.1 (January 2004): 69–104.

Boyle, Joseph M., Jr. "Artificial Provision of Nutrition and Hydration: Does the Benefit Outweigh the Burden? Affirmative Position." In *Critical Issues in Contemporary Health Care*, edited by Russell E. Smith, 111–128. Braintree, MA: Pope John Center, 1989.

Burke, Greg F. "Advanced Dementia." *Ethics & Medics* 26.3 (March 2001): 1–2.

Burroughs, T. E., B. A. Hong, D. F. Kappel, and B. K. Freedman. "The Stability of Family Decisions to Consent or Refuse Organ Donation: Would You Do It Again?" *Psychosomatic Medicine* 60.2 (March–April 1998): 156–162.

Byock, I. R. "End-of-Life Care: A Public Health Crisis and an Opportunity for Managed Care." *American Journal of Managed Care* 7.12 (December 2001): 1123–1132.

Byock, I. R. "Rediscovering Community at the Core of the Human Condition and Social Covenant." *Hastings Center Report* 33.2 suppl (March–April 2003): S40–S41.

Casarett, D. J., and J. H. Karlawish. "Are Special Ethical Guidelines Needed for Palliative Care Research? *Journal of Pain and Symptom Management* 20.2 (August 2000): 130–139.

Casarett, D. J., J. H. Karlawish, M. I. Henry, and K. B. Hirschman. "Must Patients with Advanced Cancer Choose between a Phase I Trial and Hospice?" *Cancer* 95.7 (October 1, 2002): 1061–1604.

Cataldo, Peter J. "Pope John Paul II on Nutrition and Hydration: Change of Catholic Teaching?" *National Catholic Bioethics Quarterly* 4.3 (Autumn 2004): 513–536.

Cessario, Romanus, O.P. "Catholic Considerations of Palliative Care." *National Catholic Bioethics Quarterly* 6.4 (Winter 2006): 639–650.

Chapple, H. S. "Dying to Be Rescued: American Hospitals, Clinicians, and Death." Ph.D. diss. Charlottesville, VA: University of Virginia, 2007.

Congregation for the Doctrine of the Faith. *Declaration on Euthanasia.* May 5, 1980.

Congregation for the Doctrine of the Faith. Responses to Certain Questions of the United States Conference of Catholic Bishops concerning Artificial Nutrition and Hydration. August 1, 2007. *Ethics & Medics* 32.11 (November 2007): 1–3.

Connor, S. R., B. Pyenson, K. Fitch, C. Spence, and K. Iwasaki. "Comparing Hospice and Nonhospice Patient Survival among Patients Who Die within a Three-Year Window." *Journal of Pain and Symptom Management* 33.3 (March 2007): 238–246.

Connor, S. R., M. Tecca, J. LundPerson, and J. Teno. "Measuring Hospice Care: The National Hospice and Palliative Care Organization National Hospice Data Set." *Journal of Pain and Symptom Management* 28.4 (October 2004): 316–328.

DeVita, M. A. "The Death Watch: Certifying Death Using Cardiac Criteria." *Progress in Transplantation* 11.1 (March 2001): 58–66.

Diamond, Eugene F. *A Catholic Guide to Medical Ethics: Catholic Principles in Clinical Practice.* Palos Park, IL: Linacre Institute, 2001.

Diamond, Eugene F. "Assisted Nutrition and Hydration in Persistent Vegetative State." Linacre Institute Paper. May 2004. Palos Park, IL: Linacre Institute, 2004.

Dobratz, M. C. "Issues and Dilemmas in Conducting Research with Vulnerable Home Hospice Participants." *Journal of Nursing Scholarship* 35.4 (2003): 371–376.

DuBois, James M. "Organ Transplantation: An Ethical Road Map." *National Catholic Bioethics Quarterly* 2.3 (Autumn 2002): 413–453.

DuBois, James M. and M. DeVita. "The Authors Reply [to Verheijde, Rady, and McGregor]." *Critical Care Medicine* 35.5 (May 2007): 1440.

DuBois, James M., F. L. Delmonico, and A. M. D'Alessandro. "When Organ Donors Are Still Patients: Is Premortem Use of Heparin Ethically Acceptable?" *American Journal of Critical Care* 16.4 (July 2007): 396–400.

Dworkin, Ronald, Thomas Nagel, Robert Nozick, John Rawls, Thomas Scanlon, and Judith Jarvis Thomson. "Brief as *amici curiae* in support of respondents." *Issues in Law and Medicine* 15.2 (Fall 1999): 183–198.

Emanuel, L. L. "Reexamining Death: The Asymptotic Model and a Bounded Zone Definition." *Hastings Center Report* 25.4 (July–August 1995): 27–35.

Farmer, Paul. *Pathologies of Power: Health, Human Rights and the New War on the Poor.* Berkeley: University of California Press, 2003.

Fine, P. G., and B. Jennings. "CPR in Hospice." *Hastings Center Report* 33.3 (May–June 2003): 9–10.

Furton. Edward J. "A Critique of the Five Wishes: Comments in the Light of a Papal Statement." *Ethics & Medics* 30.3 (March 2005): 3–4.

Gallagher, J. A., and J. Goodstein. "Fulfilling Institutional Responsibilities in Health Care: Organizational Ethics and the Role of Mission Discernment." *Business Ethics Quarterly* 12.4 (October 2002): 433–450.

Gawande, A. "Piecework: Medicine's Money Problem," *The New Yorker*, April 4, 2005.

Gillick, Muriel R. "Artificial Nutrition and Hydration in the Patient with Advanced Dementia: Is Withholding Treatment Compatible with Traditional Judaism?" *Journal of Medical Ethics* 27.1 (February 2001): 12–15.

Glaser, B. G., and A. L. Strauss. *Awareness of Dying.* Chicago: Aldine Publishing Co., 1965.

Glaser, John W. *Three Realms of Ethics: Individual, Institutional, Societal—Theoretical Model and Case Studies.* Kansas City, MO: Sheed & Ward, 1994.

Gummere, Peter J. "Assisted Nutrition and Hydration in Advanced Dementia of the Alzheimer's Type: An Ethical Analysis." *National Catholic Bioethics Quarterly* 8.2 (Summer 2008): 291–305.

Halpern, M. T., J. Bian, E. M. Ward, N. M. Schrag, and A. Y. Chen. "Insurance Status and Stage of Cancer at Diagnosis among Women with Breast Cancer." *Cancer* 110.2 (July 15, 2007): 403–411.

Halvorsen, Peder A., Randi Selmer, and Ivar Sønbø Kristiansen. "Different Ways to Describe the Benefits of Risk-Reducing Treatments: A Randomized Trial." *Annals of Internal Medicine* 146.12 (June 19, 2007): 848–856.

Hamel, Ronald P. and James J. Walter, eds. *Artificial Nutrition and Hydration and the Permanently Unconscious Patient: The Catholic Debate.* Washington, D.C.: Georgetown University Press, 2007.

Health and Public Policy Committee, American College of Physicians; and the Infectious Diseases Society of America. "The Acquired Immunodeficiency Syndrome (AIDS) and Infection with the Human Immunodeficiency Virus (HIV)." *Annals of Internal Medicine* 108.3 (March 1988): 460–469.

Heaney, Stephen J. "'You Can't Be Any Poorer Than Dead': Difficulties in Recognizing Artificial Nutrition and Hydration as Medical Treatments." *Linacre Quarterly* 61.2 (September 1994): 79.

Henderson, S., J. J. Fins, and E. H. Moskowitz. "Resuscitation in Hospice." *Hastings Center Report* 28.6 (November–December 1998): 20–22.

Hinkley, R. D. Michael Francis Xavier. *A Catholic Analysis of a Current Medical-Moral Dilemma in Health Care: The Moral Duty to Provide Nutrition and Hydration to Patients in the Persistent Vegetative State.* Doctoral diss. Rome: Alfonsianum, 1993.

Howsepian, A. A. "Very Quiet People: Ethical, Medical, and Theological Perspectives on Those in 'Vegetative' and Other Hypokinetic States." *Christian Research Journal* 29.1 (2006).

Hsu, F. L. K. "American Core Value and National Character." In *Psychological Anthropology: Approaches to Culture and Personality*, edited by F. L. K. Hsu, 209–229. Homewood, IL: Dorsey Press, 1961.

Hung, T. P. and S. T. Chen. "Prognosis of Deeply Comatose Patients on Ventilators." *Journal of Neurology, Neurosurgery, and Psychiatry* 58.1 (January 1995): 75–80.

Institute of Medicine. *Organ Donation: Opportunities for Action.* Washington, D.C.: National Academies Press, 2006.

Iserson, K. V. *Death to Dust; What Happens to Dead Bodies?* 2nd ed. Tucson, AZ: Galen Press, 2001.

Jennings, B. "Individual Rights and the Human Good in Hospice." In *Ethics in Hospice Care: Challenges to Hospice Values in a Changing Healthcare Environment*, edited by idem, 1–8. Philadelphia: Haworth Press, 1997.

Jennings, B., T. Ryndes, C. D'Onofrio, and M. A. Baily. "Access to Hospice Care: Expanding Boundaries, Overcoming Barriers." *Hastings Center Report* 33.2 suppl (March–April 2003): S3–7, S9–13, S15–21.

John Paul II, Pope. Address to the Participants in the International Congress on Life-Sustaining Treatments and the Vegetative State. March 20, 2004. Vatican edition. Reprinted in *National Catholic Bioethics Quarterly* 4.3 (Autumn 2004): 574–575.

John Paul II, Pope. "Building a Culture of Life." *Ad limina* Address to Bishops from California, Nevada, and Hawaii. October 2, 1998. *Origins* 28.18 (October 15, 1998): 314–316.

John Paul II, Pope. *Evangelium vitae.* March 25, 1995. Boston: Pauline Books, 1995.

John Paul II, Pope. *Salvifici doloris.* February 11, 1984. Vatican edition.

Kane, Rosalie A., and Arthur L. Caplan, eds. *Everyday Ethics: Resolving Dilemmas in Nursing Home Life.* New York: Springer, 1990.

Kass, L. R. "Death as an Event: Commentary on Robert Morison." *Science* 173.3998 (August 20, 1971): 676–756.

Katz, Paul, and Evan Catkins, eds. *Principles and Practice of Nursing Home Care.* New York: Springer, 1989.

Kaufman, S. R. *And A Time to Die: How American Hospitals Shape the End of Life.* New York: Scribner, 2005.

Koehler, S., R. Ramadan, and M. Salter. "Do-Not-Resuscitate (DNR): Analysis of the DNR Act." *Journal of the Oklahoma Medical Association* 92.7 (July 1999): 316–319.

Latkovic, Mark S. "The Morality of Tube Feeding PVS Patients: A Critique of the View of Kevin O'Rourke, O.P." In *Artificial Nutrition and Hydration: The New Catholic Debate*, edited by Christopher Tollefsen, 193–209. Dordrecht, The Netherlands: Springer, 2008.

Laureys, S., A. M. Owen, and N. D. Schiff. "Brain Function in Coma, Vegetative State, and Related Disorders." *Lancet Neurology* 3.9 (September 2004): 537–546.

Lawton, J. *The Dying Process: Patients' Experiences of Palliative Care.* New York: Routledge, 2000.

LeSage, Joan, and Diana Young Barhyte. *Nursing Quality Assurance in Long-Term Care.* Rockville, MD: Aspen, 1989.

Lindemann, Hilde, and Marian Verkerk. "Ending the Life of a Newborn: The Groningen Protocol." *Hastings Center Report* 38.1 (January–February 2008): 42–51.

Lo, Bernard, Laurie Dornbrand, Leslie Wolf, and Michelle Groman. "Sounding Board: The 'Wendland' Case—Withdrawing Life Support from Incompetent Patients Who Are Not Terminally Ill." *New England Journal of Medicine* 346.19 (May 9, 2002): 1489–1493.

Loewy, R. S. "Honouring the Age-Old Commitment to 'the Patient's Good': The Promise—and Peril—of Hospice." *Wiener Medizinische Wochenschrift (1946)* 153.17–18 (2003): 392–397.

Lofmark, R., and T. Nilstun. "Deciding Not to Resuscitate: Responsibilities of Physicians and Nurses–A Proposal." *Scandinavian Journal of Caring Sciences* 11.4 (1997): 207–211.

Lofmark, R., and T. Nilstun. "Do-Not-Resuscitate Orders: Should the Patient Be Informed?" *Journal of Internal Medicine* 241.5 (May 1997): 421–425.

Lynn, J. "Living Long in Fragile Health: The New Demographics Shape End of Life Care." *Hastings Center Report* 35.6 suppl (November–December 2005): S14–S18.

Marker, Rita. "The Right to Die Movement and the Artificial Provision of Nutrition and Hydration." In *Critical Issues in Contemporary Health Care*, edited by Russell E. Smith, 93–110. Braintree, MA: Pope John Center, 1989.

Marx, Carl F. "Medical Euthanasia." In *Ethics in Medicine: Historical Perspectives and Contemporary Concerns*, edited by Stanley J. Reiser, Arthur J. Dyck, and William J. Curran, 495–497. Cambridge, MA: MIT Press, 1977.

May, William E. "Caring for Persons in the 'Persistent Vegetative State.'" *Anthropotes* 13.2 (1997): 317–331.

May, William E. *Catholic Bioethics and the Gift of Human Life*, 2nd ed. Huntington, IN: Our Sunday Visitor, 2008.

May, William E., Robert Barry, O.P., Orville Griese, Germain Grisez, Brian Johnstone, C.Ss.R., Thomas J. Marzen, James T. McHugh, Gilbert Meilaender, Mark Siegler, and William B. Smith. "Feeding and Hydrating the Permanently Unconscious and Other Vulnerable Persons." *Issues in Law and Medicine* 3.3 (Winter 1987): 203–211.

McMahon, Kevin T. "Nutrition and Hydration: Should They Be Considered Medical Therapy?" *Linacre Quarterly* 72.3 (August 2005): 229–239.

Menikoff, J. "Doubts about Death: The Silence of the Institute of Medicine." *Journal of Law, Medicine and Ethics* 26.2 (Summer 1998): 157–165.

Mondor, E. E. "Do-Not-Resuscitate Patients in Critical Care: Moral and Ethical Considerations." *Official Journal of the Canadian Association of Critical Care Nursing* 10.1 (Spring 1999): 23–28.

Morrison, R. S., C. Maroney-Galin, P. D. Kralovec, D. E. Meier. "The Growth of Palliative Care Programs in United States Hospitals." *Journal of Palliative Medicine* 8.6 (December 2005): 1127–1134.

Multi-Society Task Force on PVS. "Medical Aspects of the Persistent Vegetative State," Part 1. *New England Journal of Medicine* 330.21 (May 26, 1994): 1499–1508.

Multi-Society Task Force on PVS. "Medical Aspects of the Persistent Vegetative State," Part 2. *New England Journal of Medicine* 330.22 (June 2, 1994): 1572–1579.

National Conference of Catholic Bishops, Committee for Pro-Life Activities. *Nutrition and Hydration: Moral and Pastoral Reflections*. Washington, D.C.: United States Conference of Catholic Bishops, April 1992.

National Hospice and Palliative Care Organization. *NHPCO Facts and Figures: Hospice Care in America*. Alexandria, VA: NHPCO, October 2008.

New York State Department of Health. *Guidelines for Determining Brain Death*. 2005.

Nuland, S. B. *How We Die: Reflections on Life's Final Chapter*. New York: Vintage, 1995.

O'Brien, Dan. "Forgoing Life Conservation: A Case Study." *Ethics & Medics* 15.10 (October 1990): 1–3.

Payne, S. K., P. Coyne, and T. J. Smith. "The Health Economics of Palliative Care." *Oncology* 16.6 (June 2002): 801–808.

Pitorak, E. F., M. Armour, and H. D. Sivec. "Project Safe Conduct Integrates Palliative Goals into Comprehensive Cancer Care." *Journal of Palliative Care* 6.4 (August 6, 2003): 645–655.

Pontifical Academy for Life and World Federation of Catholic Medical Associations. "Joint Statement on the Vegetative State." From the International Congress on Life-Sustaining Treatments and Vegetative State: Scientific Advances and Ethical Dilemmas. March 10–17, 2004. Rome.

Pontifical Council *Cor Unum*. "Questions of Ethics regarding the Fatally Ill and the Dying." June 27, 1981. In *Conserving Human Life*, edited by Russell E. Smith, 286–304. Braintree, MA: Pope John Center, 1989.

President's Commission for the Study of Ethical Problems in Medicine and Biomedical and Behavioral Research. *Defining Death: Medical, Legal, and Ethical Issues in the Determination of Death*. Washington, D.C.: U.S. Government Printing Office, 1981.

President's Council on Bioethics. *Taking Care: Ethical Caregiving in Our Aging Society*, Washington, D.C: President's Council on Bioethics, 2005.

Quill, Timothy E. "Death and Dignity: A Case of Individualized Decision Making." *New England Journal of Medicine* 324.10 (March 7, 1991): 691–694.

Quill, Timothy E., Rebecca Dresser, and Dan W. Brock. "The Rule of Double Effect: A Critique of Its Role in End-of-Life Decision Making." *New England Journal of Medicine* 337.24 (December 11, 1997): 1768–1771.

Ramsey, P. *The Patient as Person: Explorations in Medical Ethics*. New Haven: Yale University Press, 1970.

Reiser, Stanley Joel. "The Dilemma of Euthanasia in Modern Medical History: The English and American Experience." In *Ethics in Medicine: Historical Perspectives and Contemporary Concerns*, edited by Stanley J. Reiser, Arthur J. Dyck, and William J. Curran, 488–494. Cambridge: MIT Press, 1977.

Rhodes, R. L. "Racial Disparities in Hospice: Moving from Analysis to Intervention." *Virtual Mentor, American Medical Association* 8.9 (September 2006): 613–616.

Robinson, C. A., T. Hoyer, and C. Blackford. "The Continuing Evolution of Medicare Hospice Policy." *Public Administration Review* 67.1 (January/February 2007): 127–134.

Rossaro, L., C. Troppmann, J. P. McVicar, M. Sturges, K. Fisher, and F. J. Meyers. "A Strategy for the Simultaneous Provision of Pre-operative Palliative Care for Patients Awaiting Liver Transplantation." *Transplant International* 17.8 (2004): 473–475.

Shapiro, Kevin. "Lessons of the Cloning Scandal." *Commentary* (April 2006): 61–64.

Shewmon, D. Alan. "Chronic 'Brain Death': Meta-analysis and Conceptual Consequences." *Neurology* 51.6 (December 1998): 1538–1545.

Shewmon, D. Alan. "Recovery from 'Brain Death': A Neurologist's Apologia." *Linacre Quarterly* 64.1 (February 1997): 31–96.

Shewmon, D. A., and E. Seitz Shewmon. "The Semiotics of Death and Its Medical Implications." In *Brain Death and Disorders of Consciousness*, edited by C. Machado and D. A. Shewmon, 89–114. New York: Springer Science, 2004.

Shiboski, C. H., B. L. Schmidt, and R. C. Jordan. "Racial Disparity in Stage at Diagnosis and Survival among Adults with Oral Cancer in the United States." *Community Dentistry and Oral Epidemiology* 35.3 (June 2007): 233–240.

Smith, Russell E., ed. *Conserving Human Life*. Braintree, MA: Pope John Center, 1989.

Smith, William B. "Questions Answered: Vegetative State." *Homiletic and Pastoral Review* 104.9 (2004): 68–70.

Soelle, D. *Suffering*, translated by E. R. Kalin. Philadelphia: Fortress Press, 1975.

Spencer, E. M., A. E. Mills, M. V. Rorty, and P. H. Werhane. *Organization Ethics in Health Care*. New York: Oxford University Press, 2000.

Sulmasy, D. P. "Health Care Justice and Hospice Care." *Hastings Center Report* 33.2 suppl (March–April 2003): S14–S15.

Taheri, P. A. "The Cost of Trauma Center Readiness." *American Journal of Surgery* 187.1 (January 2004): 7–13.

Terminal Patients' Right to Know End-of-Life Options Act, AB 2747 (Berg-Levine), 2008 Cal. Stat. 683.

Timmermans, S. *Sudden Death and Myth of CPR*. Philadelphia: Temple University Press, 1999.

Tollefsen, Christopher, ed. *Artificial Nutrition and Hydration: The New Catholic Debate*, Catholic Studies in Bioethics, vol. 93. Dordrecht, The Netherlands: Springer, 2008.

Tomlinson, Tom, and Howard Brody. "Ethics and Communication in Do-Not-Resuscitate Orders." *New England Journal of Medicine* 318.1 (January 7, 1988): 43–46.

Torchia, Joseph, O.P. "Artificial Hydration and Nutrition for the PVS Patient: Ordinary Care or Extraordinary Intervention?" *National Catholic Bioethics Quarterly* 3.4 (Winter 2003): 719–730.

Truog, R. D. "Is It Time to Abandon Brain Death?" *Hastings Center Report* 27.1 (January–February 1997): 29–37.

U.S. Department of Health and Human Services. *Medicare & You: Medicare Made Simple—A Basic Guide for Caregivers*. Baltimore: U.S. Department of Health and Human Services, 2003.

Veatch, Robert M. "The Whole-Brain Death Oriented Concept of Death: An Outmoded Philosophical Formulation." *Journal of Thanatology* 3.1 (1975): 13–30.

Verheijde, J. L., M. Y. Rady, and J. Mcgregor. "Recovery of Transplantable Organs after Cardiac or Circulatory Death: The End Justifying the Means." *Critical Care Medicine* 35.5 (May 2007): 1439–1440.

Walter, T. *The Revival of Death*. New York: Routledge, 1994.

Whitehead, Kenneth D. "Food and Drink for the Least of These: The Pope Speaks Up for Those on Medical Death Row." *Touchstone* (December 2004).

Wijdicks, E. F. M. "Brain Death Worldwide: Accepted Fact but No Global Consensus Exists in Diagnostic Criteria." *Neurology* 58.1 (January 8, 2002): 20–25.

Wijdicks, E. F. M. "The Diagnosis of Brain Death." *New England Journal of Medicine* 344.16 (April 19, 2001): 1215–1221.

Wijdicks, E. F. M. "Electrocardiographic Activity after Terminal Cardiac Arrest in Neurocatastrophes." *Neurology* 62.4 (February 24, 2004): 673–674.

Worthley, John Abbot. *Organizational Ethics in the Compliance Context*. Chicago: Health Administration Press, 1999.

Youngner, S. J., and R. M. Arnold. "The Dead Donor Rule: Should We Stretch It, Bend It, or Abandon It?" *Kennedy Institute of Ethics Journal* 3.2 (June 1993): 263–278.

Youngner, S. J., R. M. Arnold, and E. T. Bartlett. "Human Death and High Technology: The Failure of the Whole-Brain Formulations." *Annals of Internal Medicine* 99.2 (1983): 252–258.

Zimmerman, C., R. Riechelmann, M. Krzyzanowska, G. Rodin, and I. Tannock. "Effectiveness of Specialized Palliative Care: A Systematic Review." *Journal of the American Medical Association* 299.14 (April 9, 2008): 1698–1709.

PART FIVE Selected Clinical Issues

Ackerman, Terrence F. "Why Doctors Should Intervene." In *Biomedical Ethics*, 3rd ed., edited by T. A. Mappes and J. Zembaty, 67–71. New York: McGraw-Hill, 1991. Originally published in *Hastings Center Report* 12.4 (August 1982): 14–17.

Aligheiri, Dante. *Divine Comedy*, translated by John Ciardi. New York: New American Library, 1982.

Alvarez, J., M. Gómez, J. Arias, J.I. Landa, M.J. Perez, R. Barrio, F. Martin, A. Barrientos, J.L. Balibrea. "One-Year Experience in Renal Transplantation with Kidneys from Asystolic Donors." *Transplantation Proceedings* 24.1 (February 1992): 34.

American Academy of Neurology, Quality Standards Subcommittee. "Practice Parameters for Determining Brain Death in Adults." *Neurology* 45.5 (May 1995): 1012–1014.

American Medical Association, Council on Ethical and Judicial Affairs. "The Use of Anencephalic Neonates as Organ Donors." CEJA Report 5-I-94. *Journal of the American Medical Association* 273.20 (May 24–31, 1994): 1614–1618.

Aristotle. *Nicomachean Ethics*, translated by Martin Ostwald. Upper Saddle River, NJ: Prentice Hall, 1962.

Atkinson, Gary M., and Albert S. Moraczewski, O.P., eds. *Genetic Counseling, the Church, and the Law*. St. Louis, MO: Pope John Center, 1980.

Baldwin, J.C., J.L. Anderson, M.M. Boucek, M.R. Bristow, B. Jennings, M.E. Ritsch Jr., and N.A. Silverman. "24th Bethesda Conference: Cardiac Transplantation: Task Force 2: Donor Guidelines." *Journal of the American College of Cardiologists* 22.1 (July 1993): 15–20.

Bankert, Elizabeth A. and Robert J. Amdur. *Institutional Review Board: Management and Function*, 2nd ed. Boston: Jones and Bartlett, 2006.

Bankert, Elizabeth A. and Robert J. Amdur. *Institutional Review Board: Member Handbook*, 2nd ed. Boston: Jones and Bartlett, 2007.

Busuttil, R. W. "Living-Related Liver Donation: Con." *Transplantation Proceedings* 23.1 pt 1 (February 1991): 44.

Caplan, Arthur. "Must I Be My Brother's Keeper? Ethical Issues in the Use of Living Donors as Sources of Liver and Other Solid Organs." *Transplantation Proceedings* 25.2 (April 1993): 1999.

Capron, Alexander. "The Criteria for Determining Brain Death Should Not Be Revised to Place Anencephalic Infants into the Category of Dead Bodies." *Journal of Heart and Lung Transplantation* 12.6 (1993): S375.

Cataldo, Peter J., and Albert S. Moraczewski, O.P., eds. *The Fetal Tissue Issue: Medical and Ethical Aspects*. Braintree, MA: Pope John Center, 1994.

Catechism of the Catholic Church, 2nd ed., translated by U.S. Conference of Catholic Bishops. Vatican City: Libreria Editrice Vaticana, 1997.

Cessario, Romanus, O.P. *The Moral Virtues and Theological Ethics*. Notre Dame, IN: University of Notre Dame Press, 1992.

Chevien, E.M. "Euthanasia Promises Marcus Welby, but Gives Us Jack Kevorkian." *Medical Economics* 72.1 (January 9, 1995): 25–26, 28.

Cohen, C., and M. Benjamin. "Alcoholics and Liver Transplantations." *Journal of the American Medical Association* 265.10 (March 13, 1991): 1299.

Coleman, Carl H., Jerry A. Menikoff, Jesse A. Goldner, and Nancy N. Dubler, eds. *The Ethics and Regulation of Research with Human Subjects*. Newark, NJ: Matthew Bender Properties, 2005.

Congregation for the Doctrine of the Faith. "Corrigenda." *Origins* 27.5 (September 25, 1997): 261.

Connell, S. G. "An Experimental Bone Marrow Transplant Experience." *Transplantation Proceedings* 22.3 (June 1990): 956.

Crutcher, Keith. "Fetal Tissue Research: The Cutting Edge?" *Linacre Quarterly* 60.2 (May 1993): 10–19.

Davis, Connie L., and Francis L. Delmonico. "Living-Donor Kidney Transplantation: A Review of Current Practices for the Live Donor." *American Society of Nephrology* 16 (2005): 2098–2110.

Dennison, A. R., D. Azoulay, and G. J. Maddern. "Living Related Hepatic Donation: Prometheus or Pandora's Box?" *Australia New Zealand Journal of Surgery* 63.11 (November 1993): 835–839.

Devita, M. A. "Development of the University of Pittsburgh Medical Center Policy for the Care of Terminally Ill Patients Who May Become Organ Donors after Death Following the Removal of Life Support." *Kennedy Institute Ethics* 3.2 (June 1993): 131–143.

Dietzen, John. "The Church's Position on Organ Donations." *Catholic Review*, November 3, 2005, A11.

Dixon, J. L., and M. Gene Smalley. "Jehovah's Witnesses: The Surgical/Ethical Challenge." *Journal of the American Medical Association* 246.21 (November 27, 1981): 2471–2472.

Doig, Christopher James, and Graeme Rocker. "Retrieving Organs from Non-Heart-Beating Organ Donors: A Review of Medical and Ethical Issues." *Canadian Journal of Anesthesia* 50 (2003): 1069–1076.

Dominguez-Roldán, J. M., F. Murillo-Cabezas, A. Muñoz-Sánchez, and M. A. Pérez-San-Gregorio. "Psychological Aspects Leading to Refusal of Organ Donation in Southwest Spain." *Transplantation Proceedings* 24.1 (February 1992): 25–26.

Downie, Jocelyn. "The Biology of the Persistent Vegetative State: Legal, Ethical, and Philosophical Implications for Transplantation." *Transplantation Proceedings* 22.3 (June 1990): 995–996.

Emanuel, Ezekiel J., Robert A. Crouch, John D. Arras, and Jonathan D. Moreno, eds. *Ethical and Regulatory Aspects of Clinical Research: Readings and Commentary.* Baltimore: Johns Hopkins University Press, 2003.

Evans, David Wainwright. "Seeking an Ethical and Legal Way of Procuring Transplantable Organs from the Dying without Further Attempts to Redefine Human Death." *Philosophy, Ethics, and Humanities in Medicine* 2.11 (2007).

Ghobrial, R. M. "Donor Morbidity after Living Donation for Liver Transplantation." *Gastroenterology* 135.2 (August 2008): 468–476.

Greer, D. M., P. N. Varelas, S. Haque, and E. F. Wijdicks. "Variability of Brain Death Determination Guidelines in Leading US Neurologic Institutions." *Neurology* 70.4 (January 22, 2008): 284–289.

Griese, Orville. "Reverend Humanity." *Ethics & Medics* 12.3 (March 1987): 2.

Hauet, T., and M. Eugene. "A New Approach in Organ Preservation: Potential Role of New Polymers." *Kidney International* 74.8 (October 2008): 998–1003.

Hillebrecht, J. M. "Regulating the Clinical Uses of Fetal Tissue: A Proposal for Legislation." *Journal of Legal Medicine* 10.2 (June 1989): 269–322.

Hopkin, K. "Transplanted Adult Hepatocytes Replace Diseased Liver." *Journal of NIH Research* 6.5 (1994): 50–52.

Huddle, T. S., M. A. Schwartz, F. A. Bailey, and M. A. Bos. "Death, Organ Transplantation and Medical Practice." *Philosophy, Ethics, and Humanities in Medicine* 4.3 (February 2008): 5.

Hunt, S. A., R. C. Robbins, E. B. Stinson, P. E. Dyer, N. E. Shumway, and B. A. Reitz. "A Single Center Experience with Heart Retransplantation: The 29 Year Experience at a Single Institution." In *Retransplantation: Proceedings of the 29th Conference on Transplantation and Clinical Immunology 9–11 June*, edited by J. L. Touraine et al., 229–235. Dordrecht, The Netherlands: Kluwer Academic Publishers, 1997.

Illes, R. W., G. K. Asimakis, K. Inners-McBride, and E. D. Buckingham. "Recovery of Nonbeating Donor Hearts." *Journal of Heart and Lung Transplantation* 14.3 (May–June 1995): 553–561.

International Summit on Transplant Tourism and Organ Trafficking. "The Declaration of Istanbul on Organ Trafficking and Transplant Tourism." *Clinical Journal of the American Society of Nephrology* 3.5 (September 2008): 1227–1231.

International Theological Commission. *Communion and Stewardship: Human Persons Created in the Image of God.* July 2004. Vatican edition.

John Paul II, Pope. Address to the 18th International Congress of the Transplantation Society. August 29, 2000.

John Paul II, Pope. "The Dangers of Genetic Manipulation." Address to World Medical Association Convention, Rome, October 29, 1983. *L'Osservatore Romano* (English), December 5, 1983, 10–11.

John Paul II, Pope. Discourse to the Working Group. In *Working Group on the Determination of Brain Death and Its Relationship to Human Death and Its Relationship to Human Death*, edited by R. J. White, H. Angstwurm, and I. Carrasco de Paula, 10–14. Vatican City: Pontifical Academy of Sciences, 1989.

Kaveny, M. Cathleen. "Jurisprudence and Genetics." *Theological Studies* 60.1 (March 1999): 135–147.

Keatings, M. "The Biology of the Persistent Vegetative State, Legal and Ethical Implications for Transplantation: Viewpoints from Nursing." *Transplantation Proceedings* 22.3 (June 1990): 997–999.

Kersten, Hans B., E. Douglas Thompson, and John G. Frohna. "The Use of Evidence-Based Medicine in Pediatrics: Past, Present, and Future." *Current Opinion in Pediatrics* 20.3 (2008) 326–331.

Killeen, Theresa K. "Alcoholism and Liver Transplantation: Ethical and Nursing Implications," *Perspectives in Psychiatric Care* 29.1 (January-March 1993): 7–12.

Kirchner, S. A. "Living Related Lung Transplantation: A New Dimension in Single Lung Transplantation." *AORN Journal* 54.4 (October 1991): 703–714.

Kissel, Judith Lee. "Cooperation with Evil: Its Contemporary Relevance." *Linacre Quarterly* 62 (1995): 33–45.

Koppelman, Elysa. "The Dead Donor Rule and the Concept of Death: Severing the Ties That Bind Them." *American Journal of Bioethics* 3.1 (Winter 2003): 1–9.

LaFleur, William R., Gernot Böhme, and Susumu Shimazono, eds. *Dark Medicine: Rationalizing Unethical Medical Research.* Bloomington, IN: University of Indiana Press, 2007.

Leiva, Rene. "A Brief History of Human Diploid Cell Strains." *National Catholic Bioethics Quarterly* 6.3 (Autumn 2006): 443–451.

Lysy, P. A., D. Campard, F. Smets, M. Najimi, E. M. Sokal. "Stem Cells for Liver Tissue Repair: Current Knowledge and Perspectives." *World Journal of Gastroenterology* 14.6 (February 14, 2008): 864–875.

Medearis, D. N., Jr., and L. B. Holmes. "On the Use of Anencephalic Infants as Organ Donors." *New England Journal of Medicine* 321.6 (August 10, 1989): 391–393.

Miller, G. "Parkinson's Disease: Signs of Disease in Fetal Transplants." *Science* 320.5873 (April 11, 2008): 167.

Moore, Kim, Jeanette F. Mills, and Melissa M. Thorton. "Alternative Sources of Adult Stem Cells: A Possible Solution to the Embryonic Stem Cell Debate." *Gender Medicine* 3.3 (September 2006): 161–168.

Moraczewski, Albert S., O.P. "Pastoral Hope and Genetic Medicine." In *The Bishop and the Future of Catholic Health Care: Challenges and Opportunities*, edited by Daniel P. Maher, 43–58. Braintree, MA: Pope John Center, 1997.

Moraczewski, Albert S., O.P., ed. *Genetic Medicine and Engineering.* St. Louis, MO: Catholic Health Association of America and Pope John Center, 1983.

Moss, A. H., and M. Siegler. "Should Alcoholics Compete Equally for Liver Transplantation?" *Journal of the American Medical Association* 265.10 (March 13, 1991): 1298.

Mudge, G. H. "24th Bethesda Conference: Cardiac Transplantation. Task Force 3: Recipient Guidelines/Prioritization." *Journal of the American College of Cardiology* 22.1 (July 1993): 21–31.

Muggeridge, Malcolm. *Something Beautiful for God.* New York: HarperCollins, 1971.

National Catholic Bioethics Quarterly: Ethics in Cell Research 6.3 (Autumn 2006).

National Commission for the Protection of Human Subjects of Biomedical and Behavioral Research. *The Belmont Report: Ethical Principles and Guidelines for the Protection of Human Subjects of Research.* Washington, D.C.: Department of Health, Education, and Welfare, 1979.

Nolan, Marie T., B. Walton-Moss, L. Taylor, and K. Dane. "Living Kidney Donor Decision Making: State of the Science and Directions for Future Research." *Progress in Transplantation* 14.3 (September 2004): 201–209.

Norris, M. K. "Disparities for Minorities in Transplantation: The Challenge to Critical Care Nurses." *Heart and Lung* 20.4 (July 1991): 419–420.

Osler, William. *Aequanimitas.* Philadelphia: P. Blakiston's Son, 1932.

Peabody, Joyce L., J. R. Emery, and S. Ashwal. "Experience with Anencephalic Infants as Prospective Organ Donors." *New England Journal of Medicine* 321.6 (August 10, 1989): 344–350.

Pellegrino, Edmund D. "Cooperation, Moral Complicity, and Moral Distance: The Ethics of Forensic, Penal, and Military Medicine." *International Journal of Law and Ethics* 2 (1993): 373–391.

———. "Medical Evidence and Virtue Ethics: A Commentary on Zarkovich and Upshur." *Theoretical Medicine and Bioethics* 23.4–5 (July 2002): 397–402.

Pellegrino, Edmund D., and David C. Thomasma. *For the Patient's Good.* New York: Oxford University Press, 1988.

Pellegrino, Edmund D., and David C. Thomasma. "The Four Principles and the Doctor-Patient Relationship: The Need for a Better Linkage." In *Principles of Health Care Ethics*, edited by Raanon Gillon, 353–365. New York: John Wiley & Sons, 1994.

Penslar, Robin Levin. *Institutional Review Board Guidebook* (Washington, D.C.: Office of Human Research Protections, 1993).

Pius XII, Pope. "Tissue Transplantation." In *The Human Body*, edited by the Monks of Solesmes. Boston: St. Paul Editions, 1960.

Pius XII, Pope. Address to an International Congress of Anesthesiologists. November 24, 1957. *The Pope Speaks* 4.4 (Spring 1958): 393–398.

Pontifical Academy for Life. "Moral Reflections on Vaccines Prepared from Cells Derived from Aborted Human Fetuses." June 5, 2005. Reprinted in *National Catholic Bioethics Quarterly* 6.3 (Autumn 2006): 541–549.

Potts, Michael. "Truthfulness in Transplantation: Non-Heart Beating Organ Donation." *Philosophy, Ethics, and Humanities in Medicine* 2.17 (August 24, 2007).

Reitz, N. N., and C. O. Callender. "Organ Donation in the African-American Population: A Fresh Perspective with a Simple Solution." *Journal of the National Medical Association* 85.5 (May 1993): 353–358.

Rhim, J. A., E. P. Sandgren, J. L. Degen, R. D. Palmiter, and R. L. Brinster. "Replacement of Diseased Mouse Liver by Hepatic Cell Transplantation." *Science* 263 (February 25, 1994): 1149–1152.

Ross, Lainie Friedman. "Should a PVS Patient be a Live Organ Donor?" *Medical Ethics* 13.1 (Winter 2006): 3.

Russell, S., and R. G. Jacob. "Living Related Organ Donation: The Donor's Dilemma." *Patient Education and Counseling* 21.1–2 (June 1993): 89–99.

Sanders, L. M., L. Giudice, and T. A. Raffin. "Ethics of Fetal Tissue Transplantation." *Western Journal of Medicine* 159.3 (September 1993): 400–407.

Santori G., E. Andorno, A. Antonucci, N. Morelli, G. Bottino, R. Mondello, R. Valente, et al. "Potential Predictive Value of the MELD Score for Short-Term Mortality after Liver Transplantation." *Transplantation Proceedings* 36.3 (2004): 533–534.

Saposnik, G., G. Rizzo, A. Vega, R. Sabbatiello, and J. L. Deluca."Problems Associated with the Apnea Test in the Diagnosis of Brain Death." *Neurology India* 52.3 (2004): 342–345.

Scheper-Hughes, Nancy. "The Tyranny of the Gift: Sacrificial Violence in Living Donor Transplants." *American Journal of Transplantation* 7.3 (March 2007): 507–511.

Schlotzhauer, Anna, and Bryan A. Liang. "Definitions and Implications of Death." *Hematological Oncology Clinics of North America* 16.6 (December 2002): 1397–1413.

Schyve, Paul M. "Perspective: Patient Safety—Beyond the 'Easy' Phase." *Quality Matters* 17 (April 27, 2006).

Shannon, Thomas A. "Ethical Issues in Genetics." *Theological Studies* 60.1 (March 1999): 111–123.

Shewmon, D. A., A. M. Capron, W. J. Peacock, and B. L. Schulman. "The Use of Anencephalic Infants as Organ Sources: A Critique." *Journal of the American Medical Association* 261.12 (March 14, 1989): 1773–1781.

Siminoff, L., R. H. Lawrence, and R. M. Arnold. "Comparison of Black and White Families' Experiences and Perceptions Regarding Organ Donation Requests." *Critical Care Medicine* 31.1 (2003): 146–151.

Spital, A., and M. Spital. "The Ethics of Liver Transplantation from a Living Donor." *New England Journal of Medicine* 322.8 (February 22, 1990): 549–550.

Starling, R. C. "Radical Alternatives to Transplantation." *Current Opinion in Cardiology* 12.2 (March 1997): 166–171.

Starzl, T. E., A. J. Demetris, and M. Trucco. "Matching the Black Recipient." *Transplantation Proceedings* 25.4 (August 1993): 2450–2451.

Starzl, T. E., D. Van Thiel, A. G. Tzakis, S. Iwatsuki, S. Todo, J. W. Marsh, B. Koneru, S. Staschak, A. Stieber, and R. D. Gordon. "Orthotopic Liver Transplantation for Alcoholic Cirrhosis." *Journal of the American Medical Association* 260.17 (November 4, 1988): 2542–2544.

Stevenson, L. W., S. L. Warner, M. A. Hamilton, J. D. Moriguchi, C. Chelimsky-Fallick, G. C. Fonarow, J. Kobashigawa, D. C. Drinkwater, and H. Laks. "Modeling Distribution of Donor Hearts to Maximize Early Candidate Survival." *Circulation* 86.5 suppl (November 1992): II224–230.

Truog, R. D., and J. C. Fletcher. "Anencephalic Newborns: Can Organs Be Transplanted Before Brain Death?" *New England Journal of Medicine* 321.6 (August 10, 1989): 388–391.

Ubel, Peter A., Robert M. Arnold, and Arthur L. Caplan. "Rationalizing Failure: The Ethical Lessons of the Retransplantation of Scarce Vital Organs." In *The Ethics of Organ Transplantation*, edited by Arthur L. Caplan and Daniel H. Coelho, 260–274. Amherst, MA: Prometheus Books, 1998.

U.S. Department of Health and Human Services. National Institutes of Health, and Office of Human Research Protections. *The Common Rule*, 45 *Code of Federal Regulations* 46 (Protection of Human Subjects), revised June 23, 2005; effective June 23, 2005. Washington, D.C.: DHHS, 2005.

U.S. Organ Procurement and Transplantation Network and the Scientific Registry of Transplant Recipients. *Annual Reports: Transplant Data.* (Rockville, MD: Department of Health and Human Services; Richmond, VA: United Network for Organ Sharing; Ann Arbor, MI: University Renal Research and Education Association). Yearly data available at http://www.optn.org.

Vatican Council II. *Dignitatis humanae.* December 7, 1965. Vatican edition.

Veatch, Robert M. "Abandon the Dead Donor Rule or Change the Definition of Death?" *Kennedy Institute of Ethics* 14.3 (September 2004): 261–276.

Veatch, Robert M. "The Impending Collapse of the Whole-Brain Definitions of Death." *Hastings Center Report* 23.4 (July-August 1993): 18–24.

Vegas, Annette. "Assisting the Failing Heart." *Anesthesiology Clinics* 26.3 (September 2008): 539–564.

Walter, James J. "Theological Issues in Genetics." *Theological Studies* 60.1 (March 1999): 124–134.

White, R. J., H. Angstwurm, and I. Carrasco De Paula, eds. *Working Group on the Determination of Brain Death and Its Relationship to Human Death.* Vatican City: Pontificia Academia Scientiarum, 1992.

Wijdicks, E. F. "Determining Brain Death in Adults." *Neurology* 45.5 (May 1995): 1003–1011.

PART SIX Institutional Issues

Benedict XVI. *Deus caritas est.* December 25, 2005. Vatican edition.

Berman, Harold J. "The Religion Clauses of the First Amendment in Historical Perspective." In *Religion and Politics,* edited by W. Lawson Taitte. Dallas: University of Texas Press, 1989.

Boyle, Philip, Edwin DuBose, Stephen Ellingson, David Guinn, and David McCurdy. *Organizational Ethics in Health Care: Principles, Cases, and Practical Solutions.* San Francisco: Jossey-Bass, 2001.

Carter, Stephen L. *The Culture of Disbelief: How American Law and Politics Trivialize Religious Devotion.* New York: Basic Books, 1993.

Cataldo, Peter. "Compliance with Contraceptive Insurance Mandates: Licit or Illicit Cooperation in Evil?" *National Catholic Bioethics Quarterly* 4.1 (Spring 2004): 103–130.

Cataldo, Peter. "Models of Health Care Collaboration." *Ethics & Medics* 23.12 (December 1998): 1–2.

Cataldo, Peter. "State Mandated Immoral Procedures in Catholic Facilities: How Is Licit Compliance Possible?" In *The Moral Legacy of John Paul II in Catholic Health Care,* edited by E. J. Furton, 253–267. Philadelphia: National Catholic Bioethics Center, 2006.

Cataldo, Peter J., and John M. Haas. "Institutional Cooperation: The ERDs." *Health Progress* 83.6 (November–December 2002): 49–57, 60.

Congregation for the Doctrine of the Faith. *Instruction* Dignitas personae *on Certain Bioethical Questions.* Boston: Pauline Books and Media, 2008.

Code of Canon Law: Latin–English Edition, translated by the Canon Law Society of America. Washington, D.C.: Canon Law Society of America, 1999.

Employment Division, Dept. of Human Resources of Oregon v. Smith, 494 U.S. 872 (1990).

Furton, Edward J., ed. *Urged On by Christ: Catholic Health Care in Tension with Contemporary Culture*. Philadelphia: National Catholic Bioethics Center, 2007.

Green, Thomas J. "Sanctions in the Church." In *New Commentary on the Code of Canon Law*, edited by John P. Beal, James A. Coriden, and Thomas J. Green, 1529. Mahwah, NJ: Paulist Press, 2000.

John Paul II, Pope. "The Church's Teaching in the Biomedical Field Defends the Dignity and Fundamental Rights of the Human Person." September 14, 1987. *L'Osservatore Romano* (English), September 21, 1987, 19–20.

Khushf, George. "Administrative and Organizational Ethics." *HEC Forum* 9.4 (December 1997): 299–309.

Lyons, Mary Louise, D.C. "Conscience and the Corporate Person." In *Catholic Conscience: Foundation and Formation*, edited by Russell E. Smith, 205–216. Braintree, MA: Pope John Center, 1991.

Maida, Adam J., and Nicholas P. Cafardi. *Church Property, Church Finances, and Church-Related Corporations*. St. Louis, MO: Catholic Health Association, 1984.

Moraczewski, Albert S., O.P. "How to Cooperate with Evil." *Ethics & Medics* 8.6 (June 1983): 1–3.

National Catholic Bioethics Center Ethicists. "Cooperating with Non-Catholic Partners." *Ethics & Medics* 23.11 (November 1998): 1–5.

National Health Lawyers Association. *A Looseleaf Guide to Mergers and Acquisitions: Contract Provisions and Transactional Models*. Washington, D.C.: National Health Lawyers Association, 1997.

Paul VI, Pope. *Humanae vitae*. July 25, 1968. Vatican edition.

Pellegrino, Edmund D. , and David C. Thomasma. *Helping and Healing: Religious Commitment in Health Care*. Washington, D.C.: Georgetown University Press, 1997.

Pellegrino, Edmund D. , and David C. Thomasma. "The Origins and Evolution of Bioethics: Some Personal Reflections." *Kennedy Institute of Ethics Journal* 9.1 (Winter 1998): 73–88.

Pontifical Council for Legislative Texts. "*Interpretationes Authenticae* (can. 1398)." *AAS* 80 (1988): 1818.

Potter, Robert Lyman. "On Our Way to Integrated Bioethics: Clinical/Organizational/Communal." *Journal of Clinical Ethics* 10.3 (Fall 1999): 171–177.

Schyve, Paul M. "Patient Rights and Organizational Ethics: The Joint Commission Perspective." *Bioethics Forum* 12.2 (Summer 1996): 13–20.

Singer, Lawrence E. "Realigning Catholic Health Care: Bridging Legal and Church Control in a Consolidating Market. *Tulane Law Review* 72 (1997): 159–229.

Smith, Russell E. "Duress and Cooperation." *Ethics & Medics* 21.11 (November 1996): 1–2.

Smith, Russell E. "Ethical Quandary: Forming Hospital Partnerships." In *The Gospel of Life and the Vision of Health Care*, edited by Russell E. Smith, 109–123. Braintree, MA: Pope John Center, 1996.

Smith, Russell E. "Formal and Material Cooperation." *Ethics & Medics* 20.6 (June 1995): 1–2.

Smith, Russell E. "Immediate Material Cooperation." *Ethics & Medics* 23.1 (January 1998): 1–2.

Smith, Russell E. "The Principles of Cooperation and their Application to the Present State of Health Care Evolution." In *The Splendor of Truth and Health Care*, edited by Russell E. Smith, 217–231. Braintree, MA: Pope John Center, 1995.

Tonneau, Jean, O.P. "The Teaching of the Thomist Tract on Law." *Thomist* 34.1 (1970): 13–83.

U.S. Conference of Catholic Bishops. *Married Love and the Gift of Life*. Washington, D.C: USCCB, 2006.

INDEX

gestational age, and induction of labor , 111–112, 116

gift, life as, 103–104

Gilligan, Carol, 46

Gonzalez v. Carhart (2007), 76

Good Samaritan, parable of, 276, 295

Goodwin, T. Murphy, 122

Gospel, and Catholic health care mission, 32, 64, 294, 295; and confidence in others, 20; as mandate, 294; teaching authority of, 5–6

government, and the common good, 30, 31; mandates, 159, 275–281

grief, fetal anomalies and, 115

Groningen protocol, 175

Groopman, Jerome, 200

group behavior, 58–59

guidelines, for contraceptive prescriptions from non-Catholic affiliates, 99–101; federal sentencing, 292; for health care ethics committees, 51

Hawthorne, Nathaniel, 196

health care, Catholic, conscience and, 31–34; history of, 275

health care proxy, 215–217

Health Insurance Portability and Accountability Act of 1997 (HIPAA), 292

heroism, and duty to care, 262

Hilgers, Thomas, 107, 109, 120

Hippocratic Oath, 176

HIV infection, and confidentiality, 22

Holy Spirit, as teacher, 5

hospice care, 183–190

Hospitallers of Saint John, 275

Hotel-Dieu (Paris), 275

Hsu, Francis, 184

human body, as temple of Holy Spirit, 13; totality and integrity of, 13–15

human dignity, 4; and access to health care, 295; and birth regulation, 93–94; and Catholic health care mission, 43, 61; of child, 114, 115; collaboration as offense against, 265, 270; confidentiality and, 20, 21, 23; and determination of death, 171; ethics committees and, 46,

48, 49; and euthanasia, 176, 196, 217; and hospice, 189; image of God and, 3, 13, 16; in persistent vegetative state, 204, 209; and procreation, 73, 115

Human Genome Project, 239

human immunodeficiency virus (HIV), confidentiality and, 22

human life, as God's gift, 103–104

human nature, as basis of morality, 9–10

human papilloma virus (HPV), vaccination for, 233–234

human subjects, research on, 243–245

Humanae vitae (Paul VI, 1968), 6, 29, 82, 92–93

Hwang, Woo Suk, 82

hysterectomy, 89

identity, Catholic, rooted in mission, 289–290

image of God, and human dignity, 3, 13, 16

immunization, 231–234

implantation, of human embryo, emergency contraception and, 132, 133, 153–156, 159; levonorgestrel (Plan B) and, 127, 128, 130, 135–139, 140–141 (note 18), 141–143, 143–148, 150–152; Ovral and, 129; prevention of, 73, 75; tubal, *see* ectopic pregnancy

imputability, grave, 277–270

in vitro fertilization (IVF), 3, 105–108; and abortion, 106, 107; and cloning, 77–78, 82; and prenatal diagnosis, 237–238

induced pluripotent stem cells, 81, 83

induction of labor, early, 111–118

infants, anencephalic, 114, 116–117, 223

infertility, 103–108, 109

informed consent, in clinical research, 245; for treatment decisions, 252

Institute of Medicine, 167, 171

institutional duress, 268–269

institutional review boards, 243

insurance, for civil liability, 285; genetic discrimination in, 239

integrity, and totality, principle of, 13–15, 238–239

intention, of moral act, 10–11; and principle of double effect, 24–26

minutes, of committee meetings, 55

mission, of ethics committee, 60, 61; and institutional identity, 289

models, health care, Christian versus market-driven, 293; of collaboration, 271–273

Montesquieu, Baron de, 35

Moraczewski, Albert, 119–120

moral act, nature and structure of, 10–11

moral certainty, in determination of death, 171; and emergency contraception, 153–159; in rape treatment, 137–139

"Moral Reflections on Vaccines Prepared from Cells Derived from Aborted Human Fetuses" (PAV, 2005), 233

moral theologians, on ethics committee, 60–61

morality, based on human nature, 9–10; natural law, 35–39

mother–child dialogue, in pregnancy decisions, 115–117

MRC–5 cell line, 232–233

Multi-Society Task Force on PVS, 207

Murray, John Courtney, 35

mutilation, and principle of totality and integrity, 13–15

NaProTechnology, 107

Nathanson, Bernard, 121

National Catholic Bioethics Center (NCBC), 61, 208, 271; on conscience, 32; on tube feeding, 205

National Center for the Treatment of Reproductive Disorders, 107

National Council of State Boards of Nursing, 258

National Palliative Care Research Center, 193

natural family planning (NFP), 89–90, 93–94

natural law, and abortion, 91; Church teaching and, 91–92; and contraception, 91–92; ERDs and, 91; and ethical reasoning, 35–39; in organizational ethics, 293–294

Natural Procreative Technology (NaProTechnology), 107, 109

negligence, liability through, 283–284

Netherlands, euthanasia in, 175

Neuhaus, Richard John, 203

neurological criteria, for determination of death, 167–168

non-Catholic patients, pastoral care for, 248–250

non-heart-beating organ donation, 222

nonmaleficence, in pandemic triage, 261

nurse practitioners, Catholic–affiliated, and contraceptive prescriptions (guidelines), 99–101

nutrition and hydration, assisted, 18, 202–206; in persistent vegetative state, 208–209

O'Donnell, Thomas J., 14, 89

O'Rourke, Kevin, 224, 253

object (of moral act), 10–11

objective truth, as basis for moral reasoning, 36

orders, do-not-resuscitate, 210–213

ordinary/extraordinary means, 15–18, 216

Oregon v. Smith (1990), 277

organ donation, 221–227; after cardiac death, 169–171; and determination of death, 165–166; non-heart-beating, 222; principle of totality and integrity and, 14–15

organ transplanation, 221–227

organizational ethics, 289–296

Osler, William, 251

Ovral (ethinyl estradiol/norgestrel), 75, 125, 127, 128–130

ovulation, and pregnancy prevention after rape, 125, 139, 148, 153–159

ovulation testing, clinical data, 125–130; arguments against, 134–139, 141–148, 150–152; arguments for, 153–159; protocol for, 131–133

pain management, at end of life, 194–195

palliative care, 183–190, 193–196

pandemic, duty of care during, 257–262

partial birth abortion, 76

Partial Birth Abortion Ban Act, 76

pastoral care, and abortion 248; and religious freedom, 247–250

patience, 28–29

patient rights, in long-term care, 68

patient safety, and organizational ethics, 292–293

Paul VI, Pope, 6, 82; on birth regulation, 92, 93; on contraceptive use, 278

Paul, Saint, 13, 92

Peabody, Joyce, 223

Pellegrino, Edmund, 251, 290–291, 293, 294